Medical Informatics

Medical Informatics

Computer Applications in Health Care

Edward H. Shortliffe
Leslie E. Perreault
Editors

Gio Wiederhold
Lawrence M. Fagan
Associate Editors

Section on Medical Informatics
Stanford University School of Medicine

ADDISON-WESLEY PUBLISHING COMPANY

Reading, Massachusetts • Menlo Park, California • New York
Don Mills, Ontario • Wokingham, England • Amsterdam • Bonn
Sydney • Singapore • Tokyo • Madrid • San Juan

Dedication

We dedicate this book to graduate students in medical informatics at Stanford. Their commitment to the field has challenged and enlightened us.

Library of Congress Cataloging-in-Publication Data

Medical informatics : computer applications in health care / Edward H. Shortliffe, Leslie E. Perreault, editors : Lawrence M. Fagan, Gio Wiederhold, associate editors.
    p. cm.
  Includes bibliographical references.
  ISBN 0-201-06741-2
  1. Medical informatics.   I. Shortliffe, Edward Hance.   II. Perreault, Leslie Elaine.   III. Fagan, Lawrence Marvin.   IV. Wiederhold, Gio.
R858.M397   1990
610'.285—dc20   89-18189
                                          CIP

Contributors

Ivo L. Abraham, Ph.D., R.N.
Associate Professor, School of Nursing
Associate Professor, Department of
  Behavioral Medicine and Psychiatry
School of Medicine
University of Virginia
McLeod Hall
Charlottesville, VA 22903

G. Octo Barnett, M.D.
Professor of Medicine
Harvard Medical School
Director, Laboratory of Computer
  Science
Massachusetts General Hospital
Boston, MA 02114

Marsden Scott Blois, M.D., Ph.D.
Professor of Medical Information
  Sciences and Dermatology
University of California Medical Center
San Francisco, CA 94143
(deceased)

James F. Brinkley, M.D., Ph.D.
Assistant Professor, Research
Department of Biological Structure
  SM-20
University of Washington
Seattle, WA 98195

Morris F. Collen, M.D.
Consultant
Division of Research
The Permanente Medical Group, Inc.
3451 Piedmont Avenue
Oakland, CA 94611

Martin M. Cummings, M.D.
Director-Emeritus
National Library of Medicine
8600 Rockville Pike
Bethesda, MD 20894

Alain C. Enthoven, Ph.D.
Professor of Public and Private
  Management
Graduate School of Business
Stanford University
Stanford, CA 94305

Lawrence M. Fagan, M.D., Ph.D.
Senior Research Associate
Section on Medical Informatics
Stanford University School
  of Medicine
Medical School Office Bldg X-215
Stanford, CA 94305

Reed M. Gardner, Ph.D.
Professor of Medical Informatics,
University of Utah
Codirector of Medical Computing,
LDS Hospital
8th Avenue and C Street
Salt Lake City, UT 84143

Robert A. Greenes, M.D., Ph.D.
Associate Professor of Radiology,
Harvard Medical School
Director, Decision Systems
Group,
Brigham and Women's Hospital
75 Francis Street
Boston, MA 02115

Michael C. Higgins, Ph.D.
Member of the Technical Staff
Hewlett-Packard Laboratories (28C)
1501 Page Mill Road
Palo Alto, CA 94304

Edward P. Hoffer, M.D.
Assistant Director
Laboratory of Computer Science
Massachusetts General Hospital
Boston, MA 02114

Clement J. McDonald, M.D.
Professor of Medicine
Regenstrief Institute
1001 West Tenth Street
Indianapolis, IN 46202

Alan B. McKay, Ph.D.
Associate Professor
University of Maryland School of
    Pharmacy
20 North Pine Street
Baltimore, MD 21201

Andrew B. Newman, M.D.
Clinical Assistant Professor of
    Medicine
Stanford University School of Medicine
1101 Welch Road, Suite A5
Palo Alto, CA 94304

Douglas K. Owens, M.D.
Clinical Assistant Professor of Medicine
Stanford University School of Medicine
Medical School Office Bldg X-216
Stanford, CA 94305

Judy Ozbolt, Ph.D., R.N.
Professor and Associate Dean for
    Research
Center for Nursing Research
University of Virginia School of Nursing
McLeod Hall
Charlottesville, VA 22903

Leslie E. Perreault, M.S.
Research Affiliate
Section on Medical Informatics
Stanford University School of Medicine
Medical School Office Bldg X-215
Stanford, CA 94305

Samuel Schultz II, Ph.D.
Vice President
Director, Clinical Information Network
University Hospital Consortium
One Mid America Plaza, Suite 700
Oakbrook Terrace, IL 60181

Edward H. Shortliffe, M.D., Ph.D.
Professor of Medicine and Computer
    Science
Section on Medical Informatics
Stanford University School of Medicine
Medical School Office Bldg X-215
Stanford, CA 94305

Elliot R. Siegel, Ph.D.
Assistant Director for Planning and
    Evaluation
National Library of Medicine
8600 Rockville Pike
Bethesda, MD 20894

Jack W. Smith, Jr., M.D., Ph.D.
Assistant Professor
Department of Pathology
Ohio State University
College of Medicine
571 Health Science Library
376 West 10th Avenue
Columbus, OH 43210

Harold C. Sox, Jr., M.D.
Chairman, Department of Medicine
Dartmouth-Hitchcock Medical Center
Hanover, NH 03756

Stuart M. Speedie, Ph.D.
Assistant Dean for Pharmaceutical
    Informatics
University of Maryland School of
    Pharmacy
20 North Pine Street
Baltimore, MD 21201

John R. Svirbely, M.D.
Assistant Professor
Department of Pathology
The Ohio State University College of
    Medicine
318 Doan Hall
410 West 10th Avenue
Columbus, OH 43210

Gio Wiederhold, Ph.D.
Professor (Research)
Departments of Computer Science and
  of Medicine
Margaret Jacks Hall, Rm. 438
Stanford, CA 94305

Nancy A. Wilson, R.N., M.B.A.
Consultant
Graduate School of Business
Stanford University
Stanford, CA 94305

Rose M. Woodsmall, M.L.S.
Program Analyst, Planning and
  Evaluation
National Library of Medicine
8600 Rockville Pike
Bethesda, MD 20894

Preface

Just as banks cannot practice modern banking without financial software, and airlines cannot manage modern travel planning without shared databanks of flight schedules and reservations, it is increasingly difficult to practice modern medicine without information technologies. Health professionals recognize that a large percentage of their activities relates to *information management*—for example, obtaining and recording information about patients, consulting colleagues, reading the scientific literature, planning diagnostic procedures, devising strategies for patient care, interpreting results of laboratory and radiologic studies, or conducting case-based and population-based research. It is, however, society's overriding concern for patient well-being, and the resulting need for optimal decision making, that sets medicine apart from many other information-intensive fields. That concern gives a special significance to the effective organization and management of the huge bodies of data with which health professionals must deal. It also suggests the need for specialized approaches and for skilled scientists who are knowledgeable about both medicine and information technologies.

Information Management in Medicine

Although the application of computers to medicine is recent, the clinical and research influence of medical-computing systems is already remarkably broad. Hospital information systems, which provide communication and information-management functions, are being installed in many institutions. Physicians can search entire drug indexes in a few seconds, using the information provided by a computer program to anticipate harmful side effects or drug interactions. Electrocardiograms (ECGs) often are analyzed initially by computer programs, and similar techniques are being introduced for interpretation of pulmonary-function tests and a variety of laboratory and radiologic abnormalities. Microprocessor systems routinely monitor patients and provide warnings in critical-care settings, such as the intensive-care unit (ICU) or the operating room. Both medical reserachers and clinicians regularly use computer programs to search the medical literature, and modern clinical research would be severely hampered without computer-based data-storage techniques and statistical-analysis systems. Advanced decision-support tools also are beginning to emerge from research laboratories and are likely to have a profound effect on the way medicine is practiced in the future.

Despite this growing use of computers in health-care settings, and a resulting expansion of interest in learning more about medical computing, many health students and professionals have found it difficult to obtain a comprehensive and rigorous, but nontechnical, overview of the field. Both practitioners and basic scientists are increasingly recognizing that thorough preparation for their professional futures requires that they gain an understanding of the state of the art in biomedical computing, of the current and future capabilities *and* limitations of the technology, and of the way in which such developments fit within the scientific, social, and financial context of biomedicine. In turn, the future of the medical-computing field will be largely determined by how well health professionals and other people are prepared to guide the discipline's development. This book is intended to meet this growing need for well-equipped professionals. It provides a conceptual framework for learning about computer applications in medical care, for critiquing existing systems, and for anticipating future directions that the field may take. Other recent books have surveyed medical-computing topics [Bronzino, 1982; Blum, 1986a; Javitt, 1986; Anbar, 1987; Chard, 1988], but this text differs from these in its broad coverage and in its emphasis on the field's conceptual underpinnings. Our book presumes no medical or computer-science background, but it does assume that you are interested in a comprehensive summary of the field that stresses the underlying concepts, and that introduces technical details only to the extent that they are necessary to meet the principal goal. It thus differs from an impressive early text in the field [Ledley, 1965] that emphasized technical details but did not dwell on the broader social and clinical context in which medical computing systems are developed and implemented.

Overview and Guide to Use of This Book

This book is written as a text so that it can be used in formal courses, but we have adopted a broad view of the population for whom it is intended. Thus, it may be used not only by students of medicine and of the other health professions, but also as an introductory text by future medical-computing professionals, as well as for self-study and for reference by practitioners. The book is probably too detailed for use in a 2- or 3-day continuing-education course, although it could be introduced as a reference for further independent study.

Our principal goal in writing this text is to teach *concepts* in medical informatics— the study of biomedical information and its use in decision making—and to illustrate them in the context of descriptions of representative systems that are in use today or that taught us lessons in the past. As you will see, medical informatics is more than the study of computers in medicine, and we have organized the book to emphasize that point. Chapter 1 first sets the stage for the rest of the book by providing a glimpse of the future, defining important terms and concepts, describing the content of the field, explaining the connections between medical informatics and related disciplines, and discussing the forces that have influenced research in medical informatics and its integration into medical practice.

Broad issues regarding the nature of data, information, and knowledge pervade all areas of application, as do concepts related to optimal decision making. Chapters 2 and 3 focus on these topics but mention computers only in passing. They serve as the foundation for all that follows.

Chapters 4 and 5 introduce the central notions of computer hardware and software that are important for understanding the applications described later. Also included are discussions of computer-system design and evaluation, with explanations of important issues for you to consider when you read about specific applications and systems throughout the remainder of the book.

Chapters 6 through 18 survey many of the key biomedical areas in which computers are being used. Each chapter explains the conceptual and organizational issues in building that type of system, reviews the pertinent history, and examines the barriers to successful implementations.

Chapter 19 provides a historical perspective on changes in the way society pays for health care. It discusses alternative methods for evaluating the costs and the benefits of health care, and suggests ways in which financial considerations affect medical computing. The book concludes in Chapter 20 with a look to the future—a vision of how computers one day may pervade every aspect of medical practice.

The Study of Computer Applications in Medicine

The actual and potential uses of computers in medical care form a remarkably broad and complex topic. However, just as you do not need to understand how a telephone works to make good use of it and to tell when it is functioning poorly, we believe that technical medical-computing skills are not needed by health workers who simply wish to become effective computer users. On the other hand, such technical skills are of course necessary for individuals with a career commitment to developing computer systems for medical environments. Thus, this book will neither teach you to be a programmer, nor show you how to fix a broken computer (although it might motivate you to learn how to do both). It also will not tell you about every important medical-computing system or application; we shall direct you to a wealth of literature where review articles and individual project reports can be found. We describe specific systems only as examples that can provide you with an understanding of the conceptual and organizational issues to be addressed in building systems for such uses. Examples also help to reveal the remaining barriers to successful implementations. Some of the application systems described in the book are well established, even in the commercial marketplace. Others are just beginning to be used broadly in biomedical settings. Several are still largely confined to the research laboratory.

Because we wish to emphasize the concepts underlying this field, we generally limit the discussion of technical implementation details. The computer-science issues can be learned from other courses and other textbooks. One exception, however, is our emphasis on the details of decision science as they relate to medical problem solving (Chapters 3 and 15). These topics generally are not presented in computer-science courses, yet they play a central role in the intelligent use of medical data and knowledge. Sections on medical decision making and computer-assisted decision support accordingly include more technical detail than you will find in other chapters.

All chapters include an annotated list of Suggested Readings to which you can turn if you have a particular interest in a topic, and there is a comprehensive listing of References at the end of the book. We use **boldface** print to indicate the key terms of each chapter; the definitions of these terms are included in the Glossary at the end of the book. Because many of the issues in medical informatics are conceptual, we have included Questions for Discussion at the end of each chapter. You will quickly discover that most of these questions do not have "right" answers. They are intended to illuminate key issues in the field and to motivate you to examine additional readings and new areas of research.

It is inherently limiting to learn about computer applications solely by reading about them. We accordingly encourage you to complement your studies by seeing real systems in use—ideally by using them yourself. Your understanding of system limitations and of what *you* would do to improve a medical-computing system will be greatly enhanced if you have had personal experience with representative applications. Be aggressive in seeking opportunities to observe and use working systems.

In a field that is changing as rapidly as computer science is, it is difficult ever to feel that you have knowledge that is completely current. However, the conceptual basis for study changes much more slowly than do the detailed technological issues. Thus, the lessons you learn from this volume will provide you with a foundation on which you can continue to build in the years ahead.

The Need for a Course in Medical-Computing Applications

Suggesting that new courses are needed in the curricula for students of the health professions does not increase your popularity. If anything, educators and students have been clamoring for reduced lecture time, for more emphasis on small group sessions, and for more free time for problem solving and reflection. A 1984 national survey by the Association of American Medical Colleges found that both medical students and their educators severely criticized the current emphasis on lectures and memorization. Yet the analysis of a panel on the General Professional Education of the Physician (GPEP) [Association of American Medical Colleges, 1984] specifically identified medical informatics, including computer applications, as an area in which new educational opportunities needed to be developed so that physicians would be better prepared for the practice of medicine. The report recommended the formation of new academic units in medical informatics in our medical schools.

The reason for this strong recommendation is clear: *The practice of medicine is inextricably entwined with the management of information.* In the past, practitioners handled medical information through resources such as the nearest hospital or medical-school library; personal collections of books, journals, and reprints; files of patient records; consultation with colleagues; manual office bookkeeping; and (all-too-often flawed) memorization. Although all these techniques continue to be valuable, the computer is offering new methods for finding, filing, and sorting information: online bibliographic-retrieval systems, including full-text publication; personal computers, with database software to maintain personal information and reprint files; office-practice and hospital information systems to capture, communicate, and preserve key elements of the medical record; consultation systems to provide assistance when colleagues are inaccessible or unavailable; practice-management systems to integrate billing and receivable functions with other aspects of office or clinic organization; and other online information resources that help to reduce the pressure to memorize in a field that defies total mastery of all but its narrowest aspects. With such a pervasive and inevitable role for computers in clinical practice, and with a growing failure of traditional techniques to deal with the rapidly increasing information-management needs of practitioners, it has become obvious to many people that a new and essential topic has emerged for study in schools that train medical and other health professionals.

What is less clear is how the subject should be taught, and to what extent it should be left for postgraduate education. We believe that topics in medical computing are best taught and learned in the context of health-science training, which allows concepts from both medicine and computer science to be integrated. Medical-computing novices are likely to have only limited opportunities for intensive study of the material once their health-professional training has been completed.

The format of medical-informatics education is certain to evolve as faculty are hired to develop it at more health-science schools, and as the emphasis on lectures as the primary teaching method diminishes. Computers will be used increasingly as teaching tools and as devices for communication, problem solving, and data sharing among students and faculty. In the meantime, medical informatics will be taught largely in the classroom setting. This book is designed to be used in that kind of traditional course, although the Questions for Discussion also could be used to focus conversation in small seminars and working groups. As resources improve in schools, integration of medical-computing topics into clinical experiences also will become more common. The eventual goal should be to provide instruction in medical informatics whenever this field is most relevant to the topic the student is studying. This aim requires educational opportunities throughout the years of formal training, supplemented by continuing-education programs after graduation.

The goal of integrating medicine and computer science is to provide a mechanism for increasing the sophistication of health professionals, so that they know and understand the available resources. They also should be familiar with medical computing's successes and failures, its research frontiers and its limitations, so that they can avoid repeating the mistakes of the past. Study of medical computing also should improve their skills in information management and problem solving. With a suitable integration of hands-on computer experience, computer-based learning, courses in clinical problem solving, and study of the material in this volume, health-science students will be well prepared to make effective use of computer-based tools and information management in health-care delivery.

The Need for Specialists in Medical Informatics

As mentioned, this book also is intended to be used as an introductory text in programs of study for people who intend to make their professional careers in medical informatics. If we have persuaded you that a course in medical informatics is needed, then the requirement for trained faculty to teach the courses will be obvious. Some people, however, might argue that a course on this subject could be taught by a computer scientist who had an interest in medical computing, or by a physician who had taken a few computing courses. Indeed, in the past, most teaching—and research—has been undertaken by faculty trained primarily in one of the fields and later drawn to the other. Today, however, schools are beginning to realize the need for professionals trained specifically at the interfaces among medicine, computer science, and related disciplines such as statistics, cognitive science, health economics, and medical ethics [Shortliffe, 1984b; Shortliffe and Fagan, 1989]. This book outlines a basic curriculum for students training for careers in the medical-computing field. We specifically address the need for an educational experience in which computing and information-science concepts are synthesized with biomedical issues regarding research, training, and clinical practice. It is the *integration* of the related disciplines that traditionally has been lacking in the educational opportunities available to students with career interests in medical informatics. If schools are to establish such courses and training programs (and there are already a few examples of each), they clearly need educators who have a broad familiarity with the field and who can develop curricula for students of the health professions as well as of engineering and computer science.

The increasing introduction of computing techniques into medical environments will require that well-trained individuals be available not only to teach students, but also to design, develop, select, and manage the medical-computing systems of tomorrow. There is a wide range of context-dependent computing issues that people can appreciate only by working on problems defined by the medical-care setting and its constraints. The field's development has been hampered because there are relatively few trained personnel to design research programs, to carry out the experimental and developmental activities, and to provide academic leadership in medical computing. A frequently cited problem is the difficulty a health professional and a technically trained computer scientist experience when they try to communicate with each other. The vocabularies of the two fields are complex and have little overlap, and there is a process of acculturation to medicine that is difficult for computer scientists to appreciate through distant observation. Thus, interdisciplinary research and development projects are more likely to be successful when they are led by people who can effectively bridge the medical and computing fields. Such professionals often can facilitate sensitive communication among program personnel whose backgrounds and training differ substantially.

It is exciting to be working in a field that is gradually maturing and that is having a beneficial effect on society. There is ample opportunity remaining for innovation as new technologies evolve and fundamental computing problems succumb to the creativity and hard work of our colleagues. In light of the increasing sophistication and specialization required in computer science in general, it is hardly surprising that a new discipline should arise at that field's interface with medicine. This book is dedicated to clarifying the definition and to nurturing the effectiveness of that new discipline: medical informatics.

E.H.S
L.E.P.
Palo Alto, CA
February 1990

Acknowledgments

When Larry Fagan, Gio Wiederhold, and I decided to compile the first comprehensive textbook on medical informatics, none of us predicted the enormity of the task we were about to undertake. Our challenge was to create a multiauthored textbook that captured the collective expertise of leaders in the field yet was cohesive in content and style. The concept for the book first developed in 1982. We had begun to teach a course on computer applications in health care at Stanford University School of Medicine and had quickly determined that there was no comprehensive introductory text on the subject. Although there were several collections of research descriptions and subject reviews, none had been developed with the needs of a rigorous introductory course in mind.

The thought of writing a textbook was daunting due to the diversity of topics. None of us felt sufficiently expert in the full range of important subjects to write the book alone. Yet we wanted to avoid putting together a collection of disconnected chapters containing assorted subject reviews. Thus, we decided to solicit contributions from leaders in the fields to be represented, but to provide organizational guidelines in advance for each chapter. We also urged contributors to avoid writing subject reviews, and instead to focus on the key conceptual topics in their fields and to pick a handful of examples to illustrate their didactic points.

As the draft chapters began to arrive, we realized that major editing would be required if we were to achieve our goals of cohesiveness among and a uniform orientation across all the chapters. We were thus delighted when, in 1987, Leslie Perreault, a graduate of our training program, assumed responsibility for reworking the individual chapters to make an integral whole and for bringing the project to completion. The final product is the result of many compromises, heavy editing, detailed rewriting, and numerous iterations. We greatly appreciate the cooperation of all the chapter authors who worked with us and accepted our changes to their contributions so that we all could achieve the project's goals.

The completed volume reflects the work and support of many people in addition to the editors and chapter authors. Particular gratitude is owed to Lyn Dupré, our developmental editor whose rigorous attention to detail is reflected on every page. We were also fortunate to work closely with people at Addison-Wesley throughout the project, including Nicholas Keefe, who first supported the concept of a novel publication such as this one; Peter Gordon, who subsequently supported our endeavor and tolerated the time required for us to complete the editing job; and Helen Goldstein, who kept the process moving. Janice Rohn provided invaluable assistance throughout the project, acquiring and creating many of the photographs and original figures, providing editorial assistance on earlier drafts, and coordinating the final production of the book with meticulous attention to detail. Lynne Hollander painstakingly and conscientiously compiled the index and wielded word-processing programs on many parts of the manuscript. Voy Wiederhold read thoroughly and offered comments on multiple versions of the chapters. Darlene Vian competently managed the administrative details so that we could attend to our writing. We are also grateful for the support of the SUMEX-AIM Computer Project at Stanford University, a shared national resource supported by the Division of Research Resources of the National Institutes of Health. SUMEX and its director, Tom Rindfleisch, provided us with a superb computing environment and with systems staff—notably Christopher Lane and Christopher Schmidt—who reliably provided the technical support that we needed for the book's online preparation using LATEX on Macintosh II computers.

Numerous colleagues across the country have read and critiqued the manuscript, and have contributed their insights and suggestions. Special thanks are due to Bill Brown, Bruce Buchanan, Ed deLand, Karen Duncan, Thelma Estrin, Dan Feldman, W. Edward Hammond, Allen Levy, Don Lindberg, Naomi Sager, Don Simborg, Peter Szolovits, Jan van Bemmel, and Homer Warner. We extend our appreciation to the graduate students of Stanford University's Medical Information Sciences Program. They helped us to debug the chapters we used in their courses, providing many helpful and insightful comments on the drafts. Finally, we thank our families and friends. Their support and encouragement were crucial to the completion of this project.

Contents

III. Medical Informatics in the Years Ahead   583

I

Recurrent Themes
in Medical Informatics

1

The Computer Meets Medicine: Emergence of a Discipline

Marsden S. Blois and Edward H. Shortliffe

After reading this chapter, you should know the answers to these questions:

- Why is information management a central issue in biomedical research and clinical practice?
- What are integrated information-management environments and how might we expect them to affect the practice of medicine and biomedical research in coming years?
- What do we mean by the terms *medical computer science, medical computing,* and *medical informatics*?
- Why should health professionals and students of the health professions learn about medical-informatics concepts and medical-computing applications?
- How has the development of minicomputers and microprocessors changed the nature of biomedical computing?
- How is medical informatics related to medical practice, biomedical engineering, and computer science?
- How does information in medicine differ from information in the basic sciences?
- How can changes in computer technology and the way medical care is financed influence the integration of medical computing into medical practice?

1.1 Integrated Information Management: Technology's Promise

After scientists had developed the first digital computers in the 1940s, society was told that these new machines would soon be serving routinely as memory devices, assisting with calculations and with information retrieval. Within the next decade, physicians and other health workers had begun to hear about the dramatic effect that such technology would have on medical practice. Over 3 decades of remarkable progress in computing have followed those early predictions, and many of the original prophesies have come to pass. Others, such as the routine use of computers by clinicians in their practices, are still awaiting full realization. Nonetheless, the enormous technological advances of the last decade—graphical workstations, new methods for human–computer interaction, powerful personal computers with huge memories, and remarkable innovations in mass storage of data—have all combined to make routine use of computers by all health workers and biomedical scientists inevitable if not imminent. A new world is already with us, but its greatest influence is yet to come. This book will teach you both about our present resources and accomplishments *and* about what we can expect in the years ahead.

What might that future hold for the typical practicing clinician? Let us imagine one scenario—a view of the future that presumes little in the way of new technology but that does depend, as we shall explain, on the development of an infrastructure, and of coordinated plans for medical computing and communications, that are now only beginning to be put in place. Let us consider a multispecialty group practice located close to a major hospital. The physicians in the practice have installed a *local-area network (LAN)* in their outpatient clinics,[1] and this LAN permits the computers

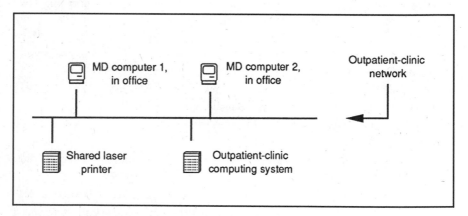

FIGURE 1.1 A local-area network for an outpatient clinic. The physicians use terminals or computers in their offices, but these machines share common resources on the network, such as printers and a machine for storing patient records. Thus, any patient's outpatient record can be accessed from any of the offices.

---

[1]LANs and basic computing concepts introduced in this scenario are discussed in Chapter 4.

in their offices to share common facilities, such as printing devices and a databank of outpatient medical records (Figure 1.1). Dr. James Robinson, an internist on the clinic staff, is working in his office between patient visits. He will soon be seeing Mr. David Jones, a middle-aged man with heart disease and a lipid disorder (excess fats in the blood). He ordered blood tests the last time Mr. Jones was seen in the office, and therefore he decides to check whether the results are available.

Dr. Robinson operates his computer system largely by selecting items of interest through use of a *mouse* pointing device, which he rolls on the desktop beside the machine. Movement of the mouse generates corresponding movement of a pointer on the screen of the computer, so Dr. Robinson can simply "point" at an item of interest, and then indicate that he wants to select that item by depressing a button on the top of the mouse. Seldom is he required to type on the keyboard—which is just as well, since he is an inordinately slow typist. On the day in question, he signs on to his computer by identifying himself on a displayed list of physicians in the practice, and by entering a password that ensures that his files are not accessed by unauthorized individuals (Figure 1.2).[2]

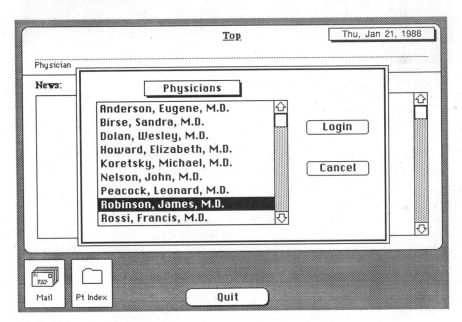

FIGURE 1.2 Dr. Robinson uses the mouse pointing device to select his name from the list of physicians who practice in his clinic. The system then requests a password before it will permit him to proceed to read messages addressed to him, or to review confidential patient information.

---

[2]The sample screens used throughout this scenario were developed using HyperCard on a Macintosh computer. They are the work of Joan Walton, a former graduate student in the Medical Informatics Program at Stanford University School of Medicine. Ms. Walton developed this prototype system as part of her exploratory work on human–computer interaction.

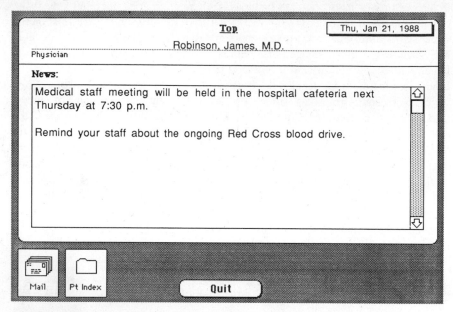

FIGURE 1.3 Once he has successfully logged on to the computer, Dr. Robinson receives recent "broadcast messages" that have been posted for reading by all his hospital's medical staff. The icons at the bottom of the display indicate that he can now read his electronic mail, review patient information, or quit (stop using the computer system).

As soon as he is logged on to his computer, Dr. Robinson sees that there are messages waiting that have been sent to him and to the other clinic physicians from the nearby hospital at which they practice (Figure 1.3). But how did such messages get to the computer in his office? Dr. Robinson does not need to know that he is actually viewing messages that are stored not on his own computer, but rather on an electronic-mail machine physically located at the hospital. His own machine queried the hospital computer for such messages and displayed any that Dr. Robinson had not previously seen. This transfer of data was made possible by a *gateway* connection between the LAN in the clinic building and a similar LAN in the hospital (Figure 1.4). The gateway is a device that connects the office network to the hospital network so that data and messages can be transferred from machines on one network to machines on the other.

In addition to such broadcast messages, which are sent to all professional staff at the hospital, Dr. Robinson has a private mailbox on the hospital computer. He accesses it by simply using the mouse to select the mail *icon,* a graphical symbol at the bottom of the screen. Among his messages is a brief note from the hospital's clinical laboratory reporting the test results for Mr. Jones' lipid panel (Figure 1.5). When Dr. Robinson ordered this test, he requested that the results be sent to him directly, rather than simply being stored in the patient's automated medical record. The laboratory computer is connected to the hospital network, and thus can send test

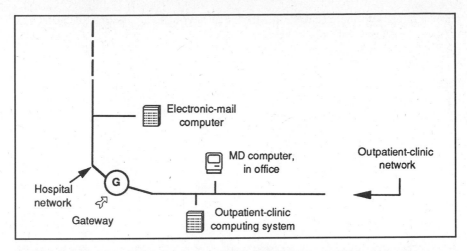

FIGURE 1.4 The broadcast messages displayed in Figure 1.3 were gathered for display by Dr. Robinson's office computer. It obtained the messages from the hospital's electronic-mail machine. For the office computer to access such information, a gateway between the clinic network and the hospital's network was required. Such gateways can be direct physical connections if the clinic is adjacent to the hospital, or they can operate via telephone lines or microwave transmission.

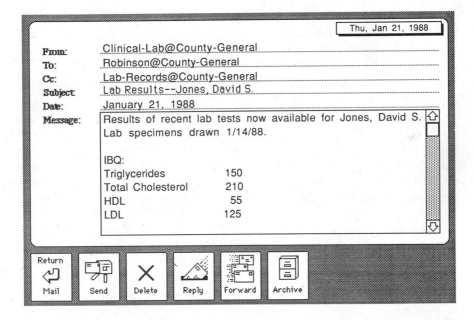

FIGURE 1.5 Dr. Robinson has checked his mail and finds that he has a message from the hospital laboratory that is reporting the results of a lipid panel for his patient, Mr. David Jones. The *scroll bar* at the right of the message window would be used to read the rest of the message if the text did not fit on a single screen. Note that the icons across the bottom of the display represent the various actions that Dr. Robinson might want to select when reading his electronic mail.

results directly to the electronic mailboxes of physicians requesting such services (Figure 1.6). The results of the tests are gratifying—Mr. Jones' total cholesterol level is finally decreasing in response to therapy.

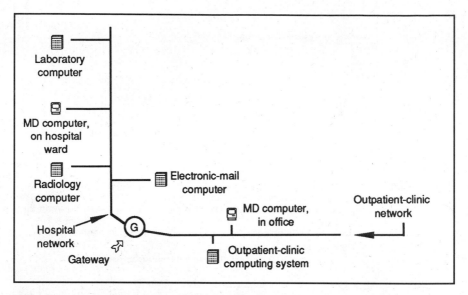

FIGURE 1.6 For the hospital's laboratory computer to send mail to Dr. Robinson's electronic mailbox, it too must be connected to the hospital network. Note that radiology and similar departmental machines are also tied to the hospital network, so that they can share results and data with other computers, as the laboratory machine did. In addition, terminals or computers on the hospital wards could be used by Dr. Robinson in much the same way that he is using the machine in his office. A uniform interface permits him to have the same functions and procedures available to him, regardless of where he happens to be located.

In preparation for the office visit with Mr. Jones, Dr. Robinson reviews the patient's electronic record. He selects the patient's name and record number from a directory (Figure 1.7), and is presented with the cover sheet for Mr. Jones' record (Figure 1.8). A variety of options is available (as indicated by the choices displayed across the bottom of the screen); Dr. Robinson is specifically interested in the clinical information in the medical record (the second icon). The medical record begins with the patient's problem list and, if relevant, a summary of critical events in the patient's medical history (surgeries, hospitalizations, biopsies, and the like; Figure 1.9). Once again, a range of options for exploring the record is displayed across the bottom of the screen; Dr. Robinson is interested in reviewing past notes, so he selects the third icon.

The patient's initial History and Physical note (Figure 1.10) is organized using the stereotypic subheadings of chief complaint (CC); history of present illness (HPI); past medical history (PMH); family medical history (FMH); social information, habits, review of systems (ROS); and physical examination (PE). Dr. Robinson can select the portion of the chart that interests him by simply selecting the appropriately labeled

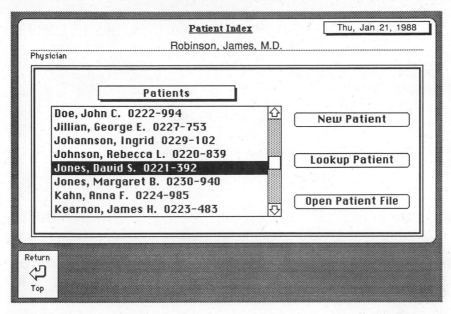

FIGURE 1.7 Dr. Robinson selects Mr. Jones' electronic chart for review. Note that he could also start a new chart for a patient who has not been seen previously in this practice.

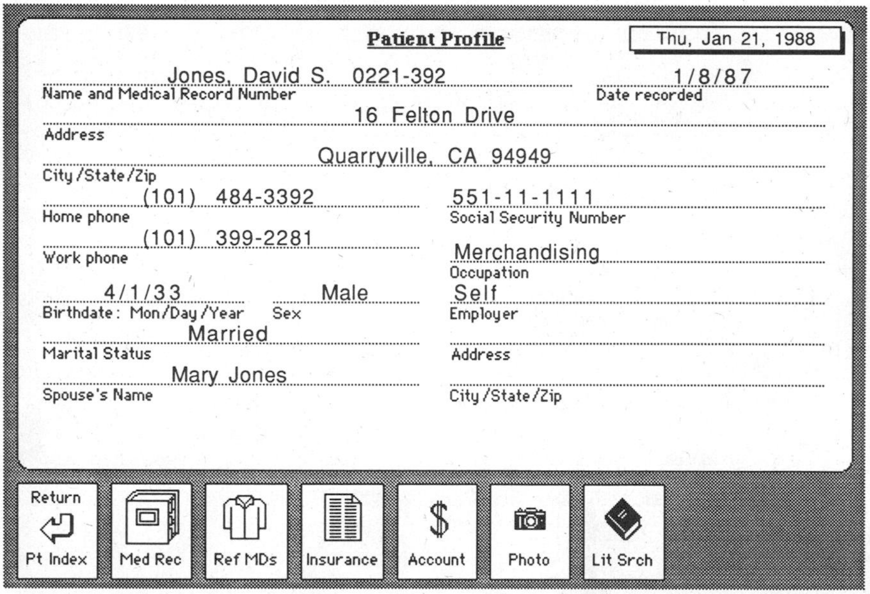

FIGURE 1.8 This patient profile corresponds to the cover sheet of the traditional medical record. The icons across the bottom of the screen show the options available to Dr. Robinson at this time. In addition to examining a list of referring physicians or financial information, he can display a digitized photograph of the patient or request assistance with a literature search (see Figure 1.16).

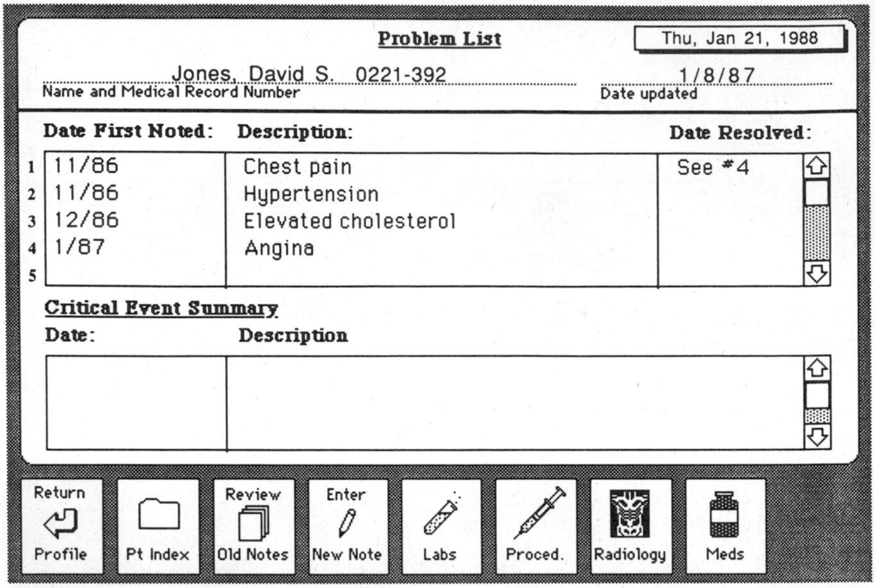

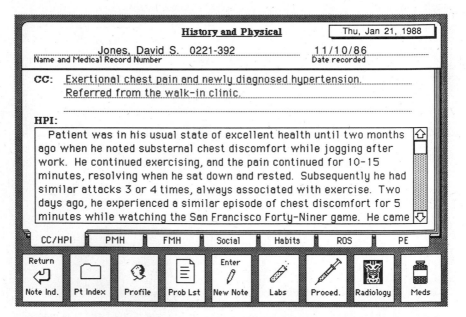

FIGURE 1.9 Dr. Robinson has requested a review of Mr. Jones' clinical record, and it begins with this display of the patient's principal problems. Note that the icons across the bottom of the display now indicate clinical options pertinent to a physician's review of a medical chart.

FIGURE 1.10 The patient's chief complaint and a portion of his presenting history are shown on this display. Note that the user can select the tabs across the bottom of the chart with the mouse, and thus can move with ease among various sections of the patient's initial history and physical examination. This approach allows straightforward browsing, because the chart does not need to be scanned sequentially.

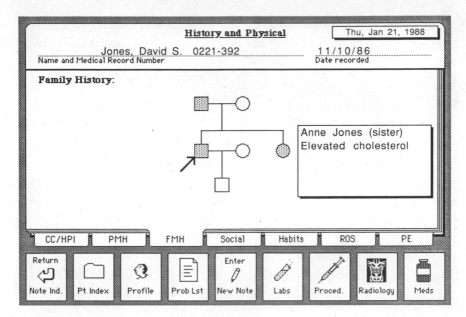

FIGURE 1.11 Modern workstations have graphical capabilities that allow computer-based records to include diagrams and pictures, much as physicians have traditionally hand-drawn such descriptive materials in paper charts. Here the family history is summarized using an interactive graphical display. Mr. Jones is indicated in the family tree with an arrow. Dr. Robinson has selected the circular icon representing the patient's sister, and pertinent history has been displayed in response.

"tab." He can review the family history by pointing at the "FMH" tab, pressing the mouse button, and then selecting, for example, the circle corresponding to Mr. Jones' sister in the family tree (Figure 1.11). Subsequent briefer clinic visits have been recorded using a condensed progress-note format (Figure 1.12), in which the tabs on the chart correspond to the patient's subjective comments (S), to the objective findings on examination or laboratory testing (O), to Dr. Robinson's assessment of the patient's status (A), and finally to the management plans that follow from that assessment (P).[3]

Dr. Robinson can review the laboratory-test results by selecting the labeled icon at the bottom of the screen. For example, Mr. Jones' lipid-panel results might well be displayed in a time-oriented table (Figure 1.13), or Dr. Robinson could ask that some of the results be plotted for increased ease of viewing (Figure 1.14). Regardless of the display format he selects, however, Dr. Robinson may well have difficulty remembering the precise guidelines for continued management of Mr. Jones' lipid

---

[3]This record-keeping system, with progress notes organized as described, is commonly used in the United States. The notes are called SOAP notes because of their four-part internal structure. The system is derived from the problem-oriented medical record, an approach originally developed by Lawrence Weed [Weed, 1969].

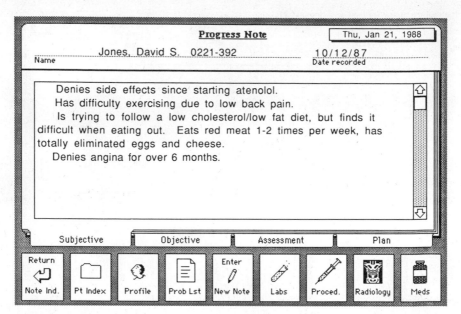

FIGURE 1.12 Progress notes are more concise than are history and physical-examination notes (Figure 1.10), so they are stored using the four-part internal organization displayed here. This is only one example of how medical data might be displayed and organized on a graphical workstation. Such systems need to be adapted to local or personal preferences.

Lipid Lab   Thu, Jan 21, 1988

Jones, David S.   0221-392

Name and Medical Record Number

Dates

Labs	Units	12/17/86	1/25/87	4/2/87	7/19/87	10/12/87	1/21/88
TG	mg/dl	250	260	240	230	235	150
TC	mg/dl	260	262	248	250	265	210
HDL	mg/dl	40	38	45	39	40	55
LDL	mg/dl	170	172	155	165	178	125

Interpret   Plot

Return — Lab Index | Pt Index | Profile | Review Old Notes | Enter New Note | Proced. | Radiology | Meds

FIGURE 1.13 When Dr. Robinson requests a display of the patient's lipid blood tests over time, he is shown the tabular summary illustrated here. If he prefers to see these results plotted, he simply selects the "Plot" icon at the right of the screen. [TG = triglycerides, TC = total cholesterol, HDL = high-density lipoprotein, LDL = low-density lipoprotein.]

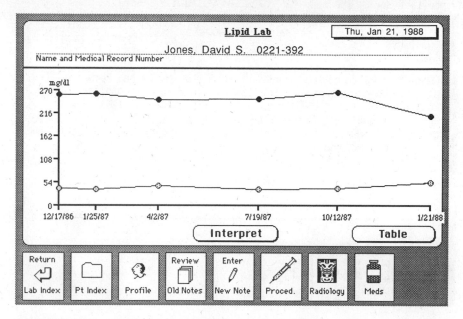

FIGURE 1.14 This is the plot of the data for total cholesterol and high-density lipoprotein from Figure 1.13. Before this graphical summary is displayed, the user is asked to select those specific tests that he would like to see plotted. Although the graphical display may be easier to interpret than the tabular version, Dr. Robinson may still be uncertain how best to proceed with this patient's lipid management. The "Interpret" icon is available to allow him to request a brief consultation from the computer regarding current management guidelines in this situation.

problems. Thus, he may choose to request an interpretation of the lipid results, selecting the "Interpret" icon on the screen and receiving a patient-specific advisory summary (Figure 1.15). At this point, Dr. Robinson may choose to follow the computer's advice or to make a different management decision based on preferences he and the patient have.

Although this scenario has shown the ease with which Dr. Robinson can review patient information and even request certain types of management advice using a computer in his office, we have not yet considered how he might request generic information from sources outside his office or hospital. Note, for example, that one of the icons at the bottom of the screen in Figure 1.8 is labeled "Lit Srch." This is the selection that permits Dr. Robinson to search the literature and other databases for information that he may need to provide patient care. Selecting this icon would result in a display such as that shown in Figure 1.16. Here, Dr. Robinson is offered several options: the ability to search and peruse clinical textbooks in their full-text format, access to the Medline database of citations and abstracts for articles in the biomedical literature, a facility to search large patient databases to find how patients around the country have fared under different treatment regimens, and a literature-assessment facility that helps him to determine whether specific studies in the literature can be appropriately applied to his specific patient's problem.

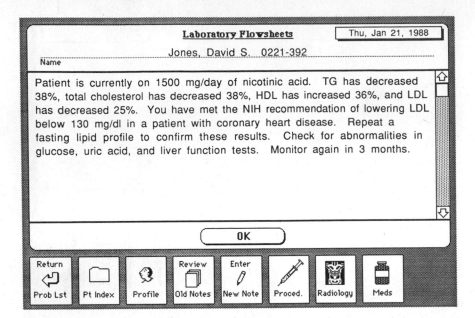

FIGURE 1.15 When Dr. Robinson requests an interpretation of Mr. Jones' current lipid results, he is given the computer-generated advice shown here. This advice is generated by an expert system for lipid management, which is linked to the patient's medical record and can give recommendations based on Mr. Jones' specific situation. The advice is only a suggestion, however, and Dr. Robinson and Mr. Jones will determine together whether to follow it.

Some of these facilities might well be provided by the biomedical library at the physician's hospital or associated medical school. Thus, the hospital network needs to be connected to the library network to allow direct access to informational resources from any terminal or computer on the network (Figure 1.17). National databases and shared communications facilities, however, require connections between the hospital's network and a nationwide biomedical communications (wide-area) network (Figure 1.18). It is this final network model, then, that illustrates the complex layers of connectivity that are required if Dr. Robinson's clinic computer is to provide the wide range of information sources that Dr. Robinson needs to practice modern medicine efficiently and with enhanced attention to quality decision making.

The vision of the future outlined here presumes little technology that is not available today. Both local- and wide-area networks are currently in use, and standards for connectivity are beginning to emerge. A few questions may arise about how some of the specific features that we illustrated would actually be provided; for example, the narrative descriptions in the patient's record need to be captured in some way. Unless we presume that physicians will actually type their observations directly into the online record, we may assume that their words will be dictated and later transcribed for the chart by other people. Alternatively, we may soon see the day when speech-recognition technology allows the physician's dictation to be understood directly by

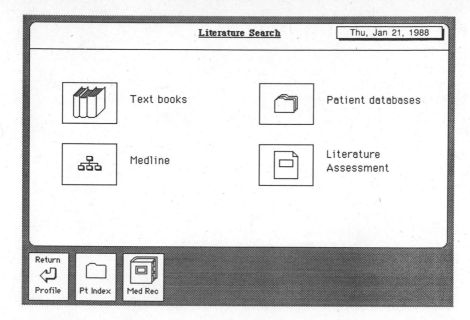

FIGURE 1.16 When Dr. Robinson requests assistance with a literature search (see Figure 1.8), he is given four choices. Although each requires access to a different computer in a different part of the country, the choices are presented as simple icons on the screen. Dr. Robinson selects the information resource that he needs, and the computer routes his request appropriately over local- or wide-area networks (see Figures 1.17 and 1.18).

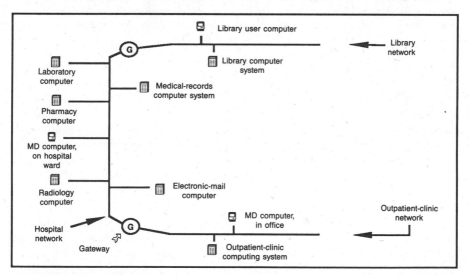

FIGURE 1.17 Library resources can be made available locally only if the hospital or medical school library is itself linked to the hospital and office-practice networks. Appropriate gateways are therefore required. Note that this arrangement also permits terminals or computers in the library to be used by clinicians to access patient information, electronic mail, or similar clinical data.

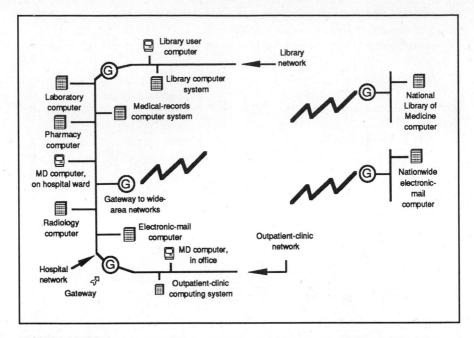

FIGURE 1.18 For information that is stored on computers in other parts of the country, the local-area networks in hospitals and offices must be linked to wide-area networks that traverse the country. Such networks typically use dedicated telephone lines or microwave and satellite links. This model imposes major requirements on the biomedical and health-care communities for agreeing on an infrastructure and on methods of coordination and cooperation that will make the implied sharing of data and information feasible.

the computer for translation into written words. We also did not illustrate the "Radiology" option shown as an icon in Figure 1.9 and in subsequent figures. Today, it would be straightforward to provide radiology reports that had been dictated by radiologists viewing conventional films, but before long, physicians will expect to see the actual X-ray pictures displayed on their computer screens as well. Once again, the technology for digital transmission of such images exists, but it is still expensive and is not yet in widespread use.

Thus, the scenario described here is meant to provide you with a glimpse of what lies ahead and to suggest the topics that need to be addressed in a book such as this one. You will find that essentially all of the chapters that follow touch on some aspect of the scenario. Before embarking on these topics, however, let us emphasize two points. First, the scenario presented in this section will become reality only if individual hospitals, academic medical centers, and national coordinating bodies provide the infrastructure that is necessary. No individual system developer, vendor, or administrator can mandate the standards for connectivity and data sharing implied by an integrated environment, such as the one illustrated in Figure 1.18. A national initiative of cooperative planning and implementation for computing and communications resources within single institutions and clinics will be required before practitioners will have routine access to information. A uniform environment is required if transitions between resources are to be facile and uncomplicated.

Second, although our scenario focused on the clinician's view of integrated information access, other workers in the field have similar needs that can be addressed in similar ways. Illustrating this point, Figure 1.19 shows the current networking environment available to biomedical researchers at one medical school. Note that the communications environment includes local shared resources (computers, printers, and specialized equipment) as well as straightforward access over existing networks to information resources and computing facilities around the country. Thus, the academic research community has already made use of much of the technology that needs to be coalesced if the clinical user in our scenario is to have similar access to data and information.

With this discussion as background, let us now consider the discipline that has led to the development of many of the facilities that need to be brought together in the integrated medical-computing environment of the future. The remainder of this

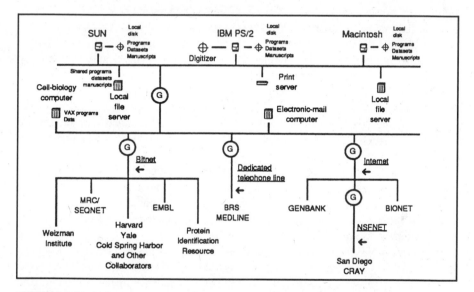

FIGURE 1.19 This diagram shows a simplified schematic summary of the networking environment available to biomedical researchers at Stanford University School of Medicine in 1989. Different personal workstations in research laboratories (top of diagram) are connected to one another and to a variety of specialized servers for printing and shared file storage. A second local network provides access to a shared computing research facility, located in the department of cell biology. In addition, connections to wide-area networks are heavily used by molecular biologists and other scientists. For example, the academic network known as Bitnet provides access to collaborators and shared databases around the world. Stanford also has installed a dedicated connection to the machine of BRS, a major vendor of the Medline database from the National Library of Medicine. Finally, the federal Internet provides access to specialized research resources (GENBANK and BIONET), as well as a connection to a supercomputer (the San Diego CRAY) over a network established by the National Science Foundation (NSF).

chapter deals with medical computing as a field and with medical information as a subject of study. It provides additional background you will need to understand many of the subsequent chapters in this book.

1.2 The Use of Computers in Biomedicine

Biomedical applications of computers is a phrase that evokes different images, depending on the nature of one's involvement in the field. To a hospital administrator, it might suggest the maintenance of medical records using computers; to a decision scientist, it might mean the assistance of computers in disease diagnosis; to a basic scientist, it might mean the use of computers for maintaining and retrieving gene-sequencing information. Many physicians immediately think of office-practice tools for tasks such as patient billing or appointment scheduling. The field includes study of all these activities, and of a great many others too. More important, it includes the consideration of various external factors that affect the medical setting. Unless you keep in mind these surrounding factors, it may be difficult to understand how medical computing can help us to tie together the diverse aspects of health care and its delivery.

To achieve a unified perspective, we might consider three related topics: (1) the applications of computers in medicine, (2) the concept of medical information (why it is important in medical practice, and why we might want to use computers to process it), and (3) the structural features of medicine, including all those subtopics to which computers might be applied. The first of these is the subject of this book. We mention the second and third topics briefly in this and the next chapter, and we provide references in the Suggested Readings section for those students who wish to learn more.

The modern computer is still a relatively young device. Because the computer as a machine is exciting, people may pay a disproportionate amount of attention to it as such—at the expense of considering what the computer can do given the numbers, concepts, ideas, and cognitive underpinnings of a field such as medicine. In recent years, computer scientists, philosophers, psychologists, and other scholars have begun *collectively* to consider such matters as what the nature of information and knowledge is, and how humans process such concepts. These investigations have been given a sense of timeliness (if not urgency) by the simple existence of the computer. The cognitive activities of physicians in practice probably have received more attention over the past few years than in all previous history. Again, the existence of the computer, and the possibilities of its extending a physician's cognitive powers, have motivated most of these studies: To develop computer-based tools to assist with decisions, we must understand more clearly such human processes as diagnosis, therapy planning, decision making, and problem solving in medicine.

1.2.1 Terminology

Ever since the 1960s, by which time almost anyone doing serious biomedical computation had access to some kind of computer system, people have been uncertain what name they should use for the medical application of computer-science concepts.

The name *computer science* was itself new in 1960, and was only vaguely defined. Even today, *computer science* is used more as a matter of convention than as an explanation of the field's scientific content.

We use the phrase **medical computer science** to refer to the subdivision of computer science that applies the methods of the larger field to medical topics. As you will see, however, medicine has provided a rich area for computer-science research, and several basic computing insights and methodologies have been derived from applied medical-computing research.

The term **information science,** which is occasionally used in conjunction with *computer science,* originated in the field of library science and is used to refer, somewhat generally, to the broad range of issues related to the management of both paper-based and electronically stored information. Much of what information science originally set out to be is now drawing renewed interest under the name **cognitive science.**

Information theory, in contrast, was first developed by scientists concerned about the physics of communication; it has evolved into what may be viewed as a new branch of mathematics. The results scientists have obtained with information theory have illuminated many processes in communications technology, but they have had little effect on our understanding of *human* information processing.

The term **biomedical computing** has been used for a number of years. It is non-descriptive and neutral, implying only that computers are employed for some purpose in biology or medicine. It often is associated with engineering applications of computers, however, in which computers are viewed more as tools for an engineering application than as the primary focus of research.

A term originally introduced in Europe is **medical informatics,** which is broader than *medical computing* (it includes such topics as medical statistics, record keeping, and the study of the nature of medical information itself), and deemphasizes the computer while focusing instead on the nature of the field to which computations are applied. Because the term *informatics* has only recently begun to be accepted in the United States, **medical information science** has often been used instead in this country; this term, however, may be confused with *library science,* and it does not capture the broader implications of the European term. As a result, the name *medical informatics* appears to have become the preferred term, even in the United States, although some people dislike the use of what they consider to be an awkward neologism. Despite this concern, we believe that the broad range of issues in biomedical information management *does* require an appropriate name, and we use *medical informatics* for this purpose throughout this book. When we are speaking specifically about computers and their use within medical-informatics activities, we use the terms *medical computer science* (for the methodologic issues) or *medical computing* (to describe the activity itself).

Although labels such as these are arbitrary, they are by no means insignificant. In the case of new fields of endeavor or branches of science, they are important both in designating the field, and in defining or restricting its contents. The most distinctive feature of the modern computer is the generality of its application. The nearly unlimited range of computer uses complicates the business of naming the field. As a result, the nature of computer science is perhaps better illustrated by examples than through attempts at formal definition. Much of this book presents examples that do just this.

In summary, we define *medical informatics* as the rapidly developing scientific field that deals with the storage, retrieval, and optimal use of biomedical information, data, and knowledge for problem solving and decision making. It accordingly touches on all basic and applied fields in biomedical science and is closely tied to modern information technologies, notably in the areas of computing and communication (medical computer science). The emergence of medical informatics as a new discipline is due in large part to advances in computing and communications technology, to an increasing awareness that the knowledge base of medicine is essentially unmanageable by traditional paper-based methods, and to a growing conviction that the *process* of informed decision making is as important to modern biomedicine as is the collection of facts on which clinical decisions or research plans are based.

1.2.2   Historical Perspective

The modern digital computer grew out of developments in the United States and abroad during World War II, and general-purpose computers began to appear in the marketplace by the mid-1950s (Figure 1.20). However, speculation about what might be done with such machines (if they should ever become available) had begun much earlier.

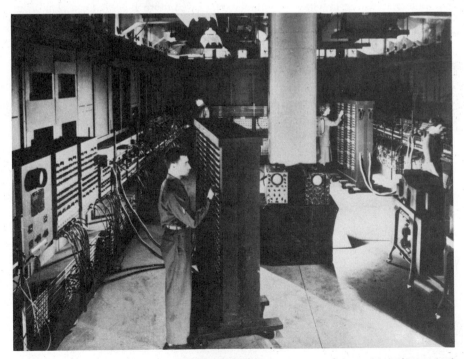

FIGURE 1.20 Early computers, such as the ENIAC, were the precursors of today's personal computers and hand-held calculators. (*Source:* Photograph courtesy of Unisys Corporation.)

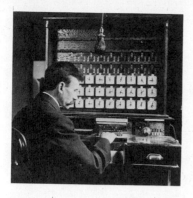

FIGURE 1.21 The Hollerith Tabulating Machine was an early data-processing system that performed automatic computation using punched cards. (*Source:* Photograph courtesy of the Library of Congress.)

Scholars at least as far back as the Middle Ages often had raised the question of whether human reasoning might be explained in terms of formal or algorithmic processes.[4] Gottfried Wilhelm von Leibnitz, a seventeenth-century German philosopher and mathematician, tried to develop a calculus that could be used to simulate human reasoning. The notion of a "logic engine" was subsequently worked out by Charles Babbage in the middle of the nineteenth century.

The first practical application of automatic computing relevant to medicine was Herman Hollerith's development of a punched-card data-processing system for the 1890 U.S. census (Figure 1.21). His methods were soon adapted to epidemiologic[5] and public-health surveys, initiating the era of electromechanical punched-card data-processing technology, which matured and was widely adopted during the 1920s and 1930s. These techniques were the precursors of the stored-program and wholly electronic digital computers that began to appear in the late 1940s [Collen, 1986].

One early activity in medical computing was the attempt to construct systems that would assist a physician in decision making (see Chapter 15). Not all medical-computing programs pursued this course, however. Many of the early ones instead investigated the notion of a total hospital information system (HIS; see Chapter 7). These projects were perhaps less ambitious in that they were more concerned with practical applications in the short term; the difficulties they encountered, however, were still formidable. The earliest work on HISs in the United States was probably that associated with the MEDINET project at General Electric, followed by work at Bolt, Beranek, and Newman in Cambridge, Massachusetts and then at the Massachusetts General Hospital (MGH) in Boston. A number of hospital application programs were developed at MGH by Barnett and his associates over 2 decades beginning in the early 1960s. Work on similar systems was undertaken by Warner at Latter Day Saints (LDS) Hospital in Salt Lake City, by Collen at Kaiser Permanente in Oakland, California, by Wiederhold at Stanford University in Stanford, California, and by scientists at Lockheed in Sunnyvale, California.[6]

---

[4] An algorithm is a well-defined procedure or sequence of steps for solving a problem.
[5] Epidemiology is the study of the incidence, distribution, and causes of disease in a population.
[6] The latter system was subsequently taken over and further developed by the Technicon Corporation (now TDS Healthcare Systems Corporation), and has now been installed in over 90 locations. The Technicon Medical Information System (TMIS) is described in Chapter 7.

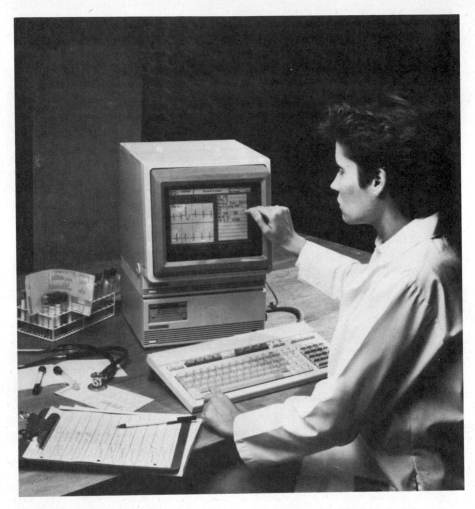

FIGURE 1.22 Hospital departments, such as the clinical laboratory, were able to implement their own custom-tailored systems when affordable minicomputers became available. Today, these departments often use microcomputers to support administrative and clinical functions. (*Source:* Photograph courtesy of Hewlett-Packard Company.)

The course of HIS applications bifurcated in the 1970s. One approach was based on the concept of an integrated or monolithic design in which a single, large, *time-shared computer* would be used to support an entire collection of applications. An alternative was a distributed design that favored the separate implementation of specific applications on smaller individual computers—minicomputers—thereby permitting the independent evolution of systems in the respective application areas. A common assumption was the existence of a single shared database of patient information. The multimachine model was not practical, however, until network technologies permitted rapid and reliable communication among distributed and (sometimes) heterogeneous types of machines. Such distributed HISs began to appear in the 1980s [Simborg et al., 1983].

Medical-computing activity broadened in scope and accelerated with the appearance of the *minicomputer* in the early 1970s. These machines made it possible for individual departments or small organizational units to acquire their own dedicated computers and to develop their own application systems (Figure 1.22). In tandem with the introduction of general-purpose software tools that provided standardized facilities to individuals with limited computer training (such as the UNIX operating system and programming environment), the minicomputer put more computing power in the hands of more medical investigators than did any other single development until the introduction of the *microprocessor,* a central processing unit (CPU) contained on one or a few chips (Figure 1.23).

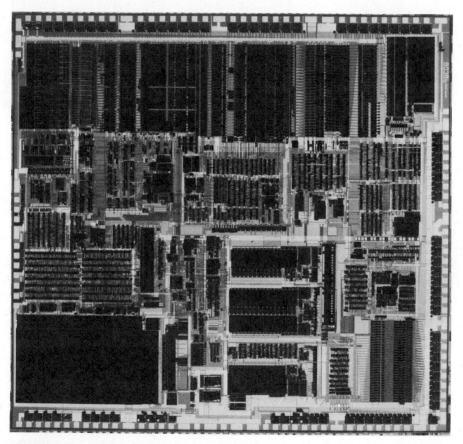

FIGURE 1.23 The microprocessor, or "computer on a chip," revolutionized the computer industry in the 1970s. By installing chips in small boxes and connecting them to a computer terminal, engineers produced the personal computer (PC)—an innovation that made it possible for individual users to purchase their own systems. (*Source:* Photograph courtesy of Intel Corporation.)

Everything changed radically beginning in the late 1970s and early 1980s, when the microprocessor and the *personal computer* (PC) or *microcomputer* became available. Not only could hospital departments afford minicomputers, but now individuals could afford microcomputers. This change enormously broadened the base of computing in our society and gave rise to a new software industry. The first articles on computers in medicine had appeared in clinical journals in the late 1950s, but it was not until the late 1970s that the first advertisements dealing with computers and aimed at physicians began to appear (Figure 1.24). Within a few years, a wide

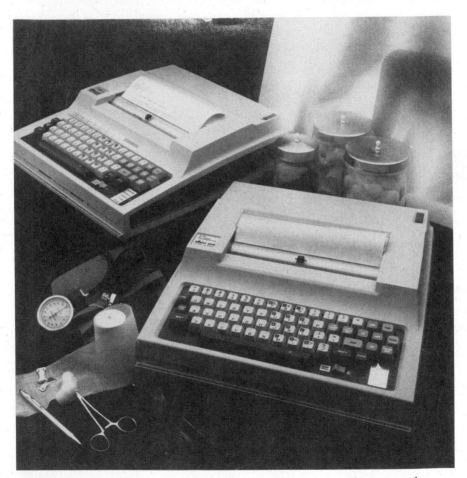

Just what the doctor ordered.

FIGURE 1.24 An early advertisement for a portable computer terminal, which appeared in general medical journals in the late 1970s. The development of compact, inexpensive peripheral devices and personal computers inspired future experiments in marketing directly to clinicians. (*Source:* Reprinted by permission of copyright holder, Texas Instruments Incorporated © 1985.)

range of computer-based information-management tools was available as commercial products; descriptions of these tools began to appear in journals alongside the traditional advertisements for drugs and other medical products. At present, individual physicians find it practical to employ microcomputers in a variety of settings, including for *limited* applications in patient care or clinical investigation. There remains, however, a serious shortage of application software for most of the professional activities in which physicians are engaged.

The stage is now set with a wide range of hardware of various sizes, types, prices, and capabilities, all of which will continue to evolve during the remainder of this century. The recent trend—reductions in size and cost of computers with simultaneous increases in power—shows no sign of slowing, although scientists are beginning to foresee the ultimate physical limitations to the miniaturization of computer circuits.

Progress in medical-computing research will continue to be tied to the availability of funding from either government or commercial sources. Because most medical-computing research is exploratory and is far from ready for commercial application, the federal government has played a key role in funding the work of the last 2 decades, mainly through the National Institutes of Health (NIH) and the National Center for Health Services Research (NCHSR). In recent years, the National Library of Medicine (NLM) (Figure 1.25) has assumed a primary role, especially with support for basic

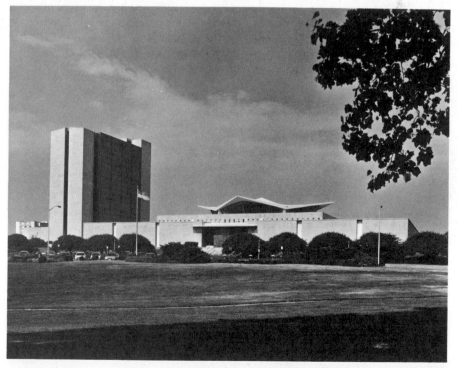

FIGURE 1.25 The National Library of Medicine (NLM) on the campus of the National Institutes of Health (NIH) in Bethesda, Maryland, is the principal biomedical library for the nation (see Chapter 14). It is also a major source of support for research in medical informatics. (*Source:* Photograph courtesy of the National Library of Medicine.)

research in the field. As increasing numbers of applications prove to be cost-effective (see Chapters 5 and 19), it is likely that more development work will shift to industrial settings and that university programs will focus increasingly on fundamental research problems viewed as too speculative for short-term commercialization.

1.3 Relationship to Medical Science and Practice

The exciting accomplishments of medical informatics, and the implied potential for future benefits to medicine, must be viewed in the context of our society and of the existing health-care system. As early as 1970, one eminent clinician suggested that computers might in time have a revolutionary influence on medical care, on medical education, and even on the selection criteria for health-science trainees [Schwartz, 1970]. The subsequent enormous growth in computing activity has been met with some trepidation by health professionals. They ask where it will all end. Will health workers gradually be replaced by computers? Will nurses and physicians need to be highly trained in computer science before they can practice their professions effectively? Will both patients and health workers eventually revolt rather than accept a trend toward automation that they believe may threaten the traditional humanistic values in health-care delivery? Will clinicians be viewed as outmoded and backward if they do not turn to computational tools for assistance with information management and decision making (Figure 1.26)?

Medical informatics is intrinsically entwined with the substance of medical science. It determines and analyzes the structure of medical information and knowledge, whereas medical science is constrained by that structure. Medical informatics melds the study of medical computer science with analyses of medical information and knowledge, thereby addressing specifically the interface between computer science and medical science. To illustrate what we mean by the "structural" features of medical information and knowledge, we can contrast the properties of the information and knowledge typical of such fields as physics or engineering with the properties of those typical of medicine (see Section 1.6).

Medical informatics is beginning to be accepted as a basic medical science. The analogy with other **basic sciences** is that medical computer science uses the results of past experience to structure and encode objective and subjective medical findings and thus to make them suitable for processing. This approach supports the integration of the findings and their analyses. In turn, the selective distribution of newly created knowledge can aid both patient care and health planning.

Medical computing is, by its nature, an experimental science. An **experimental science** is characterized by posing questions, designing experiments, performing analyses, and using the information gained to design new experiments. **Basic research** has as its goal simply the search for new knowledge. **Applications research** has as its goal the use of this knowledge for practical ends. There is a continuity between these two endeavors.

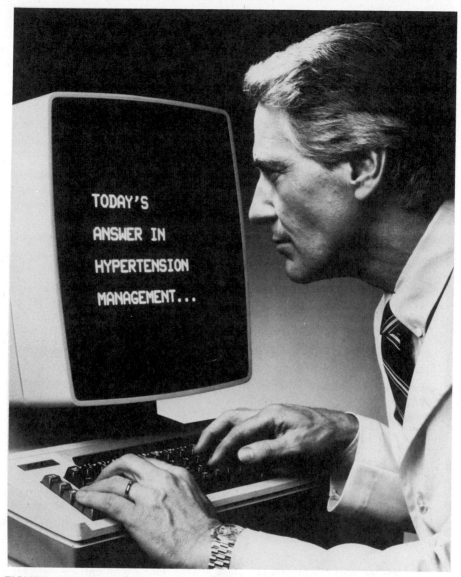

FIGURE 1.26 By the early 1980s, advertisements in medical journals began to use computer equipment as props. The suggestion in this photograph seems to be that this up-to-date physician feels comfortable using computer-based tools in his practice. (*Source:* Photograph courtesy of ICI Pharma, Division of ICI Americas, Inc.)

The scientific contributions of medical informatics also can be appreciated through its potential for benefitting the education of health professionals. For example, in the education of medical students, the various cognitive activities of physicians traditionally have tended to be considered separately and in isolation—they have been largely treated as though they are independent and distinct modules of performance.

One activity attracting increasing interest is that of formal medical decision making (see Chapter 3). The specific content of this area has not yet been defined completely, but the discipline's dependence on formal methods and its use of knowledge and information reveal that it is one aspect of medical informatics.

A particular topic in the study of medical decision making is *diagnosis*, which is often conceived and taught as though it were a freestanding and independent activity. Medical students may thus be led to view diagnosis as a process that physicians carry out in isolation before choosing therapy for a patient or proceeding to other modular tasks. Studies have shown that this model is oversimplified, and that such a decomposition of cognitive tasks may be quite misleading [Elstein et al., 1978]. Physicians seem to deal with several tasks at the same time. Although a diagnosis may be one of the first things physicians think about when they see a new patient, patient assessment (diagnosis, management, analysis of treatment results, monitoring of disease progression, and so on) is a process that never really terminates. A physician must be flexible and open-minded. It may be appropriate to alter the original diagnosis if it turns out that treatment based on it is unsuccessful, or if new information weakens the evidence supporting the diagnosis or suggests a second and concurrent disorder.

When we speak of making a diagnosis, choosing a treatment, managing therapy, making decisions, monitoring a patient, or preventing disease, these are labels for different aspects of *medical care,* an entity that has overall unity. The fabric of medical care is a continuum in which these elements are tightly interwoven. Regardless of whether we view computer and information science as a profession, as a technology, or as a science, there is no doubt about its importance to medicine. We can assume computers will be used increasingly in medical practice, in medical research, and in medical education.

1.4 Relationship to Biomedical Engineering

If medical informatics is an emerging discipline, then by contrast biomedical engineering is a well-established one. Many engineering and medical schools have formal academic programs in the latter subject, often with departmental status and full-time faculty. How does medical informatics relate to biomedical engineering, especially in an era when engineering and computer science are increasingly intertwined?

Biomedical engineering departments emerged 20 to 30 years ago, when technology began to play an increasingly prominent role in medical practice. The emphasis in such departments has tended to be research on and development of instrumentation (for example, advanced monitoring systems, transducers (see Chapter 12) for clinical or laboratory use, and image-enhancement techniques for use in radiology), with an orientation toward the development of medical devices, prostheses,[7] and specialized

---

[7]Devices that replace body parts—for example, artificial hips or hearts.

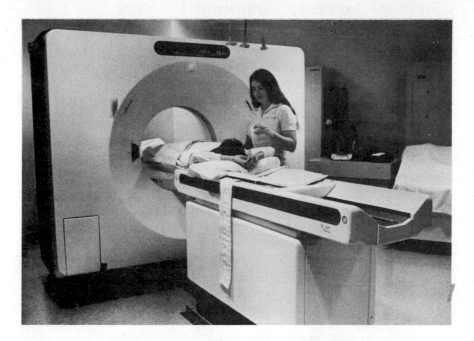

FIGURE 1.27 Computed-tomography scanners and other imaging devices used in radiology are of interest to both medical computer scientists and biomedical engineers. (*Source:* Photograph by Janice Anne Rohn.)

research tools (Figure 1.27). In recent years, computing techniques have been used both to design and build medical devices and in the medical devices themselves. For example, the "smart" devices increasingly found in most specialties are all dependent on microprocessor technology. Intensive-care monitors that generate blood-pressure records while calculating mean values and hourly summaries are examples of such "intelligent" devices.

This overlap between portions of biomedical engineering and medical computer science suggests that it would be unwise for us to draw compulsively strict boundaries between the two fields. There are ample opportunities for interaction, and there are chapters in this book that clearly overlap with biomedical-engineering topics—for example, Chapter 11 (radiology systems) and Chapter 12 (patient-monitoring systems). Even where they meet, however, the fields have differences in emphasis that can help you to understand their different evolutionary histories. In biomedical engineering, the emphasis is on medical *devices;* in medical informatics, the emphasis is on medical *information* and *knowledge,* and their management using computers. In both fields, the computer is secondary, although both use computing technology. The emphasis in this book is on the informatics end of the spectrum of medical computer science, so we shall not spend much time examining biomedical engineering topics.

1.5 Relationship to Computer Science

During its evolution as an academic entity in universities, computer science followed an unsettled course as faculty attempted to identify key topics in the field and to find the discipline's organizational place. Many computer-science programs were located in departments of electrical engineering, because major concerns of their researchers were computer architecture and design, and the development of practical hardware components. At the same time, computer scientists were interested in programming languages and software, undertakings not particularly characteristic of engineering. Furthermore, their work with algorithm design, complexity theory,[8] and other theoretical topics seemed more related to mathematics.

Medical informatics draws from all of these activities—development of hardware, software, and computer-science theory. Medical computing generally has not had a large enough market to influence the course of major hardware developments; that is, computers have not been developed specifically for medical applications. Not since the early 1960s (when health-computing experts occasionally talked about and, in a few instances, developed special *medical* terminals) have people assumed that medical-computing applications would use hardware other than that designed for general use.

The question of whether medical applications would require specialized programming languages might have been answered affirmatively a decade or so ago by anyone examining the MUMPS language (Massachusetts General Hospital Utility Multi-Programming System) [Greenes et al., 1970], which was specially developed for use in medical applications. For several years, MUMPS was the single most widely used language for certain types of medical computing, particularly those related to text processing or medical record keeping; it is still in widespread use. New implementations have been developed for each generation of mini- and microcomputers. MUMPS, however, like any programming language, is not equally useful for all computing tasks. In addition, the software requirements of medicine are better understood and no longer appear to be unique; rather, they are specific to the *kind* of task. A program for scientific computation looks pretty much the same whether it is designed for chemical engineering or for pharmacokinetic calculations.[9]

1.6 The Nature of Medical Information

From the previous discussion, you might conclude that medical applications do not raise any unique problems or concerns. On the contrary, the medical environment raises several issues that, in interesting ways, are quite distinct from those encountered

---

[8]Complexity theory provides an analytical framework for assessing the time and storage requirements of computer algorithms.

[9]Pharmacokinetics is the study of the routes and mechanisms of drug disposition over time, from initial introduction into the body, through distribution in body tissues and biotransformation, to ultimate elimination. See Chapter 10.

in most other domains of computer application. Clinical information seems to be systematically different from the information used in physics, engineering, or even clinical chemistry (which more closely resembles chemical applications generally than it does medical ones). These differences raise special problems. It is partly for this reason that some investigators suggest that medical computer science differs from conventional computer science in fundamental ways. We shall explore these differences only briefly here; for details, you can consult Blois' book on this subject (see the Suggested Readings).

Let us examine an instance of what we will call a low-level (or readily formalized) science. Physics is a natural starting point; in any discussion of the hierarchical relationships among the sciences (from the fourth-century B.C. Greek philosopher Aristotle to the twentieth-century U.S. librarian Melvil Dewey), physics will be placed near the bottom of the hierarchy. Physics characteristically has a certain kind of simplicity, or generality. The concepts and descriptions of the objects and processes of physics, however, are necessarily used in all applied fields, including medicine. The laws of physics and the descriptions of certain kinds of physical processes are essential in representing or explaining functions that we regard as medical in nature. We need to know something about molecular physics, for example, to understand why water is such a good solvent or to explain how nutrient molecules are metabolized; we talk about the role of electron-transfer reactions.

Applying a computer (or any formal computation) to a physical problem in a medical context is no different from doing so in a physics laboratory or for an engineering application. The use of computers in various **low-level processes** (such as those of physics or chemistry) is similar and is independent of the application. If we are talking about the solvent properties of water, it makes no difference whether we happen to be working in geology, engineering, or medicine. Such low-level processes of physics are particularly receptive to mathematical treatment, so using computers for these applications requires only conventional numerical programming.

In medicine, however, there are other **higher-level processes** carried out in more complex objects such as organisms (one type of which is patients). Many of the important informational processes are of this kind. When we discuss, describe, or record the properties or behavior of humans, we are using the descriptions of very high-level objects, the behavior of whom has no counterpart in physics or in engineering. The person using computers to analyze the descriptions of these high-level objects and processes encounters serious difficulties [Blois, 1984].

You might object to this line of argument by remarking that, after all, computers are used routinely in commercial applications in which humans and situations concerning them are involved, and that relevant computations are carried out successfully. The explanation is that, in these commercial applications, the descriptions of humans and their activities have been so highly abstracted that the events or processes have been reduced to low-level objects. In medicine, abstractions carried to this degree would be clinically worthless.

For example, one instance of a human in the banking business is the customer, who may deposit, borrow, withdraw, or invest money. To describe commercial activities such as these, we need only a few properties; the customer can remain an abstract entity. In clinical medicine, however, we could not begin to deal with a patient represented with such skimpy abstractions. We must be prepared to analyze most of the complex behaviors that humans display, and to describe patients as completely as possible. We must deal with the rich descriptions occurring at high levels in the hierarchy, and we may be hard pressed to encode and process this information using the tools of mathematics and computer science, which work so well at low levels. In the light of these remarks, the general enterprise known as **artificial intelligence** (AI) can be aptly described as the application of computer science to high-level, real-world problems.

Medical computer science thus includes computer applications that range from processing of very low-level descriptions, which are little different from their counterparts in physics, chemistry, or engineering, to processing of extremely high-level ones, which are completely and systematically different. When we study human beings in their entirety (including such aspects as human cognition, self-consciousness, intentionality, and behavior), we must use these high-level descriptions. We shall find that they raise complex issues to which conventional logic and mathematics are less readily applicable. In general, the attributes of low-level objects appear sharp, crisp, and unambiguous (for example, "length," "mass"), whereas those of high-level ones tend to be soft, or fuzzy, and inexact (for example, "unpleasant scent," "good").

Just as we need to develop different methods to describe high-level objects, the inference methods we use with such objects may differ from those we use with low-level ones. In formal logic, we begin with the assumption that a given proposition must be either true or false. This feature is essential because logic is concerned with the preservation of truth value under various formal transformations. It is difficult or impossible, however, to assume that all propositions have truth values when we deal with the many high-level descriptions in medicine or, indeed, in everyday situations. Such questions as "Was Woodrow Wilson a good president?" cannot be answered "yes" or "no" (unless we limit the question to specific criteria for determining the goodness of presidents). Many common questions in medicine have this same property.

1.7 Integrating Medical Computing and Medical Practice

It should be clear from the previous discussion that medical informatics is a remarkably broad and complex topic. We have argued that information management is intrinsic to medical practice and that interest in using computers to aid in information management has grown over the last 2 decades. In this chapter and throughout the book, we emphasize the myriad ways in which computers are used in medicine to ease the burdens of information processing, and the means by which new technology promises to change the delivery of health care. The rate at and degree to which such changes are realized will be determined in part by external forces that influence the costs of developing and implementing medical applications and the ability of the health-care system to accrue the potential benefits.

We can summarize several global forces that are affecting medical computing and that will determine the extent to which computers are assimilated into medical practice: (1) new developments in computer hardware and software, (2) a gradual increase in the number of professionals who have been trained in both clinical medicine and computer science, and (3) ongoing changes in health-care financing designed to control the rate of growth of medical expenditures. We touched on the first of these factors in Section 1.2.2, when we described the historical development of medical computing and the trend from mainframe computers to microcomputers and personal computers. The new hardware technology made powerful computers inexpensive and thus available to hospitals, to departments within hospitals, and even to individual physicians. The broad selection of computers of all sizes, prices, and capabilities makes computer applications both attractive and accessible. Technological advances in information-storage devices—for example, optical discs—are facilitating the inexpensive storage of large numbers of data, thus improving the feasibility of data-intensive applications, such as the all-digital radiology department discussed in Chapter 11. Standardization of hardware and advances in network technology are making it easier to share data and to integrate related information-management functions within a hospital or other health-care organization.

Computers are increasingly prevalent in all aspects of our lives, whether as an automatic bank-teller machine, as the microprocessor in a microwave oven, or as a word processor. Physicians trained in recent years may have used computer programs to learn diagnostic techniques or to manage the therapy of simulated patients. They may have learned to use a computer to search the medical literature, either directly or with the assistance of a specially trained librarian. Simple exposure to computers does not, however, guarantee an eagerness to embrace the machine. Medical personnel will be unwilling to use computer-based systems that are poorly designed, confusing, or unduly time consuming.

The second factor is the increase in the number of professionals who are being trained to understand the medical issues as well as the technical and engineering ones. Computer scientists who understand medicine are better able to design systems responsive to actual needs. Medical personnel who receive formal training in computer science are likely to build systems using well-established techniques while avoiding the past mistakes of other developers. As more professionals are trained in the special aspects of both fields, and as the programs they develop are introduced, health-care professionals are more likely to have available useful and usable systems when they turn to the computer for help with information-management tasks.

The third factor affecting the integration of computing technologies into health-care settings is the increasing pressure to control medical spending. The escalating tendency to apply technology to all patient-care tasks is a frequently cited phenomenon in modern medical practice. Mere physical findings no longer are considered adequate for making diagnoses and planning treatments. In fact, medical students who are taught by more experienced physicians to find subtle diagnostic signs by examining various parts of a patient's body nonetheless often choose to bypass or deemphasize physical examinations in favor of ordering one test after another. Sometimes, they do so without paying sufficient attention to the ensuing cost. Some new technologies replace less expensive, but technologically inferior, tests. In such cases, the use of the more expensive approach is generally justified. Occasionally, computer-related technologies have allowed us to perform tasks that previously were not possible. For example, the scans produced with computed tomography (CT; see Chapter 11) have allowed physicians to visualize cross-sectional slices of the body for the first time, and medical instruments in ICUs perform continuous monitoring of patients' body functions that previously could be checked only episodically (see Chapter 12).

Yet the development of expensive new technologies, and the belief that more technology is better, helped to fuel the rapidly escalating health-care costs of the 1970s and 1980s. Chapter 19 discusses the mechanisms that opened the door to rapid growth in health expenses and the changes in financing and delivery that were designed to curb spending in the new era of cost consciousness. Integrated computer systems potentially provide the means to capture data for detailed cost accounting, to analyze the relation of costs of care to the benefits of that care, to evaluate the quality of care provided, and to identify areas of inefficiency. Systems that can be shown to improve the quality of care while reducing the cost of providing that care clearly will be favored. The effect of cost-containment pressures on technologies that increase the cost of care while improving the quality are less clear. Medical technologies, including computers, will need to improve the delivery of medical care while either reducing costs or providing benefits that clearly exceed their costs.

Improvements in hardware and software make computers more suitable for medical applications. However, designers of medical systems must address satisfactorily many logistical and engineering questions before computers can be fully integrated into medical practice. For example, are computer terminals conveniently located? Can users complete their tasks without excessive delays? Is the system reliable enough to avoid loss of data? Can users interact easily and intuitively with the computer? In addition, cost-control pressures produce a growing reluctance to embrace expensive technologies that add to the high cost of health care. The net effect of these opposing trends will in large part determine the degree to which computers are integrated into the health-care environment.

In summary, rapid advances in computer hardware and software, coupled with an increasing computer literacy of health-care professionals, favor the implementation of effective computer applications in medical practice. Furthermore, in the increasingly competitive health-care industry, providers have a greater need for the information-management capabilities supplied by computer systems. The challenge is to demonstrate the financial and clinical advantages of these systems.

Suggested Readings

Blois, M. S. *Information and Medicine: The Nature of Medical Descriptions.* Berkeley: University of California Press, 1984.

The author analyzes the structure of medical knowledge in terms of a hierarchical model of information. He explores the notions of high- and low-level sciences and suggests that the nature of medical descriptions accounts for difficulties in applying computing technology to medicine.

Blum, B. I. *Clinical Information Systems*. New York: Springer-Verlag, 1986.
This excellent introductory book includes useful chapters on the history of computing and of the field of medical informatics.

Collen, M. F. Origins of medical informatics. *The Western Journal of Medicine,* 145:778, 1986.
This article traces the early history of the field of medical informatics and identifies the origins of the discipline's name (which first appeared in the English-language literature in 1974).

Debons, A. and Larson, A. G. (eds). *Information Science in Action: System Design* (2 Vols). The Hague: Martinus Nijhoff, 1983.
This detailed text addresses general issues in information management. It also deals with theoretical topics, such as information content and data analysis.

Elstein, A. S., Shulman, L. S., and Sprafka, S. A. *Medical Problem Solving: An Analysis of Clinical Reasoning*. Cambridge, MA: Harvard University Press, 1978.
This collection of papers describes detailed studies that have illuminated several aspects of the ways in which expert and novice physicians solve medical problems.

Pages, J. C., et al. (eds). *Meeting the Challenge: Informatics and Medical Education*. Amsterdam: North Holland, 1983.
This collection of papers was presented at a conference that assessed the international status of the use of computers in medical education, as well as the status of education about medical informatics in health-science schools.

Salamon, R., Protti, D., and Moehr, J. (eds). *Proceedings of the 1989 International Symposium of Medical Informatics and Education*. Victoria, British Columbia, Canada: School of Health Information Science, University of Victoria, 1989.
This volume is the proceedings of the third International Medical Informatics Association (IMIA) conference on medical informatics and education. It contains papers that review the status of the field in countries throughout the world, describe computer-supported approaches to medical education, and discuss curricula for medical, nursing, and dental informatics.

Questions for Discussion

1. How do you interpret the phrase "logical behavior"? Do computers behave logically? Do people behave logically? Explain your answers.
2. What do you think it means to say that a computer program is "effective"? Make a list of a dozen computer applications with which you are familiar. List the applications in decreasing order of effectiveness, as you have explained this concept. Then, for each application, indicate your estimate of how well human beings perform the same tasks (this task will require that you determine what it means for a *human* to be effective). Do you discern any pattern? If so, how do you interpret it?
3. Discuss three societywide factors that will determine the extent to which computers are assimilated into medical practice.

4. Reread the scenario in Section 1.1. Describe the characteristics of an integrated environment for managing medical information. Discuss two ways in which such a system could change medical practice.

5. Do you believe that improving the technical quality of health care entails a risk of making health-care delivery impersonal? If so, do you think such "dehumanization" would be a serious problem? Would the potential benefits of high technical quality outweigh the risk of impersonal delivery of care? Explain your reasoning.

2

Medical Data: Their Acquisition, Storage, and Use

Edward H. Shortliffe and G. Octo Barnett

After reading this chapter, you should know the answers to these questions:

- What are medical data?
- How are medical data used?
- What are the drawbacks of the traditional paper medical record?
- What is the potential role of the computer in data storage, retrieval, and interpretation?
- What distinguishes a database from a knowledge base?
- How are data collection and hypothesis generation intimately linked in medical diagnosis?
- What is the meaning of the terms *prevalence, predictive value, sensitivity,* and *specificity,* and how are they related?
- What are the alternatives for entry of data into a medical database?

2.1 What Are Medical Data?

From earliest times, the notions of ill health and its treatment have been wedded to those of the observation and interpretation of data. Whether one considers the disease descriptions and guidelines for management in early Greek literature, the shaman's response to the pattern assumed by a handful of bones thrown on the ground during a healing ceremony, or the modern physician's use of complex laboratory and X-ray studies, it is clear that gathering data and interpreting their meaning are central to the health-care process. A textbook on computers in medicine will accordingly refer time and again to issues in data collection, storage, and use. This chapter lays the foundation for this recurring set of issues that is pertinent to all aspects of the use of computers in medicine.

If data are central to all medical care, it is because they are crucial to the process of *decision making* (as is described in detail in Chapter 3). In fact, simple reflection will reveal that *all* medical-care activities involve gathering, analyzing, or using data. Data provide the basis for categorizing the problems a patient may be having, or for identifying subgroups within a population of patients. They also help in deciding what additional information is needed and what actions should be taken to gain a greater understanding of a patient's problem or to treat most effectively the problem that has been diagnosed.

It is overly simplistic to view data as the columns of numbers or monitored waveforms that are a product of our increasingly technological health-care environment. Although laboratory-test results and other numeric data are often invaluable, a variety of more subtle types of data may be just as important to the delivery of optimal care: the awkward glance to the side by a patient who seems to be avoiding a question during the medical interview, information about a patient's family or economic setting, the subjective impression of disease severity that an experienced physician will often obtain within a few seconds of entering a patient's room. No physician disputes the importance of such observations in decision making during patient assessment and management, yet the precise roles of these data and the corresponding decision criteria are so poorly understood that it is difficult to record the data in ways that convey their full meaning, even from one physician to another. It is small wonder, then, that the role of computers is inherently constrained while human cognitive and communication skills remain so poorly understood.

We shall consider a medical datum to be any single observation of a patient—for example, a temperature reading, a red-blood-cell count, a past history of rubella, or a blood-pressure reading. As this last example shows, it is sometimes a matter of perspective whether a single observation is in fact more than one datum. A blood pressure of 120/80 might well be recorded as a single data point in a setting where knowledge that a patient's blood pressure is normal is all that matters. If the difference between diastolic (while the heart cavities are filling) and systolic (while they are contracting) blood pressure is important for decision making or analysis, however, then the blood-pressure reading is best viewed as *two* pieces of information (systolic pressure = 120 mm Hg, diastolic pressure = 80 mm Hg). Human beings can glance at a written blood-pressure value and easily make the transition between its unitary view as a single data point and the decomposed information about systolic and diastolic pressure. Such dual views can be much more difficult for computers, however, unless they are specifically allowed for in the design of the method for data storage and analysis. The notion of a *data model* (see Chapter 4) for computer-stored medical data accordingly becomes an important issue in the design of medical data systems.

If a medical datum is a single observation about a patient, then medical data are a collection of such observations. Such data may involve several different observations made concurrently, the observation of the same patient parameter made at several points in time, or some combination of these. Thus, a single datum generally can be viewed as defined by four elements:

1. The *patient* in question
2. The *parameter* being observed (for example, liver size, urine sugar value, history of rheumatic fever, heart size on chest X-ray film)
3. The *value* of the parameter in question (for example, weight is *70 kg*, temperature is *98.6° F*, profession is *steel worker*)
4. The *time* of the observation (for example, 2:30 A.M., 14FEB89).

Time can particularly complicate the assessment and computer-based management of data. In some settings, the date of the observation is adequate; for example, in outpatient clinics or private offices, where a patient generally is seen infrequently, the time at which the data were collected needs to be identified with no greater accuracy than a calendar date. In others, minute-to-minute variations may be important; for example, frequent blood-sugar readings are obtained for a patient in diabetic acidosis,[1] and continuous measurements of mean arterial blood pressure are used for a patient in cardiogenic shock.[2]

It often also is important to keep a record of the circumstances under which a datum was obtained. For example, was the blood pressure taken in the arm or leg? Was the patient lying or standing? Was it obtained just after the patient exercised? Was the patient asleep? What kind of recording device was used? Was the observer reliable? These types of additional information, sometimes called "modifiers," can be of crucial importance in the proper interpretation of data.

A related issue is the *uncertainty* in the values of data. It is all too rare that an observation—even one by a skilled clinician—can be accepted with absolute certainty. Consider the following examples:

- A patient reports a childhood illness with fevers and a red rash in addition to joint swelling. Could this have been scarlet fever? The patient does not remember what his pediatrician called the disease.
- A physician listens to the heart of an asthmatic child and thinks she hears a heart murmur—but she is not certain because of the patient's loud wheezing.
- A radiologist looking at a "shadow" on a chest X-ray film is not sure whether it represents overlapping blood vessels or a lung tumor.

---

[1] Abnormally increased acidity of the blood due to poorly controlled blood sugar levels.
[2] Dangerously low blood pressure due to a heart problem.

- A confused patient is able to respond to simple questions about his illness, but the physician is uncertain how much of the history is reliable.

As we shall describe in Chapter 3, there is a variety of possible responses for dealing with the uncertainty in data and in their interpretation. One technique is to collect additional data that will either confirm or eliminate the concern raised by the initial observation. This solution is not always appropriate, however, because the *costs* of data collection must be considered. The additional observation might be expensive, risky for the patient, or wasteful of time during which treatment could have been instituted. The notion of *tradeoffs* in data collection thus becomes extremely important in guiding quality health-care decision making.

2.1.1 What Are the Types of Medical Data?

The examples in the previous section suggest that there is a broad range of data types in the practice of medicine and the allied health sciences. The range covers narrative, textual data, numerical measurements, recorded signals, and even pictures.

Narrative data account for a large component of the information that is gathered in the care of patients (Figure 2.1). For example, the patient's description of his present illness, including responses to focused questions from the physician, generally is gathered verbally and is recorded as text in the medical record. The same is true of the patient's social and family history, and the general review of systems that is part of most evaluations of new patients.

Some narrative data are loosely coded using shorthand conventions known to health personnel. This is particularly true of the physical examination, in which recorded observations reflect the stereotypic examination process taught to all practitioners. It is common, for example, to find the notation "PERRLA" under the eye examination in a patient's medical record. This encoded form indicates that the patient's "Pupils are Equal (in size), Round, and Reactive to Light and Accommodation" (accommodation is the process of focusing on near objects).

In some instances, complete phrases have become loose standards of communication among medical personnel. Examples include "mild dyspnea [shortness of breath] on exertion," "pain relieved by antacids or milk," and "failure to thrive." Such standardized expressions have become conventional notation, a form of summarization of otherwise heterogeneous conditions that characterize patients.

Many data used in medicine take on discrete numeric values. These include such parameters as laboratory-test results, vital signs (such as temperature and pulse rate), and certain measurements taken during the physical examination. In interpreting such numerical data, however, the issue of *precision* becomes important. Can a physician distinguish reliably between a 9-cm and a 10-cm liver span when examining the patient's abdomen? Does it make sense to report a serum sodium level to two-decimal-place accuracy? Is a 1-kg fluctuation in weight from one week to the next significant? Was the patient weighed on the same scale both times, or could the different values reflect variation between measurement instruments rather than changes in the patient?

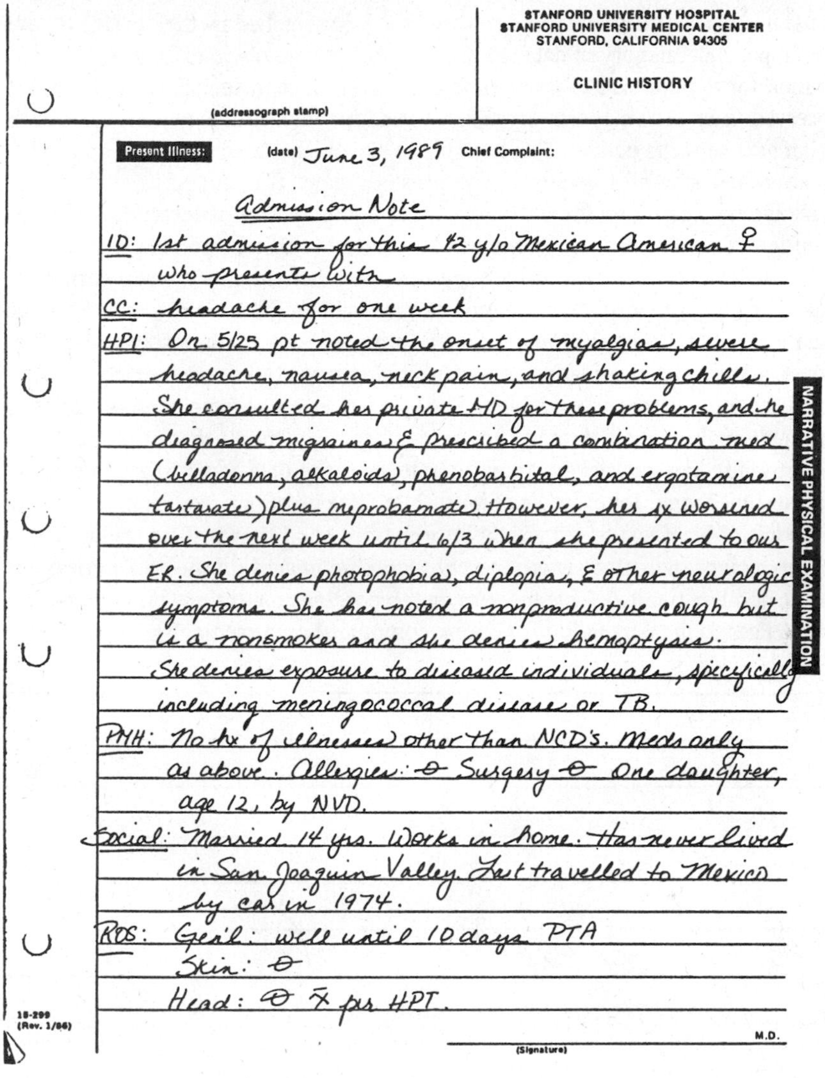

STANFORD UNIVERSITY HOSPITAL
STANFORD UNIVERSITY MEDICAL CENTER
STANFORD, CALIFORNIA 94305

CLINIC HISTORY

(addressograph stamp)

| Present Illness: | (date) June 3, 1989 | Chief Complaint: |

Admission Note

ID: 1st admission for this 42 y/o Mexican American ♀ who presents with

CC: headache for one week

HPI: On 5/25 pt noted the onset of myalgias, severe headache, nausea, neck pain, and shaking chills. She consulted her private MD for these problems, and he diagnosed migraines & prescribed a combination med (belladonna, alkaloids, phenobarbital, and ergotamine tartarate) plus meprobamate. However, her sx worsened over the next week until 6/3 when she presented to our ER. She denies photophobia, diplopia, & other neurologic symptoms. She has noted a nonproductive cough but is a nonsmoker and she denies hemoptysis. She denies exposure to diseased individuals, specifically including meningococcal disease or TB.

PMH: No hx of illnesses other than NCD's. Meds only as above. Allergies: ⊖ Surgery ⊖ One daughter, age 12, by NVD.

Social: Married 14 yrs. Works in home. Has never lived in San. Joaquin Valley. Last travelled to Mexico by car in 1974.

ROS: Gen'l: well until 10 days PTA
Skin: ⊖
Head: ⊖ x̄ per HPI.

18-299
(Rev. 1/86)

M.D.

(Signature)

FIGURE 2.1 Much of the information gathered during a physician-patient encounter is recorded textually in the medical record.

In some fields of medicine, analog data in the form of continuous signals are particularly important (see Chapter 12). Perhaps the best known example is an ECG, a tracing of the electrical activity from a patient's heart; there are many similar examples. When such data are stored in medical records, a graphical tracing frequently is included, along with a written interpretation of its meaning. There are clear challenges in determining how such data are best managed in computer storage systems.

Visual images—either acquired from machines or sketched by the physician—are another important category of data. Radiologic images are obvious examples. It also is common for a physician to draw simple pictures to represent abnormalities she has observed; such drawings may serve as a basis for comparison when she or another physician next sees the patient. For example, a sketch is a concise way of conveying the location and size of a nodule in the prostate gland (Figure 2.2).

As should be clear from these examples, the notion of *data* is inextricably bound to the notion of *data recording*. Physicians and other health-care personnel are taught from the outset that it is crucial that they not trust their memory when caring for patients. They must record their observations, as well as the actions they have taken and the rationales for those actions, for later communication to themselves and other people. A glance at a medical record will quickly reveal the wide variety of data-recording techniques that have evolved. The techniques range from hand-written text to commonly understood shorthand notation to cryptic symbols that only specialists can understand—few physicians know how to read the data-recording conventions of an ophthalmologist, for example (Figure 2.3). The notations may be highly structured records of brief text or numerical information, hand-drawn sketches, machine-generated tracings of analog signals, or photographic images (of the patient or of his radiologic or other studies). This range of data-recording conventions presents significant challenges to the person implementing computer-based medical-record systems.

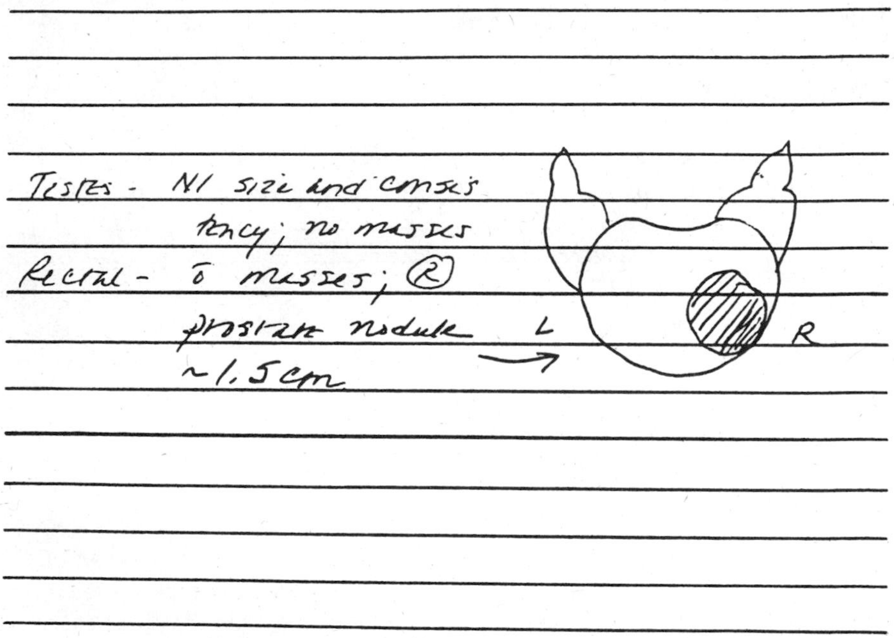

FIGURE 2.2 A physician's hand-drawn sketch of a prostate nodule. A drawing may convey precise information more easily and compactly than a textual description could.

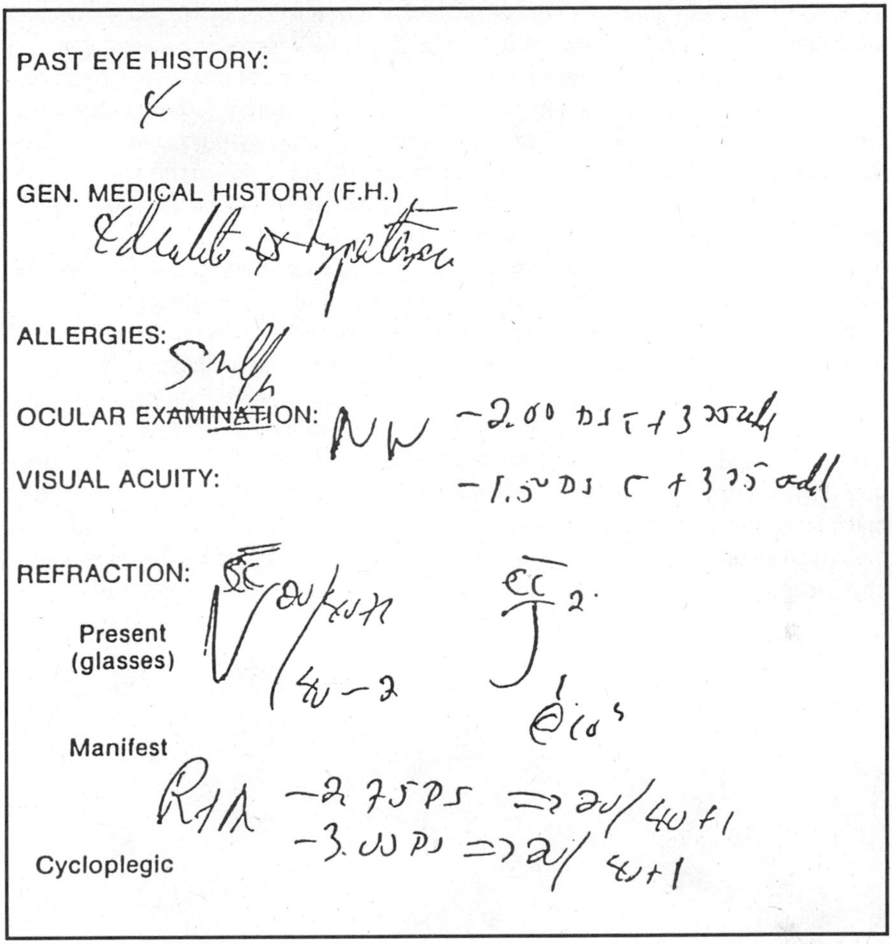

FIGURE 2.3 An ophthalmologist's report of an eye examination. Most other physicians would have difficulty deciphering the symbols the ophthalmologist has used.

2.1.2 Who Collects the Data?

Health data on patients and populations are gathered by a variety of health professionals. Although conventional notions of the "health-care team" evoke images of coworkers treating ill patients, the team has responsibilities much broader than treatment per se; data collection and recording are a central part of their task.

Physicians are key players in the process of data collection and interpretation. They converse with a patient to gather narrative descriptive data on the chief complaint, past illnesses, family and social information, and the system review. They examine the patient, collecting pertinent data and recording them during or at the end of the visit. In addition, they generally decide what additional data to collect, by ordering laboratory or radiologic studies, and by observing the patient's response to therapeutic interventions (yet another form of data that contributes to patient assessment).

In both outpatient and hospital settings, nurses play a central role in making observations and recording them for future reference. The data they gather contribute to nursing care plans as well as to the assessment of patients by physicians and other health-care staff. Thus, nurses' training includes instruction in careful and accurate observation, history taking, and examination of the patient. Because nurses spend more time with patients than physicians do, especially in the hospital setting, nurses often build caring relationships with patients that uncover information and insights that contribute to proper diagnosis, to understanding of pertinent psychosocial issues, or to proper planning of therapy or discharge management (Figure 2.4). The role of information systems in contributing to nursing tasks such as these is the subject of Chapter 8.

A variety of other health-care workers contribute to the data-collection process. Office staff and admissions personnel gather demographic and financial information. Physical or respiratory therapists record the results of their treatments and often make suggestions for further management. Laboratory personnel perform tests on biological samples such as blood and urine and record the results for later use by physicians and nurses. Radiology technicians perform X-ray examinations; radiologists

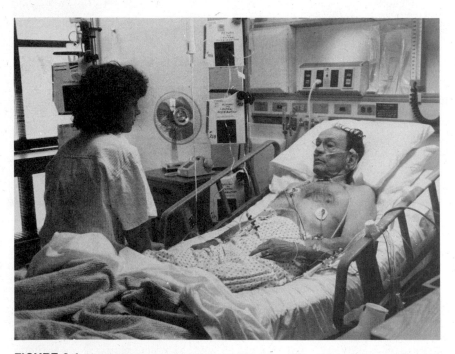

FIGURE 2.4 Nurses often develop close relationships with patients. These relationships may allow the nurse to make observations that are missed by other staff, even by the patient's own physicians. This is just one of the reasons that nursing staff play a key role in data collection and recording. (*Source:* Photograph by Janice Anne Rohn.)

interpret the resulting data and report their findings to the patient's physicians. Pharmacists may interview patients about medications or about drug allergies, and then may monitor the patients' use of prescription drugs. As these examples suggest, most people employed in health-care settings gather patient data, record them, and make use of them in their work.

Finally, there are the technological devices that generate data—laboratory instruments, imaging machines, monitoring equipment in intensive-care units, and measurement devices that take a single reading (such as thermometers, ECG machines, sphygmomanometers for taking blood pressures, and spirometers for testing lung function). Sometimes, such a device produces a paper report suitable for inclusion in a medical record. Sometimes, the device indicates on a gauge or traces a result that must be read by an operator and then recorded in the patient's chart. Sometimes, a trained specialist must interpret the output. Increasingly, however, the devices feed their results directly into computer equipment so that the data can be analyzed or formatted for electronic storage as well as reported on paper.

2.2 Uses of Medical Data

Medical data are recorded for a variety of purposes. They may be needed to support the proper care of the patient from whom they were obtained, and they also may contribute to the good of society through the aggregation and analysis of data regarding populations of individuals. One problem with traditional data-recording techniques has been that the paper record has worked reasonably well to support the proper care of individual patients but has made clinical research across populations of patients extremely cumbersome. Computer-based record keeping offers major advantages in this regard, as we shall discuss in more detail later in this chapter and in Chapters 6 and 16.

2.2.1 Form the Basis for the Historical Record

Any student of science has learned the importance of meticulous data collection and recording when carrying out an experiment. Just as a laboratory notebook provides a record of precisely what a scientist has done, what the experimental data observed were, and what the rationale for intermediate decision points was, medical records are intended to provide a detailed compilation of information about individual patients:

- What is the patient's history (development of a current illness; other diseases that coexist or have resolved; pertinent family, social, and demographic information)?
- What symptoms has the patient reported?
- What physical signs have been noted on examination?
- How have signs and symptoms changed over time?
- What laboratory results have been or are now available?
- What radiologic and other special studies have been performed?
- What interventions have been undertaken?
- What is the reasoning behind those management decisions?

Each new patient complaint and its management can be viewed as a therapeutic experiment, inherently confounded by uncertainty, and focusing on three issues:
1. What was the nature of the disease or symptom?
2. What was the treatment decision?
3. What was the outcome of that treatment?

As is true for all experiments, one purpose is to learn from experience through careful observation and recording of data. The lessons learned in a given encounter may be very individualized (for example, the physician may learn how a specific patient tends to respond to pain, or how family interactions tend to affect the patient's response to disease), or they may be best derived by pooling of data from many patients with similar problems and analysis of the results of various treatment options to determine the latter's efficacy.

Although laboratory research has contributed dramatically to our knowledge of human disease and its treatment, especially over the last 50 years, it is careful observation and recording by skilled health-care personnel that has always provided the foundation for generating new knowledge about patient care. We learn from the aggregation of information from large numbers of patients; thus, the historical record for individual patients is of inestimable importance to clinical research.

2.2.2 Support Communication Among Providers

A central function of structured data collection and recording in health-care settings is to assist in providing coordinated care to a patient over time. Most patients with significant medical conditions are seen over months or years on several occasions for one or more problems that require ongoing evaluation and treatment.

It was once common for patients to receive essentially all their care from a single provider—the family doctor who tended both children and adults, often seeing the patient over many or all the years of that person's life. We tend to picture such physicians as having especially close relationships with their patients—knowing the family and sharing in many of the patient's life events, especially in smaller communities. Such doctors nonetheless kept records of all encounters so that they would be able to refer to data about past illness and treatments as a guide to evaluating future care issues. It has long been the case that physicians have kept records *for their own use*—so that they can refer back and provide coordinated and insightful care for the same patient on future occasions.

In the world of modern medicine, the emergence of subspecialization and the increasing provision of care by *teams* of health professionals have placed new emphasis on the central role of the medical record (Figure 2.5). Now the record not only contains observations by a physician for reference on the next visit, but also serves as a communication mechanism among physicians and other health-care personnel such as physical or respiratory therapists, nursing staff, radiology technicians, social workers, or discharge planners. In many outpatient settings, patients receive care over time from a variety of physicians—colleagues covering for the primary physician on the case, or specialists to whom the patient has been referred. It is not uncommon to hear complaints from patients who remember the days when it was possible

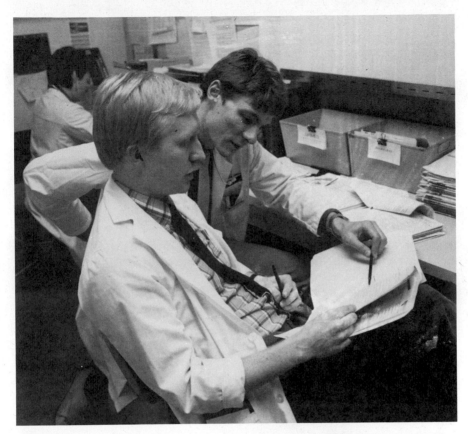

FIGURE 2.5 The medical record serves as a communication mechanism among health professionals who work together to plan patient care. (*Source:* Photograph by Janice Anne Rohn.)

to receive essentially all their care from a single physician whom they had come to trust and who knew them well. Physicians are sensitive to this issue and therefore recognize the importance of the medical record in ensuring quality and **continuity of care** through adequate recording of the details and logic of past interventions and ongoing treatment plans. This notion is of particular importance in a health-care system, such as ours in the United States, in which chronic diseases, rather than trauma or acute infections, increasingly dominate the basis for interactions between patients and their doctors.

2.2.3 Anticipate Future Health Problems

Quality medical care involves more than responding to patients' acute or chronic health problems. It also requires education of patients about the ways in which their environment and lifestyles can contribute to or reduce the risk of future development of disease. Similarly, data gathered routinely in the ongoing care of a patient may suggest that he is at high risk of developing a specific problem, even though he may feel well and be without symptoms at present. Medical data therefore are important in screening for risk factors, following patients' risk profiles over time, and providing a basis for specific patient education or preventive interventions, such as diet, medication, or exercise. Perhaps the most common examples of such ongoing risk assessment in our society are routine monitoring for excess weight, high blood pressure, and elevated serum cholesterol levels. In these cases, abnormal data may be predictive of later symptomatic disease; optimal care requires early intervention before the complications (primarily heart, kidney, and vascular diseases) have an opportunity to develop fully.

2.2.4 Record Standard Preventive Measures

The medical record also serves as a source of data on interventions that have been performed to prevent common or serious disorders. The best examples of such interventions are immunizations, the vaccinations that begin in early childhood and continue throughout life, with special treatments required when a person will be at particularly high risk (for example, injections of gamma globulin to protect people from hepatitis, administered before travel to areas where hepatitis is endemic). When a patient comes to her local hospital emergency room with a laceration, the physicians routinely check the chart for an indication of when she last had a tetanus immunization. When easily accessible in the record, such data can prevent unnecessary treatments that may be associated with risk or significant cost.

2.2.5 Identify Deviations from Expected Trends

Data often are useful in medical care only when viewed as part of a continuum over time. An example of this issue is the routine monitoring of children for normal growth and development by pediatricians (Figure 2.6). Single data points regarding height and weight generally are not useful by themselves; it is the trend in such data points observed over months or years that may provide the first clue to a medical problem. It is accordingly common for such parameters to be recorded on special charts or forms that make the trends easy to discern at a glance. Women who want to become pregnant often keep similar records of body temperature. By measuring temperature daily and recording the values on special charts, women can often identify the slight increase in temperature that accompanies ovulation, and thus may discern the days of maximum fertility. Many physicians ask patients to keep such graphical records so that they can later discuss the data with the patient and include the records in the medical chart for ongoing reference.

2.2.6 Provide a Legal Record

Another use of medical data, once they are charted and analyzed, is as the foundation for a legal record to which the courts can refer if necessary. The medical record is a legal document; most of the clinical information that is recorded must be signed

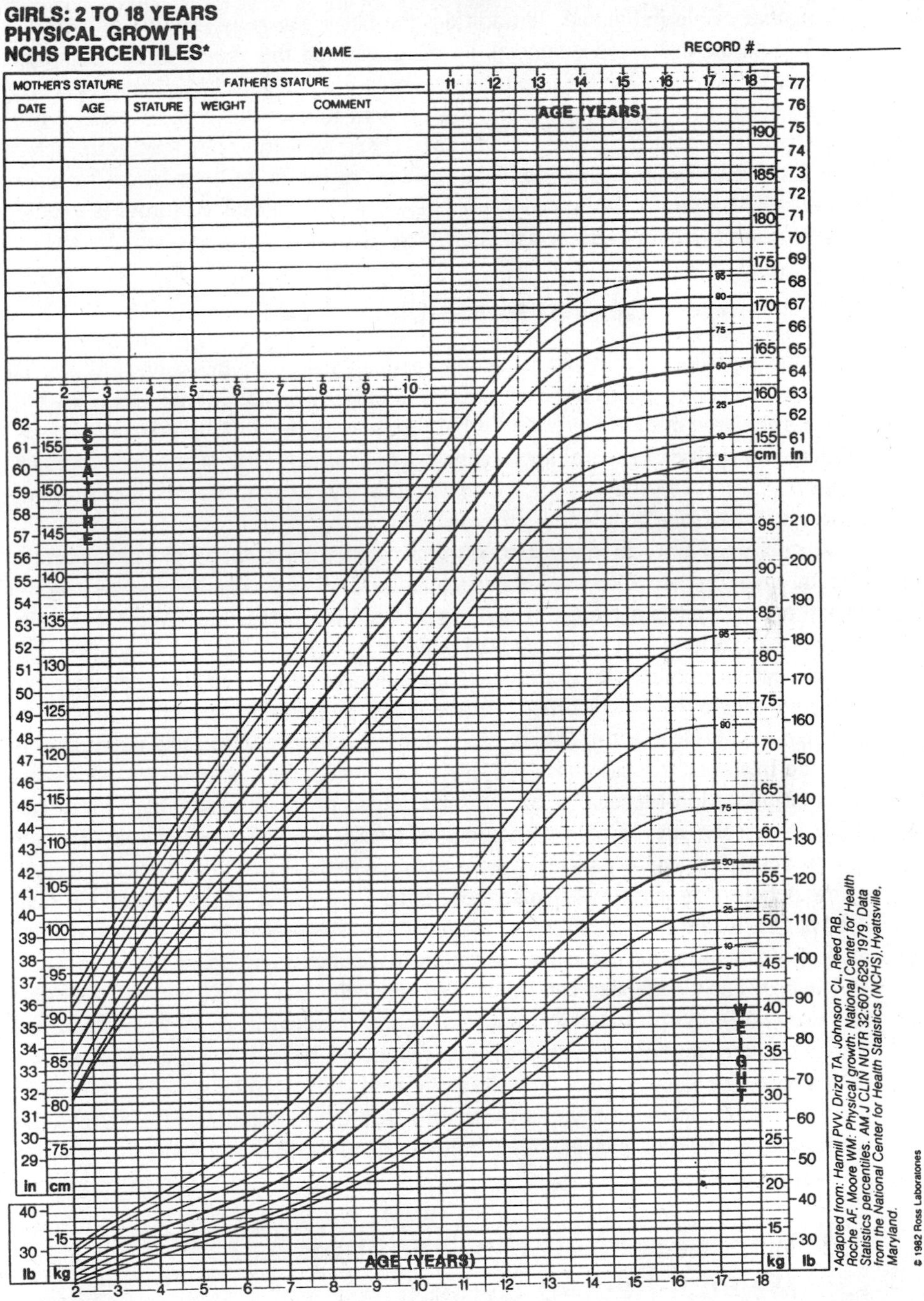

GIRLS: 2 TO 18 YEARS
PHYSICAL GROWTH
NCHS PERCENTILES*

NAME _____   RECORD # _____

FIGURE 2.6 A pediatric growth chart. Single data points would not be useful; it is the changes in values over time that indicate whether development is progressing normally. (*Source:* Used with permission of Ross Laboratories, Columbus, OH 43216.)

by the responsible individual. In addition, the chart generally should describe and justify both the presumed diagnosis for a patient and the choice of management.

We emphasized earlier the importance of recording data; in fact, data do not exist as such unless they are recorded. The legal system stresses this point as well. A provider's unsubstantiated memory of what she observed or why she took some action is of little value in the courtroom. The medical record is the foundation for determining whether proper care was delivered. Thus, a well-maintained record is a source of protection for both patients and their physicians.

2.2.7 Support Clinical Research

Although experience caring for individual patients provides physicians with special skills and enhanced judgment over time, it is only by formally analyzing data collected from large numbers of patients that researchers can develop and validate new clinical knowledge of general applicability. Thus, another use of medical data is to support clinical research through the aggregation and statistical analysis of observations gathered from populations of patients.

Randomized clinical trials (RCTs) are a common method by which specific clinical questions are addressed experimentally. They typically involve the random assignment of matched groups of patients to alternate treatments when there is uncertainty about how best to manage the patients' problem. The variables that might affect a patient's course (for example, age, gender, weight, coexisting medical problems) are measured and recorded. As the study progresses, data are meticulously gathered to provide a record of how each patient fared under treatment and precisely how the treatment was administered. By pooling such data, sometimes after years of experimentation (depending on the time course of the disease under consideration), researchers may be able to demonstrate a statistical difference among the study groups depending on the patients' precise characteristics when they entered the study or the details of how they were managed. Such results then help to define the standard of care for future patients with the same or similar problems. Computer systems to support this kind of clinical research are described in Chapter 16.

Medical knowledge also can be derived from the analysis of large patient data sets even when the patients were not specifically enrolled in an RCT. Much of the research in the field of epidemiology involves the analysis of population-based data of this type. Our knowledge of the risks associated with cigarette smoking, for example, is based on irrefutable statistics derived from large populations of individuals with and without lung cancer, other pulmonary problems, and heart disease.

2.3 Weaknesses of the Traditional Medical-Record System

The preceding description of medical data and their use has emphasized the positive aspects of information storage and retrieval in the paper record. However, all medical personnel quickly learn that the idealized view of the medical record is complicated by a bevy of logistical and practical realities that greatly limit the record's effectiveness for its intended uses.

2.3.1 Pragmatic and Logistical Issues

Recall, first, that data cannot effectively serve the delivery of health care unless they are recorded. Their optimal use is dependent on positive responses to the following questions:
- Can I find the data I need when I need them?
  - Can I find the medical record in which they are recorded?
  - Can I find the data within the record?
  - Can I do all this quickly?
- Can I read and interpret the data once I find them?
- Can I reliably update the data with new observations in a form consistent with the requirements for future access by myself or other people?

All too frequently, the traditional paper record system creates situations in which people answer such questions negatively. For example,
- The patient's chart may be unavailable when the health-care professional needs it. It may be in use by someone else at another location; it may have been misplaced despite the hospital's, clinic's, or office's record-tracking system (Figure 2.7); or it may even have been taken by someone unintentionally, and may now be lying buried on a desk.
- Once the chart is in hand, it may still be difficult to find the information required. The data may have been previously known but never recorded due to oversight by physicians or other health professionals. Poor organization in the chart may lead to the user spending an inordinate time searching for the data, especially in the charts of patients with long and complicated histories and massive paper records.
- Once the health-care professional has located the data, he may find it difficult to read them. It is not uncommon to hear one physician asking another as they peer together into a chart: "What is that word?" "Is that a two or a five?" "Whose signature is that?" Illegible and sloppy entries can be a major obstruction to effective use of the chart (Figure 2.8).
- When a chart is unavailable, the health-care professional still must provide medical care. Thus providers make do without the past data, basing their decisions instead on what the patient can tell them and on what their examination reveals. They then write a note for inclusion in the chart—when the chart is located. In a large institution with thousands of medical records, it is not surprising that such loose notes often fail to make it to the patient's chart or are filed out of sequence, so that the actual chronology of management is disrupted in the record.
- When patients with chronic or frequent diseases are seen over months or years, their records typically grow sufficiently large that they must be broken up into multiple volumes. When a hospital clinic or emergency room orders the patient's chart, only the most recent volume typically is provided. Old but pertinent data may be in early volumes that are stored offsite or are otherwise unavailable.

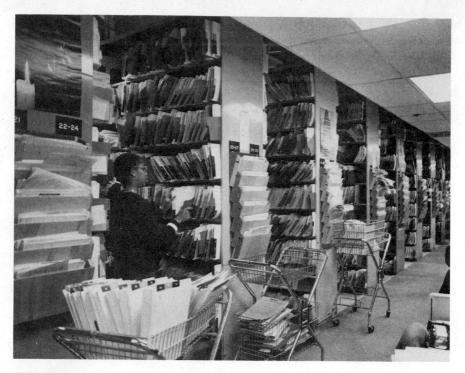

FIGURE 2.7 A typical storage room for medical records. It is not surprising that charts sometimes are mislaid. (*Source:* Photograph by Janice Anne Rohn.)

FIGURE 2.8 Written entries are standard in paper records, yet handwritten notes may be illegible. If notes cannot be interpreted by other people, this can cause delays in treatment and may even lead to inappropriate care.

As we shall describe in Chapter 6, computer-based medical-record systems offer potential solutions to all these practical problems in the use of the paper record.

2.3.2 Redundancy and Inefficiency

Partially in response to the need to be able to find data quickly in the chart, health professionals have developed a variety of techniques that provide redundant recording to match alternate modes of access. For example, the result of a radiologic study typically is entered on a standard radiology reporting form, which is filed in the portion of the chart labeled "X-ray." For complicated procedures, the same data often are summarized in a brief note by the radiologist in the narrative part of the chart, which she enters at the time of the study because she knows that the formal report will not make it back to the chart for 1 or 2 days. In addition, the study results often are mentioned in notes written by the patient's admitting and consulting physicians and the nursing staff. Although there may be good reason for recording such information multiple times in different ways and in different locations within the chart, the combined bulk of these notes accelerates the physical growth of the document and, accordingly, complicates the task of its logistical management. Furthermore, it becomes increasingly difficult to locate specific patient data as the chart succumbs to obesity. The predictable result is that someone will write yet another redundant entry, summarizing information it took hours to track down.

A similar inefficiency occurs because of a tension between opposing goals in the design of reporting forms used by many laboratories. Most health personnel prefer a consistent, familiar paper form, often with color coding, because it helps them to find information more quickly (Figure 2.9). For example, a physician may know that a urinalysis form is yellow, fills one-half of a page in a chart, and records the bacteria count halfway down the middle column of the form. This knowledge allows the physician to work backward quickly in the laboratory section of the chart to find the most recent urinalysis sheet and to check at a glance the bacterial count. The problem is that such forms typically store only sparse information. It is clearly suboptimal if a rapidly growing physical chart is filled with slips of paper that take up one-half of a page when they are pasted into position but report only a single datum.

2.3.3 Influence on Clinical Research

Anyone who has participated in a clinical research project based on chart review can attest to the tediousness of flipping through myriad medical records. For all the reasons described earlier, it is arduous to sit with stacks of patients' charts, extracting data and formatting them for structured statistical analysis, and the process is vulnerable to transcription errors. Observers often wonder how much medical knowledge is sitting untapped in medical records because there is no easy way to analyze experience across large populations of patients without first extracting pertinent data from the paper records.

Suppose, for example, that a physician notices that patients receiving a certain common oral medication for diabetes (call it drug X) seem to be more likely to have significant postoperative hypotension (low blood pressure) than do surgical patients

```
19-0505     Blood: Venous                       COLLECTED: 04/19/89   10:10 AM
       ORDERED BY: INT MED CL -- A160            RECEIVED: 04/19/89   10:51 AM
             ACCOUNT:                          ACCESSIONED: 04/19/89   10:58 AM
-----------------------------------------------------------------------------

  HEMATOLOGY                                       NORMAL RANGE
  -----------                                      ------------
     HEMOGRAM
        WBC ................        5.5   K/uL      ( 4.0 - 11.0 )
        RBC ................        4.52  MIL/uL    (Female:    3.8 - 5.2 )
                                                    (Male:      4.4 - 5.9 )
        HGB ................       14.2   gm/dl.    (Female:   11.7 - 15.7)
                                                    (Male:     13.5 - 17.7)
        HCT ................       42.8   %         (Female:     35 - 47  )
                                                    (Male:       40 - 52  )
        MCV ................       95.    fl        (  80 - 100  )
        MCH ................       31.4   pg        (  27 -  34  )
        MCHC ...............       33.1   g/dL      (  32 -  36  )
        RDW ................       13.1   %         ( less than 14.5% )

     DIFF
              POLY   BAND   META   LYMPH   MONO   EOS   BASO    REAC-LYM
               56                    27     13     2     2

              MYEL   PROM   BLAS  LYMPHOMA   OTHER  NRBC/100M    CELLS_COUNTED
                                                                  100
```

FIGURE 2.9 Laboratory reporting forms record medical data in a consistent, familiar format.

receiving other medications for diabetes. The doctor has based his hypothesis—that drug X influences postoperative blood pressure—on only a few recent observations, however, so he decides to look in existing hospital records to see whether this correlation has occurred with sufficient frequency to warrant a formal investigation. The best way to follow up on his theory from existing medical data would be to examine the hospital charts of all patients who have diabetes and also have been admitted for surgery. The task would then be to examine those charts and to note for all patients (1) whether they were taking drug X when admitted, and (2) whether they had postoperative hypotension. If the statistics showed that patients receiving drug X were more likely to have low blood pressure after surgery than were similar diabetic patients receiving alternate treatments, then a controlled trial (prospective observation and data gathering) might well be appropriate.

Note the distinction between **retrospective chart review** to investigate a question that was not a subject of study at the time the data were collected, and a **prospective study** in which the clinical hypothesis is known in advance and the **research protocol** is designed specifically to collect future data that are relevant to the question under consideration. Subjects are assigned randomly to different study groups, to help prevent researchers—who are bound to be biased, having developed the hypothesis—from unintentionally skewing the results by assigning a specific class of patients all to one group. For the same reason, to the extent possible, the studies are *double-blind;* that is, neither the researchers nor the subjects know which treatment is being administered. Such blinding is of course impractical when it is obvious to patients or physicians what therapy is being given (such as surgical procedures versus drug therapy). Prospective, randomized, double-blind studies are considered the best method for determining optimal management of disease.

Returning to our example, consider the problems in chart review that the physician would encounter in addressing the postoperative-hypotension question retrospectively. First, he would have to identify the charts of interest—a subset of medical records dealing with surgical patients who are also diabetics. In a hospital record room filled with thousands of charts, the task of chart selection can be overwhelming. Medical records departments generally do keep indexes of diagnostic and procedure codes cross-referenced to specific patients (see Section 2.4.1). Thus, it might be possible to use such an index to find all charts in which the discharge diagnoses included diabetes and the procedure codes included major surgical procedures. The doctor might be able to compile a list of patient identification numbers and have the individual charts pulled from the file room for review.

The physician's next task is to examine each chart serially to find out what treatment the patient was receiving for diabetes at the time of the surgery *and* to determine whether the patient had postoperative hypotension. Finding such information may be extremely time consuming. Where should the physician look for it? The admission drug orders might show what medications the patient received for diabetes control, but the researcher would also be wise to check the medication sheets to see whether the therapy was also administered (as well as ordered) and the admission history to see whether a routine treatment for diabetes, taken right up until the patient entered the hospital, was not administered during the inpatient stay. Information about hypotensive episodes might be similarly difficult to locate. The physician might start with nursing notes from the recovery room, or with the anesthesiologist's data sheets from the operating room, but the patient might not have been hypotensive until after leaving the recovery room and returning to the ward. So the nursing notes from the ward need to be checked too, as well as vital-signs sheets, physicians' progress notes, and the discharge summary.

It should be clear from this example that retrospective chart review is a laborious and tedious process, and that people performing it are prone to make transcription errors and to overlook key data. One of the great appeals of computer-based medical records is their potential ability to facilitate the chart-review process. Such records obviate the need to retrieve hardcopy charts; instead, researchers can use computer-based data retrieval and analysis techniques to do most of the work (finding relevant patients, locating pertinent data, and formatting the information for statistical analyses). Researchers can use similar techniques to harness computer assistance with data management in prospective clinical trials. Chapter 16 deals with this subject in further detail.

2.3.4 The Passive Nature of Paper Records

The traditional manual system has another limitation that would have been meaningless until the emergence of the computer age. A manual archival system is inherently passive; the charts sit waiting for something to be done with them. They are insensitive to the characteristics of the data recorded within their pages, such as legibility, accuracy, or implications for patient management. They cannot take an active role in responding appropriately to those implications.

Increasingly, computer-based record systems have changed our perspective on what health professionals can expect from the medical chart. Automated record systems introduce new opportunities for dynamic responses to the data that are recorded in them. As is described in many of the chapters to follow, computational techniques for data storage, retrieval, and analysis make it feasible to develop record systems that (1) monitor their contents and generate warnings or advice for providers based on single observations or logical combinations of data, (2) provide automated quality control, including the flagging of potentially erroneous data, or (3) provide feedback of patient-specific or population-based deviations from desirable standards.

2.4 The Structure of Medical Data

Scientific disciplines generally develop precise terminology or notation that is standardized and accepted by all workers in the field. Consider, for example, the universal language of chemistry embodied in chemical formulas, the precise definitions and mathematical equations used by physicists, the predicate calculus used by logicians, or the conventions for describing circuits used by electrical engineers. Medicine is remarkable for its failure to develop a standardized vocabulary and **nomenclature,** and many observers believe that a true scientific basis for the field will be impossible until this problem is addressed. Others argue that common references to the "art of medicine" reflect an important distinction between medicine and the "hard" sciences; these people question whether it is possible or desirable to introduce too much standardization into a field that prides itself in humanism.

The debate has been accentuated by the introduction of computers for data management because such machines tend to demand conformity to data standards and definitions. Otherwise, issues of data retrieval and analysis are confounded by discrepancies between the meanings intended by the observers or recorders and those intended by the individuals retrieving information or doing data analysis. What is an "upper respiratory infection"? Does it include infections of the trachea or mainstem bronchi? How large does the heart have to be before one can refer to "cardiomegaly"? How should researchers deal with the plethora of disease names based on eponyms (for example, Alzheimer's disease, Hodgkin's disease) that are not descriptive of the illness and may not be familiar to all practitioners? What do we mean by an "acute abdomen"? Are the boundaries of the abdomen well agreed on? What are the time constraints that correspond to "acuteness" of abdominal pain? Is an "ache" a pain? What about "occasional" cramping?

Imprecision and the lack of a standardized vocabulary are particularly problematic when we wish to aggregate data recorded by multiple health professionals or to analyze trends over time. Without a controlled, predefined vocabulary, data interpretation is inherently complicated and the automatic summarization of data may be impossible. For example, one physician might note that a patient has "shortness of breath." Later, another physician might note that she has "dyspnea." Unless these terms are designated as synonyms, an automated flowcharting program will fail to indicate that the patient had the same problem on both occasions.

Regardless of arguments regarding the "artistic" elements in medicine, the need for health personnel to communicate effectively is clear, both in acute-care settings and when patients are seen over long periods of time. Both quality care and scientific progress depend on *some* standardization in terminology. Otherwise differences in intended meaning or in defining criteria will lead to miscommunication, improper interpretation, and potentially negative consequences for the patients involved.

Given the lack of formal definitions for many medical terms, it is remarkable that medical workers communicate as well as they do. Only occasionally is the care for a patient clearly compromised by miscommunication. If computer-based records are to become dynamic and responsive manipulators of patient care, however, their encoded logic must be able to presume a specific meaning for the terms and data elements entered by the observers.

2.4.1 Coding Systems

We are used to seeing figures regarding the growing incidence of certain types of tumors, deaths from influenza during the winter months, and similar health statistics that we tend to take for granted. How are such data accumulated? Their role in health planning and health-care financing is clear, but if their accumulation required chart review through the process described earlier in this chapter, we would know much less about the health status of the populations in various communities.

Because of the need to know about health trends for the population, and to recognize epidemics in their early stages, there is a variety of health-reporting requirements for hospitals (as well as other public organizations) and practitioners. For example, cases of gonorrhea, syphilis, and tuberculosis generally must be reported to local public-health organizations that code the data to allow trend analyses over time. The Centers for Disease Control (CDC) in Atlanta then pools regional data and reports national as well as local trends in disease incidence, bacterial resistance patterns, and the like.

Another kind of reporting involves the coding of all discharge diagnoses for hospitalized patients, plus coding of certain procedures (for example, type of surgery) that were performed during the hospital stay. Such codes are reported to state and federal health planning and analysis agencies, and also are used internally at the institution for case-mix analysis (determining the relative frequencies of various disorders in the hospitalized population and the average length of stay for each disease category) and for research purposes. For such data to be useful, the codes must be well defined as well as uniformly applied and accepted. The government publishes a national diagnostic **coding scheme,** the current version of which is the Ninth International Classification of Disease (ICD-9) [Health Care Financing Administration, 1980; Sartorius, 1976]. ICD-9-CM, a clinical modification of ICD-9, is used by all nonmilitary hospitals in the United States for discharge coding purposes and must be reported on the bills submitted to most insurance companies (Figure 2.10). Pathologists have developed another widely used diagnostic coding scheme; originally known as SNOP

CHRONIC OBSTRUCTIVE PULMONARY DISEASE AND ALLIED CONDITIONS
(490-496)

490   Bronchitis, not specified as acute or chronic

491   Chronic bronchitis

    491.0 Simple chronic bronchitis
    491.1 Mucopurulent chronic bronchitis
    491.2 Obstructive chronic bronchitis
    491.8 Other chronic bronchitis
    491.9 Unspecified chronic bronchitis

492 Emphysema

    492.0 Emphysematous bleb
    492.8 Other emphysema

493 Asthma

    493.0 Extrinsic asthma
    493.1 Intrinsic asthma
    493.9 Asthma, unspecified

494 Bronchiectasis

495 Extrinsic allergic alveolitis

    495.0 Farmer's lung
    495.1 Bagassosis
    495.2 Bird-fanciers' lung
    495.3 Suberosis
    495.4 Malt workers' lung
    495.5 Mushroom workers' lung
    495.6 Maple bark-strippers' lung
    495.7 "Ventilation" pneumonitis
    495.8 Other specified allergic alveolitis and pneumonitis
        Cheese-washers' lung, Coffee workers' lung, Fish-meal workers' lung,
        Furriers' lung, Grain-handlers' disease or lung, Pituitary snuff-takers'
        disease, Sequoiosis or red-cedar asthma, Wood asthma
    495.9 Unspecified allergic alveolitis and pneumonitis

FIGURE 2.10 A small subset of the disease categories identified by the Ninth International Classification of Disease, Clinical Modification (ICD-9-CM). (*Source:* Health Care Financing Administration (1980). *The International Classification of Diseases, 9th Revision, Clinical Modification, ICD-9-CM.* U.S. Department of Health and Human Services, Washington, D.C. DHHS Publication No. (PHS) 80-1260.)

(Systematized Nomenclature of Pathology), it has been expanded to form SNOMED (Systematized Nomenclature of Medicine) [Coté and Robboy, 1980; American College of Pathologists, 1982]. Another coding scheme developed by the American Medical Association (AMA)—the Current Procedural Terminology (CPT) [Finkel, 1977]—is similarly widely used in producing bills for services rendered to patients. What warrants emphasis here, however, is the motivation for the codes' development:

Health-care personnel need standardized terms that can support pooling of data for analysis and can provide criteria for determining charges for individual patients.

The historical roots of a coding system reveal themselves as limitations or idiosyncrasies when the system is applied in more general clinical settings. For example, the ICD-9 code was derived from a classification scheme developed for epidemiological reporting. Consequently, it has more than 50 separate codes for describing tuberculosis infections. SNOMED permits coding of pathologic findings in exquisite detail, but contains no codes for radiologic findings such as the details of an X-ray film of the colon. In a particular clinical setting, not one of the common coding schemes is likely to be completely satisfactory. In some cases, the granularity of the code will be too coarse; a hematologist (person who studies blood diseases) may want to distinguish among a variety of hemoglobinopathies (disorders of the structure and function of hemoglobin) lumped under a single code in ICD-9. On the other hand, another practitioner may prefer to aggregate many individual codes—for example, those for active tuberculosis—into a single category to simplify the coding and retrieval of data.

Such schemes cannot be effective unless they are accepted by health-care providers. There is an inherent tension between the need for a coding system that is general enough to cover many different patients and the need for precise and unique terms that accurately apply to a specific patient and do not unduly constrain physicians' attempts to describe what they observe. Yet if physicians view the computer-based medical record as a blank sheet of paper on which any unstructured information can be written, the data they record will be unsuitable for dynamic processing, clinical research, and health planning. The challenge is to learn how to meet all these needs through a common structure that ties together the various vocabularies that have been created [National Library of Medicine, 1987]. Researchers at many institutions are currently working to develop such a Unified Medical Language System (UMLS; also see Chapter 20) [Greenes, 1988].

2.4.2 The Data-to-Knowledge Spectrum

A central focus in medical informatics is the information base that constitutes the substance of medicine. Workers in the field recently have tried to clarify the distinction between three terms frequently used to describe the content of computer-based systems: *data, information,* and *knowledge* [Blum, 1986b]. These terms are often used interchangeably. In this volume, we shall refer to a single observational point that characterizes a relationship as a **datum.** Thus, we generally regard a datum as the value of a specific parameter for a particular object (for example, a patient) at a given point in time. **Knowledge,** then, is derived through the formal or informal analysis (or interpretation) of data. Thus, it includes the results of formal studies and also commonsense facts, assumptions, heuristics (strategic rules of thumb), and models—any of which may reflect the experience or biases of people who interpret the primary data. The term **information** is more generic in that it encompasses both organized data and knowledge.

The observation that a patient Brown has a blood pressure of 180/110 is a *datum,* as is the report that the patient has had a myocardial infarction (heart attack). When researchers pool and analyze such data, they may determine that patients with high blood pressure are more likely to have heart attacks than are patients with normal or low blood pressure. This data analysis has produced a piece of *knowledge* about the world. A physician's belief that prescribing dietary restriction of salt is unlikely to be effective in controlling high blood pressure in patients of low economic standing (because these people are not likely to be able to afford special low-salt foods) is an additional personal piece of *knowledge*—a **heuristic** that guides that physician in her decision making. Note that the appropriate interpretation of these definitions depends on the context. Knowledge at one level of abstraction may be considered data at higher levels. A blood pressure of 180/110 is a raw datum; the statement that the patient has hypertension is an interpretation of that datum, and thus represents a higher level of knowledge. As input to a diagnostic decision aid, however, an indication of either the presence or absence of hypertension may be requested, in which case the presence of hypertension is treated as a data item.

A **database** is a collection of individual observations without any summarizing analysis. A computer-based medical-record system is thus primarily viewed as a database—the place in which patient data are stored. A **knowledge base,** on the other hand, is a collection of facts, heuristics, and models that can be used for problem solving. If the knowledge base provides sufficient structure, including semantic links among knowledge items, the computer itself may be able to apply that knowledge as an aid to case-based problem solving. Many decision-support systems have been called *knowledge-based systems* to reflect this distinction between knowledge bases and databases (see Chapter 15).

2.5 Strategies of Medical Data Selection and Use

It is unrealistic to conceive of a complete medical data set. All medical databases, and medical records, are necessarily incomplete because they reflect the selective collection and recording of data by the health-care personnel responsible for the patient. There can be marked interpersonal differences in both style and problem solving that account for variations in the way practitioners collect and record data for the same patient under the same circumstances. Such variations do not necessarily reflect good practices, however, and much of medical education is directed at helping physicians and other health professionals to learn what observations to make, how to make them (generally an issue of technique), how to interpret them, and how to decide whether they warrant formal recording.

An example of this phenomenon is the difference between the taking of the first medical history, performing of the physical examination, and writing of a report by a novice medical student, and the similar process undertaken by a seasoned clinician examining the same patient. Medical students tend to work from comprehensive mental outlines of questions to ask, physical tests to perform, and additional data to collect. Because they have not developed skills of selectivity, the process of taking a medical history and performing a physical examination may take more than 1 hour, after which the student writes an extensive report of what she observed and how she has interpreted her observations. It clearly would be impractical, inefficient, and inappropriate for physicians in practice to spend this amount of time assessing every new patient. Thus, part of the challenge for the neophyte is to learn how to ask only the questions that are necessary, to perform only the examination components that are required, and to record only those data that will be pertinent in justifying the ongoing diagnostic approach and in guiding the future management of the patient.

What do we mean by "selectivity" in data collection and recording? It is precisely this process that often is viewed as a central part of the "art of medicine," an element that accounts for individual styles and the sometimes marked distinctions among clinicians. As we shall discuss with the aid of numerous clinical examples in Chapter 3, the notion of selectivity implies an ongoing decision-making process that guides data collection and interpretation. Attempts to understand how expert clinicians internalize this process, and to formalize the notions so that they can better be taught and explained, are a central issue in medical-informatics research. Improved guidelines for such decision making, derived from research in medical informatics, not only are enhancing the teaching and practice of medicine, but also are providing insights that suggest methods for developing computer-based decision-support tools.

2.5.1 The Hypothetico-Deductive Approach

Studies of medical decision makers have shown that strategies for data collection and interpretation are imbedded in an iterative process known as the **hypothetico-deductive approach** [Elstein et al., 1978; Kassirer and Gorry, 1978]. As medical students learn this process, their data collection becomes more focused and efficient and their medical records become more compact. The central idea is one of sequential, staged data collection, followed by data interpretation and the generation of hypotheses, leading to hypothesis-directed selection of the next most appropriate data to be collected. As data are collected at each stage, they are added to the growing database of observations and are used to reformulate or refine the active hypotheses. This process is iterated until one hypothesis reaches a threshold level of certainty (for example, it is proven to be true, or at least the uncertainty is reduced to a satisfactory level). At that point, a management, disposition, or therapeutic decision can be made.

This process is clarified by the diagram in Figure 2.11. As shown, data collection begins when the patient presents to the physician with some complaint (a symptom or disease). The physician generally responds with a few questions that allow her to focus rapidly on the nature of the problem. In the written report, the data collected with these initial questions typically are recorded as the patient identification, chief complaint, and the initial portion of the history of the present illness. Studies have shown, however, that an experienced physician will have an initial set of hypotheses in mind after hearing the patient's response to the first six or seven questions [Elstein et al., 1978]. These hypotheses then serve as the basis for selecting additional questions. As is shown in Figure 2.11, answers to these additional questions allow the physician to refine her hypotheses (theories) about what is the source

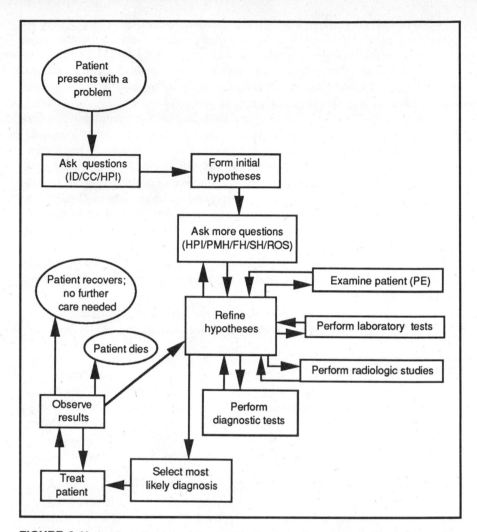

FIGURE 2.11 A schematic view of the hypothetico-deductive approach. The process of medical data collection and treatment is intimately tied to an ongoing process of hypothesis generation and refinement. See text for full discussion. [ID = patient identification, CC = chief complaint, HPI = history of present illness, PMH = past medical history, FH = family history, SH = social history, ROS = review of systems, PE = physical examination.]

of the patient's problem. Physicians refer to the set of active hypotheses as the differential diagnosis for a patient; the **differential diagnosis** comprises the set of possible diagnoses among which the physician must distinguish in order to determine how best to administer treatment.

Note that the question-selection process is inherently *heuristic;* for example, it is personalized and efficient but is not guaranteed to collect every piece of information that might be pertinent. Human beings use heuristics all the time in their decision making because it often is impractical or impossible to use an exhaustive problem-solving approach. A common example of heuristic problem solving is the playing of a complex game such as chess. Because it would require an enormous amount of time to define all the possible moves and countermoves that could ensue from a given board position, expert chess players develop personal heuristics for assessing the game at any point and then selecting a strategy for how best to proceed.

Physicians have developed safety measures, however, to help them avoid missing important issues that they might not discover when collecting data in an hypothesis-directed fashion during the history taking for the present illness [Pauker et al., 1976]. These measures tend to be focused in four general categories of questions that follow the collection of information about the chief complaint: past medical history, family history, social history, and a brief **review of systems** in which the physician asks some general questions about the state of health of each of the major organ systems in the body. Occasionally, the physician discovers entirely new problems, or finds important information that modifies the hypothesis list or modulates the treatment options available (for example, if the patient reports a serious past drug reaction or allergy).

When the physician is through asking questions, the refined hypothesis list (which may already be narrowed to a single diagnosis) then serves as the basis for a focused physical éxamination. By this time, the physician may well have expectations of what she will find on examination, or may have specific tests in mind that will help her to distinguish among still active hypotheses about diseases based on the questions she has asked. Once again, as with the question-asking process, focused hypothesis-directed examination is augmented with general tests that occasionally turn up new abnormalities and generate hypotheses that the physician did not expect on the basis of the medical history alone. In addition, unexplained findings on examination may raise issues that require additional history taking. Thus, the asking of questions generally is partially integrated with the examination process.

When the physician has completed the physical examination, her refined hypothesis list may be narrowed sufficiently that she can undertake specific treatment. It often is necessary to gather additional data, however. Such testing is once again guided by the current hypotheses. The options available include laboratory tests (of blood, urine, other body fluids, or biopsy specimens), radiologic studies (X-ray examinations, nuclear-imaging scans, computed-tomography studies, magnetic-resonance scans, sonograms, or any of a number of other imaging modalities), and other specialized tests (electrocardiograms, electroencephalograms, nerve-conduction studies, and many others). As the results of such studies become available, the physician constantly revises and refines her hypothesis list.

Ultimately, the physician is sufficiently certain about the source of a patient's problem to be able to develop a specific management plan. Treatment(s) are administered and the patient is observed. Note that the response to treatment is itself a data point that may affect the hypotheses about a patient's illness. If the patient does not respond to treatment, it may mean that the disease is resistant to that therapy and that the physician should try an alternate approach, or it may mean that the initial diagnosis was incorrect and that she should consider alternate explanations for the patient's complaint.

The patient may remain in a cycle of treatment and observation for a long time, as is shown in Figure 2.11. This is the nature of chronic-disease management, an aspect of medical care that is accounting for an increasing proportion of the health-care community's work (and an increasing proportion of the health-care dollar). Alternatively, the patient may recover and no longer need therapy, or he may die. Although the process outlined in Figure 2.11 is oversimplified in many regards, it is generally applicable to the process of data collection, diagnosis, and treatment in most areas of medicine.

Note that the hypothesis-directed process of data collection, diagnosis, and treatment is inherently *knowledge-based*. It is dependent not only on a significant fact base that permits proper interpretation of data and selection of appropriate followup questions and tests, but also on the effective use of heuristic techniques that characterize individual expertise. Another important issue, addressed in Chapter 3, is the need for physicians to balance financial costs and health risks of data collection against the perceived benefits to be gained when those data become available. It costs nothing but time to examine the patient at the bedside or to ask an additional question, but if the data collection being considered requires, for example, X-ray exposure, coronary angiography, or computed tomography of the head (all of which have associated risks and costs), then it may be preferable to proceed with treatment in the absence of full information. Differences in the assessment of cost-benefit tradeoffs in data collection often account for differences of opinion among collaborating physicians.

2.5.2 The Relationship Between Data and Hypotheses

We wrote rather glibly in the preceding section about the "generation of hypotheses from data"; now we need to ask: What precisely is the nature of that process? Researchers with a psychological orientation have spent much time trying to understand how expert problem solvers evoke hypotheses [Elstein et al., 1978; Pauker et al., 1976; Pople, 1982], but the traditional probabilistic decision sciences have much to say about the issue as well. We provide only a brief introduction to those notions here; they are discussed in greater detail in Chapter 3.

When an observation evokes an hypothesis (for example, when a clinical finding makes a specific diagnosis come to mind), the observation presumably has some close association with the hypothesis. What might be the characteristics of that association? Perhaps the finding is almost always observed when the hypothesis turns out to be true; is that enough to explain hypothesis generation? A simple example will show that such a simple relationship is *not* enough to explain the evocation process. Consider the hypothesis that a patient is pregnant and the observation that the patient is female. Clearly, all pregnant patients are female. However, when a new patient is observed to be female, the possibility that the patient is pregnant is not immediately evoked. Thus, female gender is a highly *sensitive* indicator of pregnancy (there is a 100-percent chance that a pregnant patient is female) but it is not a good *predictor* of pregnancy (most females are not pregnant). The notion of **sensitivity**—the likelihood that a given piece of data will be observed in a patient with a given disease or condition—is an important one, but it will not alone account for the process of hypothesis generation in medical diagnosis.

Perhaps the clinical manifestation seldom occurs unless the hypothesis turns out to be true; is that enough to explain hypothesis generation? This notion seems to be a little closer to the process. Suppose that a given datum is *never* seen unless a patient has a specific disease. For example, a Pap smear (a smear of cells swabbed from the cervix, at the opening to the uterus, treated with Papanicolaou's stain, and then examined under the microscope) with grossly abnormal cells (called class IV findings) is essentially never seen unless the woman has cancer of the cervix or uterus. Such tests are called **pathognomonic.** Not only do they evoke a specific diagnosis, but they also immediately prove it to be true. Unfortunately, there are very few pathognomonic tests in medicine.

More commonly, an observation is seen in one disease or disease category more frequently than it is in others, but the association is not absolute. For example, only a small number of disease entities other than infections will elevate a patient's white-blood-cell count. Certainly it is true, for example, that leukemia can raise the white-blood-cell count, as can the use of the drug prednisone, but *most* patients without infections will have normal white-blood-cell counts. An elevated white count therefore does not *prove* a patient has an infection, but it does tend to evoke or support the hypothesis that an infection is present. The word used to describe this relationship is **specificity.** An observation is highly specific for a disease if it is generally not seen in patients who do not have that disease. A pathognomonic observation is 100-percent specific for a given disease. When an observation is highly specific for a disease, it tends to evoke that disease during the diagnostic or data-gathering process.

By now, you may have realized that there is a substantial difference between a physician viewing test results that evoke a disease hypothesis and that physician being willing to act on the disease hypothesis. Yet even experienced physicians sometimes fail to recognize that, although they have made an observation that is highly specific for a given disease, it may still be more likely that the patient has other diseases (and not the suspected one) unless (1) the finding is pathognomonic, or (2) the suspected disease is considerably more common than are the other diseases that can cause the observed abnormality. This is one of the most common errors of intuition that has been identified in the medical decision-making process. To explain the basis for this confusion in more detail, we must introduce two additional terms: *prevalence* and *predictive value.*

The **prevalence** of a disease is simply a measure of the frequency with which the disease occurs in the population of interest. A given disease may have a prevalence of only 5 percent in the general population (one person in 20 will have the disease) but a higher prevalence in a specially selected subpopulation. For example, black lung disease has a low prevalence in the general population but a much higher prevalence among coal miners, who develop black lung from inhaling coal dust. The task of diagnosis therefore involves *updating* the probability that a patient has a disease from the **baseline rate** (the prevalence in the population from which the patient was selected) to a posttest probability that reflects the test results. For example, the probability that any given person in the United States has lung cancer is low (that is, the prevalence of the disease is low), but may be much higher if his chest X-ray examination shows a possible tumor. If the patient were a member of the population composed of American cigarette smokers, however, then the prevalence of lung cancer would be higher. In this case, the *same* chest X-ray report would result in an even higher updated probability of lung cancer than it would had the patient been selected from the population of all U.S. citizens.

The **predictive value** of a test is simply the posttest (updated) *probability* that a disease is present based on the results of a test. If an observation supports the presence of a disease, the predictive value will be greater than is the prevalence (also called the *pretest risk*). If the observation tends to argue against the presence of a disease, the predictive value will be lower than is the prevalence. For any test and disease, then, there is one predictive value if the test result is positive and another predictive value if the test result is negative. These are typically abbreviated PV+ (the predictive value of a positive test) and PV− (the predictive value of a negative test).

The process of hypothesis generation in medical diagnosis thus involves both hypothesis evocation *and* the assignment of a likelihood (probability) to the presence of a specific disease or disease category. The predictive value of a positive test is dependent on the test's sensitivity, specificity, and prevalence. The formula that describes the relationship precisely is

$$PV+ = \frac{(\text{sensitivity})(\text{prevalence})}{(\text{sensitivity})(\text{prevalence}) + (1 - \text{specificity})(1 - \text{prevalence})}$$

There is a similar formula for defining PV− in terms of sensitivity, specificity, and prevalence. Both formulae can be derived from simple probability theory. Note that positive tests with high sensitivity and specificity may still lead to a rather low posttest probability of the disease (PV+) if the prevalence of that disease is low. You should substitute values in the PV+ formula to convince yourself that this is true. It is this relationship that tends to be poorly understood by practitioners and often is viewed as counterintuitive (which shows that your intuition can misguide you when it is not based on solid principles). Note also that test sensitivity and disease prevalence can be ignored *only* when a test is pathognomonic (that is, when specificity is 100 percent, which mandates that PV+ be 100 percent). The PV+ formula is one of many forms of Bayes' theorem, a rule for combining probabilistic data. It is generally attributed to the work of Reverend Thomas Bayes in the 1700s. Bayes' theorem is discussed in greater detail in Chapter 3.

2.5.3 Methods for Selecting Questions and Comparing Tests

We have described the process of hypothesis-directed sequential data collection and have asked how an observation might evoke or refine the physician's hypotheses about what abnormalities account for the patient's illness. There is a complementary question: Given a set of current hypotheses, how does the physician decide what additional data should be collected? This issue also has been analyzed at length in recent years [Elstein et al., 1978; Pople, 1982] and is pertinent for computer programs that gather data efficiently to assist with diagnosis or therapeutic decision making (see Chapter 15). Because issues of test selection and data interpretation are crucial to understanding medical data and their uses, we devote the next chapter to these and related issues. In Section 3.6, for example, we shall discuss the use of decision-analytic techniques in deciding whether to treat a patient on the basis of available information or to perform additional diagnostic tests.

2.6 The Computer and Medical Data Collection

Although this chapter has not directly discussed computer systems, the potential role of the computer in medical data storage, retrieval, and interpretation should be clear to you. Much of the rest of this book deals with specific applications in which the computer's primary role is data management. One issue is pertinent to all such applications: How do you get the data into the computer in the first place?

The need for data entry by physicians has been a problem for medical-computing systems since the earliest days of the field. Awkward or nonintuitive interactions at computer terminals, particularly ones requiring keyboard typing by the physician, have probably done more to inhibit the clinical use of computers than has any other factor. Doctors, and many other health-care staff, tend simply to refuse to use computers because of the interactive requirements that accompany the systems.

A variety of approaches has been used to try to finesse this problem. One is to design systems so that clerical staff can do essentially all the data entry and much of the data retrieval as well. Many clinical-research systems have taken this approach. Physicians may be asked to fill out structured data sheets, or such sheets may be filled out by data abstractors who review patient charts, but the actual entry of data into the database is done by designated transcriptionists.

In some applications, it is possible for data to be entered automatically into the computer by the device that measures or collects them. For example, monitors in intensive- or coronary-care units, pulmonary-function or ECG machines, and measurement equipment in the clinical chemistry laboratory can interface directly with a computer in which a database is stored. Certain data can be entered directly by patients; there are systems, for example, that take the patient's history by presenting on a terminal multiple-choice questions that follow a branching logic (see Chapter 18). The patient's responses to the questions are used to generate hardcopy reports for physicians, and also may be stored directly in a computer database for subsequent use in other settings.

When physicians or other health personnel do use the machine themselves, specialized devices often allow rapid and intuitive operator–machine interaction. Most of these devices use a variant of the "point-and-select" approach; examples of such devices are touch-sensitive screens, light pens, and mouse pointing devices (see Chapter 4). When conventional terminals and keyboards are used, specialized key pads sometimes are appropriate. At the least, designers frequently try to permit logical selection of items from menus displayed on the screen so that the user does not need to learn a set of specialized commands in order to enter or review data.

These issues arise in essentially all application areas and, because they can be crucial to the successful implementation and use of a system, they warrant particular attention in system design. We encourage you to consider issues of human–computer interaction as you learn about the application areas and the specific systems described in later chapters.

Suggested Readings

van Bemmel, J. H., et al. (eds). Data, information and knowledge in medicine. *Methods of Information in Medicine,* 27(Special issue):1–373, 1988.

> *This special issue of* Methods of Information in Medicine *contains 44 articles that were previously published in the journal and that provide a historical perspective on scientific developments in medical informatics. The first section presents 10 papers on various aspects of medical data. The remaining sections are devoted to medical systems, medical information and patterns, medical knowledge and decision making, and medical research.*

Komaroff, A. L. The variability and inaccuracy of medical data. *Proceedings of the IEEE,* 67:1196, 1979.

> *This article is an excellent summary of the process of medical-data collection and the sources of variability in those data. The author provides an introduction to the notions of sensitivity and specificity in that context.*

National Library of Medicine. *NLM Long Range Plan.* Bethesda, MD: U.S. Department of Health and Human Services, Public Health Service, National Institutes of Health, 1987.

> *This series of five reports deals with many topics of relevance to this book (for example, online biomedical databases, medical informatics research, and computers in health education). Of particular pertinence to this chapter are discussions of the need for a Unified Medical Language System that would cut across medical specialties and be suitable for computer-based encoding.*

Questions for Discussion

1. You check your pulse and discover that your heart rate is 100 beats per minute. Is this normal or abnormal? What additional information do you use in making this judgment? Discuss how the *context* in which data are collected influences the interpretation of those data.
2. Given the imprecision of many medical terms, why do you think that instances of serious miscommunication among health-care professionals are not more prevalent? Why is greater standardization of terminology necessary if computers rather than humans are to manipulate patient data?
3. Based on the discussion of coding schemes for representing medical information, what problems do you foresee in attempting to construct a standardized medical terminology to be used in hospitals, physicians' offices, and research institutions throughout the United States?
4. How do you think medical practice would change if nonphysicians were to collect all medical data?
5. To decide whether a patient has a significant urinary-tract infection, physicians commonly calculate the number of bacterial organisms in a milliliter of his urine.

Physicians generally assume that a patient has a urinary-tract infection if there are at least 10,000 bacteria per milliliter. Although laboratories can provide such a quantification with reasonable accuracy, it is obviously unrealistic for the physician explicitly to count large numbers of bacteria by examining a milliliter of urine under the microscope. As a result, one recent article offers the following guideline to physicians: "When interpreting . . . microscopy of . . . stained centrifuged urine, a threshold of one organism per field yields a 95% sensitivity and five organisms per field a 95% specificity for bacteriuria [bacteria in the urine] at a level of at least 10,000 organisms per ml" [Senior Medical Review, 1987, p. 4].

a. Describe an experiment that would have allowed the researchers to determine the sensitivity and specificity of the microscopy.

b. How would you expect specificity to change as the number of bacteria per microscopic field increases from one to five?

c. How would you expect sensitivity to change as the number of bacteria per microscopic field increases from one to five?

d. Why does it take more organisms per microscopic field to obtain a specificity of 95 percent than it does to achieve a sensitivity of 95 percent?

3

Medical Decision Making: Probabilistic Medical Reasoning

Douglas K. Owens and Harold C. Sox, Jr.

After reading this chapter, you should know the answers to these questions:

- How is the concept of probability useful for understanding test results and for making medical decisions that involve uncertainty?
- How can we characterize the ability of a test to discriminate between disease and health?
- What information is necessary to interpret test results accurately?
- What is *expected-value decision making*? How can this methodology help in understanding particular medical problems?
- What is a *sensitivity analysis*? How can we use it to examine the robustness of a decision and to identify the important variables in a decision?

3.1 The Nature of Clinical Decisions: Uncertainty and the Process of Diagnosis

Because clinical data are imperfect and outcomes of treatment are uncertain, health professionals often are faced with difficult choices. In this chapter, we shall introduce the concepts of *probabilistic medical reasoning,* one approach that can help health-care providers to deal with the uncertainty inherent in many medical decisions. Medical decisions are made by a variety of methods; our approach will not be necessary or appropriate for all decisions. Throughout the chapter, however, we shall use simple clinical examples to illustrate a broad range of problems in which probabilistic medical reasoning provides valuable insight.

As we saw in the preceding chapter, medical practice *is* medical decision making. This chapter focuses on the *process* of medical decision making. Together, Chapters 2 and 3 lay the groundwork for the rest of the book. In the remaining chapters, we shall discuss ways that computers can help practitioners with the decision-making process, and we shall emphasize the relationship between information needs and system design and implementation.

The material in this chapter is presented in the context of the decisions made by an individual physician. The concepts, however, are more broadly applicable. Sensitivity and specificity are important parameters of laboratory systems that flag abnormal test results (Chapter 9), of patient-monitoring systems (Chapter 12), and of bibliographic-retrieval systems (Chapter 14). An understanding of probability and of how to adjust probabilities after the acquisition of new information will be a foundation for our study of clinical decision-support systems (Chapter 15). The importance of probability in medical decision making is hardly a new idea: " . . . good medicine does not consist in the indiscriminate application of laboratory examinations to a patient, but rather in having so clear a comprehension of the probabilities and possibilities of a case as to know what tests may be expected to give information of value" [Peabody, 1922, p. 325].

Example 1. You are the director of a large urban blood bank. All potential blood donors are tested for antibody to the human immune deficiency virus (HIV). HIV is the causative agent of acquired immune deficiency syndrome (AIDS). When exposed to the virus, a person forms antibodies that can be detected in his blood. Because AIDS is transmitted via blood, people who have been exposed to the virus must be excluded as blood donors. The screening test is positive 98 percent of the time when antibody is present, and is negative 99 percent of the time antibody is absent.[1]

If the test is positive, what is the likelihood that a donor actually has HIV antibodies? If the test is negative, how sure can you be that the antibody actually is absent? On an intuitive level, these questions do not seem particularly difficult to answer.

---

[1]The test sensitivity and specificity used in Example 1 are similar to the early reported values of sensitivity and specificity for tests used to detect antibodies to HIV [Weiss et al., 1985]. Tests with much higher sensitivity and specificity are now available.

The test appears accurate, and we would expect that, if the test is positive, the donated blood specimen is very likely to contain the antibody. Thus, we are shaken to find that, if only one in 1000 donors actually has the antibody, the test is more often mistaken than it is correct. In fact, of 100 donors with a positive test, fewer than 10 would have the antibody. *There would be 10 wrong answers for each correct result.* How are we to understand this ratio? Before we try to find an answer, consider a somewhat different example.

> **Example 2.** Mr. Jones is a 59-year-old man with coronary-artery disease (narrowing or blockage of the blood vessels that supply the heart tissue). When the heart muscle does not receive enough oxygen (hypoxia) because blood cannot reach it, the patient often experiences chest pain (angina). Mr. Jones has twice had coronary-artery bypass graft (CABG) surgery, a procedure in which new vessels, usually taken from the leg, are grafted onto the old ones such that blood is shunted past the blocked region. Unfortunately, he again begins to have chest pain that becomes progressively more severe, in spite of medication. If the heart muscle is deprived of oxygen, the result can be a heart attack (myocardial infarction), in which a section of the muscle dies.

Should Mr. Jones undergo a third operation? The medications are not working; without surgery he runs a high risk of suffering a heart attack, which may be fatal. On the other hand, the surgery is hazardous. Not only is the surgical mortality rate for a third operation higher than that for a first or second one, but also the chance that surgery will relieve the chest pain is lower than for a first operation. All choices in Example 2 entail considerable uncertainty. Further, the risks are grave; an incorrect decision may substantially increase the chance that Mr. Jones will die. The decision will be difficult even for experienced clinicians.

These examples illustrate situations in which intuition is either misleading or inadequate. A physician who uncritically accepted the test results in Example 1 would erroneously tell many people that they had been exposed to the AIDS virus, a mistake with profound emotional and social consequences. In Example 2, the decision-making skill of the physician would affect a patient's quality and length of life. Similar situations are commonplace in medicine. Our goal in this chapter is to show how the use of probability and decision analysis can help to resolve these problems.

Decision making is one of the quintessential activities of the health-care professional. Some decisions are made on the basis of deductive reasoning, or of physiological principles. Many decisions, however, are made on the basis of knowledge that has been gained through collective experience: The clinician often must rely on empirical knowledge of associations between symptoms and disease to evaluate a problem. A decision that is based on these usually imperfect associations will be, to some degree, uncertain. In this section, we shall examine decisions made under uncertainty, and shall present an overview of the diagnostic process. As Lloyd H. Smith, Jr., said, "Medical decisions based on probabilities are necessary but also perilous. Even the most astute physician will occasionally be wrong" [Smith, 1985, p. 3].

3.1.1 Decision Making Under Uncertainty

Example 3. Mr. Santos, a 33-year-old man with a history of blood clot (thrombus) in a vein in his left leg, presents with the complaint of pain and swelling in that leg for the past 5 days. On physical examination, the leg is tender and swollen to midcalf, *signs*[2] that suggest the possibility of deep-vein thrombosis. A test (venography) is performed in which radiopaque dye is injected into the veins of Mr. Santos' leg so that they are outlined on X-ray film. The veins are abnormal, but the radiologist cannot tell whether there is a new blood clot.

Should Mr. Santos be treated for blood clots? The main diagnostic concern is the recurrence of a blood clot in his leg. A clot in the veins of the leg can dislodge, flow with the blood, and cause a blockage in the vessels of the lungs, a potentially fatal event called a pulmonary embolus. Of patients with a swollen leg, only about one-half actually have a blood clot; there are numerous other causes of a swollen leg. Given a swollen leg, therefore, a physician cannot be sure that a clot is the cause. Thus, the physical findings leave considerable uncertainty. Furthermore, the most definitive test available is equivocal in Example 3, because the veins are abnormal due to an earlier clot. The treatment for a blood clot is to administer anticoagulants (drugs that inhibit blood-clot formation), which poses the risk of excessive bleeding to the patient. Therefore, the physician does not want to treat the patient unless she is fairly certain a thrombus is present.

This example illustrated an important concept: *Clinical data are imperfect.* The degree of imperfection varies, but all clinical data—including the results of diagnostic tests, the history given by the patient, and the findings on physical examination—are uncertain.

3.1.2 Probability: An Alternative Method of Expressing Uncertainty

The language physicians use to describe a patient's condition often is ambiguous, a factor that further complicates the problem of uncertainty in medical decision making. Physicians use words such as "probable" and "highly likely" to describe their beliefs about the likelihood of disease. These words have strikingly different meanings to different individuals (Figure 3.1). Because of the widespread disagreement about the meaning of common descriptive terms, there is ample opportunity for miscommunication.

The problem of expressing degrees of uncertainty is not unique to medicine. How is it handled in other contexts? Horse racing has its share of uncertainty. If experienced

---

[2]In medicine, a *sign* is an objective physical finding (something observed by the clinician), such as a temperature of 101.2 degrees Farenheit. A *symptom* is a subjective experience of the patient, such as feeling hot or feverish. The distinction may be blurred if the patient's experience also can be observed by the clinician.

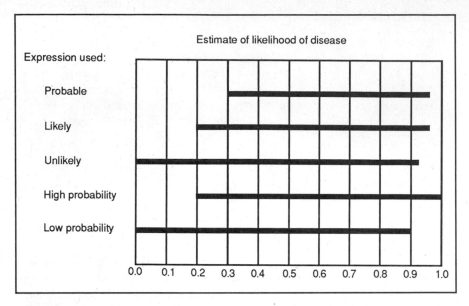

FIGURE 3.1 Probability and descriptive terms. Different physicians attach different meanings to the same terms. The bars show the wide variation in point probabilities assigned by individual physicians and other health-care workers when they were asked to interpret these terms. (*Source:* Reprinted by permission from Bryant, G. D., and Norman, G. R. Expressions of probability: Words and numbers. *The New England Journal of Medicine,* 302; 411, 1980.)

gamblers are deciding whether to place bets, they will find it quite unsatisfactory to be told a given horse has a "high chance" of winning. They will demand to know the odds.

The **odds** are simply an alternate way to express a probability. The use of probability or odds as an expression of uncertainty avoids the ambiguities inherent in common descriptive terms.

3.1.3 Overview of the Diagnostic Process

In Chapter 2, we described the hypothetico-deductive approach, a diagnostic strategy composed of successive iterations of hypothesis generation, data collection, and interpretation. We discussed how observations may evoke a hypothesis and how new information subsequently may increase or decrease our belief in that hypothesis. Here, we briefly review this process in light of a specific example. For the purpose of our discussion, we separate the diagnostic process into three stages.

The first stage involves making an initial judgment about whether a patient is likely to have a disease. After an interview and physical examination, a physician intuitively develops a belief about the likelihood of disease. This judgment may be based on previous experience or on knowledge of the medical literature. A physician's belief about the likelihood of disease usually is implicit and can be refined by explicit estimation of the probability of disease. The estimated probability, made before further information is obtained, is called the **prior probability** or **pretest probability** of disease.

> **Example 4.** Mr. Rubenstein, a 60-year-old man, complains to his physician that he has pressurelike chest pain that occurs when he walks quickly. After taking his history and examining him, his physician believes there is a high enough chance that Mr. Rubenstein has heart disease to warrant ordering an exercise stress test. In the stress test, an ECG is taken while Mr. Rubenstein exercises. Because the heart must pump more blood per stroke and must beat faster (and thus requires more oxygen) during exercise, many heart conditions are evident only when the patient is physically stressed. Mr. Rubenstein's results show abnormal changes in the ECG during exercise, a sign of heart disease.

How would the physician evaluate this patient? She would first talk to the patient about the quality, duration, and severity of his pain. Traditionally, she would then decide what to do next based on her intuition about the etiology (cause) of the chest pain. Our approach is to make this initial intuition explicit by estimating the pretest probability of disease. The clinician in this example, based on what she knows from talking with the patient, might assess the pretest or prior probability of heart disease as 0.5 (50-percent chance). We shall further explore methods to estimate pretest probability accurately in Section 3.2.

After the pretest probability of disease has been estimated, the next stage of the diagnostic process involves gathering more information, usually by performing a diagnostic test. The physician in Example 4 ordered a test to reduce her uncertainty about the diagnosis of heart disease. The positive test result supports the diagnosis of heart disease, and this reduction in uncertainty is shown in Figure 3.2(a). Although the physician in Example 4 chose the exercise stress test, there are many tests available to diagnose heart disease, and she would like to know which of these other tests she should order first. Some tests reduce uncertainty more than others do (see Figure 3.2b). The more the test reduces uncertainty, the more useful it is. In Section 3.3, we explore ways to measure how well a test reduces uncertainty, expanding the concepts of test sensitivity and specificity we introduced in Chapter 2.

Given new information provided by a test, the third step is to update the initial probability estimate. The physician in Example 4 must ask, "What is the probability of disease given the abnormal stress test?" The physician wants to know the **posttest probability,** or **posterior probability,** of disease (see Figure 3.2a). In Section 3.4, we reexamine Bayes' theorem, introduced in Chapter 2, and we discuss its use for calculating the posttest probability of disease. As we noted, to calculate posttest probability, we must know the pretest probability, as well as the sensitivity and specificity, of the test.[3]

---

[3]Note that pretest and posttest probability correspond to the concepts of prevalence and predictive value. We used the latter terms in Chapter 2 because there our discussion centered on the use of tests for screening *populations* of patients; in a population, the pretest probability of disease is simply its prevalence in that population.

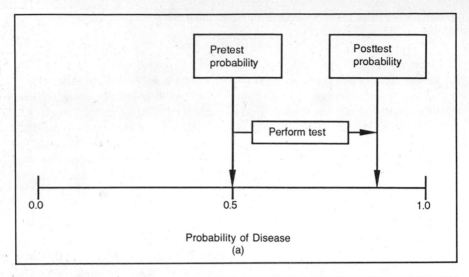

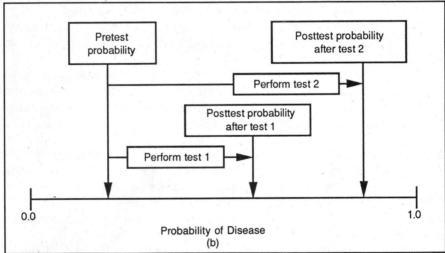

FIGURE 3.2 (a) A positive test result increases the probability of disease. (b) Test 2 reduces uncertainty about presence of disease (increases the probability of disease) more than test 1 does.

3.2 Probability Assessment: Methods to Assess Pretest Probability

In this section, we shall explore the methods physicians can use to make judgments about the probability of disease before they order tests. **Probability** is our preferred means of expressing uncertainty. In this framework, probability (p) expresses a physician's opinion about the likelihood of an event as a number between zero and one.

An event that is certain to occur has a probability of one; an event that is certain not to occur has a probability of zero.[4]

The probability of event A is written $p[A]$. The sum of the probabilities of all possible, collectively exhaustive outcomes of a chance event must be equal to one. Thus, in a coin flip,

$$p[\text{heads}] + p[\text{tails}] = 1.0.$$

The probability of event A and event B occurring together is denoted by $p[A$ and $B]$ or by $p[A,B]$.

Events A and B are considered **independent** if the occurrence of one does not influence the probability of the occurrence of the other. The probability of two independent events A and B both occurring is given by the product of the individual probabilities:

$$p[A,B] = p[A] \times p[B].$$

Thus, the probability of heads on two consecutive coin tosses is $0.5 \times 0.5 = 0.25$. (Regardless of the outcome of the first toss, the probability of heads on the second toss is 0.5.)

The probability that event A will occur given that event B is known to occur is called the **conditional probability** of event A *given* event B. This probability is denoted by $p[A|B]$, read as "the probability of A given B." Thus, a posttest probability is a conditional probability predicated on the test result or finding. For example, if 30 percent of patients with a swollen leg have a blood clot, we say the probability of a blood clot given a swollen leg is 0.3, denoted

$$p[\text{blood clot}|\text{swollen leg}] = 0.3.$$

Before the swollen leg is noted, the pretest probability is simply the prevalence of blood clots in the leg in the population from which the patient was selected, a number much smaller than 0.3.

Now that we have decided to use probability to express uncertainty, how can we estimate probability? We can do so by either subjective or objective methods; each approach has advantages and limitations.

3.2.1 Subjective Probability Assessment

Most assessments physicians make about probability are based on personal experience. The physician may do this by comparing the current problem to similar problems encountered previously, or by asking, "What was the frequency of disease in similar patients whom I have seen?"

To make these subjective assessments of probability, people rely on several discrete, often unconscious, mental processes that have been described and studied by cognitive psychologists [Tversky and Kahneman, 1974]. These processes are termed **heuristics.**

---

[4]We assume a Bayesian interpretation of probability; there are other statistical interpretations of probability.

More specifically, a cognitive heuristic is a mental process by which we learn, recall, or process information; we can think of heuristics as rules of thumb. Knowledge of heuristics is important because it helps us to understand the underpinnings of our intuitive probability assessment. Both naive and sophisticated decision makers (including physicians and statisticians) misuse heuristics and therefore make systematic, often serious, errors when estimating probability. So just as we may underestimate distance on a particularly clear day [Tversky and Kahneman, 1974], we may make mistakes in estimating probability in deceptive clinical situations.

Three heuristics have been identified as important in estimation of probability: the representativeness heuristic, the availability heuristic, and the anchoring and adjustment heuristic.

- *Representativeness.* Psychologists have shown that one way people estimate probability is to ask themselves: What is the probability that object *A* belongs to class *B*? For instance, what is the probability that this patient with a swollen leg belongs to the class of patients with blood clots? To answer, we often rely on the **representativeness** heuristic, in which probabilities are judged by the degree to which *A* is representative of, or similar to, *B*. The clinician will judge the probability of the clots (thrombosis) by the degree to which the patient with a swollen leg resembles the clinician's mental image of patients with a blood clot. If the patient has all the classical findings (signs and symptoms) associated with a blood clot, the physician judges that the patient is highly likely to have thrombosis. Difficulties occur with the use of this heuristic if the disease is rare (very low prior probability, or prevalence); if the clinician's previous experience with the disease is atypical, thus giving an incorrect mental representation; or if the patient's clinical profile is atypical.

- *Availability.* Our estimate of the probability of an event is influenced by the ease with which similar events are remembered. Events more easily remembered are judged more probable; this is the **availability** heuristic, and it is often misleading. We remember dramatic, atypical, or emotion-laden events more easily, and therefore are likely to overestimate their probability. A physician who had cared for a patient who had a swollen leg and then died from a blood clot would vividly remember thrombosis as a cause of a swollen leg. She would remember other causes of swollen legs less easily, and she would tend to overestimate the probability of a blood clot in patients with a swollen leg.

- *Anchoring and adjustment.* Another common heuristic used to judge probability is **anchoring and adjustment.** A clinician makes an initial probability estimate (the *anchor*), and then adjusts the estimate based on further information. For instance, the physician in Example 4 makes an initial estimate of the probability of heart disease as 0.5. If she then learns that all the patient's brothers had died of heart disease, the physician should raise her estimate, because the patient's strong family history of heart disease increases the probability that he has heart disease, a fact she could ascertain from the literature. The usual mistake is to adjust the initial estimate (the anchor) insufficiently in light of the new information. Instead of raising her estimate of prior probability to, say, 0.8, the physician might adjust to only 0.6.

The heuristics often introduce error into our judgments about prior probability. Errors in our initial estimates of probabilities will be reflected in the posterior probabilities, even if we use quantitative methods to derive the posterior probabilities. An understanding of heuristics is thus important for medical decision making. The clinician can avoid some of these difficulties by using published research results to estimate probabilities.

3.2.2 Objective Probability Estimates

Published research results can serve as a guide for more objective estimates of probabilities. The prevalence of disease in the population or in a subgroup of the population, or *clinical prediction rules,* can be used to estimate the probability of disease.

As we discussed in Chapter 2, the **prevalence** is the frequency of an event in a population; it is a useful starting point for estimating probability. For example, if you wanted to estimate the probability of prostate cancer in a 50-year-old man, the prevalence of prostate cancer in men of that age (5 to 14 percent) would be a useful anchor point from which you could increase or decrease the probability depending on your findings. Estimates of disease prevalence in a defined population often are available in the medical literature.

Symptoms or signs such as having a palpable prostate nodule can be used to place patients into a **clinical subgroup** in which the probability of disease is known. In patients referred to a urologist for evaluation of a prostate nodule, the prevalence of cancer is about 50 percent. This approach may be limited by difficulty in placing a patient in the correct clinically defined subgroup, especially if the criteria for classifying patients are ill defined. A recent trend has been to develop guidelines, known as clinical prediction rules, to help physicians assign patients to well-defined subgroups in which the probability of disease is known.

Clinical prediction rules are developed from systematic study of patients with a particular diagnostic problem; they define how combinations of clinical findings can be used to estimate probability. The symptoms or signs that make an independent contribution to the probability that a patient has a disease are identified, and are assigned numerical weights based on statistical analysis of the finding's contribution. The result is a list of symptoms and signs for an individual patient, each with a corresponding numerical contribution to a total score. The total score places a patient in a subgroup with a known probability of disease.

Example 5. Ms. Martin, a 65-year-old woman who recently had a heart attack, has an abnormal heart rhythm (arrhythmia), is in poor medical condition, and is about to undergo surgery.

What is the probability that Ms. Martin will suffer a cardiac complication? A clinical prediction rule has been developed to assess this risk [Goldman et al., 1977]. Table 3.1 shows a list of clinical findings and the corresponding diagnostic weights. The diagnostic weights for each of the patient's clinical findings are added to obtain

TABLE 3.1 Diagnostic Weights for Assessing Risk of Cardiac Complications from Cardiac Surgery

Clinical Finding	Diagnostic Weight
Evidence of congestive heart failure	+11
Recent documented heart attack	+10
Arrhythmia on most recent EKG	+7
> 5 PVCs/minute	+7
Age > 70 years	+5
Emergency surgery	+4
Abdominal or thoracic surgery	+3
Evidence of valvular aortic stenosis	+3
Poor medical condition	+3

PVC: premature ventricular contraction.
Source: Goldman, L., et al. Multifactorial index of cardiac risk in noncardiac surgical procedures. Reprinted, by permission of *The New England Journal of Medicine,* 297;848, 1977.

the total score. The total score places the patient in a group with a defined probability of cardiac complications, as shown in Table 3.2. Ms. Martin receives a score of 20; thus, the physician can estimate that the patient has an 11-percent chance of developing a severe cardiac complication.

Objective estimates of pretest probability are subject to error because of **bias** in the studies on which the estimates are based. For instance, published prevalences may not directly apply to a particular patient. A clinical illustration is that most clinicians thought that a patient found to have microscopic evidence of blood in the urine (microhematuria) should undergo extensive tests, because initial studies had shown that a high proportion of such patients had cancer or other serious diseases. The tests involve some risk, discomfort, and expense to the patient. Nonetheless, the approach of ordering tests for any patient with microhematuria was widely practiced for some years. Later evidence, however, suggested that the probability of serious disease in asymptomatic patients with only microscopic evidence of blood was actually very low [Mohr et al., 1986]. Before the second study was published, many patients may have undergone unnecessary tests, at considerable financial and personal cost.

What explains the discrepancy in the two estimates of disease prevalence? The initial studies that showed a high prevalence of disease in patients with microhematuria were performed on patients referred to urologists, who are specialists. The primary-care physician refers patients whom he suspects have a disease in the specialist's sphere of expertise. Because of this initial screening by primary-care physicians, the specialists seldom see patients with clinical findings that imply a low probability of disease. Thus, the prevalence of disease in the patient population in a specialist's practice often is much higher than that in a primary-care practice; studies performed with the former patients therefore almost always overestimate disease probabilities. This is an example of **selection bias.** Selection bias is common because most published studies are performed using patients referred to specialists. Thus, you may need

TABLE 3.2 Clinical Prediction Rule for Diagnostic Weights in Table 3.1

Total Score	Prevalence of Fatal Cardiac Complications (%)	Prevalence of Life-Threatening Cardiac Complications (%)
0–5	0.2	0.7
6–12	2.0	5.0
13–25	2.0	11.0
26 or greater	56.0	22.0

Source: Goldman, L., et al. Multifactorial index of cardiac risk in noncardiac surgical procedures. Reprinted, by permission of *The New England of Medicine,* 297;848, 1977.

to adjust published estimates before you use them to estimate pretest probability in other clinical settings.

We now can use the techniques we have discussed to illustrate how the physician in Example 4 might estimate the pretest probability of heart disease in her patient, Mr. Rubenstein, who has pressurelike chest pain. We begin by using the objective data that are available. The prevalence of heart disease in 60-year-old men could be used as a starting point. In this case, however, we can obtain a more refined estimate by placing the patient in a clinical *subgroup* in which the prevalence of disease is known. The prevalence in a clinical subgroup, such as in men with symptoms typical of heart disease, will predict the pretest probability more accurately than would the prevalence of heart disease in a group that is heterogeneous with respect to symptoms, such as the population at large. Assume that large studies have shown the prevalence of heart disease in men with typical symptoms to be about 0.9; this prevalence is useful as an initial estimate that can be adjusted based on information specific to the patient: Although the prevalence of heart disease in men with typical symptoms is quite high, some patients with a suggestive history do not have heart disease.

The physician might use subjective methods to adjust her estimate further based on other specific information about the patient. For example, she might adjust her initial estimate of 0.9 upward to 0.95 or higher based on information about family history of heart disease. She should be careful, however, to avoid the mistakes that can occur when using heuristics to make subjective probability estimates. In particular, she should be aware of the tendency to stay too close to the initial estimate when adjusting for additional information. By combining subjective and objective methods for assessing pretest probability, she can arrive at a reasonable estimate of the pretest probability of heart disease.

In this section, we summarized subjective and objective methods to determine the pretest probability, and we learned how to adjust the pretest probability after assessing the probability of disease in the specific subpopulation of which the patient is representative. The next step in the diagnostic process is to gather further information, usually in the form of formal diagnostic tests (laboratory tests, X-ray studies, and the like). To help you to understand this step more clearly, we shall discuss in the next two sections how to measure the accuracy of tests and how to use probability to interpret the results of the tests.

3.3 Measurement of the Operating Characteristics of Diagnostic Tests

The first challenge in assessing any test is to determine criteria for deciding whether a result is normal or abnormal. In this section, we present the issues you need to consider in making such a determination.

3.3.1 Classification of Test Results as Abnormal

Most biological measurements in a population of healthy people are continuous variables that assume different values for different individuals. The distribution of values often is approximated by the normal (Gaussian, or bell-shaped) distribution curve (Figure 3.3). Thus, 95 percent of the population will fall within two standard deviations of the mean. About 2.5 percent of the population will be more than two standard deviations from the mean at each end of the distribution. The distribution of values in individuals who are ill may be normally distributed as well. The two distributions usually overlap (see Figure 3.3).

How is a test result classified as abnormal? Most clinical laboratories report an *upper limit of normal,* which usually is defined as two standard deviations above the mean. Thus, a test result greater than two standard deviations above the mean is reported as abnormal (or positive); a test result below that cutoff is reported as normal (or negative). As an example, if the mean cholesterol concentration in the blood is 220 mg/dl, a clinical laboratory might choose as the upper limit of normal 280 mg/dl because this value is two standard deviations above the mean. Note that a

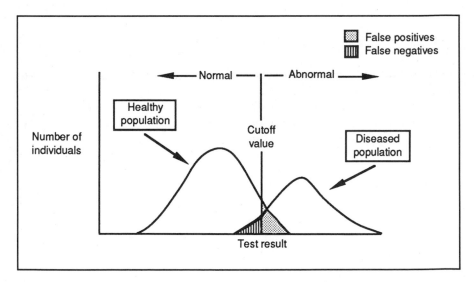

FIGURE 3.3 Distribution of test results in healthy and diseased individuals. Varying the cutoff across the continuous range of possible values will change the relative proportions of false positives and false negatives for the two populations.

cutoff that is based on an arbitrary statistical criterion may not have biological significance.

An ideal test would have no values at which the distribution of diseased and nondiseased patients overlaps. That is, if the cutoff value were set appropriately, the test would be normal in all healthy individuals, and abnormal in all individuals with disease. Few tests meet this standard. If a test result is defined as abnormal by the statistical criterion, 2.5 percent of healthy individuals will have an abnormal test. If there is an overlap in the distribution of test results in healthy and diseased individuals, some diseased patients will have a normal test (see Figure 3.3). You should be familiar with the terms used to denote these groups:

- **True positives (TP)** are positive test results obtained for patients in whom the disease is present (the test result correctly classifies the patient as having the disease).
- **True negatives (TN)** are negative test results obtained for patients in whom the disease is absent (the test result correctly classifies the patient as not having the disease).
- **False positives (FP)** are positive test results obtained for patients in whom the disease is absent (the test result incorrectly classifies the patient as having the disease).
- **False negatives (FN)** are negative test results obtained for patients in whom the disease is present (the test result incorrectly classifies the patient as not having the disease).

Figure 3.3 shows that varying the cutoff point (moving the vertical line in the figure) for an abnormal test will change the relative proportions of these groups. As the cutoff is moved further up from the mean of the normal values, the number of false negatives increases, and the number of false positives decreases.

Once we have chosen a cutoff point, we can conveniently summarize test performance—the ability to discriminate disease from nondisease—in a 2 × 2 **contingency table,** as shown in Table 3.3. The table summarizes the number of patients in each group—TP, FP, TN, and FN. Note that the sum of the first column is the total number of diseased patients, TP + FN. The sum of the second column is the total number of nondiseased patients, FP + TN. The sum of the first row, TP + FP, is the total number of patients with a positive test result. Likewise, FN + TN gives the total number of patients with a negative test result.

TABLE 3.3 A 2 × 2 Contingency Table for Test Results*

Results of Test	Disease		Total
	Present	Absent	
Positive Result	TP	FP	TP + FP
Negative Result	FN	TN	FN + TN
	TP + FN	FP + TN	

*TP: true positive; TN: true negative; FP: false positive; FN: false negative.

A perfect test would have no FN or FP results. Erroneous test results do occur however, and the 2 × 2 contingency table can be used to define the measures of test performance that reflect these errors.

3.3.2 Measures of Test Performance

Measures of test performance are of two types: measures of agreement between tests, or *measures of concordance,* and measures of disagreement, or *measures of discordance.* Two types of *concordant* test results occur in the 2 × 2 table in Table 3.3: TPs and TNs. The relative frequency of these results forms the basis of the measures of concordance. These correspond to the notions of the sensitivity and specificity of a test, which we introduced in Chapter 2. We shall define each measure in terms of the 2 × 2 table, and in terms of conditional probabilities.

The **true-positive rate (TPR)** or **sensitivity** is the likelihood that a diseased patient has a positive test. In conditional-probability notation, sensitivity is expressed as the probability of a positive test given that disease is present:

p[positive test|disease].

Another way to think of the TPR is as a ratio. The likelihood that a diseased patient has a positive test is given by the ratio of diseased patients with a positive test to all diseased patients:

$$TPR = \frac{\text{number of diseased patients with positive test}}{\text{total number of diseased patients}}.$$

We can determine these numbers for our example from the 2 × 2 table (Table 3.3). The number of diseased patients with a positive test is TP. The total number of diseased patients is the sum of the first column, TP + FN. So,

$$TPR = \frac{TP}{TP + FN}.$$

The **true-negative rate (TNR)** or **specificity,** is the likelihood that a nondiseased patient has a negative test result. In terms of conditional probability, specificity is the probability of a negative test given that disease is absent:

p[negative test|no disease].

Viewed as a ratio, the TNR is the number of nondiseased patients with a negative test, divided by the total number of nondiseased patients:

$$TNR = \frac{\text{number of nondiseased patients with negative test}}{\text{total number of nondiseased patients}}.$$

From the 2 × 2 table (Table 3.3),

$$TNR = \frac{TN}{TN + FP}.$$

The measures of discordance—the false-positive rate and false-negative rate—are defined similarly. The **false-negative rate (FNR)** is the likelihood that a diseased patient has a negative test result. As a ratio,

$$FNR = \frac{\text{number of diseased patients with negative test}}{\text{total number of diseased patients}} = \frac{FN}{FN + TP}.$$

The **false-positive rate (FPR)** is the likelihood that a nondiseased patient has a positive test result:

$$FPR = \frac{\text{number of nondiseased patients with positive test}}{\text{total number of nondiseased patients}} = \frac{FP}{FP + TN}.$$

Example 6. Consider again the problem of screening blood donors for the antibody to HIV. In actual practice, the test currently used to screen blood donors for HIV antibody is an enzyme-linked immunosorbent assay (ELISA). To measure the performance of the ELISA, the test is performed on 400 patients; the hypothetical results are shown in the 2 × 2 table in Table 3.4.[5]

To determine test performance, we calculate the TPR (sensitivity) and TNR (specificity) of the ELISA antibody test. The TPR, as defined previously, is

$$\frac{TP}{TP + FN} = \frac{98}{98 + 2} = 0.98.$$

Thus, the likelihood that a patient with the antibody will have a positive test is 0.98. If the test were performed on 100 patients who truly had antibody, we would expect two of the patients to receive incorrect, negative results, a false-negative rate of 2 percent. (You should convince yourself that the sum of TPR and FNR by definition must be equal to one: TPR + FNR = 1.)

TABLE 3.4 A 2 × 2 Contingency Table for HIV Antibody ELISA*

ELISA Test Result	Antibody		Total
	Present	Absent	
Positive	98	3	101
Negative	2	297	299
	100	300	400

*ELISA: enzyme-linked immunosorbent assay

---

[5]This example assumes that we have a perfect method (different from ELISA) for determining the presence or absence of antibody. We discuss the notion of *gold-standard tests* in Section 3.3.4.

The TNR is

$$\frac{TN}{TN + FP} = \frac{297}{297 + 3} = 0.99.$$

The likelihood that a patient without antibody will have a negative test is 0.99. Therefore, if the ELISA test were performed on 100 individuals who had not been exposed to AIDS, it would be negative in 99, and incorrectly positive in 1. (Convince yourself that the sum of TNR and FPR also must be equal to one: TNR + FPR = 1.)

3.3.3 Implications of Sensitivity and Specificity: How to Choose Among Tests

It may be clear to you already that the calculated values of sensitivity and specificity for a continuous-valued test are dependent on the particular cutoff value chosen to distinguish normal and abnormal results. In Figure 3.3, note that increasing the cutoff level (moving it to the right) would significantly decrease the number of false-positive tests, but it also would increase the number of false-negative tests. Thus, the test would have become *more* specific but *less* sensitive. Similarly, a lower cutoff value would increase the false positives and decrease the false negatives, thereby increasing sensitivity while decreasing specificity. Whenever a decision is made about what cutoff to use in calling a test abnormal, there is an inherent philosophic decision being made about whether it is better to tolerate false negatives (missed cases of abnormality) or false positives (normal people inappropriately classified as abnormal). The choice of cutoff depends on the disease in question and on the purpose of testing. If the disease is very serious and if life-saving therapy is available, then we should try to minimize the number of false-negative results. On the other hand, if the disease is not very serious and the therapy is dangerous, we should set the cutoff value so as to minimize false-positive results.

We stress the point that sensitivity and specificity are characteristics not of a test per se, but rather of the test *and* a criterion for when to call that test's results abnormal. Varying the cutoff in Figure 3.3 has no effect on the test itself (the way it is performed, or the specific values for any particular patient); instead, it trades off specificity for sensitivity. Thus, the best way to characterize a test is by the range of values of sensitivity and specificity that it can take on over a range of possible cutoffs. The typical way to show this relationship is to plot the test's sensitivity against 1 minus specificity (that is, the true-positive rate against the false-positive rate) as the cutoff is varied and the two test characteristics are traded off against each other (Figure 3.4). The resulting curve, known as a **receiver operating characteristic (ROC) curve,** was originally described by researchers investigating methods of electromagnetic-signal detection and later applied to the field of psychology [Swets, 1973; Peterson and Birdsall, 1953]. Any given point along an ROC curve for a test corresponds to the test sensitivity and specificity for a given threshold of "abnormality."

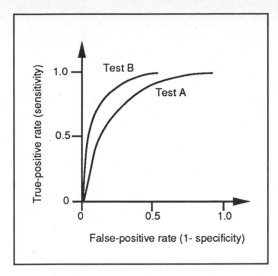

FIGURE 3.4 Receiver operating characteristic (ROC) curves for two hypothetical tests. Test B is better (has greater discriminating power) than test A is because its curve is higher (for example, the false-positive rate for test B is lower than the false-positive rate for test A is at any value of true-positive rate). The better test may not always be preferred in clinical practice, however (see text).

Similar curves can be drawn for *any* test used to associate observed clinical data with specific diseases or disease categories. For example, a radiologist who looks at 100 chest X-ray films of patients with possible pneumonias generally will misclassify some percentage of them [Komaroff, 1979]. A sensitivity and specificity for his interpretations could thus be calculated. If he looks at the same 100 films a second time, he may not classify all the films the same way that he did the first time. Thus, another sensitivity and specificity could be calculated. If he were to read the same 100 films many times and a false-positive and false-negative rate were calculated after each set of readings, an ROC curve could be plotted to correspond to his readings of the films.

Suppose a new test were introduced to compete with the current way of screening for the presence of a disease. For example, suppose a new radiologic procedure for assessing the presence or absence of pneumonia became available. This new test could be assessed for tradeoffs in sensitivity and specificity, and an ROC curve could be drawn. As is shown in Figure 3.4, a test is better than a competing test (that is, it has greater discriminating power) if its ROC curve lies above the inferior test. In other words, test B is better than test A when its specificity $(1 - \text{FPR})$ is greater than test A's specificity for any level of sensitivity (and when its sensitivity is greater than test A's sensitivity for any level of specificity).

ROC curves are important in understanding issues of test selection and data interpretation. However, physicians should not necessarily always choose the test with the best ROC curve. Issues of cost, risk, discomfort, and delay also are important in choosing what data to collect and which tests to perform. When you must choose among several available tests, you should select the test with the highest sensitivity and specificity, *provided* other factors, such as cost and risk to the patient, are equal. The higher the sensitivity and specificity of a test, the more the test will reduce uncertainty about probability of disease.

3.3.4 Design of Studies of Test Performance

In Section 3.3.2, we discussed measures of test performance—the test's ability to discriminate disease from nondisease. When we classify a test result as TP, TN, FP, or FN, we assume that we know with certainty whether a patient is diseased or healthy. Thus, the validity of any test's results must be measured against some gold standard— against a test that reveals the patient's true disease state, such as a biopsy of diseased tissue, or a surgical operation. A **gold-standard test** is a procedure that is used to define unequivocally the presence or absence of disease. The test whose discrimination is being measured is called the **index test.** The gold-standard test usually is more expensive, riskier, or more difficult to perform than is the index test (otherwise, the less precise test would not be used at all).

The performance of the index test is measured in a small, select group of patients enrolled in a study. We are more interested, however, in how the test performs in the broader group of patients in which it will be used in actual practice. The test may perform differently in the two groups, so we make the following distinction: The **study population** comprises those patients (usually a subset of the clinically relevant population) in whom test discrimination is measured and reported; the **clinically relevant population** comprises those patients in whom a test typically is used.

3.3.5 Bias in the Measurement of Test Characteristics

We mentioned earlier the problem of *selection bias.* Published estimates of disease prevalence (derived from a study population) may differ from the prevalence in the clinically relevant population because diseased patients are more likely to be included in studies than are nondiseased patients. Similarly, published values of sensitivity and specificity are derived from study populations that may differ from the clinically relevant populations in terms of average level of health and disease prevalence. These differences may affect test performance so the reported values may not apply to many patients in whom a test is used in clinical practice.

> **Example 7.** In the early 1970s, a blood test, the carcinoembryonic antigen (CEA), was developed and touted as a screening test for colon cancer. Reports of early investigations indicated the test had a high sensitivity and specificity. Subsequent work, however, proved the CEA to be completely valueless as a screening blood test for colon cancer. Screening tests are used in unselected populations, and the differences between the study and clinically relevant populations were partly responsible for the original miscalculations of the CEA's TPR and TNR [Ransahoff and Feinstein, 1978].

The experience with CEA has been repeated with numerous tests. Early measures of test discrimination are overly optimistic and subsequent test performance is disappointing. Problems arise when the TPR and TNR, as measured in the study population, do not apply to the clinically relevant population. These problems usually are the result of bias in the design of the initial studies, notably spectrum bias, test-referral bias, or test-interpretation bias.

Spectrum bias occurs when the study population includes only individuals with advanced disease (the "sickest of the sick") and healthy volunteers, as is often the case when a test is first being developed. Advanced disease may be easier to detect than is early disease. For example, it is easier to detect cancer when it has spread throughout the body (metastasized) than when it is localized to a small portion of the colon. The clinically relevant population will contain more cases of early disease that are more likely to be missed by the index test (FNs), compared to the study population. Thus, the study population will have an artifactually low FNR, which produces an artifactually high TPR (TPR = 1 − FNR). In addition, healthy volunteers are less likely than are actual patients to have other diseases that may cause false-positive results;[6] the study population will have an artificially low FPR, and therefore the specificity will be overestimated (TNR = 1 − FPR). Inaccuracies in early estimates of the TPR and TNR of the CEA were partly due to spectrum bias.

Test-referral bias occurs when a positive index test is a criterion for ordering the gold-standard test. In clinical practice, patients with negative index tests are less likely to undergo the gold-standard test than are patients with positive tests. In other words, the study population, comprising individuals with positive index-test results, has a higher percentage of patients with disease than does the clinically relevant population. Therefore, patients with TN and FN test results will be underrepresented in the study population. The result is overestimation of the TPR and underestimation of the TNR in the study population.

Test-interpretation bias develops when the interpretation of the index test affects that of the gold-standard test, or vice versa. This bias causes an artificial concordance between the tests (the results are more likely to be the same) and spuriously increases measures of concordance—the sensitivity and specificity—in the study population. (Remember, the relative frequencies of TPs and TNs are the basis for measures of concordance.)

To counter these three biases, you may need to adjust the TPR and TNR when they are applied to a new population. All the biases result in a TPR that is higher in the study population than it is in the clinically relevant population. Thus, if you suspect bias, you should adjust the TPR (sensitivity) downward when you apply it to a new population.

Adjustment of the TNR (specificity) depends on which type of bias is present. Spectrum bias and test-interpretation bias result in a TNR that is *higher* in the study population than it will be in the clinically relevant population. Thus, if these biases are present, you should adjust the specificity downward when you apply it to a new population. Test-referral bias, on the other hand, produces a measured specificity in the study population that is *lower* than it will be in the clinically relevant population.

---

[6]Volunteers are often very healthy, whereas patients in the clinically relevant population often have several diseases *in addition* to the disease for which a test is designed. These other diseases may cause false-positive test results. For example, patients with benign (rather than malignant) enlargement of their prostate glands are more likely than are healthy volunteers to have false-positive elevated levels of a blood enzyme called acid phosphatase. The level of this enzyme often is elevated in patients with prostate cancer, and its measurement has been used to help confirm that diagnosis.

If you suspect test-referral bias, you should adjust the specificity upward when you apply it to a new population.

This section has dealt with the second step in the diagnostic process, acquisition of further information with diagnostic tests. We have learned how to characterize the performance of a test with the sensitivity (TPR) and specificity (TNR). These measures reveal the probability of a test result given the true state of the patient. But this probability is not the answer to the clinically relevant question posed in the opening example: Given a positive test, what is the probability of disease? To answer this question, we must learn methods to calculate the posttest probability of disease.

3.4 Posttest Probability: Bayes' Theorem and Predictive Value

The third stage of the diagnostic process (see Figure 3.2a) is to adjust our probability estimate to take account of the new information gained from diagnostic tests by calculating the posttest probability.

3.4.1 Predictive Value of a Test

In Chapter 2, we presented a formula for calculating the positive predictive value of a test (PV+) based on the sensitivity, specificity, and prevalence of the disease:

$$PV+ = \frac{(\text{sensitivity})(\text{prevalence})}{(\text{sensitivity})(\text{prevalence}) + (1 - \text{specificity})(1 - \text{prevalence})} .$$

To gain insight into this formula, we recall that the **positive predictive value** of a test is the likelihood that a patient with a positive test has disease. Thus, PV+ also can be calculated directly from a 2 × 2 contingency table:

$$PV+ = \frac{\text{number of diseased patients with a positive test}}{\text{total number of patients with a positive test}} .$$

From the 2 × 2 contingency table in Table 3.3,

$$PV+ = \frac{TP}{TP + FP} .$$

The **negative predictive value** (PV−) is the likelihood that a patient with a negative test does not have disease:

$$PV- = \frac{\text{number of nondiseased patients with a negative test}}{\text{total number of patients with a negative test}} .$$

This value is obtained from Table 3.3 as

$$PV- = \frac{TN}{TN + FN} .$$

Example 8. We can calculate the predictive value of the ELISA test from the 2×2 table we constructed in Example 6 (Table 3.4):

$$PV+ = \frac{98}{98 + 3} = 0.97,$$

$$PV- = \frac{297}{297 + 2} = 0.99.$$

The probability that antibody is present in a patient with a positive index test (ELISA) in this study is 0.97; about 97 of 100 patients with a positive test actually will have antibody. The likelihood that a patient with a negative test index does *not* have antibody is about 0.99.

It is worth reemphasizing the difference between predictive value and sensitivity and specificity, as both are calculated from the 2×2 table and they often are confused. The sensitivity and specificity give the probability of a particular test result in a patient who has a particular disease state. The predictive value gives the probability of true disease state once the patient's test result is known.

The positive predictive value calculated from Table 3.4 is 0.97, so we expect 97 of 100 patients with positive index text actually to have antibody. Yet, in Example 1, we found that less than one of 10 patients with a positive test were expected to have antibody. What explains the discrepancy in these examples? The sensitivity and specificity in the two examples are identical. The discrepancy is due to an extremely important and often-overlooked characteristic of predictive value: The predictive value of a test depends on the prevalence of disease in the population in which the test is used. The predictive value cannot be generalized to a new population, because the prevalence of disease may differ between the two populations.

The difference in predictive value of the ELISA in Example 1 and of that in Example 6 is due to a difference in the prevalence of disease in the example populations. The prevalence of antibody was given as 0.001 in Example 1, and as 0.25 in Example 6 (the prevalence can be calculated from Table 3.4 as TP + FN divided by the total number of patients).

At last we can understand the surprising result of the opening example: Highly sensitive and specific tests may have poor predictive value if the prevalence of disease in the population is low.

3.4.2 Bayes' Theorem

As we emphasized earlier in this chapter, the notions of posttest probability and predictive value of a test are identical. In the preceding discussion, we used disease prevalence in the patient population to represent the pretest risk of disease. Once a physician begins to accumulate information about a patient, however, he revises his estimate of the probability of disease. The revised estimate (rather than the disease prevalence in the general population) becomes the pretest probability for the next test he performs. Thus, we need formulae for PV+ and PV− (posttest probability) that are more general—that are based on the pretest probability derived using all previously available information about the patient. The pertinent mathematical formulation for such calculations is known as Bayes' theorem.

Bayes' theorem is a quantitative method for calculating posttest probability using the pretest probability and the sensitivity and specificity of the test. The theorem is derived from the definition of conditional probability and the properties of probability (see the Appendix at the end of this chapter for the derivation).

Recall that a conditional probability is the probability that event A will occur, given that event B is know to occur (see Section 3.2). In general, we want to know the probability that disease is present (event A), given that the test is known to be positive (event B). We will denote the presence of disease as D, its absence as $-$D, a test result as R, and the pretest probability of disease as $p[D]$. The probability of disease, given a test result is written $p[D|R]$. Bayes' theorem is

$$p[D|R] = \frac{p[D] \times p[R|D]}{p[D] \times p[R|D] + p[-D] \times p[R|-D]}.$$

We can reformulate this general equation in terms of a positive test, $(+)$, by substituting $p[D|+]$ for $p[D|R]$, $p[+|D]$ for $p[R|D]$, $p[+|-D]$ for $p[R|-D]$, and $1 - p[D]$ for $p[-D]$. From Section 3.3, recall that $p[+|D] = $ TPR and $p[+|-D] = $ FPR. Substitution provides Bayes' theorem for a positive test:

$$p[D|+] = \frac{p[D] \times \text{TPR}}{p[D] \times \text{TPR} + (1 - p[D]) \times \text{FPR}}.$$

Recall that PV+ is an alternative notation for $p[D|+]$, and substitute prevalence for $p[D]$. Note that the formula for PV+ given in Section 3.4.1 follows directly from this derivation.

We can use a similar derivation to develop Bayes' theorem for a negative test:

$$p[D|-] = \frac{p[D] \times \text{FNR}}{p[D] \times \text{FNR} + (1 - p[D]) \times \text{TNR}}.$$

Example 9. We are now able to calculate the clinically important probability in Example 4: the posttest probability of heart disease after a positive exercise test. At the end of Section 3.2, we estimated the pretest probability of heart disease to be 0.95, based on the prevalence of heart disease in men who have typical symptoms of heart disease and on the prevalence in people with a family history of heart disease. Assume that the TPR and FPR of the exercise stress test are 0.65 and 0.20, respectively. Substituting in Bayes' formula for a positive test, we obtain the probability of heart disease given a positive test result:

$$p[D|+] = \frac{0.95 \times 0.65}{0.95 \times 0.65 + 0.05 \times 0.20} = 0.98.$$

Thus, the positive test raised the posttest probability to 0.98 from the pretest probability of 0.95. The change in probability is modest because the pretest probability was high (0.95), and because the FPR also is high (0.20). If we repeat the calculation with a pretest probability of 0.75, the posttest probability is 0.91. If we assumed the FPR of the test to be 0.05 instead of 0.20, a pretest probability of 0.95 would change to 0.996.

3.4.3 The Odds-Ratio Form of Bayes' Theorem

Although the formula for Bayes' theorem is straightforward, it is awkward for mental calculations. We can develop a more convenient form of Bayes' theorem by expressing probability as *odds* and by using a different measure of test discrimination.

Probability and odds are related as follows:

$$\text{odds} = \frac{p}{1 - p} ,$$

$$p = \frac{\text{odds}}{1 + \text{odds}} .$$

Thus, if the probability of rain is 0.75, the odds are 3:1. We should expect rain to occur three times for each time it does not occur.

The measures of test discrimination discussed earlier can be combined to give one number that characterizes the discriminatory power of a test: the **likelihood ratio (LR):**

$$\text{LR} = \frac{\text{probability of result in diseased persons}}{\text{probability of result in nondiseased persons}} .$$

We can use the likelihood ratio to characterize clinical findings (such as a swollen leg) or a test result. We describe either by two likelihood ratios, one corresponding to a positive test result (or the presence of a finding) and the other corresponding to a negative test (or absence of a finding). These are abbreviated LR+ and LR−, respectively.

$$\text{LR+} = \frac{\text{probability that test is positive in diseased persons}}{\text{probability that test is positive in nondiseased persons}}$$

$$= \frac{\text{TPR}}{\text{FPR}} .$$

In a test that discriminates well between disease and nondisease, the TPR will be high, the FPR will be low, and thus LR+ will be much greater than one. A likelihood ratio of one means the probability of a test result is the same in diseased and nondiseased individuals; the test has no value. Similarly,

$$\text{LR−} = \frac{\text{probability that test is negative in diseased persons}}{\text{probability that test is negative in nondiseased persons}}$$

$$= \frac{\text{FNR}}{\text{TNR}} .$$

A desirable test will have a very low FNR and a high TNR; therefore, the LR− will be much less than one.

A simple relationship exists between pretest odds and posttest odds:

posttest odds = pretest odds × LR,

or

$$\frac{p[D|R]}{p[-D|R]} = \frac{p[D]}{p[-D]} \times \frac{p[R|D]}{p[R|-D]} \, .$$

This is the **odds-ratio form** of Bayes' theorem.[7] It can be derived in a straight-forward fashion from the definitions of Bayes' theorem and conditional probability that we provided earlier. Thus, to obtain the posttest odds, we simply multiply the pretest odds by the likelihood ratio for the test in question.

Example 10. We can calculate the posttest probability for a positive exercise stress test in a 60-year-old man whose pretest probability is 0.75. The pretest odds are

$$\text{Odds} = \frac{p}{1-p} = \frac{0.75}{1-0.75} = \frac{0.75}{0.25} = 3, \text{ or } 3{:}1.$$

The likelihood ratio for the stress test is

$$\text{LR+} = \frac{\text{TPR}}{\text{FPR}} = \frac{0.65}{0.20} = 3.25.$$

We can calculate the posttest odds of a positive test result using the odds-ratio form of Bayes' theorem:

posttest odds = 3 × 3.25 = 9.75:1.

We can then convert the odds to a probability:

$$p = \frac{\text{odds}}{1 + \text{odds}} = \frac{9.75}{1 + 9.75} = 0.91.$$

As expected, this result agrees with our earlier answer (see the discussion of Example 9).

The odds-ratio form of Bayes' theorem allows rapid calculation, so you can determine the probability at, for example, the bedside. The likelihood ratios of many diagnostic tests are available [Sox et al., 1988]. If you know the pretest odds, you can calculate the posttest odds in one step.

3.4.4 Implications of Bayes' Theorem

In this section, we explore the implications of Bayes' theorem for test interpretation. These ideas are extremely important, yet they often are misunderstood.

---

[7]Some authors refer to this expression as the **odds-likelihood form** of Bayes' theorem.

Figure 3.5 illustrates one of the most essential concepts in this chapter: The post-test probability of disease increases as the pretest probability of disease increases. Figure 3.5(a) was produced by calculation of the posttest probability after a positive test result for all possible pretest probabilities of disease. Figure 3.5(b) was similarly derived for a negative test result.

The 45-degree lines in the two parts of Figure 3.5 denote a test in which the pretest and posttest probability are equal (likelihood ratio = 1)—a test that is useless. The curve in Figure 3.5(a) relates pretest and posttest probabilities in a test with a sensitivity and specificity of 0.9. Note that, at low pretest probabilities, the posttest probability after a positive test result is much higher than is the pretest probability. At

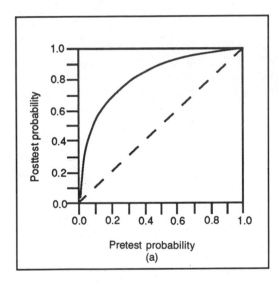

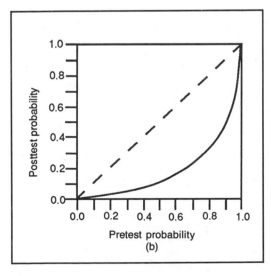

FIGURE 3.5 Relationship between pretest probability and posttest probability of disease. The dotted lines correspond to a test that has no effect on the probability of disease. Sensitivity and specificity of the test were assumed to be 0.90 for the two examples. (a) The posttest probability of disease corresponding to a *positive* test result (solid curve) was calculated with Bayes' theorem for all values of pretest probability. (b) The posttest probability of disease corresponding to a *negative* test result (solid curve) was calculated with Bayes' theorem for all values of pretest probability. (*Source:* Adapted from Sox, Jr., H. C. Probability theory in the use of diagnostic tests: Application to critical study of the literature. In Sox, Jr., H. C. (ed), *Common Diagnostic Tests: Use and Interpretation.* Philadelphia: American College of Physicians, 1987, p. 1–17. Reproduced with permission from the American College of Physicians.)

high pretest probabilities, the posttest probability is only slightly higher than the pretest probability.

Figure 3.5(b) shows the relationship between the pretest and posttest probabilities after a negative test result. At high pretest probabilities, the posttest probability after a negative test result is much lower than is the pretest probability. A negative test, however, has little effect on the posttest probability if the pretest probability is low.

This discussion emphasizes another key idea of this chapter: The interpretation of a test result depends on the pretest probability of disease. If the pretest probability is low, a positive test has a large effect, and a negative test has a small effect. If the pretest probability is high, a positive test has a small effect, and a negative test has a large effect. In other words, when the clinician is almost certain of the diagnosis prior to testing (pretest probability nearly zero or nearly one), a confirmatory test has little effect on the posterior probability (see Example 9). If the pretest probability is intermediate or if the result contradicts a strongly held clinical impression, the test result will have a large effect on the posttest probability.

Note from Figure 3.5(a) that, if the pretest probability is very low, a positive test result can raise the posttest probability into only the intermediate range. Assume that Figure 3.5(a) represents the relationship between the pretest and posttest probabilities for the exercise stress test. If the clinician believes the pretest probability of coronary-artery disease is 0.1, the posttest probability will be about 0.5. Although there has been a large change in the probability, the posttest probability is in an intermediate range, which leaves considerable uncertainty as to the diagnosis. Thus, if the pretest probability is low, it is unlikely that a positive test result will raise the probability of disease far enough for the clinician to make that diagnosis with confidence. Similarly, if pretest probability is very high, it is unlikely that a negative test result will lower the posttest probability enough to exclude a diagnosis.

Figure 3.6 illustrates another important concept: Test specificity affects primarily the interpretation of a positive test; test sensitivity affects primarily the interpretation of a negative test. In both parts (a) and (b) of Figure 3.6, the top family of curves corresponds to positive test results, and the bottom family to negative test results. Figure 3.6(a) shows the posttest probabilities for tests with varying specificities (TNR). Note that changes in the specificity produce large changes in the top family of curves (positive test results). That is, an increase in the specificity of a test markedly changes the posttest probability if the test is positive, but has relatively little effect on the posttest probability if the test is negative. Thus, if you are trying to *rule in* a diagnosis,[8] you should choose a test with high specificity. Figure 3.6(b) shows the posttest probabilities for tests with varying sensitivities. Note that changes in sensitivity produce large changes in the bottom family of curves (negative test results), but have little effect on the top family of curves. Thus, if you are trying to *rule out* a disease, you should choose a test with a high sensitivity.

---

[8]In medicine, to *rule in* a disease is to confirm that the patient *does* have the disease; to *rule out* a disease is to confirm that the patient does *not* have the disease. A doctor who strongly suspects that her patient has a bacterial infection orders a culture to *rule in* her diagnosis. Another doctor is almost certain his patient has a simple sore throat, but orders a culture to *rule out* streptococcal infection (strep throat).

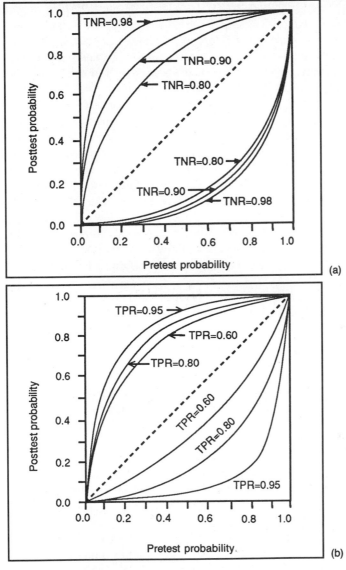

(a)

(b)

FIGURE 3.6 Effect of test sensitivity and specificity on posttest probability. Parts (a) and (b) are similar to parts (a) and (b) of Figure 3.5, except that the calculations have been repeated for several values of the sensitivity (TPR, true-positive rate) and specificity (TNR, true-negative rate) of the test. In (a), the sensitivity of the test was assumed to be 0.90, and the calculations were repeated for several values of test specificity. In (b), the specificity of the test was assumed to be 0.90, and the calculations were repeated for several values of the sensitivity of the test. In both graphs, the top family of curves corresponds to positive test results, and the bottom family of curves corresponds to negative test results. (*Source:* Adapted from Sox, Jr., H. C. Probability theory in the use of diagnostic tests: Application to critical study of the literature. In Sox, Jr., H. C. (ed), *Common Diagnostic Tests: Use and Interpretation*. Philadelphia: American College of Physicians, 1987, p. 1–17. Reproduced with permission from the American College of Physicians.)

3.4.5 Cautions in the Application of Bayes' Theorem

Bayes' theorem provides a powerful method for calculating posttest probability. You should be aware, however, of the possible errors you can make when you use it. Four common problems are inaccurate estimation of pretest probability, faulty application of test-performance measures, and violation of the assumptions of conditional independence and of mutual exclusivity.

Bayes' theorem provides a means to adjust an estimate of pretest probability to take account of new information. The accuracy of the calculated posttest probability is limited, however, by the accuracy of the estimated pretest probability. Accuracy of estimated prior probability is aided by proper use of published prevalence rates, heuristics, and clinical prediction rules, and usually can be made acceptable. In a decision analysis, as we shall see, a *range* of prior probability often is sufficient. Nonetheless, if the pretest probability assessment is unreliable, Bayes' theorem will be of little value.

A second potential mistake you can make when using Bayes' theorem is to apply published values for the test sensitivity and specificity without paying attention to the possible effects of bias in the studies in which the test performance was measured (see Section 3.3.5).

A third potential problem arises when you use Bayes' theorem to interpret a *sequence* of tests. If a patient undergoes two tests in sequence, you can use the posttest probability after the first test result, calculated with Bayes' theorem, as the pretest probability for the second test. Then, you use Bayes' theorem a second time, to calculate the posttest probability after the second test. This approach is valid, however, only if the two tests are conditionally independent. Tests for the same disease are **conditionally independent** when the probability of a particular result on the second test does not depend on the result of the first test, *given* (conditioned on) the disease state. Expressed in conditional-probability notation, for the case in which the disease is present, p[second test positive | first test positive and disease present] = p[second test positive | first test negative and disease present] = p[second test positive | disease present]. If you apply Bayes' theorem sequentially in situations in which conditional independence is violated, you will obtain inaccurate posttest probabilities.

The fourth common problem arises when you assume that all test abnormalities result from one (and only one) disease process. The Bayesian approach, as we have described it, generally presumes that the diseases under consideration are **mutually exclusive**. If they are not, Bayesian updating must be applied with great care.

We have shown how to calculate posttest probability. In the next section, we shall turn to the problem of decision making when the outcomes of a physician's actions (for example, treatments) are uncertain.

3.5 Expected-Value Decision Making

Medical decision-making problems often cannot be solved by reasoning based on pathophysiology. For example, clinicians need a method for choosing among treatments when the outcome of a treatment is unpredictable, as are the results of a surgical operation. You can use the ideas developed in the preceding sections to solve such difficult decision problems. We shall discuss two methods: the decision tree, a method for representing and comparing the expected outcomes of each decision alternative; and threshold probability, a method for deciding whether new information can change a management decision. These techniques help you to clarify the decision problem and thus to choose the alternative that is most likely to help the patient.

3.5.1 Comparing Uncertain Prospects

Like most biological events, the outcome of an individual's illness is unpredictable. How can a physician determine which course of action has the greatest chance of success?

> **Example 11.** There are two available treatments for a fatal illness. The length of a patient's life after either treatment is unpredictable, as illustrated by the frequency distribution shown in Figure 3.7 and summarized in Table 3.5. Each treatment is associated with uncertainty: Regardless of which treatment a patient receives, he will die by the end of the fourth year, but there is no way to know which year will be the patient's last. Figure 3.7 shows that survival until the fourth year is more likely with treatment B, but the patient might die in the first year with treatment B or might survive to the fourth year with treatment A.

Which of the two treatments is preferable? This example demonstrates a significant fact: A choice among treatments is a choice among gambles. How do we usually choose among gambles? More often than not, we rely on hunches or on a sixth sense. How *should* we choose among gambles? We shall propose a method for

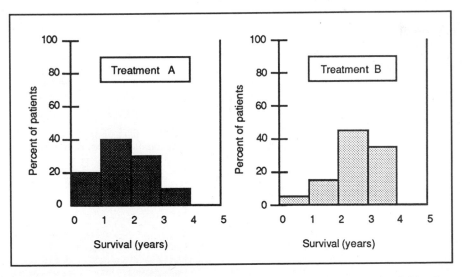

FIGURE 3.7 Survival after treatment for a fatal disease. Two treatments are available; the results of either are unpredictable.

TABLE 3.5 Distribution of Probabilities for the Two Treatments in Figure 3-7

Years after Treatment	Probability of Death	
	Treatment A	Treatment B
1	0.20	0.05
2	0.40	0.15
3	0.30	0.45
4	0.10	0.35

choosing called **expected-value decision making:** Characterize each gamble by one number and use that number to compare the gambles.[9] In Example 11, treatment A and treatment B are both gambles with respect to duration of life after treatment. We want to assign a measure (or number) to each treatment that summarizes the outcomes such that we can decide which treatment is preferable.

The ideal criterion for choosing a gamble should be a number that reflects preferences for the outcomes of the gamble. **Utility** is the name given to a measure of preference that has a desirable property for decision making: The gamble with the highest utility should be preferred. We shall only touch briefly on utility, but you can pursue this topic and the details of decision analysis in other textbooks (see the Suggested Readings at the end of this chapter).[10] We shall use the average duration of life after treatment (survival) as a criterion for choosing among treatments, but you should remember that this is an oversimplified model, used here for discussion only. Later, we shall consider other factors, such as the quality of life.

Because we cannot be sure of the duration of survival in any given patient, we characterize a treatment by the mean survival (average length of life) that would be observed in a large number of patients after they were given the treatment. The first step we take in calculating the mean survival for a treatment is to divide the population receiving the treatment into groups of patients who have similar survival rates. Then, we multiply the survival time in each group[11] by the fraction of the total population in that group. Finally, we sum these products over all possible survival values.

We can perform this calculation for the treatments in Example 11. Mean survival for treatment A = $(0.2 \times 1.0) + (0.4 \times 2.0) + (0.3 \times 3.0) + (0.1 \times 4.0) = 2.3$ years. Mean survival for treatment B = $(0.05 \times 1.0) + (0.15 \times 2.0) + (0.45 \times 3.0) + (0.35 \times 4.0) = 3.1$ years.

Survival after a treatment is under the control of chance. Treatment A is a gamble characterized by an average survival equal to 2.3 years. Treatment B is a gamble characterized by an average survival of 3.1 years. If length of life is our criterion for choosing, we should select treatment B.

---

[9]Expected-value decision making had been used in many fields before it was first applied to medicine.
[10]A more general term for expected-value decision making is *expected-utility* decision making. Because a full treatment of utility is beyond the scope of this chapter, we have chosen to use the term *expected value.*
[11]For this simple example, death during an interval is assumed to occur at the end of the year.

3.5.2 Representing Choices with Decision Trees

The choice between treatments A and B is represented diagrammatically in Figure 3.8. Events that are under the control of chance can be represented by a **chance node.** By convention, a chance node is shown as a circle from which several lines emanate. Each line represents one of the possible outcomes. Associated with each line is the probability of the outcome occurring. For a single patient, only one outcome can occur. Some physicians object to using probability for just this reason: "You cannot rely on population data because each patient is an individual." In fact, we often *must* use the frequency of the outcomes of many patients experiencing the same event to inform our opinion about what might happen to an individual. From these frequencies, we can make patient-specific adjustments and thus estimate the probability of each outcome at a chance node.

A chance node can represent more than just an event governed by chance. The outcome of a chance event, unknowable for the individual, can be represented by the **expected value** of the chance node. The concept of expected value is very important and is easy to understand. We can calculate the mean survival that would be expected if many patients had the treatment depicted by the chance node in Figure 3.8. This average length of life is called the *expected survival,* or, more generally, the *expected value at the chance node.* We calculate expected value at a chance node by the process just described: We multiply the survival value associated with each possible outcome by the probability that it will occur. We then sum the product of probability times survival over all outcomes. Thus, if several hundred patients were assigned to receive either treatment A or treatment B, the expected survival would be 2.3 years for treatment A and 3.1 years for treatment B.

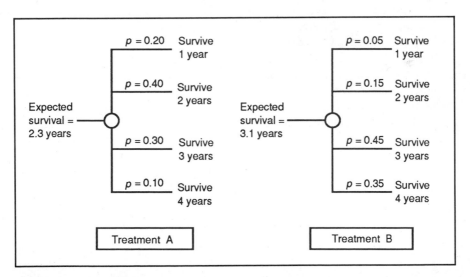

FIGURE 3.8 A chance-node representation of survival after the two treatments in Figure 3.7. The probabilities are multiplied by the corresponding years of survival and summed to obtain the total expected survival.

We have just described the basis of expected-value decision making. The term *expected value* is used to characterize a chance event, such as the outcome of a treatment. If the outcomes of a treatment are measured in units of duration of survival, sense of well-being,[12] or dollars, then the treatment is characterized by, respectively, expected duration of survival, expected sense of well-being, or expected monetary cost it will confer on the patient.

To use expected-value decision making, we follow this strategy when there are treatment choices with uncertain outcomes: (1) calculate the expected value of each decision alternative, then (2) pick the alternative with the highest expected value.

3.5.3 Performing a Decision Analysis

We shall clarify the concepts of expected-value decision making by discussing an example. First, note that there are four steps in decision analysis:

1. Create a decision tree; this step is the most difficult step, because it requires formulating the decision problem, assigning probabilities, and measuring outcomes
2. Calculate the expected value of each decision alternative
3. Choose the decision alternative with the highest expected value
4. Use sensitivity analysis to test the conclusions of the analysis

Many health professionals balk when they first learn about the technique of decision analysis, because they recognize the opportunity for error in assigning values to both the probabilities and the utilities in a decision tree. They reason that the technique encourages decision making based on small differences in expected values that are estimates at best. The defense against this concern, which also has been recognized by decision analysts, is a technique known as sensitivity analysis. We shall discuss this important fourth step in a decision analysis in Section 3.5.4.

The first step in a decision analysis is to create a **decision tree** that represents the decision problem. Consider the following clinical problem.

Example 12. The patient is Mr. Danby, a 66-year-old man who has been crippled with arthritis of both knees severe enough that he can get about the house with the aid of two canes but otherwise must use a wheelchair. His other major health problem is emphysema, a disease in which the lungs lose their ability to exchange oxygen and carbon dioxide between blood and air, which in turn causes shortness of breath (dyspnea). He is able to breathe comfortably when he is in a wheelchair, but the effort of walking with canes makes him breathe heavily and feel uncomfortable. Several years ago, he seriously considered knee-replacement surgery but decided against it, largely because his internist told him that there was a serious risk that he would not survive the operation because of his lung disease. Recently, however, Mr. Danby's wife had a stroke that left her partially paralyzed; she now requires a degree of assistance that the patient cannot supply given his present

---

[12]If utility is used as a measure of preference for the outcomes, the process is termed *expected-utility decision making.*

state of mobility. He tells his doctor that he is reconsidering knee-replacement surgery.

Mr. Danby's internist is familiar with decision analysis. She recognizes that this problem is filled with uncertainty: Mr. Danby's ability to survive the operation is in doubt, and the surgery sometimes does not restore mobility to the degree required by this patient. Furthermore, there is a small chance that the prosthesis (the artificial knee) will become infected, and Mr. Danby then would have to undergo a second risky operation to remove it. After removal of the prosthesis, Mr. Danby would never again be able to walk, even with canes. The possible survival outcomes of knee replacement include death from the first procedure, and death from a second procedure if the prosthesis becomes infected (which we shall assume occurs in the immediate postoperative period, if it occurs at all). Possible functional outcomes include recovery of full mobility, or continued, and unchanged, poor mobility. Should Mr. Danby choose to undergo knee-replacement surgery, or should he accept the status quo?

Using the conventions of decision analysis, the internist sketches the decision tree shown in Figure 3.9. She uses a square box to denote a **decision node,** and lines emanating from a decision node to represent an action that could be taken.

According to the methods of expected-value decision making, the internist first must assign a probability to each branch of each chance node. To accomplish this task, the internist asks several orthopedic surgeons for their estimate of the chance of recovering full function after surgery (p[full recovery] = 0.60) and the chance of developing infection in the prosthetic joint (p[infection] = 0.05). She uses her subjective estimate of the probability that the patient will die during or immediately after knee surgery (p[operative death] = 0.05).

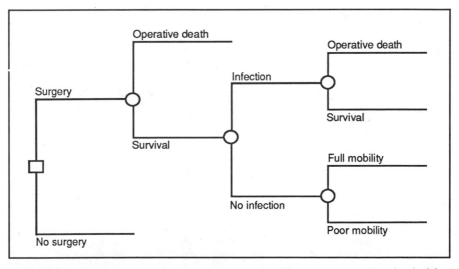

FIGURE 3.9 Decision tree for knee-replacement surgery. The square represents the decision node (whether to have surgery). The circles represent chance nodes.

TABLE 3.6 Outcomes for Example 12

Survival (years)	Functional Status	Years of Full Function Equivalent to Outcome
10	Full mobility (successful surgery)	10
10	Poor mobility (status quo or unsuccessful surgery)	6
10	Wheelchair-bound (the outcome if a second surgery is necessary)	3
0	Death	0

Next, she must assign a value to each outcome. To accomplish this task, she first lists the outcomes. As you can see from Table 3.6, the outcomes differ in two dimensions: length of life (survival) and quality of life (functional status). To characterize each outcome accurately, the internist must develop a measure that takes into account these two dimensions. Simply using duration of survival is inadequate, because Mr. Danby values 5 years of good health more than he values 5 years of poor health. The internist can account for this tradeoff factor by converting outcomes with two dimensions into outcomes with a single dimension: duration of survival in good health. The resulting measure is called a **quality-adjusted life-year (QALY)**.[13] She can convert years in poor health into years in good health by asking Mr. Danby to indicate the shortest period in good health (full mobility) that he would accept in return for his full expected lifetime (10 years) in a state of poor health (status quo). Thus, she asks Mr. Danby, "Many people say they would be willing to accept a shorter life in excellent health in preference to a longer life with significant disability. In your case, how many years with normal mobility do you feel is equivalent in value to ten years in your current state of disability?" She asks him this question for each outcome. The patient's responses are shown in the third column of Table 3.6. The patient decides that 10 years of limited mobility are equivalent to 6 years of normal mobility, whereas 10 years of wheelchair confinement are equivalent to only 3 years of full function. Figure 3.10 shows the final decision tree—complete with probability estimates and utility values for each outcome.[14]

The second task the internist must undertake is to calculate the expected value, in healthy years, of surgery and of no surgery. She calculates the expected value at each chance node, moving from right (the tips of the tree) to left (the root of the tree). Let us consider, for example, the expected value at the chance node represent-

---

[13]Quality-adjusted life-years commonly are used as measures of utility in medical decision analysis and in health-policy analysis (see, for example, the discussion of cost-effectiveness analysis in Chapter 19).

[14]In a more sophisticated decision analysis, the physician also would adjust the utility values of outcomes that require surgery, to account for the pain and inconvenience associated with surgery and rehabilitation.

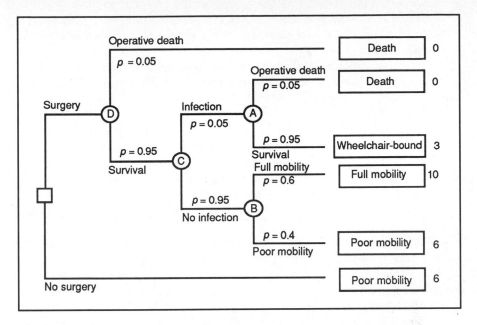

FIGURE 3.10 Decision tree for knee-replacement surgery. Probabilities have been assigned to each branch of each chance node. The patient's valuations of outcomes (measured in years of perfect mobility) are assigned to the tips of each branch of the tree.

ing the outcome of surgery to remove an infected prosthesis (node *A* in Figure 3.10). The calculation requires three steps:

1. Calculate the expected value of operative death after surgery to remove an infected prosthesis. Multiply the probability of operative death (0.05) by the QALY of the outcome—death (0 years): $0.05 \times 0 = 0$ (QALY).
2. Calculate the expected value of surviving surgery to remove an infected knee prosthesis. Multiply the probability of surviving the operation (0.95) by the number of healthy years equivalent to 10 years of being wheelchair bound (3 years): $0.95 \times 3 = 2.85$ (QALY).
3. Add the expected values calculated in step 1 (0 QALY) and step 2 (2.85 QALY) to obtain the expected value of developing an infected prosthesis: $0 + 2.85 = 2.85$ (QALY).

Similarly, the expected value at chance node *B* is calculated: $(0.6 \times 10) + (0.4 \times 6) = 8.4$ (QALY). To obtain the expected value of surviving knee-replacement surgery (node *C*), we proceed as follows:

1. Multiply the expected value of an infected prosthesis (already calculated as 2.85 QALY) by the probability that the prosthesis will become infected (0.05): $2.85 \times 0.05 = 0.143$ (QALY).
2. Multiply the expected value of never developing an infected prosthesis (already calculated as 8.4 QALY) by the probability that the prosthesis will not become infected (0.95): $8.4 \times 0.95 = 7.98$ (QALY).

3. Add the expected values calculated in step 1 (0.143 QALY) and step 2 (7.98 QALY) to get the expected value of surviving knee replacement surgery: 0.143 + 7.98 = 8.123 (QALY).

This process, called **averaging out at chance nodes,** is performed for node *D* as well, working back to the root of the tree, until the expected value of surgery has been calculated. The outcome of the analysis is as follows. For surgery, Mr. Danby's average life expectancy, measured in years of normal mobility, is 7.7. What does this value mean? It does not mean that Mr. Danby is guaranteed 7.7 years of mobile life by accepting surgery. One look at the decision tree will show that some patients die in surgery, some develop infection, and some do not gain any improvement in mobility after surgery. So, an individual patient has no guarantees. However, if the physician had 100 similar patients who underwent the surgery, the *average* number of mobile years would be 7.7. We can understand what this value means for Mr. Danby only by examining the alternative, no surgery.

In the analysis for no surgery, the average length of life, measured in years of normal mobility, is 6.0, which Mr. Danby considered equivalent to 10 years of continued poor mobility. Not all patients will experience this outcome; some will live longer than, and some will live less than, 10 years with poor mobility. The average length of life, however, expressed in years of normal mobility, will be 6. Because 6.0 is less than 7.7, *on average* the surgery will provide an outcome with higher value to the patient. Thus, the internist recommends performing the surgery.

The key insight of expected-value decision making should be clear from this example: Decision analysis cannot guarantee a good outcome. Decision analysis can help the physician to identify the treatment that will give the best results when averaged over many similar patients. The decision analysis is tailored to a specific patient in that both the utility functions and the probability estimates are adjusted to the individual. Nonetheless, the results of the analysis represent the outcomes that would occur *on the average* in a population of similar patients. Given the unpredictable outcome in an individual, the best choice for the individual is the alternative that gives the best result on the average in similar patients.

3.5.4 Performing Sensitivity Analysis

Sensitivity analysis is a test of the validity of the conclusions of an analysis over a wide range of assumptions about the probabilities and the values, or utilities. The probability of an outcome at a chance node may be the best estimate that is available, but there often is a wide range of "reasonable" probabilities that a physician could use with nearly equal confidence. We use sensitivity analysis to answer this question: Do my conclusions regarding the preferred choice change when the probability and outcome estimates are assigned values that lie within a reasonable range?

The knee-replacement decision in Example 12 illustrates the power of sensitivity analysis. If the conclusions of the analysis (surgery is preferable to no surgery) remain the same despite a wide range of assumed values for the probabilities and outcome measures, the recommendation is trustworthy. Figures 3.11 and 3.12 show the expected survival in healthy years with surgery and without surgery under varying

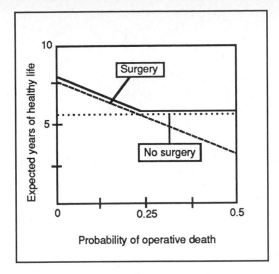

FIGURE 3.11 Sensitivity analysis of the effect of operative mortality on length of healthy life (Example 12). As the probability of operative death increases, the relative values of *surgery* versus *no surgery* change. The point at which the two lines cross represents the probability of operative death at which *no surgery* becomes preferable. The solid line represents the preferred option at a given probability.

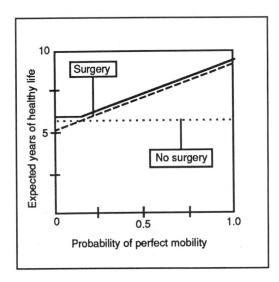

FIGURE 3.12 Sensitivity analysis of the effect of a successful operative result on length of healthy life (Example 12). As the probability of a successful surgical result increases, the relative values of *surgery* versus *no surgery* change. The point at which the two lines cross represents the probability of a successful result at which *surgery* becomes preferable. The solid line represents the preferred option at a given probability.

assumptions of the probability of operative death and the probability of attaining perfect mobility, respectively. Each point (value) on these lines represents one calculation of expected survival using the tree in Figure 3.9. Figure 3.11 shows that expected survival is higher with surgery over a wide range of operative mortality rates. Expected survival is lower with surgery, however, when the operative mortality rate exceeds 25 percent. Figure 3.12 shows the effect of the probability that the operation will lead to perfect mobility. The expected survival, in healthy years, is higher for surgery as long as the probability of perfect mobility exceeds 20 percent, a much lower figure than is expected from previous experience with the operation. (In Example 12, the consulting orthopedic surgeons estimated the chance of full recovery at 60 percent.)

Thus, the internist can proceed with confidence to recommend surgery. Mr. Danby cannot be sure of a good outcome, but he has valid reasons for thinking that he is more likely to do well with surgery than he is without surgery.

Another way to state the conclusions of a sensitivity analysis is to indicate the range of probabilities over which the conclusions apply. The point at which the two lines in Figure 3.11 cross is the probability of operative death at which the two treatment options have the same expected survival. If expected survival is to be the basis for choosing treatment, the internist (and the patient) should be indifferent between surgery and no surgery when the probability of operative death is 25 percent.[15] When the probability is lower, they should select surgery. When it is higher, they should select no surgery. The probability at which the preferred treatment changes (the point at which the lines for the alternate choices cross) is called the *treatment-threshold probability*. This concept is useful for decision making, as we shall see in the next section.

3.6 Treat, Test, or Do Nothing?

The physician who faces a diagnostic challenge and has evaluated one of a patient's symptoms must then choose among the following actions:
1. Do nothing further (neither perform additional tests nor treat the patient)
2. Obtain additional diagnostic information (test) before choosing whether to treat
3. Treat without waiting for more information

This decision is simplified when the physician knows the patient's true state; testing is unnecessary, and the doctor needs only to assess the tradeoffs among therapeutic options (as in Example 12). Learning the patient's true state, however, usually requires costly, time-consuming, and often risky or uncomfortable diagnostic procedures. Therefore, physicians often are willing to consider treating a patient even when they are not absolutely certain about a patient's true state. There are risks in this course: The physician may withhold treatment from a person who has the disease of concern, or he may administer treatment to someone who does not have the disease yet may suffer undesirable side effects of treatment.

Deciding among treating, testing, and doing nothing sounds difficult, but you have already learned all the principles you need to solve this kind of problem. There are three steps:
1. Determine the treatment-threshold probability of disease
2. Determine the pretest probability of disease
3. Decide whether a test result could affect your decision to treat

The **treatment-threshold probability** of disease is the probability of disease at which you should be indifferent between treating and not treating. Below the treatment threshold, you should not treat. Above the treatment threshold, you should treat (Figure 3.13).

---

[15]An operative mortality rate of 25 percent may seem high; however, this value is correct when one uses QALY as the basis for choosing treatment. A decision maker performing a more sophisticated analysis could use a utility function that reflects the degree of the patient's aversion to risking death. See the Suggested Readings for discussions of utility functions.

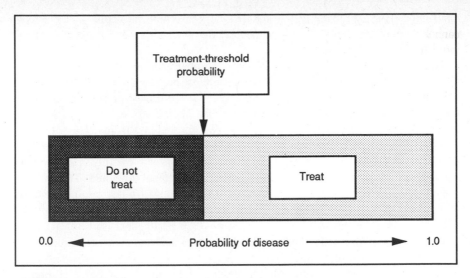

FIGURE 3.13 Depiction of the treatment-threshold probability.

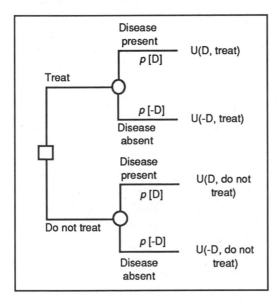

FIGURE 3.14 Decision tree with which to calculate the treatment-threshold probability of disease. By setting the utilities of the *treat* and *do not treat* choices to be equal, we can compute the probability at which the physician should be indifferent to the choice. Recall that $p[-D] = 1 - p[D]$.

Whether to treat when the diagnosis is not certain is a problem you can solve with a decision tree, such as is shown in Figure 3.14. You can use this tree to learn the treatment-threshold probability of disease by leaving the probability of disease as an unknown, setting the expected value of surgery equal to the expected value for medical (that is, nonsurgical, such as drugs or physical therapy) treatment, and solving for the probability of disease. (In this example, surgery corresponds to the "treat" branch of the tree in Figure 3.14, and nonsurgical intervention corresponds to the "do not treat" branch.) Because you are indifferent between medical treatment and surgery at this probability, it is the treatment-threshold probability. This determination completes step 1. In practice, people often determine the treatment threshold intuitively rather than analytically.

Once you know the pretest probability, you know what to do in the absence of further information about the patient. If the pretest probability is below the treatment threshold, you should not treat the patient. If the pretest probability is above the threshold, you should treat the patient. This determination completes step 2.

One of the guiding principles of medical decision making is this: Do not order a test unless it could change your management of the patient. In our framework for decision making, this principle means that you should order a test only if a test result could cause the probability of disease to cross the treatment threshold. Thus, if the pretest probability is above the treatment threshold, a negative test result must lead to a posttest probability that is below the threshold. Conversely, if the pretest probability is below the threshold probability, a positive result must lead to a posttest probability that is above the threshold. In either case, the test result would alter your decision whether to treat the patient.

To decide whether a test could alter management, we simply use Bayes' theorem. Calculate the posttest probability following the test result (positive or negative) that would move the probability of disease toward the treatment threshold. If the pretest probability is above the treatment threshold, calculate the probability of disease if the test result is negative. If the pretest probability is below the treatment threshold, calculate the probability of disease if the test result is positive. This calculation completes step 3.

Example 13. You are a pulmonary medicine specialist. You suspect that a patient of yours has a pulmonary embolus (blood clot lodged in the vessels of the lungs). The usual approach is to do a radionuclide lung scan, a test in which tiny radioactive particles are injected into a vein. These particles flow into the small vessels of the lung. A scanning device detects the radiation from the particles. The particles cannot go to a part of the lungs that is supplied by a vessel that is blocked by a blood clot. Unfortunately, there are other causes of blank areas in the scan, so that you cannot be sure that a blood clot is present when there is a blank area. Thus, if the scan is abnormal (shows a blank area), you must perform a definitive test to confirm the diagnosis. Such a test is a pulmonary arteriogram, in which radiopaque dye is injected into the arteries in the lung, and an X-ray image is obtained. The procedure involves some risk, discomfort, and substantial cost to the patient. If the scan is negative, you do no further tests and do not treat the patient.

To decide whether this strategy is correct, you take the following steps:
1. Determine the treatment-threshold probability of pulmonary embolus
2. Estimate the pretest probability of pulmonary embolus
3. Decide whether a test result could affect your decision to treat for an embolus

First, assume you decide that the treatment threshold should be 0.10 in this patient. What does it mean to have a treatment-threshold probability equal to 0.10? If you could obtain no further information, you would treat for pulmonary embolus if the pretest probability was above 0.10 (that is, if you believed that there was greater than a one-in-10 chance that the patient had an embolus), and would withhold treatment if the pretest probability was below 0.10. A decision to treat when the pretest probability is at the treatment threshold means that you are willing to treat nine patients without pulmonary embolus to be sure of treating one patient who has pulmonary embolus. This approach may be reasonable, because someone with pulmonary embolus (which could be fatal) benefits a great deal from treatment, whereas there is only a relatively small danger in treating someone who does not have pulmonary embolus. This reasoning completes step 1.

You estimate the pretest probability of pulmonary embolus to be 0.05. Because the pretest probability is lower than the treatment threshold, you should do nothing unless a positive lung-scan result could raise the probability of pulmonary embolus to above 0.10. This reasoning completes step 2.

To decide whether a test result could affect your decision to treat, you must decide whether a positive lung-scan result would raise the probability of pulmonary embolism to more than 0.10, the treatment threshold. You review the literature and learn the true-positive rate of the lung scan is 0.75, and the false-positive rate is 0.25.

A negative lung-scan result will move the probability of disease away from the treatment threshold and will be of no help in deciding what to do. A positive result will move the probability of disease toward the treatment threshold and could alter your management decision if the posttest probability was above the treatment threshold. You therefore use Bayes' theorem to calculate the posttest probability of disease if the lung-scan result is positive:

$$p[D|+] = \frac{p[D] \times \text{TPR}}{p[D] \times \text{TPR} + (1 - p[D]) \times \text{FPR}}$$

$$= \frac{0.05 \times 0.75}{0.05 \times 0.75 + 0.95 \times 0.25} = 0.14.$$

Because the posttest probability of pulmonary embolus is higher than the treatment threshold, a positive lung-scan result would change your management of the patient, and you should order the lung scan. This result completes step 3.

This example is especially useful for two reasons. First, it demonstrates one method for making decisions. Second, it shows how the concepts that were introduced in this chapter all fit together in a clinical example of medical decision making.

3.7 The Role of Probability and Decision Analysis in Medicine

After reading this chapter, you still may be wondering how probability and decision analysis might be integrated smoothly into medical practice. An understanding of probability and measures of test performance will prevent any number of misadventures. In Example 1, we discussed a hypothetical test that, on casual inspection, appeared to be an accurate way to screen blood donors for previous exposure to the AIDS virus. Our quantitative analysis, however, revealed that the test results were misleading more often than they were helpful, because the prevalence of HIV antibodies in the clinically relevant population was low.[16]

The need for knowledgeable interpretation of test results is widespread. In the mid-1980s the federal government instituted a policy of drug screening for civil employees in "sensitive" positions, and many companies now screen employees for drug use. These policies have reached lofty levels indeed: In 1986, President Reagan submitted his urine to be tested for drugs. If the drug test used by an employer had a sensitivity and specificity of 0.95, and if 10 percent of the employees actually used drugs, one-third of the positive tests would be false positives. (Had this been the case at the White House, the president, if he tested positive, would have had a 33 percent chance of a false-positive result.) An understanding of these issues should be of great interest to the public; health-professionals should be prepared to answer the questions of their patients.

Although we should interpret every kind of test result accurately, decision analysis has a more selective role in medicine. Not all decisions clinicians make require decision analysis. Some decisions depend on physiologic principles or deductive reasoning. Other decisions involve little uncertainty. Nonetheless, many decisions must be based on imperfect data, and they will have outcomes that cannot be known with certainty at the time the decision is made. Decision analysis provides a technique for managing these situations.

A full decision analysis often strikes health-care professionals as an unwieldy approach to problems that are difficult but must be solved very quickly. This misgiving is legitimate. Some decisions warrant a full decision analysis, but many do not. A complete decision analysis, including a review of the literature to obtain necessary probabilities and an assessment of the patient's utilities, can be time consuming.

For many problems, simply drawing a tree that denotes the possible outcomes explicitly will clarify the question enough to allow you to make a decision. When time is limited, even a "quick and dirty" analysis may be helpful. By using expert clinicians' subjective probability estimates and guessing what the patient's utilities might be, you can perform an analysis quickly and learn which probabilities and utilities are the important determinants of the decision. You can spend time in the library or at the bedside getting accurate estimates of these important probabilities and utilities. You can solve other decision problems once, and then use the decision trees as often as the need arises, by changing the variables to fit the particular patient. Journals such as *Medical Decision Making* contain decision analyses that you can adapt to fit a specific patient. Once you have performed the first quantitative analysis, you often find that some of the variables in the tree have an insignificant effect on the decision. Therefore, in any further analyses regarding that problem, you will not need to give those variables much attention.

---

[16]We emphasize that the sensitivity and specificity of currently available HIV tests are significantly better than the sensitivity and specificity used in our example. In practice, all positive tests are confirmed by a highly specific second test; the use of a sequence of tests markedly attenuates the problem of false-positive test results [Burke et al., 1988].

Health-care professionals sometimes are reluctant to use decision analysis because the analysis may depend on probabilities that must be estimated, such as the pretest probability. A thoughtful decision maker will be concerned that the estimate may be in error, particularly because the information needed to make the estimate often is difficult to obtain from the medical literature. We argue, however, that uncertainty in the clinical data is a problem for *any* decision-making method and that the effect of this uncertainty is made explicit with decision analysis. The means to this end is sensitivity analysis: We can examine any variable to see whether its value is critical to the final recommended decision. Thus, we can determine, for example, whether a change in pretest probability from 0.6 to 0.8 makes a difference in the final decision. In so doing, we often discover that it is necessary to estimate only a range of probabilities for a particular variable, rather than a precise value. In some cases, we need to know only whether the variable is above or below the treatment threshold. Thus, with a sensitivity analysis, we can decide whether uncertainty about a particular variable should concern us.

Computers have not been mentioned in this chapter, but they can simplify many aspects of decision analysis (see Chapter 15). MEDLINE and other bibliographic retrieval systems (see Chapter 14) make it easier to obtain published estimates of disease prevalence and test performance. Computer programs for performing statistical analyses can be used on data collected by hospital information systems. Decision-analysis software, available for personal computers, can help physicians to structure decision trees, to calculate expected values, and to perform sensitivity analyses. Eventually, clinical consultation systems that evaluate patient data and provide diagnostic or treatment recommendations will be widely available.

Medical decision making often involves uncertainty for the physician and risk for the patient. Most health-care professionals would welcome an opportunity to reduce the uncertainty in their decisions. There are important, difficult medical problems for which decision analysis can offer that opportunity.

Appendix: Derivation of Bayes' Theorem

Bayes' theorem is derived as follows. We denote the conditional probability of disease, D, given a test result, R, by $p[D|R]$. The prior (pretest) probability of D is $p[D]$. The formal definition of conditional probability is

$$p[D|R] = \frac{p[R,D]}{p[R]} . \tag{3.1}$$

The probability of a test result ($p[R]$) is the sum of its probability in diseased patients and its probability in nondiseased patients:

$$p[R] = p[R,D] + p[R,-D].$$

Substituting in (3.1), we obtain

$$p[D|R] = \frac{p[R,D]}{p[R,D] + p[R,-D]} . \tag{3.2}$$

Again, from the definition of conditional probability,

$$p[R|D] = \frac{p[R,D]}{p[D]} \text{ and } p[R|-D] = \frac{p[R,-D]}{p[-D]} .$$

These expressions can be rearranged

$$p[R,D] = p[D] \times p[R|D], \tag{3.3}$$

$$p[R,-D] = p[-D] \times p[R|-D]. \tag{3.4}$$

Substituting (3.3) and (3.4) in (3.2), we obtain Bayes' theorem:

$$p[D|R] = \frac{p[D] \times p[R|D]}{p[D] \times p[R|D] + p[-D] \times p[R|-D]} . \tag{3.5}$$

Suggested Readings

Goldman, L., et al. Multifactorial index of cardiac risk in noncardiac surgical procedures. *New England Journal of Medicine*, 297:845, 1977.

> *This article describes the development of a clinical prediction rule used to estimate the probabilities of life-threatening complications and cardiac death in patients undergoing noncardiac surgery.*

Raiffa, H. *Decision Analysis: Introductory Lectures on Choices Under Uncertainty.* Reading, MA: Addison-Wesley, 1970.

> *This book provides an advanced, nonmedical introduction to decision analysis, utility theory, and decision trees.*

Sox, Jr., H. C. Probability theory in the use of diagnostic tests. *Annals of Internal Medicine,* 104:60, 1986.

> *This article is written for physicians; it contains a summary of the concepts of probability and test interpretation.*

Sox, Jr., H. C., Blatt, M. A., Higgins, M. C., and Marton, K. I. *Medical Decision Making.* Boston, MA: Butterworths, 1988.

> *This introductory textbook covers the subject matter of this chapter in greater detail, as well as discussing many other topics. An appendix contains the likelihood ratios of 100 common diagnostic tests.*

Tversky, A. and Kahneman, D. Judgment under uncertainty: Heuristics and biases. *Science,* 185:1124, 1974.

> *This article provides a clear and interesting discussion of the experimental evidence for the use and misuse of heuristics in situations of uncertainty.*

Weinstein, M. C. and Fineberg, H. V. *Clinical Decision Analysis.* Philadelphia, PA: W. B. Saunders, 1980.

> *This textbook provides a clinical perspective of decision analysis. It addresses in greater detail all the topics introduced in this chapter, and covers utility assessment (including quality-adjusted life-years) and cost-effectiveness analysis.*

Questions for Discussion

1. Calculate the following probabilities for a patient about to undergo CABG surgery (see Example 2).
   a. The only possible, mutually exclusive outcomes of surgery are death, relief of symptoms (angina, dyspnea), or continuation of symptoms. The probability of death is 0.02, and the probability of relief of symptoms is 0.80. What is the probability the patient will continue to have symptoms?
   b. Two known complications of heart surgery are stroke and heart attack, with probabilities of 0.02 and 0.05, respectively. The patient asks what chance he has of having *both* complications. Assume the complications are conditionally independent, and calculate your answer.
   c. The patient wants to know the probability that he will have a stroke given that he has a heart attack as a complication of his surgery. Assume that one in 500 patients has *both* complications, that the probability of heart attack is 0.05, and that the events are independent. Calculate your answer.
2. The results of a hypothetical study to measure test performance of the ELISA antibody test for HIV (see Example 1) are shown in the 2 × 2 table in Table 3.7.
   a. Calculate the sensitivity, specificity, disease prevalence, positive predictive value, and negative predictive value.
   b. Use the TPR and TNR calculated in part (a) to fill in the 2 × 2 table in Table 3.8. Calculate the disease prevalence, positive predictive value, and negative predictive value.
3. You are asked to interpret an ELISA HIV (AIDS) antibody test in an asymptomatic man whose test was positive when he volunteered to donate blood. After taking his history, you learn that he is an intravenous-drug user. You know that the overall prevalence of antibodies to the HIV virus in your community is one in 500, and that the prevalence of antibodies in intravenous-drug users is 20 times as high as in the community at large.
   a. Estimate the pretest probability that this man has HIV antibodies.
   b. The man tells you that two people with whom he shared needles subsequently died of AIDS. Which heuristic will be useful in making a subjective adjustment to the pretest probability in part (a)?
   c. Use the sensitivity and specificity that you worked out in Question 2(a) to calculate the posttest probability of the patient having HIV antibody after a positive and negative test. Assume the pretest probability is 0.10.

TABLE 3.7 A 2 × 2 Contingency Table for the Hypothetical Study in Problem 2

ELISA Test	Gold-Standard Test		Total
	Positive	Negative	
Positive	2	47	49
Negative	48	8	56
Total	50	55	105

TABLE 3.8 A 2 × 2 Contingency Table to Complete for Problem 2b

ELISA Test	Gold-Standard Test		Total
	Positive	Negative	
Positive	X	X	X
Negative	100	99,900	X
Total	X	X	

    d. If you wanted to increase the posttest probability of disease given a positive test result, would you change the TPR or TNR of the test?

4. You have a patient with cancer who has a choice between surgery or chemotherapy. If the patient chooses surgery, she has a 2-percent chance of dying from the operation (life expectancy = 0), a 50-percent chance of being cured (life expectancy = 15 years), and a 48-percent chance of not being cured (life expectancy = 1 year). If the patient chooses chemotherapy, she faces a 5-percent chance of death (life expectancy = 0), a 65-percent chance of cure (life expectancy = 15 years), and a 30-percent chance the cancer will be slowed but not cured (life expectancy = 2 years). Create a decision tree and calculate the expected value of each option in terms of life expectancy.

5. You are concerned that a patient with a sore throat may have a bacterial infection that would require antibiotic therapy (as opposed to a viral infection, for which no treatment is available). Your treatment threshold is 0.4, and based on the examination you estimate the probability of bacterial infection as 0.8. A test is available (TPR = 0.75, TNR = 0.85) that indicates the presence or absence of bacterial infection. Should you perform the test? Explain your reasoning.

6. What are the three kinds of bias that can influence measurements of test performance? Explain what each bias is, and state how you would adjust the posttest probability to compensate for it.

7. How could a computer system ease the task of performing a complex decision analysis? Look at the titles of the chapters in Part 2 of this text (applications). What role could each kind of system play in the medical-decision process?

8. When you search the medical literature to find probabilities for patients similar to one you are treating, what is the most important question to consider? How should you adjust probabilities in light of the answer to this question?

9. Why do you think physicians sometimes order tests even if the results will not affect their management of the patient? Do you think the reasons you identify are valid? Are they valid in only certain situations? Explain your answers.

10. Develop a decision tree for an important choice you must make in your personal life. What insights do you gain while you are constructing the decision tree?

4

Essential Concepts
for Medical Computing

Leslie E. Perreault and Gio Wiederhold

After reading this chapter, you should know the answers to these questions:

- How are medical data stored and manipulated in a computer?
- Why does a computer system have external memory? What are the relative advantages and disadvantages of magnetic disk, magnetic tape, and optical disc?
- How can data be entered into a computer effectively?
- How can information be displayed clearly?
- What are the functions of a computer's operating system?
- What advantages do database-management systems provide compared to programmed methods of file management?
- What are local-area networks? How can they facilitate data sharing and communication within hospitals and other health-care institutions?

4.1 An Overview of Computer Hardware and Software

Health professionals encounter computers of a variety of sizes and capabilities. In some hospitals, physicians and nurses can order drugs and laboratory tests, review test results, and record medical observations using a hospital information system that runs on a large, mainframe computer or on a network of smaller machines. Most hospitals and many outpatient clinics have a computer to help manage financial and administrative information. Many physicians in private practice have purchased personal computers to allow them to access and search the medical literature, and to help their office staff with the tasks of billing and word processing.

Computers differ in size, speed, and cost; in the number of users they can support; and in the types of applications programs they can run. On the surface, the differences among computers can be bewildering, and, as we shall discuss in Chapter 5, the selection of appropriate software and hardware is crucial to the success of a computer system. Despite external differences, however, most computers use the same basic mechanisms to store and process information. At the conceptual level, the similarities among machines greatly outweigh the differences. In this chapter, we shall discuss the central concepts related to computer hardware and software, and the use of these tools in medical computing. Our aim is to provide you with a simple overview of the most essential topics, to give you the background necessary for understanding the technical aspects of the applications discussed in later chapters. If you already have a basic understanding of computers and how they work, you may want to skim this chapter.

4.1.1 Hardware

The first computers were expensive to purchase and operate. They were space and energy consuming, and they required specially trained personnel to program, operate, and maintain them. Consequently, only very large institutions could acquire a computer. Sometimes, smaller institutions bought computer time to meet their processing needs. In the 1960s, the integration of circuits on silicon chips (ICs) resulted in dramatic increases in computing power per dollar. During the 1970s and 1980s, computer hardware became smaller, more powerful, and more reliable, while decreasing in price from 25 to 40 percent per year. The result is the enormous diversity of computers available today.

Traditionally, general-purpose computers have been classified into three types: mainframe computers, minicomputers, and microcomputers. This distinction reflects several parameters, primarily size (related to cost and power) and style of usage. **Mainframe computers** are large, multiuser machines that are operated and maintained by professional computing personnel. A mainframe might handle the information-processing needs of a large hospital. Often, mainframes are used to manage large databases and are oriented to data-processing tasks, such as billing and report generation. At the other end of the spectrum are the **microcomputers,** or **personal computers (PCs)**—small, relatively inexpensive, single-user machines.

Typically, the processors for these computers are contained entirely on one or a few chips. The speed of the processor and the size of memory determine the types of applications for which PCs can be used. **Minicomputers** are multiuser machines of moderate size and cost. Typically, they support multiple users carrying out similar or related tasks. Thus, a minicomputer might be used to automate a clinical laboratory or a small group practice.

The distinctions among classes of computers have blurred as smaller computers have become more powerful and less expensive. Physical size no longer is a valid indication of computing power. Furthermore, a host of special-purpose machines has been developed to meet specific computing needs, such as the microprocessor-based patient-monitoring systems discussed in Chapter 12, the specialized **workstations** that are used by professionals in their problem-solving and information-management tasks, and the graphics computers that are used for three-dimensional modeling of molecules and anatomical regions.

The basic **hardware** (physical equipment) and organization of most computers are similar; the most common computer **architectures** are organized according to principles expressed by John von Neumann in 1945. Figure 4.1 illustrates the configuration of a simple **von Neumann machine,** in which the computer is composed of a single processing unit (the **central processing unit,** or **CPU**) that performs computation, computer **memory** that stores programs and data that are being used actively by the CPU, and an electrical pathway called a **data bus** that transports data between CPU and memory. In addition, a computer system has devices for the input and output of data, and typically includes auxiliary data-storage devices. Architectures based on models other than von Neumann's model are possible but are still relatively uncommon. In recent years, however, researchers have gained interest in **parallel processing**—using multiple processors running in parallel to solve complex problems.

Central Processing Unit

Although complete computer systems appear to be complex, the underlying principles are simple. In fact, computer systems provide a prime example of how simple components can be combined carefully to create systems with impressive capabilities. The structuring principle is that of *hierarchical organization:* Primitive units (electronic switches) are combined to form basic units that can store letters and numbers, add digits, and compare values with one another. The basic units are assembled into **registers** capable of storing and manipulating text and large numbers. These registers in turn are assembled into the large functional units that make up a computer—the CPU and the memory.

The atomic element for all digital computers is the *binary digit* or **bit.** Each bit can assume one of two values: 0 or 1. A single bit value is stored by an electronic switch that can be set to either of two states. (Think of a light switch that can be either on or off.) These primitive units are the building blocks of computer systems.

Sequences of bits (implemented as sequences of switches) are used to represent numbers, text, and program instructions. For example, four switches can store 2^4, or 16, values. Because each unit can have a value of either 0 or 1, there are 16

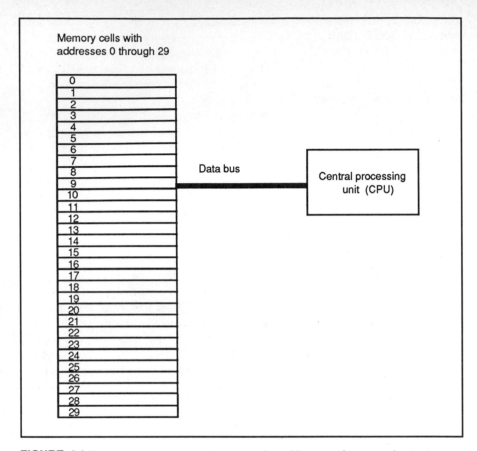

FIGURE 4.1 The von Neumann model is the basic architecture of most modern computers. The computer comprises a single central processing unit, an area for memory, and a data bus for transferring data between the two.

combinations of 4-bit values: 0000, 0001, 0010, 0011, 0100, 0101, 0110, and so on, to 1111. Thus, 4 bits can represent any decimal value from 0 to 15; for instance, the sequence 0101 is the binary (base 2) representation of the decimal number 5 ($0 \times 2^3 + 1 \times 2^2 + 0 \times 2^1 + 1 \times 2^0 = 5$). A **byte** is a sequence of 8 bits (and therefore can take on $2^8 = 256$ values).

Bits and bytes can represent not only decimal integers, but also fractional numbers, alphanumeric characters (upper- and lower-case letters, digits, and punctuation marks), and instructions to the CPU. Figure 4.2 shows the **American Standard Code for Information Interchange (ASCII),** a common scheme for representing alphanumeric characters using 7 bits. Mainframe computers manufactured by the International Business Machines Corporation (IBM) use a different internal code, the **External Binary Coded Decimal Interchange Code (EBCDIC),** which represents each character using 8 bits of information.

Characte	Binary code	Character	Binary code	Character	Binary code
blank	010 0000	@	100 0000	`	110 0000
!	010 0001	A	100 0001	a	110 0001
"	010 0010	B	100 0010	b	110 0010
#	010 0011	C	100 0011	c	110 0011
$	010 0100	D	100 0100	d	110 0100
%	010 0101	E	100 0101	e	110 0101
&	010 0110	F	100 0110	f	110 0110
'	010 0111	G	100 0111	g	110 0111
(	010 1000	H	100 1000	h	110 1000
)	010 1001	I	100 1001	i	110 1001
*	010 1010	J	100 1010	j	110 1010
+	010 1011	K	100 1011	k	110 1011
,	010 1100	L	100 1100	l	110 1100
-	010 1101	M	100 1101	m	110 1101
.	010 1110	N	100 1110	n	110 1110
/	010 1111	O	100 1111	o	110 1111
0	011 0000	P	101 0000	p	111 0000
1	011 0001	Q	101 0001	q	111 0001
2	011 0010	R	101 0010	r	111 0010
3	011 0011	S	101 0011	s	111 0011
4	011 0100	T	101 0100	t	111 0100
5	011 0101	U	101 0101	u	111 0101
6	011 0110	V	101 0110	v	111 0110
7	011 0111	W	101 0111	w	111 0111
8	011 1000	X	101 1000	x	111 1000
9	011 1001	Y	101 1001	y	111 1001
:	011 1010	Z	101 1010	z	111 1010
;	011 1011	[	101 1011	{	111 1011
<	011 1100	\	101 1100			111 1100
=	011 1101	]	101 1101	}	111 1101
>	011 1110	^	101 1110	~	111 1110
?	011 1111	_	101 1111	null	111 1111

FIGURE 4.2 The American Standard Code for Information Interchange (ASCII) is a standard scheme for representing alphanumeric characters using 7 bits. The upper- and lowercase alphabet, the decimal digits, and common punctuation characters are shown here with their ASCII representations.

The CPU works on data it retrieves from memory, placing them in working registers. By manipulating the contents of its registers, the CPU performs the mathematical and logical functions that are basic to information processing: addition, subtraction, and logical comparison ("is greater than," "is equal to," "is less than"). In addition to registers that perform computation, the CPU also has registers that it uses to store instructions (a **computer program** is a set of such instructions) and to control processing. In essence, a computer is an instruction follower; it fetches an instruction from memory, then executes the instruction, which usually is an operation that requires the retrieval, manipulation, and storage of data into memory or registers. The processor performs a simple loop, fetching and executing each instruction of a program in sequence. Some instructions can direct the processor to begin fetching instructions from a different point in the program. Such a transfer of control provides flexibility in program execution.

Memory

The computer's working memory stores the programs and data currently being used by the CPU. Working memory has two parts: **read-only memory (ROM)** and **random-access memory (RAM).** ROM, or fixed memory, is permanent and unchanging. It can be read, but it cannot be altered or erased. It is used to store programs that do not change and that must be available at all times. One such program is the **bootstrap,** a set of initial instructions that is executed each time the computer is started (often called *booting* the machine). ROM also is used to store programs that must run quickly—for example, the graphics programs that run the Macintosh interface.

RAM, or **variable memory** (sometimes called **core memory**) can be both read and written into. It is used to store the intermediate results of computation and the programs and data that are in current use. RAM is much larger than ROM. Its size is one of the primary parameters used to describe a computer. For example, we speak of a 640K personal computer. A 640K memory can store 655,360 bytes of information. (The symbol K, for kilobytes, represents 2^{10} or 1024 bytes.)

A sequence of bits that can be accessed as a unit is called a **word.** The word size is a function of the computer's design, but it typically is an even number of bytes. Thus, computers with a word size of 8 or 16 bits are common; fast microcomputers today are 32-bit machines that can access 4 bytes of information at a time. The CPU accesses each word in memory by specifying its location, or **address.**

The computer's working memory is relatively expensive; therefore, it is limited in size—the amount of information we would like to save and process in many medical applications exceeds greatly the memory capacity of most computers. The contents of working memory are not retained when a program finishes running.

Auxiliary Storage

Programs and data typically must persist over long periods so that they can be reused. They are stored in the less expensive **auxiliary memory** provided by peripheral storage devices, and they are loaded into working memory when needed. Conceptually, auxiliary memory can be divided into two types. **Active storage** is used to store data with long-term validity that may need to be retrieved with little delay (in a few seconds or less)—for example, the medical record of a patient who currently is being treated within the hospital. **Archival storage** is used to store data for documentary or legal purposes.

Currently, **magnetic disks** are the most common medium for active storage (Figure 4.3). Each magnetic disk is a round, flat plate of material that can accept and store magnetic charge. The disk spins beneath a read-write head, much like a phonograph record spinning beneath a needle. As the disk spins, data are stored by the read-write

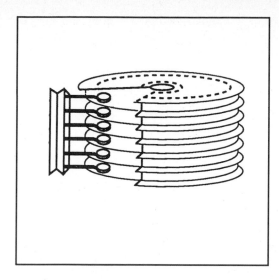

FIGURE 4.3 A cutaway illustration of a disk unit with six platters (10 magnetic surfaces). Physical movement of the read-write heads interleaved between the platters allows data to be stored and retrieved from the concentric tracks of each disk's surface.

head, which places a sequence of magnetic charges on the disk's surface along circular tracks. Similarly, the read-write head reads data by detecting the presence or absence of charge along the tracks. A disk unit consists of one or more disks—either fixed or removable, a drive system to rotate the disk, a movable read-write head to access the data, and a mechanism to position the read-write head over the surface. Disks can be either *hard* or *floppy.* Floppy disks are inexpensive relative to hard disks and frequently are used for information archival and transport through the mail.

Magnetic disks are less expensive than main memory is, but data retrieval is much slower. Whereas the CPU can quickly access any data element in RAM by addressing the memory location directly, it must access externally stored data in two time-consuming steps. First, it must mechanically position the read-write head over the track that stores the data. Then it must search through that track sequentially, following the track as the disk rotates. Once the read-write head has been positioned correctly, blocks of data can be transferred rapidly. Whereas data in working memory can be accessed in microseconds, access times for data stored on disk can reach several tenths of a second.

The most common medium for archival storage is **magnetic tape,** a ribbon of plastic covered with material that can accept and store magnetic charge. Like the disk drive, a tape drive has a read-write head that places or detects magnetic charges along the tracks of the tape. Magnetic tape currently is the least expensive means for storing information. Retrieval of archived data, however, is slow. A computer operator must locate the tape and physically mount it on a tape drive, a procedure that can produce delays of minutes or hours. The tape then must be scanned linearly from the beginning until the information of interest is located.

Optical storage is a relatively new technology that is growing rapidly in popularity. The main advantage of using **optical discs** is that huge numbers of data can be stored compactly—the high wavelength of light permits a much higher density of data-carrying spots on the surface than can be achieved by magnetic techniques. **Compact-**

disc read-only memory (CD-ROM) stores prerecorded information, which is read by a finely focused semiconductor laser that detects reflections from the disc. Such compact discs have become a common medium for recording and playing music. The first medical applications of optical-disc technology have been the storage of large bodies of reference material. For example, portions of the MEDLINE database of medical literature (see Chapter 14) now are available on CD-ROM.

Although rewritable discs are becoming available, most optical-recording devices are limited to recording information once, and reading it as often as desired, but never changing it subsequently. Such discs are called WORMs (write once, read many [times]). Data are recorded on an optical disc by a finely focused laser that marks the plastic or metallic surface. When the data are to be read, the laser is set to a lower intensity level and the absence or presence of a reflection indicates whether the surface was deformed previously. In the future, optical storage may become attractive for applications such as distributing text literature, storing permanent medical records, and archiving digitized X-ray images (see Chapter 11). A major obstacle to overcome is the lack of a fast and economical means for indexing and searching the huge amount of information that can be stored.

The choice of storage medium has a major effect on the performance and cost of a computer system. Data that are needed rapidly must be kept in more expensive active storage (for example, hard disks), whereas less time-critical data can be archived on less expensive media (for example, tapes or floppy disks). Because data often have to be shared, the designer must consider who will be expected to read the data, and how the data will be read. Devices that can handle standard tapes or floppy disks allow sharing of data among sites—the data are copied and are physically transported to a destination with a compatible drive. The compatibility of storage devices is less important when computers are linked into communication networks that can transport data from site to site by wire, rather than by physical movement of a storage medium (see Section 4.3).

Input Devices

Data entry remains the most costly and awkward aspect of medical data processing. Some data can be acquired automatically; for example, many laboratory instruments provide electronic signals that can be transmitted to computers directly. Furthermore, redundant data entry can be minimized if data are shared among computers over networks or across direct interfaces. For example, if a clinic's computer can acquire data from a laboratory computer directly, clinic personnel will not have to reenter into the computer-based medical record the information displayed on printed reports of laboratory-test results. Currently, however, a relatively small fraction of the data in the medical record is acquired automatically. Most data are entered manually by data-entry clerks or other health-care personnel.

The most common instrument for data entry is the typewriter-style **keyboard** of a **video display terminal (VDT).** Typically, as characters are typed by an operator on the keyboard, they are echoed back for viewing on the **display monitor,** an output device that is logically distinct from the keyboard. A highlighted or blinking element, called the **cursor,** indicates the current position on the screen. Although clerical personnel often are comfortable with this mode of data entry, many health professionals lack typing skills and are not motivated to learn them. Thus, systems developers have experimented with a variety of alternate input devices that minimize or eliminate the need to type.

With a **light pen,** a user can *select* an item displayed on the screen by pointing at the item and depressing a button on the pen. With a **touch screen,** a user can select items simply by pointing; when the user's finger touches the screen, it identifies a position in the grid that crosses the screen, thus pinpointing the item of interest. Alternatively, a **mouse** or a **joystick** can be used to position the cursor on the screen. The user moves the mouse on a flat surface, or on a special mouse pad, until the cursor is located over the item of interest, then selects the item by depressing a button on the mouse. Similarly, the movement of a joystick controls the movements of the cursor.

Often, these input devices are used in conjunction with **menus,** which are lists of items from which users can make selections (Figure 4.4). Thus, users can enter

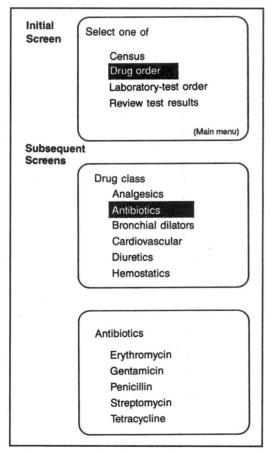

FIGURE 4.4 Initial and subsequent screens of a menu-driven order-entry system. The highlighted entry indicates which item was selected (with a mouse, light pen, or finger) to display the subsequent screen.

data simply by choosing relevant items, rather than by typing characters. By listing all (and only) valid options, menus also facilitate coding and can enforce the use of a standardized vocabulary. Typically, menus are arranged hierarchically; for example, to order a treatment, a physician might first select *drug order* from a menu of alternative actions, then the appropriate *drug class* from a submenu, and finally an individual *drug name* from the next screen menu. If there are still many alternatives, the drug list might be divided further; for example, the drugs might be grouped alphabetically by name. Menu selection is efficient; an experienced user can select several screens per second. Typing the drug name is more time consuming and carries the risk of misspelling.

Graphical display monitors provide system developers with more flexibility to create interesting and attractive interfaces to their programs. For example, the input screens of the ONCOCIN system, a decision-support system that provides physicians with advice on cancer-treatment protocols (see Chapter 15), look just like the paper flowcharts physicians have used for years. Physicians enter patient data into the database directly by using a mouse to select values from menus (Figure 4.5). In addition, graphical displays have opened the door for entirely new forms of data entry; for instance, images are used to record information, and **icons** are used to specify

Lymphoma Flow Sheet									
Mass / X-ray									
Disease Activity									
WBC x 1000	8.6	9.0	1.5	4.2	9.0	3.6	5.6	3.3	?
% polys	71	93	29						
% lymphs			43						
PCV	29.6	32.9	33.7	33.6	30.9	31.6	28.4	29.3	
Hemoglobin	10.1	11.1	11.3	11.6	10.4	10.5	9.4	9.9	?
Platelets x 1000	562	511	516	592	436	255	500	345	?
Sed. Rate	100								
% total granulocytes	75	93	39	82.6	83.4	90.3	80.3	70.1	?
Granulocytes	6.45		.585		7.506		4.4968		
Chemotherapy									
Radiotherapy									
Symptom Review									
Toxicity							?		
Physical Examination									
Chemistry							?		
To order: Labs and Procedures									
To order: Nuclear Medicine and Tomography									
Scheduling									
Day	28	03	10	17	24	30	7	14	21
Month	May	Jun	Jun	Jun	Jun	Jun	Jul	Jul	Jul
Year	87	87	87	87	87	87	87	87	87

326

7 8 9   erase
4 5 6   n/a
1 2 3   clear
0   abort
        done

FIGURE 4.5 The data-entry screen of the ONCOCIN consultation system is a computer-based representation of the familiar paper flowchart on which physicians normally record information regarding their cancer patients. The physician can enter the platelet count into the database by selecting digits from the numerical menu displayed in the upper-right corner of the figure. Only the hematology section of the flowchart currently is visible. The physician can view data on disease activity, chemotherapies, and so on, by selecting from the alternative section headings. (*Source:* Courtesy of Section on Medical Informatics, Stanford University.)

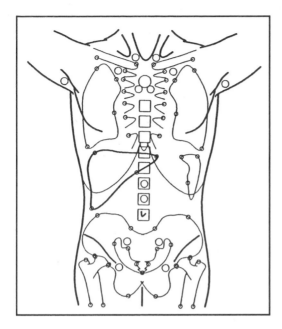

FIGURE 4.6 Bit-mapped displays and images provide an alternative means of entering data. Rather than describing the location of a tumor in words, a physician using the ONCOCIN consultation system can indicate the location of a lesion by selecting regions on a torso. In this figure, the physician has indicated involvement of the patient's liver. (*Source:* Courtesy of Section on Medical Informatics, Stanford University.)

commands. Physicians can use images to indicate the location of an injury, the size of a tumor, the area to be covered by radiation therapy, and so on (Figure 4.6). Because of the imprecision of medical language, a graphical indication of the affected body parts can be a valuable supplement to coded or textual descriptions.

Much medical information is available in narrative text form—for example, physician-transcribed visit notes, hospital discharge summaries, and all the medical literature. Text-scanning devices now are available that can scan lines or entire pages of typewritten text and convert each character into its ASCII-coded binary format. These devices reduce the need to retype information that previously was typed, but they cannot capture handwritten information.

Physicians are comfortable with dictating their notes; therefore, researchers have investigated the possibility of using voice input for data entry. The simplest method for capturing voice data is to record messages directly from a microphone. The voice signal then is encoded in digital form (see Section 4.2), identified as a textual message, and stored and transmitted with the other computer data. When the data are retrieved, the message simply is played back through a speaker. Using a more sophisticated technology for voice-data input, the computer recognizes the digitized voice signals by matching the sound patterns to the patterns of a vocabulary of known words. The speech input is then stored as ASCII-coded text. Currently, systems exist that can interpret sequences of discrete words, but researchers have had limited success with systems that can recognize continuous speech, in which the sounds run together. In neither case does the computer *understand* the content of the messages. This same lack of understanding applies to most (uncoded) textual data, which are entered, stored, retrieved, and printed without any analysis of their meaning.

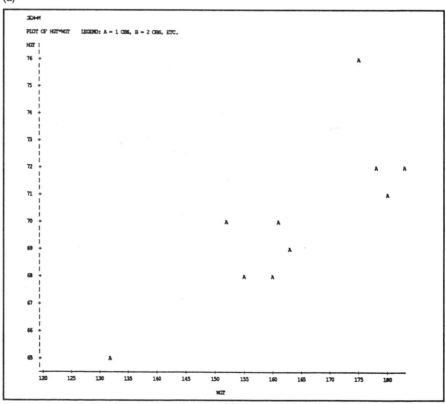

(a)

(b)

FIGURE 4.7

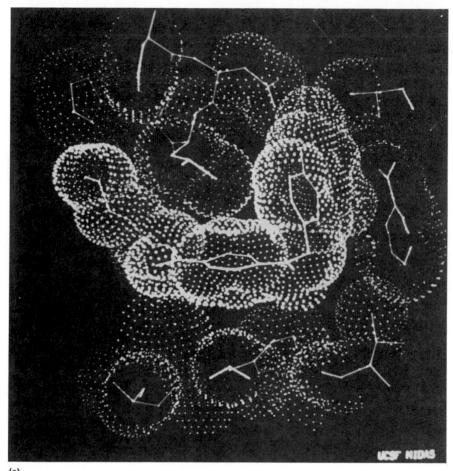

(c)

FIGURE 4.7 (a) Bit-mapped displays allow onscreen presentation of digitally encoded pictures. With a little creativity, the user can display graphical output using (b) character-based screens and printing devices, or (c) vector-based displays. Compared to the bit-mapped displays of modern graphics monitors, however, the results of the older character-based or vector technologies are unsatisfactory for many applications. (*Source:* (a) Courtesy of Vesalius, Inc., and of Williams and Wilkins, Baltimore, MD; (c) Courtesy of the Computer Graphics Laboratory, University of California, San Francisco.)

Output Devices

The *presentation* of results, or **output,** is the final step in the processing of medical data. Many systems compute information that is transmitted to health-care providers and immediately displayed on VDTs so that action can be taken. Another large volume of output consists of reports, which are printed or simply are kept available to document the actions taken. Chapter 6 describes various reports and messages that commonly are used to present patient information. Here, we describe the devices that are used to convey these outputs.

Most immediate output appears at its destination on a display screen, such as the **cathode-ray tube (CRT)** display of a VDT. If the results require urgent attention, a signal such as a ringing bell may alert personnel to the data's arrival. More routinely, results are placed in storage and are automatically retrieved when the patient's record is accessed by an appropriate provider. Important findings may be highlighted on the screen.

A CRT is driven by local memory, which holds at least as many characters as can be displayed on its screen (typically 25 lines of 80 characters). Each character is represented by a byte. Thus, for a character-oriented display, the CRT's memory holds 2000 bytes or $2000 \times 8 = 16{,}000$ bits of information. The device generates the actual image by converting the bytes to a pattern of dots on the lines. These lines are written using a television-type **raster scan.** Within the memory, additional characters may be stored that indicate formatting choices and display modes, such as color, boldface type, or blinking presentation. Sometimes, users can edit the data displayed on the screen prior to transferring the data to the computer. Terminals that are able to perform processing of this type are called **intelligent terminals.** Note that, although intelligent terminals are equipped to perform limited processing related to data input and output, they are not computers. Be sure you understand the difference between a *personal computer (PC),* which is a standalone computer, and a *terminal,* which is a device used to communicate with a computer at a remote site; both have a keyboard and a display monitor.

Graphical output is essential for summarizing and presenting the information derived from voluminous data. There are three alternative technologies for providing graphics: bit-mapped, character-based, and vector displays. The decreasing cost of memory has made **bit-mapped displays** the only practical alternative for producing graphics. Most PCs and many modern terminals support this technology, which provides the capability of displaying *pictures* on the screen or of printing pictures on special printers (Figure 4.7a). Bit-maps can be used to display even digitally encoded X-ray images.

The graphics screen is divided into a grid of picture elements, called **pixels.** Each pixel is associated with 1 or more bits in memory. In a black-and-white monitor, the value of each pixel on the screen is associated with a single bit of information. The value of the bit indicates whether that spot on the display is on (black) or off (white). If the monitor supports multiple levels of intensity, or **gray scale,** several bits are needed to indicate the value of each pixel. For example, 2 bits can distinguish four values: black, white, and two intermediate shades of gray. Similarly, multiple bits are necessary to specify the color of pixels on color graphics monitors. The number of bits per pixel determines the **contrast resolution** of an image. The number of pixels per square inch determines the **spatial resolution** of the image (Figure 4.8). As we shall discuss in Chapter 11, both parameters determine the requirements for storing images. A display with high spatial resolution requires an array of about 1000×1000 pixels, whereas a 400×400 array might suffice for a textual display. A simple color display needs 3 bits per pixel; to obtain a full range of shades, the bit map records for each pixel the intensity of each of the three basic colors (red, green, and blue).

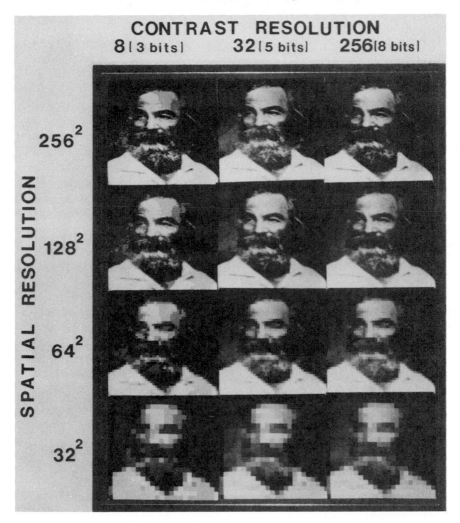

FIGURE 4.8 Varying the number of pixels and number of bits per pixel affects the spatial and contrast resolution of a digital image. The image in the upper-right corner was displayed using a 256 × 256 array of pixels, 8 bits per pixel; the subject (Walt Whitman) is easily discernable. (*Source:* Reproduced, with permission, from Price, R. R., and James, A. E. Basic principles and instrumentation of digital radiography. In Price, R. R., et al. (eds), *Digital Radiography: A Focus on Clinical Utility.* Orlando, FL: W. B. Saunders, 1982.)

Bit-mapped graphics technology has made the alternative methods for producing graphics obsolete. However, many health-care facilities installed computer systems before bit-maps became practical, and they continue to use hardware based on the older technologies. Character-oriented display terminals can produce primitive graphics by arranging text characters to form plots or pictures. Bars and slashes (/ \ − |) are arranged to produce horizontal, vertical, and diagonal lines; infrequently used characters (@ # % $) are used to fill different areas in graphs or plots.

Graphic images produced in this manner look stilted (Figure 4.7b). Vector-based displays can produce arbitrary lines and are used in many medical sites to display patient measurements from instruments (Figure 4.7c).

Sometimes, visual display is not convenient to use, and output is *printed* on paper. Printing information is slower than is displaying it on a screen, so, whenever possible, printing is done in advance of need. In a clinic, relevant portions of the patient record may be printed on high-volume printers the night before a scheduled visit. Low-volume output can be produced using typewriter-like *impact printers*. These printers provide highly legible output, but are slow and noisy. Multiple-sheet forms require impact printers to produce the carbon copies. *Dot-matrix printers* print small dots on paper similar to the way that the CRT forms characters on a screen from small dots. These printers can be fairly fast (120 characters per second), but those that operate at high speed often produce poor output that may become illegible when it is photocopied.

Laser printers use an electronically controlled laser beam to generate an image on a xerographic drum, which then is used to produce paper copies, just as is done in a regular photocopier. Many laser printers permit the user to select from a variety of fonts and typefaces, and some also can produce graphics. Laser-produced graphics can be finely detailed, because the laser beam can be set to any one of several hundred lines per inch (about 10,000 lines per page), producing a finer resolution than is possible on a bit-mapped display. Laser printers are relatively quiet, so they are particularly suitable for hospital environments.

4.1.2 Software

All the functions performed by the hardware of a computer system—data acquisition from input devices, transfer of data and programs to and from working memory, computation and information processing by the CPU, formatting and presentation of results—are directed by computer programs, or **software.**

Programming Languages

In the previous section, we explained that a computer processes information by manipulating words of information in registers. Instructions that tell the processor which operations to perform also are sequences of 0s and 1s, a binary representation called **machine language,** or *machine code*. Machine-code instructions are the only directives that a computer can process without translation. These binary patterns, however, are difficult or impossible for people to understand and manipulate. People can think symbolically. Thus, a first step toward making programming easier and less error-prone was the creation of an assembly language. **Assembly language** replaces the strings of numbers of machine-language programs with words and abbreviations meaningful to humans; a programmer instructs the computer to LOAD from memory, STORE into memory, ADD an amount to the contents of a register, and so on. A program called an **assembler** translates these instructions into binary machine-language representation prior to execution of the code.

In most cases, there is a one-to-one correspondence between instructions in assembly and machine languages. An assembly-language programmer must consider problems on a hardware-specific level, instructing the computer to transfer data between registers and memory and to perform primitive operations, such as incrementing registers and comparing characters (see Figure 4.9). On the other hand, the problems that the users of a computer wish to solve are on a higher conceptual level. Users are concerned with real-world problems. They need to instruct the computer to perform tasks such as to retrieve the latest serum-creatinine test result, to monitor the status of a hypertensive patient, or to compute a patient's current account balance. To make communication with computers more understandable and less tedious, computer scientists developed higher-level, user-oriented symbolic programming languages.

Using a higher-level language, such as FORTRAN, Pascal, BASIC, COBOL, MUMPS, or LISP, a programmer can create variables to represent higher-level entities and can specify arithmetic and symbolic operations without worrying about the details of how the hardware performs these operations. The complexity of the

---

Assembly-language program:

```
      ORG  0        /Origin of program is location 0
      LDA A         /Load operand from location A
      ADD B         /Add operand from location B
      STA C         /Store sum in location C
      HLT           /Halt
A,    DEC  3        /Location A contains decimal 3
B,    DEC  15       /Location B contains decimal 15
C,    DEC  0        /Location C contains decimal 0
      END           /End of program
```

Machine-language program:

Location	Instruction code
0	0010 0000 0000 0100
1	0001 0000 0000 0101
10	0011 0000 0000 0110
11	0111 0000 0000 0001
100	0000 0000 0000 0011
101	0000 0000 0000 1111
110	0000 0000 0000 0000

FIGURE 4.9 An assembly-language program and a corresponding machine-language program to add two numbers and to store the result.

operation of the hardware is hidden from the user, who can specify with a single statement an operation that may translate to tens or hundreds of machine instructions. A **compiler** is used to translate automatically a high-level program into machine code. Some languages are *interpreted* instead of compiled. An **interpreter** converts and executes each statement before moving to the next statement, whereas a compiler translates all the statements at one time, creating a binary program, which then can be executed. MUMPS is an interpreted language, LISP may be either interpreted or compiled, and FORTRAN routinely is compiled prior to execution.

Each statement of a language is characterized by **syntax** and **semantics.** The syntactic rules describe how the statements, declarations, and other language constructs are written—they define the language's grammatical structure. Semantics is the meaning given to the various syntactic constructs. The following three statements (written in Pascal, FORTRAN, and LISP) all have the same semantics:

```
C:= A + B;
C = A + B
(SETQ C (PLUS A B))
```

These statements instruct the computer to add the values of variables A and B, then assign the result to variable C. Each language, however, has a distinct syntax for indicating which operations to perform. Regardless of the particular language in which a program is written, the computer responds by manipulating sequences of 0s and 1s within its registers.

Programmers can work in successively higher levels of abstraction by writing, and later invoking, standard functions and subroutines. Built-in functions and subroutines create an environment in which users can perform complex operations by specifying single commands. For example, users can search and retrieve data from large databases using the query language of a database-management system (which we shall describe later). They can perform extensive statistical calculations, such as regression analysis and correlation, using prewritten programs from a statistical package, such as the Statistical Analysis System (SAS) or the Statistical Package for the Social Sciences (SPSS). Or they can use a spreadsheet program, such as Lotus 1-2-3, to record and manipulate data in a spreadsheet. In each case, the physical details of the data-storage structures and the access mechanisms are hidden from the user. Each of these programs provides its own specialized language for instructing a computer to perform desired high-level functions.

Operating Systems

Users interact with the computer through the **operating system,** a program that supervises and controls the execution of all other programs and that directs the operation of the hardware. The operating system is one of a group of **system programs,** software that is included with a computer system and that makes it possible to use the system. Typically, system software also includes utility programs, such as **text editors** and **debuggers;** compilers that make it possible to write programs in higher-level languages rather than in machine language; libraries of standard routines, such as sorting programs and programs to perform complex mathematical functions; and diagnostic programs to help maintain the computer system. The intervening layer of system software runs in the background and handles the details of file management, memory allocation, communication among hardware components, and so on.

The kernel of the operating system resides in memory at all times and supervises the other programs running in the computer. It loads programs for execution, allocates memory, manages the transfer of data from input devices and to output devices, and manages the creation, opening, reading, writing, and closing of data files. In shared systems, it allocates the resources of the system among the competing users. The operating system insulates programmers from much of the complexity of handling these processes. Thus, they are able to concentrate on higher-level problems of information management. They can write **application programs** to store and organize data, to facilitate the integration and communication of information, to perform bookkeeping functions, to monitor patient status, to aid in education—to perform all the functions provided by medical computing systems (see Chapter 5).

There are two primary modes of operation for a *multiuser* system, in which multiple users share a single processor: batch mode and time-sharing mode. In **batch mode,** users communicate with the computer only to initiate processing and to obtain results on completion. They submit their programs for execution. The operating system **queues** the jobs and, after execution, returns the results in files stored on disk, or on hardcopy printouts. If there are many users, those who have jobs near the end of the queue may have to wait a long time before their work is processed. In **time-sharing mode,** on the other hand, all users have simultaneous access to the computer; users communicate *interactively* with a central computer that switches rapidly among all the jobs that are running. The operating system allocates to each job a slice of time. The CPU processes a job until it is complete, or until the time slice runs out; in the latter case, the job is requeued for future execution. Because people work slowly compared to computer processing speeds, the computer can respond to multiple users, seemingly at the same time. Thus, each user has the illusion that she has the full attention of the machine. The CPU expends some time for queuing, switching, and requeuing jobs. Therefore, the system breaks down if the demand is too high—high loads produce a relatively high overhead and slow the service for everyone.

The basic concept common to both batch and time-sharing modes is **multiprogramming.** In a multiprogramming system, several application programs reside in main memory simultaneously. Because the computer works with several programs in sequence, all its parts are kept busy, thus reducing the time each resource is idle. Multiprogramming permits the effective use of multiple devices; while the CPU is executing one program, another program may be receiving input from external storage, and another may be printing results on the laser printer. If each program ran start to finish before another was started, much inefficiency would result. In **multiprocessing systems,** several processors are used in a single computer system, thus increasing the processing power of the system. Note, however, that multiprogramming does not imply multiprocessors.

In large multiuser systems, memory management is particularly important. Main memory is small relative to the total need; when multiple programs must reside in main memory simultaneously, the *complete* programs and data often will not fit. Thus, the operating system splits users' programs and data into *pages,* which are brought into main memory as they are needed. Large computer systems also support a **virtual memory** to further increase memory capacity. Virtual memory uses space on a peripheral disk to produce the illusion that main memory can hold many more pages than it actually can. Thus, users can write programs that require more memory than is available in main memory. Each address that is referenced by the CPU goes through an address mapping from the *virtual address* to an actual address in main memory (Figure 4.10). This mapping is handled automatically by the hardware.

Most microcomputers today have been designed to be workstations for a single user. Users are in sole control of their workstations; they work **online,** controlling the steps of processing interactively. Single-user operation simplifies memory management and other tasks of the operating system. For example, the systems can execute only one program at a time and often can perform no other work while the CPU is compiling a program, while it is receiving input from the keyboard, or while a file

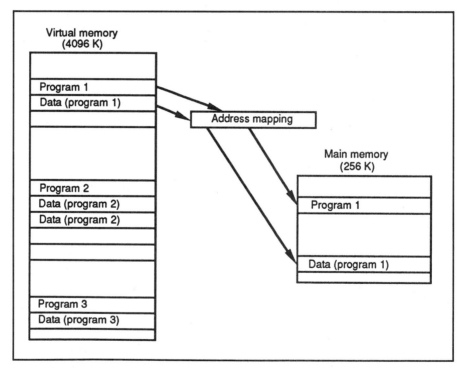

FIGURE 4.10 Virtual memory provides users with the illusion that they have many more addressable memory locations than there are in real memory—in this case, 16 times as many. Programs and data stored on peripheral disks are swapped into main memory when they are referenced; logical addresses are translated automatically to physical addresses by the hardware.

is being printed out. Thus, PCs usually have only a single-process operating system (sometimes called the monitor, supervisor, or executive program). The falling price of memory and the increasing computing power of small machines have made available PCs that provide functionality more like that of larger machines. The operating systems of some modern PCs allow a single user to run multiple processes simultaneously; some microcomputers can support even multiple users.

Database-Management Systems

Throughout this book, we shall continue to emphasize the importance to good medical decision making of timely access to large numbers of data from diverse sources. Computers provide the means for organizing and accessing these data; however, the programs to provide these functions are complex and are difficult to write. Programming is particularly difficult when multiple users share data (and thus may try to access data simultaneously), when users must search large numbers of data rapidly and at unpredictable times, and when the relationships among data elements are complex (and thus require complex data-storage structures). For health-care applications, it is important that the data be complete and error-free. Furthermore, the need for long-term reliability makes it unwise to entrust a medical database to locally written programs, because the programmers tend to move from project to project. Database technology supports the integration and organization of data and assists users with data entry, storage, and retrieval.

Not only the individual data, but also their meanings and their relationships with other data must be stored. For example, an isolated data element (say, the number 99.7) is useless unless we know what that number represents (say, body temperature in degrees Fahrenheit) and other information that is necessary to interpret its value (say, the value pertains to a particular patient who is identified by a unique medical record number, the observation was taken at a certain time [02:35, 7FEB90] in a certain way [orally], and so on). To avoid loss of descriptive information, clusters of related data elements must be kept together throughout processing.

The meaning of data elements and the relationships among those elements are captured in the structure of the database. **Databases** are collections of data, typically organized into fields, records, and files (Figure 4.11). The **field** is the most primitive element; each field represents one data element. For example, the database of a hospital information system typically has fields for the patient's identification number, name, date of birth, gender, admission date, admitting diagnosis, and so on. Fields are grouped together to form **records;** usually, a record is uniquely identified by one or more **key fields**—for example, patient-identification number and observation time. Records that contain similar information are grouped in **files.** In addition to files related to patients (diagnoses, treatments, and drug therapies), the database of a hospital information system (HIS) will have separate files containing information about charges and payments, personnel and payroll, inventory, and so on.

Once programmers know the structure and format of a data file, they can write programs to access the data directly. For example, if they know that a patient's identification number is stored in the first field of each record as a string of 10 alphanumeric

Record-number	Name	Sex	Date-of-birth
22-546-998	Adams, Clare	F	11Nov88
62-847-991	Barnes, Tanner	F	07Dec87
47-882-365	Clark, Laurel	F	10May88
55-202-187	Davidson, Travis	M	10Apr86

FIGURE 4.11 A simple patient data file containing records for four pediatric patients. The key field of each record contains the medical-record number that uniquely identifies the patient. The other fields of the record contain demographic information.

characters, they can write programs to read each record, to extract the contents of that field, and to store the value in a variable, PATIENT-ID. If, however, the structure of the database changes—for example, because new fields are added to a record—it will be necessary to modify all such existing programs. The desire for **data independence** is a key reason for building a database-management system.

A **database-management system (DBMS)** is an integrated set of programs created to help users to store and manipulate data more easily and efficiently. The conceptual (logical) view of a database provided by a DBMS allows users to specify *what* the results should be without worrying too much about *how* those results will be obtained; the DBMS handles the details of managing and accessing data. A DBMS features a **schema,** a machine-readable definition of the contents and organization of the records of a data file. Programs are insulated from changes in the way data are stored, because the programs access data by field name rather than by location—the schema file of the DBMS must be modified to reflect changes in record format, but the application programs that use the data do not need to be altered. A DBMS also provides facilities for entering, editing, and retrieving data. Often, fields are associated with lists or ranges of valid values; thus, the DBMS can detect and request correction of some data-entry errors, thereby improving database integrity.

Typically, users retrieve data from a database in either of two ways. Users can query the database directly using a *query language* to extract information in an ad hoc fashion—for example, to retrieve the records of all male hypertensive patients ages 45 to 64 years for inclusion in a retrospective study. Figure 4.12 shows the syntax for such a query using Structured Query Language (SQL). Query formulation can be difficult, however; users must understand the contents and underlying structure of the database to construct a query correctly. Often, database programmers formulate the requests for health professionals. On the other hand, many database queries are routine requests—for example, the resource-utilization reports used by health-care administrators, and the end-of-month financial reports generated for business offices. Thus, DBMSs often provide an alternative, simpler means for formulating such queries, called *report generation.* Users specify their data requests on the input screen of the report-generator program. The report generator then produces the actual query program using information stored in the schema. The reports are formatted so that

SELECT   Patient-ID, Name, Age, Systolic

FROM   Patients

WHERE   Sex = 'M' and
               Age >= 45 and
               Age <= 64 and
               Systolic > 140

FIGURE 4.12 An example of a simple database query written in Structured Query Language (SQL). The program will retrieve the records of males whose age is between 45 and 64 years and whose systolic blood pressure is greater than 140 mm Hg.

they can be distributed without modification. The report-generation programs can extract header information from the schema.

Many DBMSs support multiple **views,** or models of the data. The data stored in a database have a single physical organization, yet different user groups can have different perspectives on the contents and structure of a database. For example, the clinical laboratory and the finance department might use the same underlying database, but each might have available only the data relevant to its individual application area. Basic patient information will be shared; the existence of other data is hidden from groups that do not need them. Application-specific descriptions of a database are stored in subschemas. Through the subschemas, a DBMS controls access to data and supports data security. It might limit access to sensitive data to only a privileged class of users—for example, only managers might be able to view salary information. Other data might be read by any user, but edited only by users in the group that owns them, and so on. Thus, a DBMS facilitates the integration of data from multiple sources and avoids the expense of creating and maintaining multiple files containing redundant information. At the same time, it accommodates the differing needs of multiple users. Modern database technology, combined with communications technology (see Section 4.3), will enable health-care institutions to attain the benefits both of independent, specialized applications and of large integrated databases.

A variety of structures can be used to organize data files and to implement databases. The Suggested Readings provide sources for further reference. Blum's book summarizes concisely the most common organizations for data files and the corresponding methods for locating, adding, and deleting information. The Korth and Silberschatz text provides a detailed study of the technical details of file management and DBMSs, and discusses the three alternative models for structuring traditional DBMSs: the relational, hierarchical, and network models. Wiederhold's book discusses the organization and use of databases in health-care settings.

4.2 Data Acquisition and Signal Processing

A prominent theme of this book is that capturing and entering data into the computer is difficult and expensive. **Real-time acquisition** of data directly from the source by direct electrical connections to instruments can overcome these problems. Direct acquisition of data avoids the need for people to measure, encode, and enter the data manually. Sensors attached to a patient convert biological signals—such as blood pressure, pulse rate, mechanical movement, and electrical activity—into electrical signals, which are transmitted to the computer. Tissue density can be obtained by scanning X-ray transmission. The signals are sampled periodically and are converted to digital representation for storage and processing. Automated data-acquisition and signal-processing techniques are particularly important in patient-monitoring settings (see Chapter 12). Similar techniques also apply to the acquisition and processing of human voice input.

Most naturally occurring signals are **analog signals**—signals that vary continuously. The first bedside monitors, for example, were wholly analog devices. Typically, they acquired an analog signal (such as that measured by the ECG) and displayed its level on a dial or other continuous display (see, for instance, the continuous signal recorded on the ECG strip shown in Figure 12.9).

The computers we deal with are digital computers. A **digital computer** stores and processes values in discrete units. Before processing is possible, analog signals must be converted to discrete units. The conversion process is called **analog-to-digital conversion (ADC).** You can think of ADC as *sampling and rounding*—the continuous value is observed at some instant and rounded to the nearest discrete unit (Figure 4.13). You need 1 bit to distinguish between two levels (for example, on or off). If you wish to discriminate among four levels, you need 2 bits (because $2^2 = 4$), and so on.

Two parameters determine how closely the digital data represent the original analog signal: the precision with which the signal is recorded and the frequency with which the signal is sampled. The **precision** describes the degree of accuracy of a sample observation of the signal. It is determined by the number of bits used to represent a signal and their correctness; the more bits, the greater the number of levels that can be distinguished. Precision also is limited by the accuracy of the equipment that converts and transmits the signal. Ranging and calibration of the instruments, either manually or automatically, is necessary for signals to be represented with as much precision as possible. Improper ranging will result in loss of information. For example, a change in a signal that varies between 0.1 and 0.2 volts will be undetectable if the instrument has been set to record changes between 0.0 and 1.0, in 0.25-volt increments (see Figure 4.14 for another example of improper ranging).

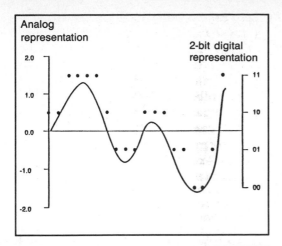

FIGURE 4.13 Analog-to-digital conversion is a technique for transforming continuous-valued signals to discrete values. In this example, each sampled value is converted to one of four discrete levels (represented by 2 bits).

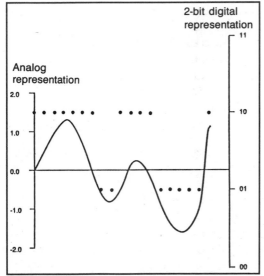

FIGURE 4.14 The amplitude of signals from sensors must be *ranged* to account for individual patient variation (for example, due to obesity). As illustrated here, the details of the signal may be lost if the signal is amplified insufficiently. On the other hand, overamplification will produce clipped peaks and troughs.

The **sampling rate** is the second parameter that affects the correspondence between an analog signal and its digital representation. A sampling rate that is too low relative to the rate at which a signal changes value will produce a poor representation (see Figure 4.15). On the other hand, oversampling increases the expense of processing and storing the data. As a general rule, you need to sample at least twice as frequently as the highest-frequency component needed from a signal. For instance, looking at an ECG (see Figure 12.9), we find that the basic repetition frequency is at most a few per second, but that the QRS wave contains useful frequency components on the order of 150 cycles per second. Thus, the data sampling rate should be at least 300 measurements per second. This rate is called the **Nyquist frequency.**

Another aspect of signal quality is the amount of **noise** in the signal—the component of the acquired data that is *not* due to the specific phenomenon being measured.

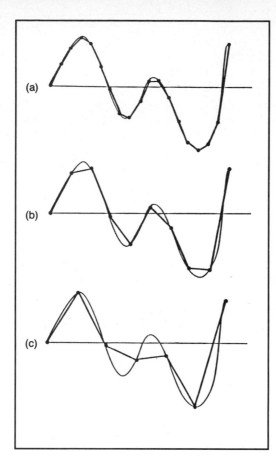

FIGURE 4.15 The higher the sampling rate, the more closely the sampled observations will correspond to the underlying analog signal. The sampling rate in (a) is highest; that in (b) is lower. When the sampling rate is low (c), the results of the analog-to-digital conversion can be misleading. Note the degradation of the quality of the signal from (a) to (c). (Figure 12.7 illustrates the effects of varying sampling rate on the quality of an ECG signal.)

A primary source of noise is the electrical or magnetic signals produced by nearby devices and power lines. Once the signal has been obtained from a sensor, it must be transmitted to the computer. Often, the signal has to leave a laboratory and pass through other equipment. Enroute, the analog signals are susceptible to electromagnetic interference. Inaccuracies in the sensors, poor contact between sensor and source (for example, the patient), and disturbances from signals produced by processes other than the one being studied (for example, respiration interferes with recording of the ECG) are other common sources of noise.

Three techniques, often used in combination, minimize the amount of noise in a signal:

1. *Shielding, isolation, and grounding* of cables and instruments carrying analog signals reduce electrical interference. Often, two twisted wires are used to transmit the signal, one to carry the actual signal, the other to transmit the ground voltage at the sensor. At the destination, a differential amplifier measures the difference. Most interference affects both wires equally; thus, the difference should reflect the true signal. The use of glass fiberoptic cables instead of copper wires for signal

transmission eliminates interference from electrical machinery, because optical signals are not affected by electrical or magnetic fields.

2. For robust transmission over long distances, analog signals can be *converted* into a frequency-modulated (FM) representation, or into digital form. An FM signal represents changes of the signal as changes of frequency, not of amplitude. FM reduces noise greatly, because interference disturbs directly only the amplitude of the signal. As long as the interference does not create amplitude changes near the high carrier frequency, no loss of data will occur during transmission.

    Conversion of analog signals to digital form provides the most robust transmission. The nearer to the source the conversion occurs, the more effective this technique is. Digital transmission of signals is inherently noise-free; interference rarely is great enough to change a 1 value to a 0 value, or vice versa. Furthermore, digital signals can be coded to permit detection and correction of faults. Placement of a microprocessor near the signal source is now the most common way to achieve such a conversion. The development of digital signal processing (DSP) chips— also used for computer voice mail—will accelerate this trend.

3. *Filtering algorithms* can be used to reduce the effect of noise. Usually, these algorithms are applied to the data once the latter have been stored in memory. A characteristic of noise is its relatively random pattern. Repetitive signals, such as an ECG, can be integrated over several cycles, thus reducing the effects of random noise. When the noise pattern differs from the signal pattern, Fourier analysis can be used to filter the signal; a signal is decomposed into its individual components, each with a distinct period and amplitude. (Wiederhold and Clayton's article, described in the Suggested Readings, explains Fourier analysis in greater detail.) Unwanted components of the signal are assumed to be noise and are eliminated. Some noise (such as the 60-cycle interference caused by a building's electrical circuitry) has a regular pattern. In this case, the portion of the signal that is known to be caused by interference can be filtered out.

Once the data have been acquired and filtered, they typically are processed to reduce their volume and to abstract information for use by interpretation programs. Often, the data are analyzed to extract important parameters, or *features,* of the signal—for example, the duration or intensity of the ST segment of an ECG. The computer also can analyze the shape of the waveform, by comparing the signal to models of known patterns, or templates. In speech recognition, the voice signals can be compared to stored profiles of spoken words. Further analysis is necessary to determine the meaning or importance of the signals—for example, to allow automated ECG-based cardiac diagnosis or speech understanding.

4.3 Data Communications and Network Technology

The transmission of data from sensor to computer is one type of data communication. On a much larger scale is the transmission of data among independent computer systems to allow the sharing of information, computer programs, and hardware among multiple users. As we shall see in Chapter 7, data communication and integration are critical functions of HISs. The trend over the last 2 decades has been away from centralized architectures—in which all applications run on a single, large machine and share a central database—to federated systems, which are affiliations of relatively independent distributed subsystems.

Distribution offers flexibility in choice of software and hardware. Specialized computer systems can better fulfill the diverse needs of health professionals in the laboratory, the pharmacy, the intensive-care unit, the business office, and so on. The primary disadvantage of distribution, however, is that sharing information among independent users on different types of systems is difficult. Instead of being directly accessible in a common storage system, sharable information may have to be sent to several participating computers, via a communication network. The development of technology to allow linking of independent computers in networks promises the best of both worlds—independent, local systems that communicate with one another easily, sharing data and other resources. In this section, we shall introduce the important concepts that underlie network technology.

The most common method for communicating computer information is to use the telephone lines. A **modem** (modulator-demodulator) converts the digital data generated by a keyboard or a computer to analog signals in the voice range. It then transmits the tones over the telephone lines—a conversation between computers occurs. At the receiving end, the tones are reconverted to the original digital signals by another modem.

Different modems can support different **baud rates,** or rates of information-transfer. The standard transmission rate for data entry supports up to 300 baud—an information-transfer rate equivalent to 300 bits per second (bps), or 30 characters per second. This speed is adequate for transmitting data as they are typed, but too slow for input of scanned documents or for transmitting results as they are reproduced by a computer. For these purposes, modems of at least 1200 baud are needed; to communicate information for viewing on VDTs, a baud rate of 2400 or 4800 is desirable. At high speeds, data signals become unacceptably noisy. Dedicated telephone lines suitable for transmitting data, and modems that can handle an information-transfer rate of up to 19,200 baud, are available. Currently, they are expensive, but their price is falling rapidly. Nonetheless, it can be more advantageous for an institution to invest in its own local-area network.

A **local-area network (LAN)** links multiple computer **nodes**, rather than just two at a time (recall the opening scenario in Chapter 1). Thus, it simplifies the sharing of resources—data, software, and equipment—among multiple users. Users working at individual workstations can retrieve data and programs from network **file servers**—computers dedicated to storing files, both shared and private. They can process information locally, then save the results over the network to the file server or send output to a printer for hardcopy. Communication within the network is accomplished via transmission of messages bundled as packets of data; each packet contains the data to be sent and the network addresses of the sending and receiving nodes. Typically, all the nodes connected by a LAN are owned and maintained by the same organization and operate within a geographical area of at most a few miles. Government or commercially operated **wide-area networks** connect computers owned by independent users and institutions and distributed over long distances (Figure 4.16).

One type of LAN is the **private branch exchange (PBX)**, an extension of an organization's internal telephone system; the telephone wires are used to transfer both voice signals and data. Digital data are converted to analog signals and can be transmitted to any location where the telephones are connected. PBXs are configured such that they will not introduce interference into the transmission, even at fairly high transmission rates, such as at 9600 baud.

More rapid transmissions can be supported by dedicated LANs. Most LANs operate in the range of 1 million to 10 million bps. At 10 million bps, the entire contents of this book could be transmitted in a few seconds. LANs can be based on either broadband or baseband technology. **Broadband** is adapted from the technology for transmitting cable television. A broadband LAN can transmit multiple signals simultaneously, so it provides a unified environment for sending computer data, voice messages, and images. Each signal is sent within an assigned frequency range (channel). **Baseband** is simpler; it transmits digital signals over a single coaxial wire, one packet at a time.

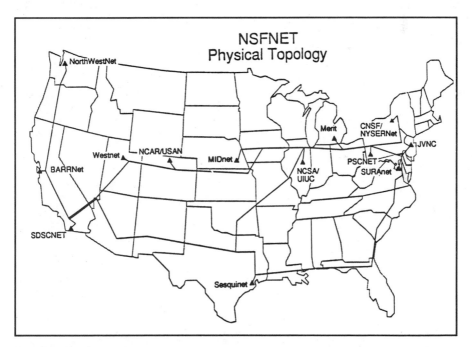

FIGURE 4.16 The NSFNET built by the National Science Foundation comprises several cross-country backbones and gateways into regional computer networks (shown as triangles). By 1990 it had replaced the Advanced Research Projects Agency Network (ARPANET), operated by the Defense Communications Agency, as the major communications network connecting research institutions throughout the United States. (*Source:* Courtesy of The Merit Computer Network.)

The nodes of a LAN are interconnected by some type of communications medium—the physical material on which data are transmitted. Most commercial LANs use *coaxial cable* as the communication medium. It is reliable, is relatively inexpensive, and has a high **bandwidth** (capacity for information transmission)—up to 100 million bps. On the other hand, coaxial cable is susceptible to electrical and radio-frequency interference. An alternate medium, *fiberoptic cable,* offers the highest bandwidth (up to 1 billion bps) and a high degree of reliability, because it does not suffer from problems of interference. The use of fiberoptic cable has the potential to increase transmission speeds and distances by at least 1 order of magnitude. In addition, fiberoptic cable is lightweight and easy to install. Currently, however, switches and connectors for the cable are expensive. Messages also can be transmitted through the air by microwave, satellite signal, or line-of-sight light transmission, but these modes have limited application for LANs.

The configuration, or shape, of the physical connections among the nodes of a LAN is the **network topology.** The most common topologies are the star, ring, and bus (Figure 4.17). In a *star network,* all communication passes through a central node enroute to any other node. For example, the switching device of a PBX data system serves as the central node of a star LAN. The main advantage of a star network is its simplicity. The central computer may act as the communication controller, as well as a common database for storage and retrieval of information. It is relatively easy to connect a new device to the network by establishing a connection between the new node and the central device. A disadvantage of the star topology is that the central node is a potential communication bottleneck. Furthermore, it is a single point of failure for the entire network.

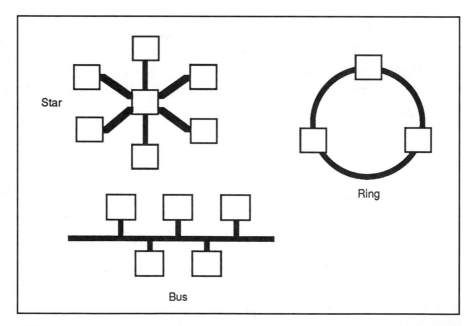

FIGURE 4.17 The star, ring, and bus are the most common topologies for local-area networks.

Ring networks link all nodes in a closed circle. Message packets are passed from node to node around the ring until they reach their destinations. Like a star network, a ring is simple in that each device receives all messages from a single source and passes on all messages to only one other source. A disadvantage of the ring network is that the failure of any one node will break the ring, thus bringing down the entire network.

Each node in a *bus network* is connected to a common communication line or cable. A message sent from any device on the network is heard directly by all other devices. If the packet is addressed to the host, the message is accepted. Otherwise, the message is ignored. Thus, bus networks are particularly well suited for transmitting broadcast messages intended for many users. Bus networks are less subject to a single point of failure than are either ring or star networks. A disadvantage of the bus, however, is the complexity of the software for controlling network access to ensure equitable and orderly use.

The exchange of data within a LAN is controlled by a set of rules, a **network protocol** that specifies how messages are prepared and transmitted electronically. If two people are to communicate effectively, they must agree on the meaning of the words they are using, the style of the interaction (lecture versus conversation), a procedure for handling interruptions, and so on. The **RS-232-C standard** defines the protocol for data interfaces among electronic devices (for example, CPUs, printers, modems, and medical instruments). The protocol of the LAN settles these issues on the level of computer communication.

The International Standards Organization (ISO) has organized protocol rules into seven layers (Figure 4.18). At the lowest levels, protocols define the physical connections, the packet formats, and the means for detecting and correcting errors. Higher levels define the method of addressing packets, and the timing and sequencing of transmission. Each layer serves the layer above it and expects certain functions or

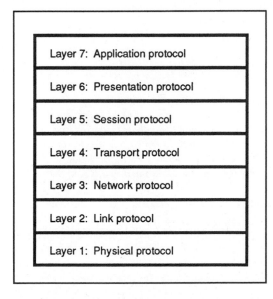

FIGURE 4.18 The Open Systems Interconnection (OSI) Reference Model developed by the International Standards Organization (ISO) specifies seven layers of network protocols at successively higher levels of abstraction. Each layer serves the layer above it and expects particular functions or services from the layer below it.

services from the layer below it. This Open Systems Interconnection (OSI) Reference Model was used as a framework for establishing various protocol standards for specific layers. For example, the Ethernet protocol developed jointly by Xerox, Intel, and Digital Equipment Corporation (DEC) is now an Institute of Electrical and Electronics Engineers (IEEE) standard, after having been widely adopted in the private sector. This baseband protocol operates at 10 million bits per second. The token ring developed by International Business Machines and the token bus supported by General Motors—the other standard LAN protocols approved by the IEEE—also use the OSI model as a frame of reference.

Several LANs can be interconnected to allow communication among machines that are more widely dispersed geographically or that are owned by separate institutions. Two independent computer systems on connected networks can send messages through **gateways,** special computers that reside on both networks and that are equipped to forward and to translate the packets, if the two networks run different protocols. The linking of LANs to wide-area networks such as the ARPANET and the BITNET make it possible to share data and resources among independent users and institutions coast to coast and around the world. Network users can access shared patient data (such as a hospital's medical records) or nationwide databases (such as the bibliographic databases of scientific literature citations). They can read electronic bulletin boards to obtain information and programs, and they can exchange mail electronically.

As we have seen in this chapter, the synthesis of such large-scale information systems is accomplished through the careful construction of hierarchies of hardware and software. Each successive layer is more abstract and hides many of the details of the preceding layer. Without worrying much about the technical details, users can access a wealth of computational resources, and can perform complex information management tasks, such as information storage and retrieval, communication, and the other information-processing functions described in the next chapter. Thus, simple methods for storing and manipulating bits of data ultimately produce complex information systems with powerful capabilities.

Suggested Readings

Blum, B.I. *Clinical Information Systems.* New York: Springer-Verlag, 1986.
> *The first five chapters of this book cover many of the topics we presented here; they include an overview of hardware and software, an introduction to databases, and a survey of programming languages. The first chapter provides a brief summary of the development of computing from the invention of the earliest computational tools in the 1600s, to the experiments with early electronic computers (such as the Mark I and ENIAC), to the advent of today's microprocessors.*

Korth, H. F. and Silberschatz, A. *Database System Concepts.* New York: McGraw-Hill, 1986.
> *This introductory-level textbook on database systems describes the four major database models: the entity-relationship, relational, network, and hierarchical models. Other chapters discuss the theory of relational-database design, file organization, data-access techniques, distributed databases, and databases for artificial-intelligence applications.*

McDonald, C. J. (ed). *Tutorials.* New York: Springer-Verlag, 1988.

> *The third in a series of* M.D. Computing: Benchmark Papers, *this volume contains 17 tutorials originally published in* M.D. Computing, *including articles on computer hardware, LANs, operating systems, and programming languages. The collection will be of interest to computing novices who wish to understand how computers work, or who would like to learn elementary programming skills.*

Mano, M. M. *Computer System Architecture,* 2nd ed. Englewood Cliffs, NJ: Prentice-Hall, 1982.

> *This technical book provides an in-depth explanation of the physical and conceptual underpinnings of computer hardware and operation. It is suitable for technically oriented readers who want to understand the details of computer architecture.*

Simborg, D. W., et al. Local area networks and the hospital. *Computers and Biomedical Research,* 16:247, 1983.

> *This article first summarizes the information needs of hospitals, then discusses a local-area communications network that is well suited to meeting these needs. It briefly explains alternative network topologies (geometric configurations for linking computers) and the ISO's layered network-protocol model.*

Tanenbaum, A. S. *Computer Networks,* 2nd ed. Englewood Cliffs, NJ: Prentice-Hall, 1988.

> *This heavily revised edition of a classic textbook on computer communication is well organized, clearly written, and easy to understand. The introductory chapter describes network architectures and the ISO OSI Reference Model. Each of the remaining chapters discusses in detail one layer of the ISO model.*

Wiederhold, G. *Databases for Health Care.* New York: Springer-Verlag, 1981.

> *This book uses a health-care perspective to introduce the concepts of database technology. It describes the structure and functions of databases and discusses the scientific and operational issues associated with the use of databases, including the problems of missing data and the conflict between data sharing and data confidentiality. The appendices describe examples of COSTAR (see Chapter 6), ARAMIS (see Chapter 16), and other databases currently used in health-care settings.*

Wiederhold, G. and Clayton, P. D. Processing biological data in real time. *M.D. Computing,* 2(6):16, 1985.

> *This article discusses the principles and problems of acquiring and processing biological data in real time. It covers much of the material discussed in the signal-processing section of this chapter, and provides more detailed explanations of analog-to-digital conversion and Fourier analysis.*

Questions for Discussion

1. Why do computer systems use magnetic disks and other auxiliary storage media to store data and programs, rather than keeping everything in main memory where it could be accessed much more quickly? What are two key considerations in deciding whether to keep data in active versus archival storage?
2. Explain how system programs (a computer system's *software layer)* insulate users from hardware changes.
3. The trend in computer-system architectures over the last 2 decades has been to move away from centralized systems toward distributed systems. Discuss the ad-

vantages and disadvantages of time-shared access to mainframe computers versus online access to individual workstations linked in a LAN.

4. Define the terms *data independence* and *database schema*. How do database-management systems facilitate data independence?

5. What are high-level and low-level computer languages? What are the advantages and disadvantages of each? Why have so many different computer languages been developed?

6. *Computer viruses* are programs that are loaded into a computer without the user's knowledge when legitimate programs and data are transferred. Such virus programs may be benign—for example, they may display a single greeting. However, they also may modify or destroy data and programs, or allow unauthorized users to gain access to the infected system. Keeping in mind the analogy to biological viruses, discuss potential mechanisms for protecting a system against computer viruses.

5

System Design and Evaluation

Leslie E. Perreault and Gio Wiederhold

After reading this chapter, you should know the answers to these questions:

- What functions do medical computer systems perform?
- Why is communication between medical personnel and computing personnel crucial to the successful design and implementation of a medical information system?
- What are the tradeoffs between purchasing a *turnkey system* and developing a *custom-designed system*?
- What design features affect a system's acceptance by users?
- Why is evaluation an essential activity during all phases of system design, development, and operation?
- What ethical issues arise when computers are used in medical settings?

5.1 Computer Systems: Functions and Use

In Chapter 4, we introduced basic concepts related to computer hardware and software. In this chapter, we shall see how computer systems created from these components can be used by health professionals to support the health-care delivery process. We shall describe the basic functions performed by medical computer systems, and shall discuss important issues in system design, implementation, and evaluation. You should keep these concepts in mind as you read about the various medical computing applications in the chapters that follow. Think about how each system meets (or fails to meet) the needs of its users, and about what are the practical reasons why some systems have been accepted for routine use in patient care, whereas other systems have failed to make the transition from the research environment to the real world.

At a minimum, a system's success depends on the selection of appropriate hardware and the implementation of efficient data-storage and data-processing methods. We shall not discuss, however, the technical issues related to specific hardware and software choices—those determinations are beyond the scope of this book. Instead, we shall provide a general introduction to practical issues in the design and implementation of systems. In particular, we shall stress the importance of designing systems that not only meet users' requirements for information, but also fit smoothly into their everyday routines. A central theme of this chapter is the importance of communication between health-care and computing professionals in defining problems and developing workable solutions. With this perspective, we shall explore the factors that create a need for automation, and shall discuss important issues in the design, development, and evaluation of medical information systems.

5.1.1 Concept of a System

Until now, we have referred freely to *medical information systems* and *computer systems.* What do we mean when we refer to a *system?* In the most general sense, a **system** is an organized set of procedures for accomplishing a task. It can be described in terms of (1) the problem to be solved, (2) the data and knowledge required to address the problem, and (3) the internal process for transforming the available **input** into the desired **output** (see Figure 5.1). When we talk about systems in this book, we usually mean *computer-based* systems. A **computer system** combines both manual and automated processes; people and machines work in concert to manage and use information. A computer system has three components:

1. *Hardware*—the physical equipment, including CPU, data-storage devices, terminals, and printers
2. *Software*—the computer programs that direct the hardware to process input data and stored information; such programs usually are accompanied by manuals that instruct users regarding the procedures for system operation and maintenance
3. *Users*—the people who interact with the software and hardware of the system

Often, we think of a computer system as a complete and independent entity. It is important to realize, however, that every input used by the system must be supplied

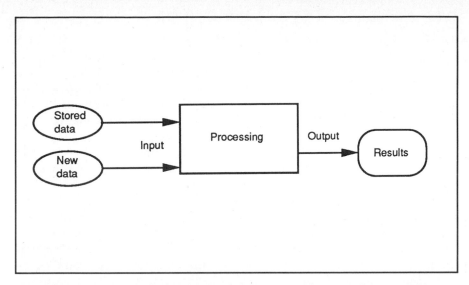

FIGURE 5.1 A computer system applies automated and manual procedures to produce desired outputs from the available input data.

by a user or by another computer system. Likewise, output information is produced because it is needed by a health-care professional or as input to another computer system. In other words, a medical computer system functions within the context of the greater health-care delivery system.

The overall health-care system determines not only the need for the computer system (for example, which data must be processed and which reports must be generated), but also the requirements for the system's operations (for example, the necessary degree of reliability and timeliness of access to information). Acquisition of a computer system has implications for the organization of an institution. Who controls the information? Who is responsible for the accuracy of the data? How will the system be financed? The installation of a computer system may have sociological consequences as well. The introduction of a new system alters the work routines of health-care workers. Furthermore, it may affect the traditional roles of these workers, and the existing relationships among groups of individuals—for example, between physicians and nurses, between nurses and patients, and between physicians and patients.

In addition, the introduction of computers into health-care settings raises important ethical and legal questions related to the confidentiality of patient information, the appropriate role of computers in patient care, especially in the medical decision-making process, and the responsibility of developers and users for ensuring the correct operation of the system. Although the technical issues of system development are important subjects of research, the organizational, sociological, ethical, and legal factors often are the crucial determinants of the success of a computer system within an institution and of the ease with which successful technology can be transferred to other institutions.

5.1.2 Functions of a Computer System

Computers have been used in every aspect of health-care delivery, from the simple processing of business data, to the collection and interpretation of physiological data, to the education of physicians and nurses. Each chapter in Part 2 of this book describes an important area for the application of computers in medicine. The unique characteristics of each problem area create special requirements for system builders to address. The underlying motivation for each of these diverse applications, however, is the computer's ability to help health professionals in some aspect of information management. We identify eight topics that define the range of basic functions that may be provided by medical computer systems: (1) data acquisition, (2) record keeping, (3) communication and integration, (4) surveillance, (5) information storage and retrieval, (6) data analysis, (7) decision support, and (8) education. Table 5.1 indicates the primary functions provided by each of the types of systems addressed in later chapters. Notice that most systems assist with several tasks. In addition, although decision support is noted as a primary function for only two categories of applications, essentially all uses of computers in medicine can be viewed as helping to support improved decision making in some way.

TABLE 5.1 The Primary Functions Provided by Medical Computer Systems in Each of the Application Areas Discussed in Part 2

Chapter	Data Acquisition	Record Keeping	Communication and Integration	Surveillance	Information Storage and Retrieval	Data Analysis	Decision Support	Education
6. Medical-Record Systems			X	X	X	X		
7. Hospital Information Systems		X	X	X				
8. Nursing Information Systems			X				X	
9. Laboratory Information Systems	X	X		X				
10. Pharmacy Systems		X		X				
11. Radiology Systems	X	X						
12. Patient-Monitoring Systems	X			X			X	
13. Office Systems		X					X	
14. Bibliographic-Retrieval Systems					X			
15. Clinical Decision-Support Systems							X	X
16. Clinical Research Systems						X	X	
17. Medical Education Systems								X
18. Health-Assessment Systems	X	X						

Data Acquisition

Health professionals require assistance with data acquisition when the number of data that must be collected and processed overwhelms human capabilities. One of the first uses of computers in a medical setting was the automatic analysis of specimens of blood and other body fluids. As we shall see in Chapter 9, laboratory technicians using manual techniques could not keep up with the growing demand for laboratory testing. Thus, researchers developed automated instruments for measuring chemical concentrations and for counting cells and organisms. Computer-based patient-monitoring systems that collect physiological data directly from patients were another early application of computing technology (see Chapter 12). The use of patient-monitoring systems ensures that vital signs, ECGs, and other indicators of patient status are measured frequently and consistently. More recently, researchers have developed the sophisticated medical imaging applications described in Chapter 11, including computed tomography, magnetic resonance imaging, and digital-subtraction angiography. These computationally intensive procedures cannot be performed manually because they require the collection and manipulation of millions of individual bits of information.

Computer systems that perform data acquisition often are self-contained medical instruments or measurement devices. This characteristic, however, is not essential. For instance, we consider computer-based history-taking systems (one component of the health-assessment systems described in Chapter 18) to be data-acquisition systems because they free health professionals from the need to collect and enter routine demographic and history information.

Record Keeping

Given the data-intensive nature of health-care delivery, it is no surprise that record keeping is a primary function of many medical computer systems. Computers are well suited to performing tedious and repetitive data-processing tasks, such as collecting and tabulating data, transcribing those data from one form to another, and formatting and producing reports. They are particularly useful for processing large volumes of data. Thus, an automated billing system is a natural application of computers in health-care settings, and typically is the first component installed when a hospital, clinic, or private practice decides to use computer technology.

Individual departments within a hospital have similar needs for automated data processing. Today, most clinical laboratories use computer-based information systems to keep track of orders and specimens and to report test results; many pharmacy and radiology departments also have acquired computers to perform analogous functions. By automating administrative processing in areas such as these, health-care facilities are able to speed up data processing, to reduce direct labor costs, and to reduce the number of errors. When computers are not available, the costs of these activities often are prohibitive.

Communication and Integration

In hospitals and other distributed health-care environments, myriad data are collected by multiple health professionals working in a variety of settings; each patient receives care from a host of providers—nurses, physicians, technicians, pharmacists, and so on. Communication among the members of the team is essential for effective health-care delivery. Data must be available to decision makers when and where they are needed; computers help by storing, transmitting, and displaying information. As we describe in Chapters 2 and 6, the medical record is the primary vehicle for communication of clinical information. A critical limitation of the traditional medical record, however, is the concentration of information in a single location, which prohibits simultaneous access by multiple people. HISs and automated medical-record systems allow decentralization of many activities, such as admission, appointment, and resource scheduling; review of laboratory-test results; and inspection of patient records.

Sometimes, not all the information necessary for decision making is available within a single computer system. For example, in many institutions, clinical and financial activities are supported by separate systems. Under current reimbursement schemes, however, hospital administrators must integrate clinical and financial information to analyze costs and to evaluate the efficiency of the health-care delivery process. Similarly, clinicians may need to review data collected at other institutions, or they may wish to consult online databases of biomedical information. The emergence of local-area networks (LANs) for sharing information among independent computers and wide-area networks (WANs) for exchanging information among geographically distributed sites promises increased communication and greater integration of information among distributed users.

Surveillance

Data overload is as detrimental to good decision making as is insufficient access to data. Sometimes, health professionals have available the data necessary for appropriate action, but they overlook those data. Surveillance and monitoring systems can help health professionals to cope with the enormous numbers of data relevant to patient management by calling attention to significant events—for example, by reminding doctors of the need to order screening tests and other preventive-health-care measures (see Chapter 6), or by warning them when a dangerous event or constellation of events has been detected.

Laboratory systems routinely identify and flag abnormal test results. Similarly, when patient-monitoring systems in intensive-care units detect a significant abnormality in a patient's status, they sound alarms to alert nurses and physicians to this potentially dangerous situation. A pharmacy system that maintains computer-based drug profile records for patients can screen incoming drug orders and warn physicians who order a drug that interacts with another drug the patient is receiving, or a drug to which the patient has a known allergy. By correlating data from multiple sources, an integrated HIS can monitor for even more complex events, such as interactions among patient diagnosis, drug regimen, and physiological status (indicated by laboratory-test results).

Information Storage and Retrieval

Storage and retrieval of information is essential to all computer systems. This function, however, is foremost in systems that serve as information archives. One reason for installing medical-record systems, for example, is the desire to archive patient data in a way that allows effective retrieval of those data. The query languages provided by many automated medical-record and clinical research systems assist researchers in retrieving pertinent records from among the many saved in the large databases of patient information. As we shall discuss in Chapter 14, bibliographic-retrieval systems now are essential to effective searching of the medical literature.

Data Analysis

Systems that aid decision makers in data analysis present information in a form that is more understandable than are the raw data. They may present data graphically to facilitate trend analysis, or they may compute secondary parameters (means, standard deviations, rates of change, and so on) from the primary data. Clinical research systems have modules for performing sophisticated statistical analyses of large sets of patient data, and typically provide facilities for graphically displaying data and results for easier interpretation.

Decision Support

In a sense, all the functions described here support decision making by health professionals. The distinction between decision-support systems and systems that monitor events and issue alerts is not clear-cut; the two differ primarily in the degree to which they interpret data and recommend patient-specific action. The best-known examples of decision-support systems are the clinical consultation systems that use population statistics or encode expert knowledge to assist physicians in diagnosis and treatment planning. Similarly, some nursing information systems help nurses to evaluate the needs of individual patients, and thus assist the nurses in allocating nursing resources. In Chapter 15, we shall discuss computer-based systems that use algorithmic, statistical, or artificial-intelligence techniques to provide advice about patient care.

Education

Rapid growth in biomedical knowledge and in the complexity of therapy management has produced an environment in which students cannot learn all they need to know during training—they must learn how to learn and make a lifelong educational commitment. Today, physicians and nurses have available a broad selection of computer programs designed to help them acquire and maintain the knowledge and skills they need to care for their patients. The simplest programs are of the drill and practice variety; more sophisticated programs can help students to learn complex problem-solving skills, such as diagnosis and therapy management (see Chapter 17). Computer-aided instruction provides a valuable means by which health professionals can gain experience and learn from mistakes without endangering real patients. Clinical decision-support systems and other systems that can explain their recommendations also perform an educational function. In the context of real patient cases, they can suggest actions and explain the reasons for those actions.

5.1.3 Identification and Analysis
of the Need for a Computer System

The first step in the introduction of computers in health-care settings is to identify a clinical, administrative, or research need—an inadequacy or inefficiency in the delivery of health care. The decision to acquire a computer system may be based on a desire to improve the *quality* of care, to lower the *cost* of care, to improve *access* to care, or to collect the information needed to document and evaluate the health-care delivery process itself. Sometimes, a computer-based system will correct defects in the old system; for example, more accurate record keeping can reduce the level of drug-administration errors. Other computer systems can provide functions not possible with manual systems—for example, they allow simultaneous access to patient records. In some cases, a computer system simply duplicates the capabilities of the manual system, but at lower cost.

It will become apparent in the following chapters that the number and sophistication of medical computer systems have increased substantially since the late 1950s and early 1960s, when computers were first applied to the problems of health-care delivery. The developers of new systems usually have made progress by building on lessons learned from past experiments, emulating the successes and trying to avoid the mistakes of other researchers in the field. As the discipline has matured, researchers have gained a better understanding both of the types of problems computer systems can solve and of the requirements for system success.

Clearly, computers can facilitate many aspects of health-care delivery. Installing a computer system, however, is not a panacea—for example, an information system cannot aid in decision making if critical information does not exist or if health professionals do not know how to apply the information once they have it. Similarly, a computer will not transform a poorly organized system into one that operates smoothly—automating a defective system may well make matters worse, not better. Performing a careful analysis prior to attempting a computer-based solution allows the system developers to clarify the requirements for change and may allow them to identify correctable deficiencies in the current system.

Ideally, we first recognize a *need,* then search for techniques to address it. At times, this logical sequence has been inverted; the development of new hardware or computing methodologies may encourage system developers to apply the state of the art in a medical context. Development that is driven by technology, however, often fails. The adoption of any new system requires users to learn and to adjust to a new routine; given the time constraints under which health professionals operate, users may be unwilling to discard a working system unless they perceive a clear reason to change.

Once health professionals have recognized a need for a computer system, the next step is to identify the function or combination of functions that fulfills that need. There usually are many possible solutions to a broadly defined problem. A precise definition of the problem narrows the range of alternative solutions. Is the problem one of access to data? Do health professionals have the data they need to make informed decisions? Is the problem an inability to analyze and interpret data? As we explained in the previous section, computer systems perform a variety of functions, ranging from simply displaying relevant information to aiding actively in complex decision making.

The natural temptation is to minimize this important first step of problem definition and to move directly to the solution phase. This approach is dangerous, however, and may result in the development of an unacceptable system. Consider, for example, a situation in which physicians desire improved access to patient data. Health-care personnel may seek assistance from technologists to implement a specific technical solution to the perceived problem. They may request that each patient's medical history be stored in a computer. When that is achieved, however, they may find that the relevant information is hidden among the many irrelevant data and is more tedious to access than before. If the system developers had analyzed the problem carefully, they might have realized that the raw medical data simply were too voluminous to be informative. A more appropriate solution also might include filtering or other data processing, so that only essential information or easy-to-read summaries are displayed.

The development of information systems requires a substantial commitment in terms of labor, money, and time. Once health professionals have clearly defined the need for a system, the question of worth inevitably arises. Scarce resources devoted to this project are unavailable for other potential projects. The administrator of a health-care institution, who works within a fixed budget, must decide whether to invest in a computer system or to spend the money in other ways—for example, an institutional decision maker may prefer to purchase new laboratory equipment, or to expand the neonatal intensive-care unit.

To assess the value of a medical information system relative to competing needs, the administrator must estimate the costs and the benefits attributable to the system. Some benefits are relatively easy to quantify. If admission clerks can process each admission twice as fast using the new system as they could using the old one, an institution will pay for fewer clerk-hours to process the same amount of work—a measurable savings in labor costs. Many benefits, however, are less easily quantified. For example, how can we quantify the benefits due to reduced patient mortality, increased patient satisfaction, or reduced stress and fatigue among the staff? In Chapter 19, we discuss various approaches to valuing life and health, and introduce cost-benefit and cost-effectiveness analyses, two methodologies decision makers can use to help assess the worth of a computer system relative to alternative investments.

5.2 Development and Implementation of Medical Information Systems

Whether they aim to produce a sophisticated HIS for a 500-bed hospital, a medical-record system for a small clinic, or a simple billing program for a physician in private practice, system developers should follow the same basic process. In the initial phase of system development, the primary task is to define the problem. The goal is to produce a clear and detailed statement of the system's objectives—that is, of what the system will do and what conditions it must meet if it is to be accepted by its users.

The systems analysts also must establish the relative priorities of multiple, sometimes conflicting, goals—for example, low cost, high efficiency, easy maintenance, and high reliability.

Once analysts have clearly specified the goals of the system, they must choose among alternative approaches for meeting those goals. Ideally, a commercial system exists that provides all the desired functions, but it may be necessary to custom-design a new system. Following acquisition or development of a system, the next step is to establish the system within the organization. Major activities at this stage include training users, and installing and testing the system; after the system is operational, it must be continually evaluated and maintained.

We frame the discussion of this section in terms of institutional system planning and development. Many of the same issues, however, apply to the development of smaller systems, albeit on a correspondingly smaller scale of complexity. Blum's article, described in the Suggested Readings, briefly examines issues of system development that are particularly relevant for practitioners who wish to build their own systems.

5.2.1 An Illustrative Case Study

In addition to identifying functional requirements, a **requirements analysis** must be sensitive to the varying needs and probable concerns of the system's intended users. These *human* aspects of computer system design often have been overlooked, and the results can be devastating. Consider, for example, the following hypothetical case, written by Shortliffe, that embodies many of the issues that are the subject of this chapter.[1] It provides a glimpse of some of the tasks that computer systems now perform in health-care settings. It also illustrates many of the problems that can and do arise when a new system perturbs the familiar routines of its users.

Three months ago, a major teaching hospital purchased and installed a large computer system that assists the physicians with ordering drugs and laboratory tests, the clinical laboratories with reporting laboratory-test results, the head nurses with creating nursing schedules, and the admissions staff with monitoring hospital occupancy. Personnel access the system using the VDTs located in each nursing unit. There also are printers associated with each unit, so that the computer can generate reports for the patient charts and worksheets used by the hospital staff. The HIS depends on a large, dedicated computer, which is housed in the hospital complex and is supported by several full-time personnel. It has modules to assist hospital staff with both

---

[1]This case study is adapted from one written by E. H. Shortliffe and appearing in "Coming to terms with the computer," in Reiser, S. J. and Anbar, M. (eds). *The Machine at the Bedside: Strategies for using technology in patient care.* Cambridge, England: Cambridge University Press, 1984, pp. 235–239 [Shortliffe, 1984a]. It is used here by permission from Cambridge University Press.

administrative and clinical duties. The following four modules are the primary subsystems used in patient care:

1. *The pharmacy system.* Using this component of the HIS, physicians order drugs for their patients; the requests are displayed immediately in the hospital pharmacy. Pharmacists then fill the prescriptions and affix computer-printed labels to each bottle. The drugs are delivered to the ward by a pneumatic-tube system. The computer keeps a record of all drugs administered to each patient; when new prescriptions are ordered, it warns physicians about possible drug interactions.

2. *The laboratory system.* Using this component, physicians order laboratory tests for their patients. The requests are displayed in the relevant clinical laboratory, and worksheets are created to assist laboratory personnel in planning blood-drawing schedules and performing tests. As soon as test results are available, health professionals can display them on the screen of any system terminal; in addition, paper summaries are printed on the wards for inclusion in the patients' charts.

3. *The bed-control system.* The admissions office of the hospital, in conjunction with the various ward administrators, uses this component to keep track of the location of patients within the hospital. When a patient is transferred to another ward, the computer is notified so that physicians, telephone operators, and other personnel can locate him easily. The system also is used to identify patients whose discharge has been ordered; thus, the system aids the admissions office in planning bed assignments for new patients.

4. *The diagnosis system.* To help physicians reach correct diagnoses for their patients, this component provides a clinical consultation program. Physicians enter their patient's signs and symptoms, laboratory-test results, and X-ray–examination results. Based on these data, the system suggests a list of likely diagnoses.

Despite the new capabilities provided by the HIS, the system received mixed reviews about its effectiveness. Most of the people who raised concerns were involved in patient care. A consulting expert was called in to assess the computer system's strengths and weaknesses. She interviewed members of the hospital staff and noted their responses.

A **nurse** said, "I like the system a lot. I found it hard to get used to at first (I never have been a very good typist), but once I got the hang of it, I found that it simplified much of my work. The worst problem has turned out to be dealing with doctors who don't like the system; when they get annoyed, they tend to take it out on us, even though we're using the system exactly as we've been trained to do. For instance, I can't log on to the computer as a physician to log verbal orders in someone else's name, and that makes some of the doctors furious. The only time I personally get annoyed with the computer is when I need to get some work done and the other nurses are using all the ward terminals. They ought to have a few more terminals available."

One **medical resident** was less than enthusiastic about the new HIS: "I wish they'd rip the darn thing out! It is totally unrealistic in terms of the kinds of things it asks us to do or won't allow us to do. Did the guys who built it have any idea what it is like to practice medicine in a hospital like this? For example, the only way we used to be able to keep our morning ward rounds efficient was to bring the chart rack with us and to write orders at the bedside. With the new system, we have to keep sending someone back to the ward terminal to log orders for a patient. What's worse, they won't let the medical student order drugs, so we have to send an intern. Even the nurses aren't allowed to log orders in our name—something to do with the 'legality' of having all orders entered by a licensed physician—but that was never a problem with paper order sheets as long as we eventually countersigned the orders. Some of the nursing staff are doing everything by the book now, and sometimes they seem to be obstructing efficiency rather than aiding it. And the designers were so hung up on patient confidentiality that we have a heck of a time cross-covering patients on other services at night. The computer won't let me write orders on any patient that isn't 'known' to be mine, so I have to get the other physicians' passwords from them when they sign out to me at night. And things really fall apart when the machine goes down unexpectedly. Everything grinds to a halt, and we have to save our management plans on paper and transcribe them into the system when it finally comes up. I should add that the system always seems to be about three hours late in figuring out about patient transfers. I'm forever finding that the computer still thinks a patient is on the first floor when I know he's been transferred to the intensive-care unit.

"In addition, the 'diagnosis system' is a joke. Sure, it can generate lists of diseases, but it doesn't really understand what the disease processes are, can't explain why it thinks one disease is more likely than another, and is totally unable to handle patients who have more than one simultaneous disease. I suppose the lists are useful as memory joggers, but I no longer even bother to use that part of the system.

"And by the way, I still don't really know what all those buttons on the terminal keyboard mean. We had a brief training session when they first installed the system, but now we're left to fend for ourselves. Only a couple of the house staff seem to know how to make the system do what they want reliably. What's the best part of the system? I guess it is the decrease in errors in orders for drugs and lab tests, and the improved turnaround time on those orders—but I'm not sure the improvement is worth the hassle. How often do I use the system? As rarely as possible!"

A **hospital pharmacist** said, "The HIS has been a real boon to our pharmacy operation. Not only can we fill new orders promptly because of the improved communication, but also the system prints labels for the bottles and has saved us the step of typing them ourselves. Our inventory control also is much improved; the system produces several useful reports that help us to anticipate shortages and to keep track of drugs that are soon to expire. The worst thing about the system, from my point of view, is the effect it has had on our interaction with the medical staff. We used to spend some of our time consulting with the ward teams about drug interactions, for example. You know, we'd look up the relevant articles and report back at ward rounds the next day. Now our role as members of the ward teams has been reduced by the system's knowledge about drugs. Currently, a house officer finds out about a potential drug interaction at the moment he is ordering a treatment, and the machine even gives references to support the reported incompatibility."

One member of the **HIS computing staff** expressed frustration: "Frankly, I think the doctors have been too quick to complain about this system. It has been here for only three months, and we're still discovering problems that will take some time to address. What bothers me is the gut reaction many of them seem to have; they don't even *want* to give the system a chance. Every hospital is a little different, and it is unrealistic to expect any HIS package to be right for a new institution on the first day. There has to be a breaking-in period. We're trying hard to respond to the complaints we've heard through the grapevine. We hope that the doctors will be pleased when they see that their complaints are being attended to and new features are being introduced."

This example, although hypothetical, does not exaggerate the kinds of reactions that computer systems have sometimes evoked in clinical settings. The case was inspired in part by Shortliffe's experience with a pharmacy system that was implemented in several teaching wards of the hospital where he served his medical internship. The initial version of the system failed to account for key aspects of the way in which health professionals practiced medicine, just as in the case study. The physicians objected loudly, and the system was subsequently removed. Although the system was later redesigned to remedy the earlier problems, it was never reimplemented, at least in part because of persistent negative bias caused by the failure of the earlier version.

Likewise, the introduction of a new blood-bank system at another institution instigated disputes between physicians and nurses over responsibility for the entry of blood orders. In this case, the system was designed to encourage direct order entry, but also allowed nurses to enter orders. Given the option, physicians continued to write paper orders and relied on nurses for order entry. Nurses, however, balked at performing this task, which they perceived as being the physicians' responsibility. Even matters that at first seem trivial can cause problems if work habits and requirements are not taken into account. At the same institution, for example, objection by surgeons was one factor in the decision to use passwords rather than machine-readable identification cards to control system access; surgeons typically do not carry personal belongings when wearing surgical garb and thus would have been unable to log on to the system [Gardner, 1989].

These cases help to emphasize the importance of careful design, of responsiveness to needs *as they are perceived by the intended users,* and of awareness of different users' varying perspectives when a system is intended to meet both clinical and administrative goals. The key considerations include (1) deciding whether to purchase from a commercial system vendor, (2) analyzing the system for software development, (3) designing for use, (4) involving users during development, and (5) planning for change. We shall discuss these five topics in detail in the remainder of this section.

5.2.2 The Decision of Whether to Purchase or to Build

Once an organization has decided to acquire a new computer system, it faces the choice of buying a commercial system or building a system in house. The primary tradeoff between purchasing a **turnkey system** (a vendor-supplied system that requires only installation and "the turn of a key" to make it operational) and developing a **custom-designed system** is one of functional compatibility versus expense and delay. In general, if an institution can find a commercial system that approximately meets its needs, then it should purchase that system. A vendor-supplied system usually is less expensive than is a custom-designed system, because the vendor can spread the costs of development over multiple clients. It also is available immediately, whereas a new system may take years to design and develop. Often, a turnkey system includes all the hardware, software, and technical support necessary to operate the system.

Unfortunately, the functions supplied by a turnkey system rarely match perfectly an institution's information-management needs. The system may not perform all the desired functions, may provide superfluous features, or may require some reorganization and modification of responsibilities and established flows of information within the institution. It also is important to consider carefully the reputation of the vendor and the terms of the contract, and to answer questions such as, "What is the extent of the support and maintenance?" and "To what extent will the vendor tailor the system to the institution (for example, by modifying the format of screens, the vocabulary used in coding classifications, and the like)?" If no available commercial system is adequate, then the institution may choose to build its own system or to make do with the current system; the option of keeping the current system always should be considered as one of the possible alternatives.

Before embarking on an ambitious project, administrators must assess whether the institution possesses the resources necessary for success. For example, do members of the inhouse staff have the knowledge and experience to implement a new system, or can outside consultants and technical staff be hired to assist in development? If outside consultants are used and if they succeed, will they continue to support the system, or will they provide for successors?

An important cost consideration is the time necessary to complete the project. Some simple tasks require a short development period of several months, but other projects may require years to complete. Successful systems may exist in research settings; however, developers should not underestimate the difficulty of transferring the technology to a working environment. A rule of thumb used by some researchers is that it will require *seven* times the work needed to develop an academically successful demonstration of a new computing technology to transform the system to a practical implementation. Furthermore, if the new technology has to be integrated with an existing computer system, the time already estimated must be multiplied by an additional factor of 3 or 4. During integration, computing personnel must modify the existing system, develop interfaces, and retrain system users. Even though many of the changes made during integration may be minor, the breadth of these changes means they will cost a great deal. The difficulty of technology transfer has been a significant obstacle to the growth of medical computing.

5.2.3 The Software-Development Process

If the institution is prepared to custom-tailor a computer system to meet its needs, system developers can employ a variety of software-engineering tools to organize and manage the development process. Such tools include formal approaches to system analysis, techniques of **structured programming,** and testing methodologies, as well as methodologies for managing the project and metrics for assessing the performance of the product and of the software-development process itself. The field of **software engineering** had its beginnings in the late 1960s and early 1970s. As the systems being developed grew more complex, teams of programmers, analysts, and managers replaced individual programmers working in isolation, and the software-development process grew increasingly complex and costly. At the same time, the costs of hardware and computing time (which previously dominated the total cost of a system) declined rapidly. It became imperative to produce correct, understandable, and modifiable systems in a timely and cost-effective manner.

Figure 5.2 depicts a classic model of the software-development process, from requirements analysis, through design, implementation, testing, and maintenance. In general, the tasks at one step must be completed before moving to the next step. As the figure suggests, however, there is feedback and iteration between successive steps. Although the *waterfall* model provides a traditional view of the software lifecycle, the inflexibility of the standard development process makes it inappropriate for many applications and developers have experimented with alternative models. Artificial-intelligence systems, for example, typically are designed to solve poorly structured problems. In these cases, problem definition and system design are entwined, and a strategy of rapid prototyping and iterative refinement may be more appropriate.

The design phase can be decomposed into two steps. First, systems analysts must specify the system's behavior precisely and concisely—the specific tasks the system must accomplish, the data it requires, the results it will produce, the performance requirements for speed and reliability, and so on. It is at this phase of development that system developers answer questions such as, "What are the sources of necessary

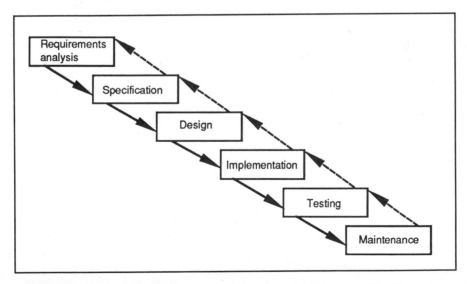

FIGURE 5.2 The waterfall model is the oldest and most well-known model of the system-development process. According to this model, system development proceeds through sequential phases.

information?" and "What are the existing mechanisms for communication in the current system?" Once the functional design has been developed, it can be expanded into a detailed design that can be implemented.

For all but the tiniest systems, developers need to create models to help them to understand the functions of the system. Systems can be partitioned into subsystems, subsystems into smaller components, and so on, until the whole has been decomposed into manageable chunks (Figure 5.3). What we consider a system versus a subsystem, however, often is a matter of perspective, and the boundaries delimiting related systems may not be clear-cut. Notice in Figure 5.3, for example, that a hospital information system (HIS) can be viewed as a hierarchy of nested and interrelated subsystems. In general, a system has strong internal linkages relative to its linkages with the external world.

Earlier in the chapter, we described a system in terms of *data* and *processes* for transforming input to output. In *structured analysis,* one classic approach to system design, developers view systems in terms of such processes.[2] A graphical representation called the data-flow diagram (DFD) provides a succinct way to describe such a partitioning of the system. It represents the sources and destinations of data, the processes for transforming the data, and the points in the system where long- or short-term data storage is required. The DFD in Figure 5.4(a) is a model of a simple laboratory information system. It illustrates the flow of laboratory-test orders and

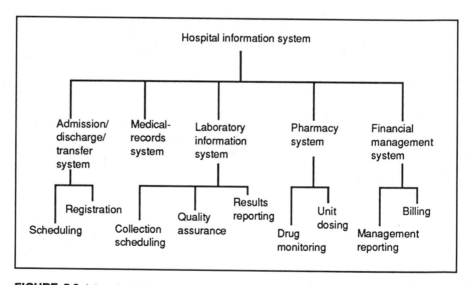

FIGURE 5.3 A hospital information system comprises interrelated subsystems that serve individual departments. In turn, each subsystem comprises multiple functional subcomponents.

---

[2]The structured-analysis approach is only one of various software engineering methodologies that are currently in use. New variations of this method are continually being developed, and alternative design approaches that model a system in terms of the data it uses, rather than in terms of processes, also have been developed.

results and the basic functions of the proposed system: (1) creation of specimen-collection schedules, (2) analysis of results, (3) reporting of test results, and (4) performance of quality-assurance activities. The designer can describe each higher-level process in the DFD by creating a more detailed DFD (Figure 5.4b).

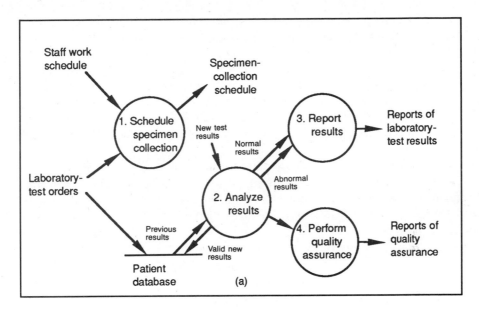

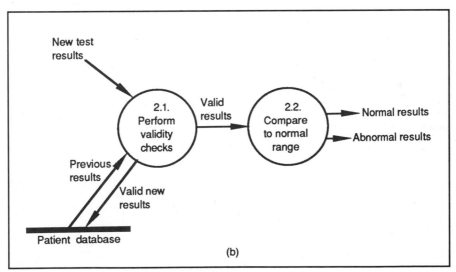

FIGURE 5.4 A data-flow diagram (DFD) graphically represents the processes and data flows within a laboratory information system. (a) *Bubbles* depict processes (or functions), *vectors* depict data flows, and *straight lines* depict databases. (b) Often, DFDs are layered to show greater detail within higher-level processes. This second-level DFD decomposes the process of analyzing test results into two lower-level processes. Note that the net inputs and outputs of this DFD match the inputs and outputs of the higher-level process in (a).

Many informal mechanisms for data communication and storage that exist in manual systems disappear when computers are used to process data. Health professionals trade much valuable information in hallways and at nursing stations; for example, they will discuss a baffling case to help develop new insights and approaches. Some crucial information never enters the formal record, but is noted on scraps of paper or stored in people's memories. Such informal methods of information management serve health care well, and are easily overlooked in a formal analysis. System designers must take care to identify and replace such mechanisms. The absence of even minor functions can produce errors in health-care delivery and will be perceived as a failure of the system, thus leading to resistance by the users. Recall from the hypothetical case, for example, the friction between physicians and nurses that occurred when the new system failed to allow for verbal orders. Often, technologists discount resistance as an unwillingness to keep up with progress, but they should interpret it as a signal that something is wrong with the new system.

Information-systems development is a political as well as a technical process. Health institutions, just like all other organizations, are composed of different groups of individuals, and often these groups have conflicting priorities, objectives, and values. Health administrators, physicians, nurses, ancillary personnel, and patients have different needs that the computer system should meet. Information systems can alter relationships among these people—they affect patterns of communication, perceived influence, authority, and control. A strategy for implementation must recognize and deal with these political forces. A new system should disrupt the organizational infrastructure as little as possible. Keen's article listed in the Suggested Readings discusses the political aspects of system development and implementation in greater detail.

5.2.4 The Match Between Design and Use

The success of a system depends not only on the system's ability to meet the informational needs of its users, but also on the manner in which human and machine interact. The resident's complaints in the hypothetical example illustrate an important point: The disruption of effective and established routines and the inconvenience often associated with computer information systems can cause users to work around the system and thus to fail to use its features. Studies of the attitudes of medical personnel regarding computer-based clinical consultation systems have shown that successful programs not only must provide expert-level advice, but also must be integrated into the daily routines of physicians and other users [Teach and Shortliffe, 1981; Friedman and Gustafson, 1977]. Computer-based information systems should acknowledge the hectic schedules of health professionals, and should demystify and simplify the mechanics of the human–computer interface. By involving users in system design, developers can avoid many of the impediments to widespread success.

The following parameters of computer systems are among the most important to consider during system design:

- *Quality and style of interface.* From a user's point of view, a system's interface *is* the system. In the past, the developers of medical computer systems have paid insufficient attention to the quality of the interface between users and computers.

With the growth of interactive computing and the trend toward the use of computers by nontechnical users, computing personnel have begun to realize the importance of developing user-friendly interfaces; there is a growing body of research related to the psychology of the human–machine interaction. Physicians' reluctance to communicate with computers by typing at a keyboard is well known. Thus, system developers have used a number of alternative devices for interaction, including light pens, touch screens, and mouse pointing devices. Other researchers are investigating speech recognition and natural-language understanding with the hope that someday talking with computers will be as natural and easy as talking with humans is now. Menus, graphics, and the use of color all help to make systems more attractive and simpler to learn and use, and online help is invaluable for teaching new procedures. In systems that perform decision support and offer advice about patient care, the style of communication is particularly important. Is the system too terse or too verbose? Does it project a helpful attitude, or does it seem pedantic or judgmental? Can it justify its recommendations?

- *Convenience.* Users must have convenient access to the system. The number and placement of terminals and printers are important considerations if the system is to be assimilated into users' routines. For example, if a medical-record system is intended to replace the traditional medical record, it must be accessible wherever and whenever health professionals need to look up patient data—in the physician's office, in the nursing station, possibly at the bedside, and so on. Enough terminals should be available that users do not have to wait long to use the system, even during times of peak use.

- *Speed.* System developers must choose hardware that has sufficient capacity to handle users' demands for information during peak hours, and they must design software that allows users timely access to the data, in the correct form. Health professionals are understandably reluctant to use systems that are tedious or unduly time consuming.

- *Reliability.* Health personnel must resort to manual procedures if they are to continue to work in the event of hardware or software failure. Frequent data backup and redundant hardware can minimize the loss of data and the amount of time that the system is unavailable.

- *Security.* The confidentiality of sensitive medical data is an important issue in the design of medical information systems. The system should be easily accessible to authorized personnel, yet inaccessible to unauthorized users. These goals, however, are difficult to achieve. The most common compromise solution is to assign an account with a password to each user. Variable access to the data then can be controlled for individual users or for classes of users. Some operations may be restricted to particular terminals. For example, the ability to modify patient charges might be restricted to financial personnel working from terminals located in the accounting office.

- *Integration.* The integration of independent systems eliminates some of the difficulties and enhances the benefits of using computer systems. If, for example, a laboratory system and a pharmacy system are independent and incompatible, health professionals must access two separate systems (possibly from different terminals) to view a single patient's data. If the two systems need to share data, people will have to collect output from the first and reenter it into the second system. The development of LANs to allow exchange of information among independent systems will reduce the need for redundant entry and storage of critical information (a time-consuming process that also is a source of errors).

5.2.5 Involvement of Users During Development

Although the central focus of this chapter is *computer*-based information systems, you should realize that people are a critical component of these systems: People identify the need for systems; people develop, implement, and evaluate the systems; and, eventually, people operate the systems. A successful system must take into account both the needs of the intended users and the constraints under which these users function.

Even the most perceptive and empathetic developer cannot anticipate all the needs of all users. Thus, the success of a system depends on interaction between health and technical personnel. Effective communication among the participants, however, potentially is difficult because these people are likely to have widely varying backgrounds, education, and experience.

A major barrier to communication is attributable to a difference between the health-care and general scientific paradigms. In Section 1.6, we discussed the ways in which clinical information differs from the information used in the basic sciences (recall the difference between low-level and high-level sciences), and we examined reasons why some medical computer scientists suggest that medical computing differs fundamentally from basic computer science. In medical practice, as in other human tasks, we expect that a person who can deal with a certain type of problem can, with little incremental effort, extrapolate to handle similar and related problems. In the formal mathematical sciences, however, the ability to solve problems can depend critically on what appear to be relatively minor differences in basic assumptions.

The rigor of the mathematical approach also is reflected in computer systems; computer systems never are as flexible as people are. Although it is easy to imagine that a computer program that deals with one class of problems embodies sufficient concepts to deal with other (seemingly) similar problems, the work required to adapt or extend the program often costs as much as, and sometimes costs much more than, the original development. Occasionally, adaptation is impossible. The problems of extrapolation often are not well appreciated by health-care professionals, because most of these people's interactions are with humans rather than with machines.

Empathy for the differences in the two approaches to problem solving can minimize some problems. Medical informatics specialists—people trained in both computer science and health science—can facilitate communication and mediate discussions. They can ease the process of specifying accurately and realistically the need for a system, and of designing workable solutions to satisfy that need. One objective of this book is to provide basic material for people serving this intermediary role.

5.2.6 Creation of Plans for Change

Many medical information systems, particularly custom-designed systems, take a long time to develop. This delay can be problematic; without effective communication, it is difficult for the medical establishment to perceive what is being done by the system development staff, and the development staff receives no feedback on the correctness of the assumptions on which they are basing their design. The involvement of users through demonstrations, training sessions, and incremental installation of the system can build the enthusiasm and support of users and provide computing personnel an invaluable means for evaluating progress.

Prototype systems—working models that exhibit the essential features of the system under development—facilitate communication between computing personnel and users. Users develop a realistic idea of how the system will look, how it will work, and what it will do. Developers receive feedback and can modify the system in response to users' comments, thus improving the likelihood that the final system will be deemed acceptable. A good prototype provides a realistic demonstration of the method of interaction with the system and should be able to deal with most of the common varieties of data input. Much simplification, however, is possible when reliability and data permanence can be ignored, as they can in a prototype system that is intended only for demonstration and discussion purposes.

Formal training courses also can help to dispel the mystery of a new system. Without adequate reinforcement, however, people are apt to forget what they learn. A training program should start slowly and should extend over a long period. At first, teachers should clarify basic concepts and initiate users to the general operational environment. When system installation is imminent, health professionals should receive specific and intensive training in the use of the system. Experience with the Apple Macintosh interface suggests that the development of intuitive interfaces and systems that allow users to experiment and explore their capabilities can reduce the need for formal training.

The problems associated with a major change can be greatly ameliorated by **phased installation.** For instance, a schedule in which the components of an HIS are installed at 3-month intervals permits the staff to gain familiarity gradually. Phased installation also permits the implementors to deal with problems incrementally, rather than all at once. The feedback provided to the developers during successive phases helps to ensure that problems will not be repeated or multiplied as the system nears completion.

Training is simplified if part of the system is operational. Users can see real examples of the system in action, and thus are less likely to develop overly ambitious expectations. Because those parts of the system that are installed first usually are less problematic, users often view the initial phase as a success. Furthermore, the attitude generated by initial success can enhance the acceptance of the system in other areas, including in those locations that inherently are more difficult to address using computer-based techniques. In hospitals, for instance, computer systems often are used first in the admissions office, where the applications are relatively straightforward, and later are expanded for use on medical wards, where the user community is particularly diverse and demanding.

Gradual installation also decreases the risk of failure, because developers can adapt the system in response to criticism generated from earlier phases. If early components of the total system are judged to be failures, additional system development and installation can be abandoned, thus avoiding major loss. There have been a number of cases in which complete systems were developed and installed, and subsequently were found to be unacceptable. In these institutions, later computer-system developers first had to overcome the staff's negative feelings that had been generated by the earlier projects. A similar problem arises if an early stage of a phased installation fails, but at least fewer people need to be converted to cooperate with developers of subsequent phases.

5.3 Evaluation of Medical Information Systems

The goal of system design is to combine the functions of data acquisition and storage, information processing, and information display to create a system that effectively meets users' informational needs. How well does a system meet this goal? Continued expenditure of resources, or the decision to adopt a system for widespread use, requires an answer to this question. But issues of evaluation are complex, especially because there are so many variables one could choose to measure. In fact, many workers in medical computing believe that new methods for **staged evaluation** of systems are themselves worthy of attention by researchers [National Library of Medicine, 1986b].

Evaluation should continue throughout the lifetime of a system. The goals and formality of an evaluation study should depend, however, on the system's stage of development. We discussed how incremental feedback and informal evaluation during development help to keep a project on track and to alert developers to the need for midcourse correction. As a system reaches the final phases of development, more formal evaluations are appropriate to test whether the system performs correctly, is acceptable to users, and is cost-effective.

There are at least eight steps in evaluating a developing system:

1. Define the measures of success and the study methodology
2. Demonstrate the feasibility of the design
3. Run informal test cases to gain feedback from users
4. Formally evaluate performance
5. Formally evaluate acceptability to users
6. Evaluate the system in a limited test site
7. Evaluate the system in its intended environment
8. Continually reevaluate the operational system to identify errors, necessary modifications, and desired enhancements

The results of each successive evaluation guide further development and aid the interpretation of future studies [Shortliffe and Buchanan, 1984]. For example, if users fail to accept a system, but previous analyses of the system's performance showed positive results, researchers can focus on the user interface or logistical problems as the cause of poor acceptance.

Evaluation is particularly important during the maintenance phase if a system is to be flexible and responsive to changes in users' needs. An estimated 60 to 80 percent of software costs are incurred during the maintenance phase of system operation. During this phase, the support staff modifies the system to correct defects and to enhance capabilities. They also assess the system's performance in light of changing requirements for information, evolving user expectations, and advancing technology.

5.3.1 Performance

Formal evaluation consists of collecting and analyzing measures of system performance, and generating recommendations. Typically, measures are quantifiable, facilitating comparison among institutions or with the same institution over time. A natural place to start when evaluating a medical information system is to ask, "Does the system meet the clinical or administrative need that it was intended to satisfy?"

In the case of clinical systems, we often classify evaluation parameters in two general categories: process measures and outcome measures. **Process measures** describe the effects of the computer system in terms of changes to the way the overall health-care delivery system functions. For example, one objective of installing a pharmacy system often is to reduce the incidence of medication errors that can occur when drug orders are not kept current. Comparison of rates of medication errors before and after installation of the computer system thus provides a useful process measure for evaluating system performance. **Outcome measures** for a clinical system reflect the health status of the relevant population—for example, the changes in mortality and morbidity rates correlated with use of the system. Useful outcome measures for a pharmacy system might be the hospital length of stay or the rate of drug-related complications experienced by patients.

In general, outcome measures are more difficult to collect and compare than are process measures. In addition, they often are affected by external factors, independent of the computer system, or provide a measure that must be interpreted with great care. For instance, although a reduction in the rate of medication errors should reduce the average length of time that patients stay in the hospital, a well-run hospital should not have such a high error rate that length of stay will be significantly affected by a reduction in the number of errors. Furthermore, many medication errors will not increase the length of stay, and errors that result in patient death actually may *decrease* the average length of stay! Note also that the distinction between process and outcome is not always clear. For example, hospital length of stay could be considered a process variable—it measures the health of a patient only indirectly.

The ideal objective always is to determine the system's effect on outcome, even though one may have to measure process variables that proxy for patient outcome. In the pharmacy example, we believe that medication errors do affect outcome, but if the relationship between process and outcome is not well established, we could be misled by parameters that have little relationship to our objectives. Stated in a slightly different way, it is important to keep our top-level outcome objectives in mind when designing evaluation studies; obtaining good process measurements must not emerge as the objective of the system just because process variables are relatively easy to measure.

Let us illustrate this concept by continuing our pharmacy example. The system records the time of day that medications are administered. An overly rigid evaluation criterion might classify as a nursing error the administration of a medication more than 1 hour before or after the scheduled time; one process measure might be the rate of occurrence of such administration-timing errors. In practice, waking the patient to administer routine medication precisely on time might be more harmful to health and recovery than delaying the medication would be. If the hospital administration pressured nurses to reduce this type of error, patient morbidity might increase.

5.3.2 Cost-Effectiveness

Cost reduction due to labor saved in performing clerical tasks often is a primary motivation for implementing a medical information system. As we shall discuss in Chapter 19, changes in the financial forces acting on health institutions have resulted in greater cost-consciousness in the health industry. Computer systems represent large commitments in resources for health institutions, but their potential to reduce labor costs, to increase productivity, and to improve the quality of patient care make them economically reasonable and even necessary features of the health-care environment. Thus, studies to measure the cost-effectiveness of computer systems are of interest to institutions that have installed systems, to institutions that are contemplating adding a system, and to the funding agencies that support experimental system development.

Financial systems, such as those that handle billing and payroll, and the administrative components of laboratory information systems clearly are cost-effective. These systems dramatically increase the productivity of workers in processing large volumes of information. Evaluating the cost-effectiveness of less circumscribed systems that perform many functions, however, has proved to be both difficult and expensive.

Drazen summarized and critiqued 11 cost studies of automated HISs designed to manage patient data [Drazen, 1980]. Most of the studies focused on direct-cost variables such as changes in productivity and the effect of these changes on personnel costs. Drazen concluded that the studies' assumptions tended to overstate cost savings and to understate the costs of installing and operating a system, thus producing unrealistic estimates of the net effect of an HIS on costs. In the original studies, the researchers did little to assess direct costs and benefits to patients or indirect benefits such as improved quality of care, decreased data loss, and improved turn-around times for test ordering and results reporting.

The most extensive evaluation of a hospital information system was funded by the National Center for Health Services Research and was conducted by the Battelle Memorial Institute [Barrett et al., 1979]. The study concluded that the Technicon Medical Information System (TMIS; see Chapter 7) produced a 5-percent savings in nursing costs per patient, and that costs grew more slowly at El Camino Hospital than at comparable hospitals once the system was installed. From the perspective of total hospital costs, however, the results were not definitive.

5.3.3 User Acceptance

Evaluators often view an information system in terms of that system's functionality. Does it provide accurate information? Does it improve productivity? Does it reduce costs? Most formal evaluations have examined these aspects of system performance. Yet, the criteria for system success are broader, encompassing both functional performance and acceptability to users.

The case study we described early in this chapter illustrated many of the problems that arise when a hospital tries to integrate automated and manual systems— problems that stem from the disruption of normal routines and those related to the convenience and ease of system use. The low acceptability of many systems to users is one of the major barriers to widespread adoption of computer technology in health-care settings. Furthermore, resistance by unhappy users can reduce or eliminate anticipated cost savings.

We reemphasize the importance of designing systems that can be integrated with health professionals' existing information-management routines. Providing time-saving features (for example, the automatic generation of routine reports that previously were created manually) will help to counterbalance increased inconvenience in other areas (for example, data entry). Furthermore, the coordination of subsystems within an institution and information sharing using network technology will help users to reach the critical point at which the benefits exceed the large fixed costs of acquiring a new system. Equally important is the need to involve users in the development of systems and to support them with ample training, so that they can understand both the reasons for change and the methods for achieving change effectively.

Actual use patterns provide the ultimate and the most realistic evaluation; if a system is accepted by its end users and functions adequately in the real world, then it is a success. Here a pragmatic question is whether the users are paying real money for the services provided. If the system is free or subsidized, then acceptance is not an adequate indication that the benefits exceed the cost. In other instances, system usage is imposed from above; users may work with the system, but they may be dissatisfied. If the system is innovative, then the transfer of a system or technology to other sites is another indication of success.

5.3.4 Safety

The most problematic evaluation issues are the ethical and legal issues related to the safe and appropriate use of computer-based systems. Such systems always will be subject to errors, albeit subtle ones, in both design and implementation. Furthermore, the consequences of computer errors in health-care environments are potentially serious, and could result in increased patient morbidity or mortality. Understandably, safety is a major concern, and the testing and evaluation of medical computer systems is an important issue. When is a computer system "safe" for use in caring for patients?

Systems that perform straightforward data-reporting and record-keeping functions can be evaluated for correctness by rigorous testing in a variety of situations. The **validation** of systems that interpret data and provide patient-specific advice or affect patient care directly, however, poses serious conceptual problems. For example, in the evaluation of a program that assists physicians in diagnosis or therapy planning, the most serious conceptual problem is that of establishing a *gold standard* for correctness—what is the *correct* answer (see Chapters 2 and 15)? Often, medical experts disagree about a patient's diagnosis, or about the preferable way to treat the patient. Should the system be considered correct only when it determines the actual diagnosis (if the experts agree on what that diagnosis is)? What if it reaches the same (incorrect) diagnosis as the experts do? What is an acceptable level of performance? Given the degree of uncertainty inherent in diagnosis and therapy management, even experts are sometimes wrong.

Another question is how often a decision-support program must be updated to reflect advances in medical knowledge. New findings in medical science may invalidate conclusions that previously were considered to be correct. Furthermore, due to unanticipated interactions between program code and the data it manipulates, modifications that correct deficits in one part of the system can introduce errors into other parts that were correct before the changes were made.

Government regulation of medical software has been a topic of intense study in recent years. How much of a role should the government play in the premarket regulation of medical computer systems? After much discussion, the Food and Drug Administration (FDA) concluded that the analogy between computer information systems and other sources of medical information—textbooks, for example—is valid (also see Chapter 15). The FDA's current policy is *not* to regulate medical software designed to be used by a trained practitioner who assesses the program's advice before following its recommendations [Young, 1987]. Therefore, the only software systems that currently fall under FDA regulation are medical devices and instruments that directly control a patient's treatment, such as computer-controlled drug-infusion pumps and respirators; the developers of these types of computer systems must demonstrate the safety and efficacy of their products prior to releasing those products on the market.

To what type of liability are the designers, developers, distributors, and users subject if a defect in the medical software, or misuse of the clinical decision-support system, results in harm to a patient? As yet, no formal legal precedents have been set. A pivotal concern is whether the courts will apply negligence law (which requires only that a system meet reasonable expectations for safety) or product liability law (which requires that a product cause no harm) [Miller et al., 1985]. The resolution of legal and ethical issues related to the use of medical computer systems will affect the degree to which clinical decision-support systems and other medical software evolve from experimental prototypes and are incorporated into health-care settings.

Computer systems potentially can facilitate many aspects of information management as this subject relates to the delivery of health care. Each of the chapters in Part 2 discusses some aspect of medical practice where computers are used. How well the systems achieve their potential depends on how well they are designed; as we have seen, state-of-the-art computer hardware and software technology are not enough. System designers must be ingenious in building systems that respond to the needs of the users and fit in with the constraints of the medical environment.

Computer systems have been used in health-care settings for over 2 decades, yet today, relatively few health-care institutions employ the full range of automation possible, and many clinical information systems remain in the realm of research. In the past, some of the barriers to widespread implementation have been related to the limited capabilities of the hardware and software techniques. Although technical considerations still are significant, we now better understand how to overcome the major problems of data storage and retrieval, multiuser environments, networking, and so on. Many of the remaining barriers have to do with people—these issues generally have not been addressed adequately. We now have an improved understanding of the needs of the people who use medical computer systems; next, we must work to build systems that meet those needs.

Suggested Readings

Anderson, J. G. and Jay, S. J. (eds). *Use and Impact of Computers in Clinical Medicine.* New York: Springer-Verlag, 1987.

This collection of papers presents research on the factors that affect the adoption, diffusion, and use of clinical information systems in hospitals. It includes chapters on the attitudes of health professionals toward computers and the likely effects of clinical systems on aspects of medical practice, such as the role of physicians, the relations between doctors and patients, and the organization of the health-care delivery system.

Blum, B. How to implement systems. *M.D. Computing,* 4:50, 1987.

This article reviews the system-development process, data-flow diagrams, and structured coding techniques for health professionals who wish to design and develop their own software systems.

Charette, R. N. *Software Engineering Environments.* New York: McGraw-Hill, 1986.

This book discusses the high cost of software, the great variation in software-development practices, and the low productivity of developers—three major problems that plague current software development. It describes each phase of system development in detail, and introduces general techniques of software engineering and system development.

Keen, P. G. W. Information systems and organizational change. *Communications of the ACM,* 24:24, 1981.

This paper emphasizes the pluralistic nature of organizations. It discusses the changes in patterns of communication, influence, and control that often occur when new information systems are implemented, and suggests strategies for minimizing social inertia and resistance.

Miller, R. A., Schaffner, K. F., and Meisel, A. Ethical and legal issues related to the use of computer programs in clinical medicine. *Annals of Internal Medicine,* 102:529, 1985.

This article raises provocative questions. For example, in what situations is it appropriate to use medical computer programs? How can society determine whether a program is safe for human use? What is the legal status of a program that provides medical advice? Is it possible to achieve a proper balance between the needs for confidentiality of patient information and for shared access to medical records by health personnel?

Orthner, H. F. and Blum, B. I. (eds). *Implementing Health Care Information Systems.* New York: Springer-Verlag, 1989.

This book provides an overview of health-care applications for information systems. It introduces important issues that must be addressed by system developers, and reviews system-development techniques that have been used in health-care settings.

Reiser, S. J. and Anbar, M. (eds). *The Machine at the Bedside: Strategies for using technology in patient care.* Cambridge, England: Cambridge University Press, 1984.

> *This book discusses the theory and use of health-care technologies—such as cardiac arrhythmia monitoring, diagnostic imaging, and electronic fetal monitoring—in the context of legal, ethical, economic, and social concerns. It contains 23 case studies that depict the benefits and limitations of using these technologies.*

Shortliffe, E. H. and Buchanan, B. G. The problem of evaluation. In Buchanan, B. G. and Shortliffe, E. H. (eds). *Rule-Based Expert Systems.* Reading, MA: Addison-Wesley, 1984, pp. 571–588.

> *This article summarizes the lessons learned during three evaluation studies of the MYCIN expert system. It discusses in greater detail the concept of staged evaluations and the issues that arise when researchers are deciding what aspects of a clinical consultation system to evaluate and how to perform the studies. Most of the discussion is relevant to the evaluation of any medical computer system.*

Questions for Discussion

1. Reread the hypothetical case in Section 5.2.1.
   a. What are the primary benefits of the HIS? What are the primary disadvantages?
   b. Do you think that the benefits of the HIS outweigh the problems? Are there adequate noncomputer solutions to the problems the HIS was designed to help people solve?
   c. How would you change the HIS? Among the topics you might address are the effect of the computer on hospital routine, the reliability of the computer system, the availability of terminals, and the adequacy of user training programs.
2. Describe an outpatient clinic's billing system in terms of inputs, outputs, and processes. Sketch a simple data-flow diagram that represents your model of the system.
3. Discuss the inherent tension between protecting the confidentiality of patient records and providing health professionals with rapid and convenient access to clinical information. What level of system security do you believe provides an appropriate balance between these conflicting goals?
4. Discuss three barriers to technology transfer among health-care institutions.
5. Explain the difference between *outcome* and *process* measures of system performance. Identify two outcome and two process parameters that you might use to evaluate the performance of a clinical consultation system that assists physicians in diagnosing disease. Describe an experiment that you could perform to evaluate the effect of the system on one of these parameters. What potential difficulties can you foresee in conducting the experiment?
6. In what ways is the use of a clinical consultation system similar to the use of human consultants or static sources of medical information such as textbooks? In what ways is it different? Do you agree or disagree with the FDA's current policy for regulating medical software? Why or why not?

II

Medical Computing Applications

6

Medical-Record Systems

Clement J. McDonald and G. Octo Barnett

After reading this chapter, you should know the answers to these questions:

- What are the primary functions of a medical record?
- What are the advantages and disadvantages of a computer-stored medical record?
- How do automated ambulatory medical-record systems differ from hospital information systems?
- What are the options for entering into a computer the data collected by physicians?
- What are the common types of computer-generated output reports?
- What are query and surveillance systems, and how do they facilitate the provision of medical care?

6.1 What Is the Medical Record?

The preceding chapters introduced the conceptual basis for the field of medical computing. A central theme in these chapters is the notion of modern health professionals as information managers who collect and analyze data from myriad sources in caring for their patients. We devoted a large part of Chapter 2 to discussing the various types and uses of these medical data. The repository for this information is the medical record, an abstracted, filtered account of a patient's encounter with the health-care system.

For many years, the paper medical record served physicians well, but, as we also noted in Chapter 2, logistical and practical limitations reduce the effectiveness of traditional records for storing and organizing great numbers of diverse data. In this chapter, we shall see how computer-based medical-record systems offer potential solutions to many of these limitations.

6.1.1 Purposes of a Medical Record

Lawrence Weed [Weed, 1969] was perhaps the first person to analyze seriously the purposes of the medical record. We can now divide these purposes into three classes of functions: The medical record facilitates patient care, serves as a financial and legal record, and aids clinical research. Because the medical record is a human artifact, however, its purposes are not immutable. We can expect the functions of the medical record to change as new technologies provide alternative methods for recording and analyzing data, and as financial and legal institutions impose new requirements for documentation and reporting.

Patient Care

The main purpose of the medical record is to facilitate patient care. The record summarizes a patient's history and documents the observations, diagnostic conclusions, and plans of health-care personnel. In a sense, it serves as an external memory to which health-care providers can refer when they think about a patient at a later time.

The medical record also provides a means of communication between specialists and referring physicians, between physicians and nurses, and so on. In a hospital, it is the main conduit for action. Physicians initiate diagnostic and therapeutic actions by recording orders on the medical chart. The people who complete the orders, in turn, record their actions and observations; for example, technicians record the results of laboratory tests, pharmacists keep records of the medications they dispense, and nurses note the details of their interactions with patients.

The hospital medical record is the primary mechanism for ensuring **continuity of care** during a patient's hospitalization. The **ambulatory medical record** helps to ensure continuity *across* outpatient visits. As life expectancy increases and the population ages, the focus of ambulatory medicine shifts to emphasize preventive medicine and the treatment of chronic illness rather than that of acute illness. The ambulatory medical record enables health-care professionals to view data collected over time, and thus to track the course of problems and diseases [Bleich et al., 1985].

Legal and Financial Requirements

The medical record is the foundation for determining whether a patient received proper care. The chart often contains information concerning a health-care professional's actions and the justifications for those actions. For the health-care provider involved in litigation, the contents may either protect or incriminate. Apart from meeting legal requirements, the medical record provides the basis for professional and institutional quality assurance; professional-standards review organizations (PSROs; see Chapter 19) and hospital-accreditation organizations judge the appropriateness of the care delivered from the information recorded in medical records. Legal requirements influence the handling of records, as well as their content. Records must be resistant to change, and must be available for at least seven years after a patient's last visit. Records of children must be preserved until they are adults, and many experts recommend maintaining patient records for a person's entire life *plus* seven years.

Medical record keeping also affects the fiscal health of an institution. Information needed to classify patients into diagnosis-related groups (DRGs; the basis for Medicare payments; see Chapter 19) is abstracted from the medical record. Third-party carriers (insurance companies) disallow charges for procedures not documented in the medical record. When third-party carriers contest lump-sum (unitemized) drug bills, for example, hospital administrators rely on the medical record to provide a detailed breakdown of drug orders. From the other side, hospitals scrutinize medical records to find procedures performed by health-care personnel but not charged to the patient.

Research Support

Medical records have long been a source of new medical knowledge. Retrospective studies based on medical-record reviews have identified important medical relationships—for example, that smoking increases the risk of cancer, and that taking birth-control pills increases the risk of venous thrombosis and pulmonary embolism. Much epidemiological research is based on retrospective analysis of large sets of patient records (see Chapter 16).

6.1.2 Use of a Computer-Stored Medical Record

In Chapter 2, we discussed the disadvantages of the traditional paper medical record. Here we see how computer-stored medical-record systems can remedy many of these shortcomings.

Advantages

Inaccessibility is a common drawback of paper records. In large hospitals, the traditional record may be unavailable for days because it is being used in the business office, or is stashed away waiting for a discharge transcription by the attending physician. With computer-stored records and a nearby terminal, physicians can access patient data in seconds rather than waiting the minutes or hours required to retrieve a paper record. Computer-based records permit **remote access**; for example, a doctor can access data from her home. They also permit **simultaneous access**; for example, an office nurse can review a patient's blood pressures, while in another room the physician reviews the patient's laboratory results—a feat impossible with the paper chart.

Computer-based systems provide more legible and better organized reports—the reports are more legible because they are not handwritten, and are better organized because computers impose structure on the data they contain. The computer can improve the completeness and quality of entered data by automatically applying validity checks (see Section 6.3.1). Moreover, an interactive system can prompt the user for additional information—a feature that even the best static form cannot provide. Finally, the computer can help the data-entry process in more sophisticated ways, such as by managing the flow of input reports or verifying that needed reports have been completed.

Computer-based medical records can report their content on media ranging from video display terminals (VDTs) to paper. Of course, a computer-stored record does not imply the absence of paper—a subject to which we shall return later in this chapter. In addition, with a computer system, the same information can be reported in many formats; a visit note, a letter to a referring physician, and a physician's narrative report contain much the same information. The format and content of computer-generated reports can be tailored to the purpose of the report, thus reducing the need for redundant recording of data. Moreover, information from many patients can be aggregated, a useful feature for clinical research and practice management.

A computer-stored record has the great benefit that it can make decisions automatically about the data it captures and reports. As we noted previously, the system can ask for important missing information. More important, it can analyze the data and assist health-care personnel in making diagnostic and therapeutic decisions.

The degree to which a particular medical-record system will have these advantages depends on four factors:

1. The system's *informational scope*. Does it contain results from only the outpatient setting or from all care sites? Does it contain only drug and laboratory data, or does it also include physicians' clinical observations?

2. The system's *duration of use*. A record that has accumulated patient data over 5 years will be more valuable in many situations than is one that contains records of only those visits made during 1 specific month.

3. The *representation of data* in the system. Medical data that are stored simply as narrative text entries will be more legible and accessible than are similar entries in a paper medical record. Uncoded information, however, is not standardized (see Section 6.3.1), and inconsistent use of medical terminology limits the ability to retrieve data. Only if a controlled, predefined vocabulary is used is it possible to aggregate and summarize data provided by different physicians or by the same physician at different times. Thus, an unstructured online record cannot aid users actively in decision making or medical research.

4. The *geographic dispersion of terminals* that access the system. A system that is used by many people and is accessible from only a few sites will be less valuable

than if it is accessible from hundreds of terminals around the hospital, or even from private offices and physicians' homes.

Disadvantages

A computer-stored medical-record system also has some disadvantages. It requires a larger initial investment than its paper counterpart because of hardware, software, and training costs. Key personnel may have to spend a week or more away from their practice to learn the system, after which they must spend additional time training other staff. Existing personnel may not adapt to the computer procedures; personnel turnover and practice disruption can be the consequence. Furthermore, there are delays between the installation of the computer-stored record and the appreciation of its full benefits—which occur when most active patients have accumulated a computer record of substance. The importance of maintaining confidentiality of electronically stored data adds to the work of using the computer and to the cost of managing it.

Computer-based systems have the potential for subtle as well as catastrophic failures. If the computer hardware fails, stored information may be unavailable for hours or days. Thus, alternative manual procedures must be maintained. Furthermore, because disk failures can cause a loss of stored data, system developers must implement and maintain procedures for backing up and restoring data. When data are hand written by health-care providers and then are entered by an operator, transcription errors can result, and faulty software can alter even correctly entered data.

Most of these problems can be avoided with appropriate hardware and software. System developers must be aware of these potential pitfalls, and must design systems that minimize them (see Chapter 5). For example, they can reduce the costs of data entry and training by using graphics and color to clarify what users should do, and by having online instructions available. Duplicate equipment, if properly configured, reduces the chance that data will be destroyed or will be temporarily unavailable due to hardware failure.

Finally, there is the central problem of capturing physician-collected data for a computer-stored record. The decisional content of directly observed clinical information is low; physicians often use a great deal of information to make one small decision. The cost of entering all the data a physician uses to make a decision thus can be high relative to the value of the decision assistance a computer could provide. New techniques to facilitate direct physician entry of such information (for example, speech input) can reduce this problem.

6.2 Historical Development of Medical-Record Systems

The historical development of the medical record parallels the development of science in clinical care. The Flexner report on medical education was the first formal statement made about the function and contents of the medical record [Flexner, 1910]. In advocating a scientific approach to medical education, it also encouraged physicians to keep a patient-oriented medical record.

The contents of medical records in hospitals became the object of scrutiny in the 1940s, when hospital-accrediting bodies began to insist on the availability of accurate, well-organized medical records as a condition for accreditation. Since then, these organizations also have required that hospitals abstract certain information from the medical record and submit it to national data centers. Such discharge abstracts contain (1) demographic information, (2) admission and discharge diagnoses, (3) length of stay, and (4) major procedures performed. The national centers produce statistical summaries of these case abstracts; an individual hospital can then compare its own statistical profile with that of similar institutions.

In the 1960s, computer-based hospital information systems (HISs) began to emerge. These systems were intended primarily for communication. They collected orders from nursing stations, routed the orders to various parts of the hospital, and, in the process, identified all chargeable services. These usually were only order-entry and results-reporting systems. Although they contained some medical information—for example, drug orders and results of many diagnostic studies—their major purpose was charge capture, not clinical care. Most optimized rapid transmission and display, and thus used text-storage techniques that made it easy to display information. As we discussed in Chapter 2, however, narrative data are difficult to interpret automatically. Furthermore, it is expensive to store voluminous text online.

The introduction of the **problem-oriented medical record** (POMR) by Lawrence Weed [Weed, 1969] influenced medical thinking about both manual and automated medical records. Weed was among the first to recognize the importance of the internal structure of the medical record, whether stored on paper or in a computer. He suggested that the primary organization of the medical record should be by the medical problem; all diagnostic and therapeutic plans should be linked to a specific problem. The computer-stored version of the POMR (PROMIS; see Chapter 7) displayed advisory information as physicians recorded their notes and orders. It introduced many technical innovations—for example, touch-screen data entry, high-speed transaction processing, and minicomputer networking.

The ambulatory medical record has received less attention than has the hospital record because of differences in government and regulatory requirements. Moreover, ad hoc approaches to the storage of outpatient information and the small income associated with each clinic visit compared to each hospital stay precluded the kind of investment in abstracting and review that is common to inpatient services.

Thirty years ago, a single family physician provided almost all of an individual's medical care. Today, however, responsibility for ambulatory care is shifting to teams of health-care professionals in outpatient clinics and health-maintenance organizations (HMOs; see Chapter 19). Ambulatory records may contain lengthy notes written by many different health-care providers, large numbers of laboratory-test results, and a diverse set of other data elements, such as X-ray examination and pathology reports and hospital discharge summaries. Accordingly, the need to use computer technology to facilitate ambulatory practice has increased.

In 1972, the National Center for Health Services Research and Development and the National Center for Health Statistics sponsored a conference to develop a more systematic approach to the ambulatory medical record. A few years later, analysts surveyed a number of computer-based ambulatory-record systems that were under development [Henley et al., 1975]. A followup to this study, conducted in 1981, summarized the developmental progress of many of these same systems [Kuhn et al., 1982]. In Section 6.4, we describe three systems that survived this early evolution: COSTAR, the Regenstrief Medical Record System (RMRS), and The Medical Record (TMR).

6.3 Fundamental Issues for Computer-Stored Medical-Record Systems

The objectives of all medical-record systems are the same, regardless of whether the system is automated or manual. The mechanism for accomplishing these objectives differs, however. From a user's perspective, the two approaches differ fundamentally in the way data are entered into and information is extracted from the record. In this section, we explore the issues and alternatives related to data entry, then describe the options for displaying and retrieving information from a computer-based medical record.

6.3.1 Data Entry

The timely and accurate transfer of patient information into the computer is the most difficult and labor-intensive step in the maintenance of a computer-stored medical record. Yet this step tends to be overlooked by developers and potential buyers of such systems, perhaps because responsibility for entry of data into the manual record is spread among many different health professionals, and because the task is such a habitual part of their daily routines that it is almost invisible.

The transfer of data from its source to the computer requires two separate procedures: (1) data capture, and (2) data input.

Data Capture

If the *scope* of the medical record is restricted to the variables under the control of the organization maintaining the record, then **data capture** is trivial; an office practice can easily obtain both data collected internally and the results of diagnostic studies ordered. On the other hand, capture of comparable information collected during a patient's hospitalization, visit to the emergency room, or visit to a consulting physician in an independent practice, can be difficult or impossible. Relevant information may go unnoticed (for example, the patient fails to mention a recent hospitalization); it may be illegible (for example, the data recorded on the third carbon of the emergency room visit form are illegible); or it may be available in insufficient detail (for example, the consulting physician reports that all the patient's test results were normal, but does not specify the tests' actual values). Solutions require personal negotiations with sites that frequently provide care to a practice's patients and extra work on the part of the practice.

It may be necessary to restrict the scope of the medical record to information that is returned to the practice—but such restrictions can limit the computer program's ability to provide intelligent feedback about patient care. A computer system in a medical clinic, for example, cannot make accurate recommendations about the need for cervical Pap testing if most cervical Pap results are requested by, and returned to, a consulting gynecologist. The clinic would need to develop special procedures to obtain copies of those reports for entry into the medical-clinic computer. Similarly, inpatient medical-record systems are constrained in their ability to generate alerts and reminders if data collected in one department are inaccessible to another department. The trend toward larger, more integrated, and more self-contained health-care systems (see Chapter 7) will tend to diminish the problem of data capture.

Data Input

The data-input step is burdensome because of the personnel time required. People must interpret or translate the data as well as enter them into the computer. Data may be entered in **free-text** form, in coded form, or in a form that combines both free text and code. In Chapter 2, we described alternative schemes for classifying diagnoses and medical procedures. The major advantage of coding is that data are classified and standardized, thus facilitating research, billing, and selective retrieval of medical records. Coding lets the computer "understand" the data, and thereby process them more intelligently. In addition, coded data usually can be stored more compactly than uncoded data can be—and when the codes are few, information can be entered with only a few keystrokes via selection from menus.

The major disadvantage of coding is the cost of translating the source text into the valid codes. It takes time to classify source text by code class, especially when the text is unusual and seems to fit none of the classifications. In addition, time is required to train data-entry personnel and to maintain the coding dictionary that describes the mapping between individual observations and their coded classifications. There also is the potential for coding errors—which, in contrast to errors in free-text entry, can be difficult to detect because coded information lacks the internal redundancy of most text data. For example, a transposition error causing a substitution of code 392 for 329 may not be detected unless the computer displays the associated text and the data-entry operator notices the error.

There are tradeoffs between coding and free-text data entry. The more coding, the greater the interpretation time; the more free text, the greater the typing time. Coding is favored when the number of individual codes is few, or when data-entry personnel are medically well educated and remain in their jobs long enough to understand, and to apply effectively, more complex classification schemes. Conversely, free text is favored when the number of codes is high, and when data-entry personnel cannot be trained easily to perform the complicated translations. A medical-record system can balance these tradeoffs by using codes for common diagnoses and findings and free text for the remainder of the record.

The coding of hand-written physicians' notes presents special difficulties because of legibility problems. As we shall discuss later in this section, the use of **structured encounter forms** can facilitate this activity greatly. Using such a form, and placing a strict limit on the entry of free-text notes, a rheumatology-clinic system was able to capture all the information in physicians' hand-written visit notes [Whiting-O'Keefe et al., 1985].

The availability of electronically encoded patient data from a computer's laboratory and pharmacy systems simplifies the entry of clinical data into a computer. It eliminates the need to type in the data and can reduce, but usually does not eliminate, the coding work. Coding remains a problem because the coding scheme used by a source computer system, such as a laboratory reporting system, rarely is congruent with that of the destination medical-record system. For example, one laboratory might report the result of a test on a scale from 1 to 4, whereas another might report the result as normal or abnormal. Dates, times, and patient identifiers often are reported in incompatible formats. Thus, the personnel who use medical-record systems often must translate even coded information into a common internal code to facilitate retrieval and flowcharting.

The major barriers to the widespread usage of medical-records systems are the cost, delay, and potential for error inherent in manual data entry. These barriers will be eliminated if data can be captured directly from their sources in machine-readable form. However, standardization of data formats, and to some degree the schemes for encoding information, are necessary before this potential becomes reality. Such standards currently are being developed by the American Society for Testing and Materials (ASTM) [McDonald and Hammond, 1989; American Society for Testing and Materials, 1988].

Error Prevention

Because of the chance of transcription errors when clinical information is entered into the computer, computer-stored medical-record systems must apply **validity checks** scrupulously. A number of different kinds of checks can be used for clinical data [Schwartz et al., 1985]. *Range checks* can detect or prevent entry of values that are out of range (for example, a serum-potassium level of 50.0—the normal range for healthy individuals is 3.5 to 5.0 meq/l). *Pattern checks* can verify that the entered data have a required pattern (for example, the three digits, hyphen, and four digits of a local telephone number). *Computed checks* can verify that values have the correct mathematical relationship (for example, white-blood-cell differential counts [reported as percentages] must sum to 100). *Consistency checks* can detect errors by comparing entered data (for example, the recording of cancer of the prostate as the diagnosis for a woman). *Delta checks* warn of large and unlikely differences between the value of a new result and the previous observation (for example, a recorded weight that changes by 100 pounds in 2 weeks). *Spelling checks* verify the spelling of individual words.

Physician-Entered Data

Physician-gathered patient information requires special comment because it presents the most difficult problem to those people who develop and operate medical-record systems. Physicians record four kinds of information:

1. The patient's reports, such as of medical history or of present symptoms
2. The physician's physical findings
3. The physician's differential diagnosis
4. The physician's treatment plan

Some information (for example, the history that is ordinarily collected by physicians) can be obtained by other means, such as through questionnaires, nurse interviews, and computer interviews [Slack, 1984]. In one study, however, history data gathered by questionnaire and by nurse interview were much less predictive of the correct diagnoses than were comparable data gathered by physicians [Hickam et al., 1985b]. Thus, we cannot assume that data of equivalent form that are collected by different mechanisms have equivalent content.

Physicians' notes can be entered via one of three mechanisms: transcription of dictated or written notes, entry of data recorded on structured encounter forms, or direct data entry by physicians. **Transcription** of physicians' notes is especially pertinent when the practice has already invested in dictation services, because then the cost of keying already has been absorbed. If physicians follow a standard form in their dictation, a transcriptionist can enter that dictation into a modestly structured computer record [Park, 1982]. For example, if the physician dictates the report using the standard format of present illness, past history, physical examinations, and treatment plan, the transcriptionist can enter these components into corresponding fields displayed on a screen.

The second data-entry method is to have physicians use a **structured encounter form** from which their notes are transcribed (and possibly encoded) by support personnel. This has been the most successful approach to date. Examples of highly tailored turnaround encounter forms are shown in Figures 6.1 through 6.4. Encounter forms often contain checklists of common signs, symptoms, and diagnoses; fields where required information may be filled in; and space for free-text comments.

The third alternative is the **direct entry** of data, by a physician, via a VDT. Physicians do enter orders directly in some hospitals. Direct order entry has been most readily accepted by surgeons, because these doctors can create a few standard order batteries to cover the requirements of most of their patients. Such batteries can be entered with a few keystrokes—which is faster than equivalent manual order writing. General internists, family practitioners, and other physicians who see patients with a greater variety of clinical problems have been less willing to enter their orders directly into a computer because of the greater time required to enter the data, and because data entry often has required typing, a skill that many physicians are reluctant to acquire [Anderson and Jay, 1983]. Direct entry of the patient's history, physical findings, and progress notes has been even less accepted by physicians than has direct entry of orders, largely because of the lengthy dialogue needed to enter such information into the computer [Lundsgaarde et al., 1981].

Resistance is likely to diminish with the introduction of dedicated microcomputer workstations, high-resolution displays, pointing devices such as trackballs and mice, and voice input [Carl et al., 1978; McDonald and Tierney, 1986a]. The last technique offers great promise, because physicians already are familiar with, and tend to prefer, dictating patient data. Commercial systems already exist that will record a

SUMMARY TIME ORIENTED RECORD (STOR) -- PART A

NAME:

UNIT #: 082 12 90-2   BIRTHDATE: 09/04/1945   CLINIC: DIAB
ACE: 44   PHONE #1:   DATE: 8-9-88

DATE CLINIC PROVIDER			8-9-88 DIAB	6-12-88 10 6-20-88	6-6-88 DIAB AO61	4-27-88 10 5-3-88	4-18-88 DIAB AO61	4-11-88 DIAB Y483	3-28-88 DIAB AO61
PROBLEMS/MANIFESTATIONS	**ONSET**	**UNITS**							
2 VITAL SIGNS:	VS								
3 WEIGHT	WT	LBS			182.1		181.3	181	181
4 BLOOD PRESSURE (HYPERTENSION BY HX)	BP	MM HG			110/80			132/82	132/82
5 PULSE RATE	PULS	#/MIN			80			88	88
36 DIABETIC NEPHROPATHY (S/P TRANSPLANT X 2)	DHE	1972							
19 DIABETES MELLITUS I.D.D.M.	DM	1965					IMPROVED CONTROL		POOR CONTROL
17 SELF TEST BLOOD GLU.	SHBG				230-280		140-200	200++	200-300
21 ROUTINE CARE (RN POD. DIET. OPTH.)	RCRP	R P D O			O P			RN	
15 PERIPHERAL NEUROPATHY (SEVERE)	PN	REMOTE			SLOWLY PROGRES.			STABLE	
17 RETINOPATHY BLIND SINCE 1980	RETI	1972	0-3 SCALE						
38 RECURR. ABSCESS/ULCERS	RCAU	ABT 1982							
39 CHRONIC ANKLE ULCERS	CAU	11-3-86	0-3 SCALE		STABLE		ACTIVE		
41 FINGER ULCERS	FNBL	11-19-87	0-3 SCALE		GETTING BETTER			SEE NOTE	3+
37 R GREAT TOE INFECTION R/O OSETOMYELITIS	RGTI	6-1-88							
18 CHRONIC DIARRHEA (DIABETIC OVERGROWTH)	CHDI	1985	#STOOLS		1-2/DAY		1-2/DAY IMPROVED	1-3/DAY KEFLEX	3-5 ON
34 BORDERLINE MALABSORPT. (SEE GI NOTE 6-26-87)	BRML	6-87							

THERAPIES		ROUTE	UNITS						
3 IMODIUM (FOR DIARRHEA)	IMOD	PO	MG		2MG PRN X12/DAY				
3 IMURAN	IMRN	PO	MG		50 QD			50 QD	50 QD
8 PREDNISONE	PRED	PO	MG		8 QD			8 QD	5 QD
8 REGULAR INSULIN	REG	SUBCUT	UNITS		12/10 AM/PM/HS		12/16/0 AM/PM/HS	12/16/ AM/PM/HS	12/ 12 AM/PM/HS
9 NPH INSULIN	NPH	SUBCUT	UNITS		12/16 AM/PM/HS		12/0/10 AM/PM/HS	12/ 12 AM/PM/HS	
12 KEFLEX	KFLX	PO	MG		250 QID			250 QID	250 QID
11 CODEINE	CODE	PO	MG						QTC

LABORATORY			UNITS						
25 WBC COUNT	WBC		K/MCL		9.4	7.3	6.2		8.3
5 UREA NITROGEN	BUN		MG/DL		12.	14.	14.		14.
6 CREATININE	CR		MG/DL		1.0	0.9	0.9		1.0
16 PROTEIN ,UR	PRUA		MG/DL			30	300		
10 GLUCOSE ,UR	CLUA		MG/DL			250	500		
17 KETONES ,UR	KEUA		MG/DL			NEG	15		
19 WBCS ,UR	WBCU		/HPF				<3		
20 RBCS ,UR	RBCU		/HPF				<3		
30 GLUCOSE	CLR		MG/DL		309.	262.	315.	170	213	213
7 GLUCOSE, FASTING	FBS		MG/DL		300.		222.		
38 GLYCOSYLATED HGB	HBA1		PERCENT						12.2

THE FOLLOWING ITEMS HAVE BEEN BUMPED TO PART B: L-TRIG L-CHOL

FIGURE 6.1 Part A of the encounter form of the University of California at San Francisco's STOR system is a time-oriented flowsheet of signs, symptoms, therapies, and laboratory-test data. Physicians use one of the columns of the flowsheet to record data collected during the current visit. (*Source:* Courtesy of University of California, San Francisco Medical Center.)

```
                        SUMMARY TIME ORIENTED RECORD (STOR) -- PART B

NAME:                              UNIT #: 082 12 90-2    BIRTHDATE: 09/04/1943    CLINIC: DIAB
                                   AGE: 44                PHONE #1:                DATE:   8-8-88
ADDR:
                                                          PRVD: RAMBERG

============================================================================================
  REPORTS
============================================================================================

UCSF       HOSPITALIZATION: 6-6-88 to 6-16-88                        JEWETT, DON L
              DIAGNOSES: 1.  Cellulitis, right great toe.
                         2.  Insulin-dependent diabetes mellitus.
                         3.  Neuropathy.

XRAY    MAG EXAM (IND PRO) : 6-7-88                                  GENANT, HARRY
                         1.  No evidence of osteomyelitis.
                         2.  Marked soft tissue swelling of the 1st, 2nd and 3rd toes. Infection cannot be ruled
                             out as a cause of this.

MICRO             TAKEN: 6-6-88 12:30P, PVT        ACCN #:            DR JEWETT, DON L (ORDER MD)
               RECEIVED: 6-6-88 3:45P
                 SOURCE: SKIN WOUND, RT GREAT TOE; TRANS SWAB
              PROCEDURE: AEROBIC & ANAEROBIC CULTURE
                RESULTS:    SMEAR:  FEW GRAM POS COCCI IN PAIRS
                            CULTURE: MOD STAPHYLOCOCCUS EPIDERMIDIS GROUP

DIAB              VISIT: 6-6-88                             RAMBERG, MARILYN E   A061:Z204
                         CONTROL REMAINS A PROBLEM BECAUSE OF CHRONIC ULCERS AND LOW GRADE INFECTIONS. THE
                         PATIENT HAS A NEW ULCER/CELLULITIS ON THE R GREAT TOE. I WILL CONSULT WITH ORTHOPEDICS
                         REGARDING POSSIBLE OSTEOMYELITIS. CONTINUE ALL CURRENT MEDS.

DIAB              VISIT: 4-18-88                            RAMBERG, MARILYN E   A061:Z204
                         RIGHT INDEX FINGER DEBRIDED IN ORTHO CLINIC 4/11/88. X-RAY SHOWS ONLY DEMINERALIZATION
                         OF DISTAL TUFF. FITTED WITH PROTECTIVE BRACE. FS NOW IN THE 140-200 RANGE. THESE
                         ULCERS AND ABSCESSES CONTINUE TO BE A MAJOR PROBLEM. F/U IN ORTHO. CONTINUE KEFLEX.
```

PROBLEMS/MANIFESTATIONS		ONSET/ RESOLVED	UNITS	LAST DATA	DATE	LOC/ PRVD	COMMENT	NEW DATA
8 PAST MEDICAL HISTORY:	(PMH)							
33 RECTAL WALL ABSCESS STAPHYLOCOCCUS AUREUS	(RCWA)	7-1-85 7-12-85				P768		
9 SURGERIES:	(SURG)							
31 RENAL TRANSPLANT (LIVING, SISTER DONOR)	(RNTR)	2-8-83				P768	UNCOMPLICATED SISTER DONATED TRANSPLANT AFTER PREVIOUS CADAVER RT FAILED.	
14 RENAL TRANSPLANT (CADAVER)	(RT)	1-21-80 4-9-82			11-2-87	DIAB A061		
36 CO2 LASER EXCISION VASCULAR HEMANGIOMA	(C2LE)	6-26-87				A061		
10 HOSPITALIZATIONS:	(HOSP)							
32 GANGRENE (RIGHT GREAT TOE)	(GNGR)	9-7-82 9-20-82						
42 SOFT TISSUE ABSCESS (LEFT THIGH, ? BUG)	(STA)	9-21-87				Y483	RESPONDED TO INPATIENT ANTIBIOTICS	

LABORATORY		UNITS	DATA	DATE	LOW-HIGH		COMMENT
5 UREA NITROGEN	(BUN)	MG/DL	12.	6-20-88	10-24	LAST	
6 CREATININE	(CR)	MG/DL	1.0	6-20-88	0.5-1.4	LAST	
1 SODIUM	(NA)	MEQ/L	133.	6-20-88	135-145		
2 POTASSIUM	(K)	MEQ/L	4.5	6-20-88	3.5-5		
3 CHLORIDE	(CL)	MEQ/L	101.	6-20-88	102-113		
26 SEDIMENTATION RATE	(ESR)	MM/HR	42	6-12-88	0-10		
7 GLUCOSE, FASTING	(FBS)	MG/DL	300.	6-12-88	60-115	LAST	
30 GLUCOSE	(CLR)	MG/DL	262.	6-8-88	6-115		
36 T4, TOTAL	(T4)	MCG/DL	6.5	12-26-87	5-12	LAST	
35 T4 INDEX	(T4I)		2.8	12-26-87	1.5-4.2	LAST	
34 T3, TOTAL	(T3)	MG/DL	62	12-26-87	85-185	LAST	
60 CHOLESTEROL	(CHOL)	MG/DL	152.	9-4-87	-240	BUMP	
61 TRIGLYCERIDES	(TRIG)	MG/DL	101.	9-4-87	25-150	BUMP	
36 T4, TOTAL	(T4)	MCG/DL	6.4	6-2-87	5-12	FIRST	BY NUCLEAR MED.
70 TSH/THYROTROPHIN	(TSH)	MCU/ML	3.93	6-2-87	0.4-4.8	HOLD	THYROID RESEARCH

FIGURE 6.2 Part B of the STOR system's encounter form is divided into sections that summarize patients' clinic visits, hospitalizations, and ancillary-test results (radiology examinations, microbiology cultures, and so on), as well as important problems, therapies, and laboratory data that are not reported in the flowsheet portion (part A) of the encounter form (Figure 6.1). (*Source:* Courtesy of University of California, San Francisco Medical Center.)

```
THE NEPHROLOGY SERVICE                      PATIENT
Category: HYPERTENSIVE/            RV
  Primary MD: LEE A. DALY         WWS        12 BYTE ST
  Occupation: CONSTRUCTION,RET               DURHAM, NC   27705
    Employer:                              919-999-9999
                                             Birthdate: 04/01/23
                                           999-99-9999

                                             62 yo wh  male
08/09/85 11:53                    ---------------------------------


  ONSET  RESOLVED SEEN CODE    ALL PROBLEMS
11/15/83 _____  __    88 RENAL ARTERY STENOSIS (UNIL) - RT
??/??/73 _____  __     1   HYPERTENSION-DIASTOLIC
04/26/83 _____  __   401   POLYCYTHEMIA - INC. RBC MASS /C NL PLASMA VOL
07/18/85 _____  __   216   NEPHRECTOMY - RIGHT
01/30/84 _____  __   251   PULMONARY EMBOLUS
04/21/83 _____  __   374   MICROSCOPIC HEMATURIA
04/21/83 _____  __   128   PYURIA
05/09/83 _____  __   127   PROTEINURIA - 188MG/24HR
??/??/?? _____  __   273 DEGENERATIVE JOINT DISEASE
12/12/83 _____  __   257 THROMBOPHLEBITIS - SUPERFICIAL R THIGH
01/27/84 _____  __   357 S/P B/L FEM-POP

_____ _____  __  ____ _____


  SUBJ/PHY         LAST VALUE            TODAY'S VALUE
T58-1                        |  TEXT   _____
T58-3                        |  TEXT   _____
FATIGUE                 N|      MLD;MOD;SEV;NO
SLEEP DIST                   |  TEXT   _____
POSTURAL SX             N|      TEXT   _____
HACHE GEN               N|      MLD;MOD;SEV;NO
CHEST PAIN                   |  TEXT   _____
PALPITAT                N|      YN
DYSPNEA                      |  REST;MIN-EX;MOD-EX;HEAVY-EX;NO
PND                          |  YN
ORTHOPD                      |  ↑ PILLOW
CLAUDICAT               N|      REST;MIN-EX;MOD-EX;HEAVY-EX;NO
NAUSEA                  N|      YN   _____
IMPOTENCE                    |  YN
WT                    76.6|     ↑ KG  _____
TEMP                         |  ↑ C   _____
PUL SUP                 64|     ↑ MIN _____
PUL SIT                      |  ↑ MIN
PUL STA                 72|     ↑ MIN _____
BP SUP              134/86|     ↑/↑ MM  _____
BP SIT                       |  ↑/↑ MM
BP STA              106/80|     ↑/↑ MM
ART NAR                MOD|     MLD;MOD;SEV;NO
AV NICK                MLD|     MLD;MOD;SEV;NO
HEMORRHAGE                   |  TEXT   _____
EXUDATE                      |  TEXT   _____
PAPILL                       |  RT;LT;BILAT;NO
```

FIGURE 6.3 An encounter form produced for the Duke University nephrology service by the TMR system summarizes recent clinical findings and treatments. Note that the appropriate answers are suggested in the area for entering today's data. (*Source:* Courtesy of Duke University Medical Center.)

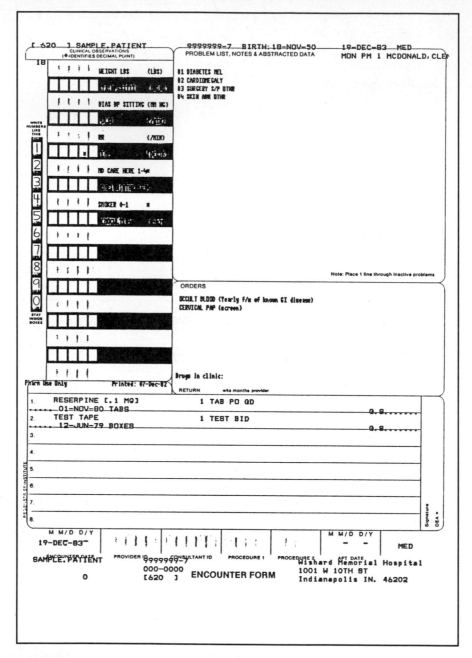

FIGURE 6.4 The patient-specific encounter form of the Regenstrief Medical Record System displays a list of problems and a list of active prescriptions. It also provides areas to record data, to order laboratory tests, and to order drugs. The form has been designed for automatic entry by a character-recognition system. (*Source:* Courtesy of Regenstrief Institute.)

radiologist's voice report of an examination, and then will play it over a telephone to other personnel who need to know the results quickly. When computers can accept vocal messages, physicians will be able to encode the common observations and statements with menu selection, and to dictate the remainder directly into the computer. Computer *interpretation* of voice input has even greater promise, since it could permit the computer to "understand" oral commands and to translate them into the appropriate codes or text. An early trial in a clinical environment (radiology), however, was not successful because of high transcription error rates [Leeming et al., 1981]. Later systems have been more successful. The newer Kurzweil system has achieved a recognition rate of 95 percent, but it cannot recognize continuous speech. Furthermore, users are restricted to using a predefined vocabulary when composing reports [Robbins et al., 1987].

6.3.2 Alternative Methods for Displaying Information

Manual charts have but one organization—that of the physical relationships of their pages. To present data in more than one format, you must enter them more than once—and this is the common practice. Physicians record their medication plans in the progress notes, then write them again on the order sheet or prescription pad. Technicians paste laboratory reports into the charts, and physicians then copy selected results to their notes, flowsheets, and discharge summaries. There are many other examples of duplicate recording of the medical information.

In contrast, data stored once in the computer can be presented in numerous formats without further entry work. In addition, computer-stored records can be produced in novel formats that are unavailable in manual systems.

Paper Versus Video Display Terminal

A VDT has many advantages. It presents data almost instantaneously, compared to the seconds or minutes required for a printer to produce a report. Video displays can change dynamically in response to users as they review information. Moreover, terminals are quiet and require no tending for ribbon or paper changes.

Paper, despite the hubbub over a "paperless" office, does have some advantages. Today's low-priced printers can present four times as much information on a single page as can a standard 24-row by 80-column video display. Moreover, the formatting capabilities of printers generally are superior to those of comparably priced VDTs. People can easily carry a paper report in a pocket, annotate it, and use it without special training. Moreover, humans can read a paper report 25 percent faster and 10 percent more accurately than they can read a comparable report on a VDT [Gould and Grischkowsky, 1984].

Large-format, high-resolution graphics terminals will increase the advantage of VDTs over paper and will speed the day when the manila folder and its contents are historical relics. We doubt, however, that they will completely eliminate paper from the office; physicians probably will choose to produce paper copies of the medical record for specific uses for some time to come [Gould et al., 1986].

Computer Versions of Manual Reports

Computer-based medical-records systems produce most of the reports contained in manual systems; examples of such reports are visit notes (Figure 6.5), back-to-work notes, letters to referring physicians, specimen labels, and flowsheets.

The **flowsheet** format organizes data according to the time they were collected, thus emphasizing change over time. For example, a flowsheet used to monitor patients in a weight-loss program might contain values for weight, blood pressure, skinfold thickness, and other pertinent information recorded at each visit. Fries reported that physicians can find information in a structured flowsheet four times faster than they can on a standard paper record [Fries, 1974]. Computer-stored medical records can present much or all of the record as a flowsheet (Figures 6.1 and 6.6). Flowsheet programs may permit choices of destination (should the report go to the printer or to the VDT?), or orientation (which results are presented in which order, and how are they grouped?), and of temporal granularity (what is the time interval between observations?).

The last category needs explanation. When a patient is in the intensive-care unit (ICU), minute-to-minute changes in his state may be of interest. An outpatient's physician is more likely to want to know how that patient's data changed over weeks or months. For convenience of human review, the temporal granularity should be appropriate to the intensity of care. Thus, 25 blood-gas values (for oxygen, carbon dioxide, and other gases in the blood) obtained in a single hospital stay should not all be presented in an outpatient flowsheet showing the 2-year course of an emphysema patient, because they would obscure the long-term patterns.

```
                              VISIT  NOTE
     PROV:   JONES,WILLIAM J                              UN: DEMO-017
     SITE 1                                               EXAMPLE,CASE

     DATE OF VISIT:   3/18/83                  (M)   57 YRS  (4/22/28)

     MAJOR PROBLEMS
        ASTHMA
            MINIMAL UPPER RESP INFECTION LAT WEEK; SOME DEGREE OF
            WHEEZING.

     PHYSICAL EXAMINATION
        CHEST:
            MINIMAL WHEEZING IN LOWER BASE POSTERIOR

     LABORATORY TESTS
        HEMATOLOGY
            WHITE BLOOD CELL COUNT              * 9400

     CHANGE IN THERAPIES AND RENEWALS
        TETRACYCLINE CAPSULES
            250 MG PO 4ID TAKE WITH MEALS
            QTY: 50 REFILL: 0
```

FIGURE 6.5 A COSTAR visit note summarizes important information for one clinic visit, including diagnoses, results of the physical examination and laboratory tests, and medication orders. (*Source:* Courtesy of Massachusetts General Hospital.)

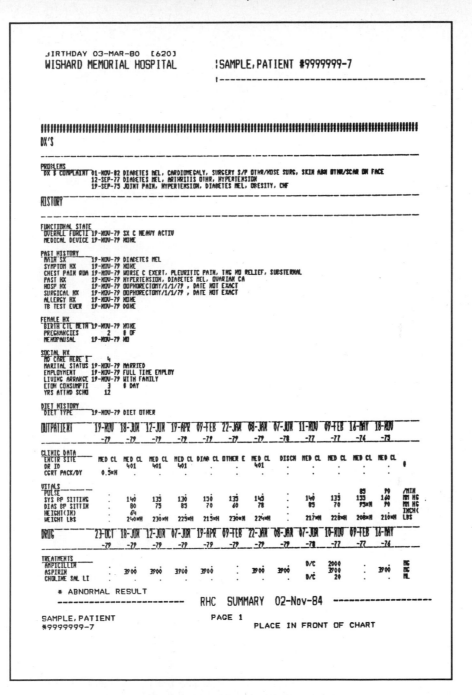

FIGURE 6.6 The Regenstrief medical-record flowsheet is a time-oriented summary of the patient database. The form is subdivided into related sections to improve readability. (*Source:* Courtesy of Regenstrief Institute.)

When large numbers of observations are presented in a single flowsheet, there are tradeoffs between formatting them as one large matrix or as many submatrices. A single large matrix has the advantage of ease of comparisons of dates across parameters, but makes it difficult to compare sequential results of tests ordered infrequently. Moreover, the report will tend to contain large amounts of whitespace. Consequently, it usually is better to break a large flowsheet into smaller subflowsheets, as shown in Figure 6.6.

Summaries and Abstracts

Computer-based medical records can highlight their important components in smaller, more digestible reports. The usual strategy is to select specific classes of observation: active allergies, active problems, active treatments, and recent observations. The COSTAR case-status summary (Figure 6.7) is a good example. In the future, we can expect more sophisticated summarizing strategies, such as detection of significant changes in observations, or aggregation of abnormal observations with a similar meaning (for example, elevated SGOT, elevated alkaline phosphatase, and elevated bilirubin, all of which are indicators of liver dysfunction) into a summary diagnostic statement. We also shall see reports that distinguish abnormal changes that have been treated from those that have not, and displays that dynamically organize the supporting evidence for existing problems (see Figures 6.8 and 6.9). Eventually, computers should be able to produce concise and flowing summary reports much like an experienced physician's hospital discharge summary.

Turnaround Documents

Turnaround documents are computer-tailored reports that both present information to and ask questions of the user. They are the paper equivalent of an input screen on a VDT. Visit encounter forms (see Figures 6.1 through 6.4, and 6.7) and superbills (described in Chapter 13) are turnaround documents produced by most medical-records systems.

A well-structured turnaround document can make it possible to capture clinical information directly from physicians in many environments. Paper turnaround documents are familiar materials; people can use them with little training. Obviously, turnaround documents have their greatest application in outpatient care, where there is sufficient time to prepare them prior to patient visits. They also have been used in ward services—for example, to gather drug-administration information and notes from nurses, and as request forms for diagnostic studies.

Dynamic Displays

Anyone who has tried to review a patient's chart knows how difficult it can be to find a particular piece of information, such as the interpretation of the last CT scan—or whether one ever was done. (Examinations such as a CT scan are performed only rarely, but the results may be critical to diagnosis.) Physicians may ask hundreds of

```
                          CASE SUMMARY
PRIMARY PROV: LIMBO,NO ONE,MD            UN: DEMO-017
IMA-8                                    EXAMPLE,CASE
LAST VISIT: 2/8/85
ADDR: 121 LONGVIEW RD                    (M) 57 YRS  (4/22/28)
     APT 345                             PH: 756-1111
     DORCHESTER,MA 02124                 OTHER PH: 793-9999 WK

DATE:_____ PROVIDER:_____ SITE:_____
VISIT TYPE: [ ]NEW PT [ ]SCHED RTN [ ]UNSCHED RTN [ ]MED REFILL [ ]NO SHOW

PERSONAL DATA AND OVERALL HEALTH: (2/8/85)

REASON FOR VISIT:_____


HEALTH MAINTENANCE
   TETANUS TOXOID INJECTION   0.5CC IM                    3/8/83
   INFLUENZA VACCINE                                      9/10/82
   RECTAL GUAIAC   NEGATIVE                               5/1/81

   CHECK & PROVIDE RESULTS IF DONE:

   GUAIAC:_____

   PNEUMOVAX:_____

   FLU VACCINE:_____


ALLERGIES/SENSITIVITIES                  DATE FIRST ENTERED
* DRUG ALLERGY                                   2/8/85
       /PENICILLIN.
* PENICILLIN ALLERGY                            10/3/81
       AS CHILD, DETAILS VAGUE

MAJOR PROBLEMS
   DIABETES MELLITUS                             2/8/85
   ASTHMA                                       10/3/81
       MINIMAL UPPER RESP INFECTION LAT WEEK: SOME DEGREE OF
       WHEEZING.                                [3/18/83]

   HYPERTENSION                                 10/3/81
       CONTINUES TO HAVE ELEVATED BP. NO HEADACHES. SEEMS TO BE
       CONCERNED ABOUT STARTING MEDICATION . WILL KEEP CAREFUL
       NOTE OF EYE GROUNDS, MAY BE A THIRD HEART SOUND - CAN'T
       TELL.                                    [3/17/83]

   OBESITY                                      10/3/81
       SIGNED UP WEIGHT-WATCHERS                [3/8/83]

   COUGH  [S/P]                                  2/8/85




STATUSES: M/MAJOR    I/INACT    H/HO    R/RO    Y/SP    P/PRESUM
              D/DO NOT DISPLAY    S/SHORT TERM PROBLEM
```

FIGURE 6.7 The COSTAR case summary portrays the patient's current medical status. In contrast to the visit note shown in Figure 6.5, the case summary contains information from multiple visits. (*Source:* Courtesy of Massachusetts General Hospital.)

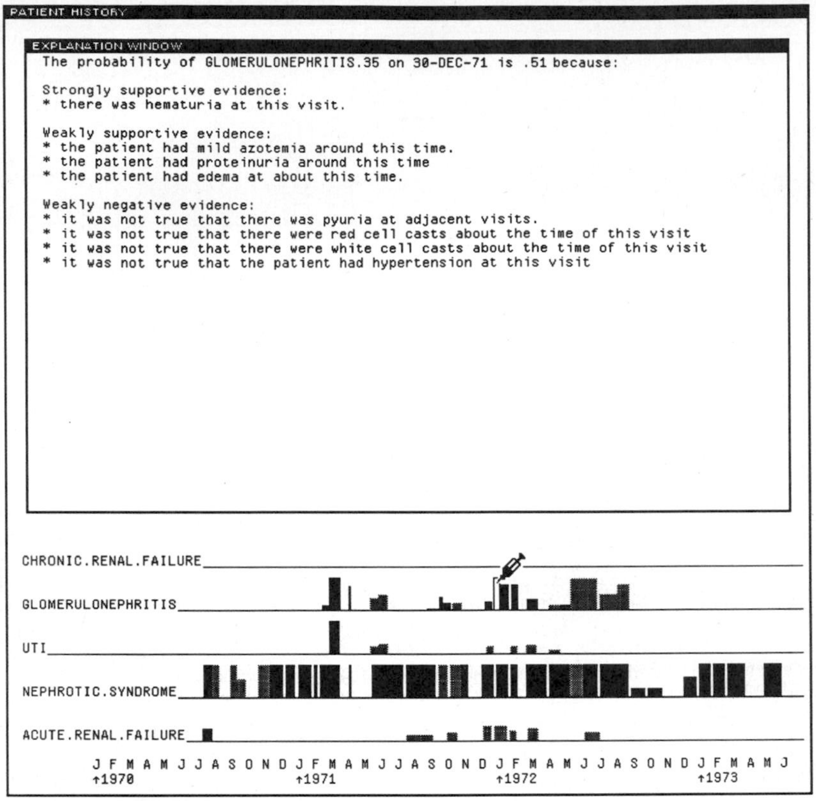

PATIENT HISTORY

EXPLANATION WINDOW
The probability of GLOMERULONEPHRITIS.35 on 30-DEC-71 is .51 because:

Strongly supportive evidence:
* there was hematuria at this visit.

Weakly supportive evidence:
* the patient had mild azotemia around this time.
* the patient had proteinuria around this time
* the patient had edema at about this time.

Weakly negative evidence:
* it was not true that there was pyuria at adjacent visits.
* it was not true that there were red cell casts about the time of this visit
* it was not true that there were white cell casts about the time of this visit
* it was not true that the patient had hypertension at this visit

CHRONIC.RENAL.FAILURE

GLOMERULONEPHRITIS

UTI

NEPHROTIC.SYNDROME

ACUTE.RENAL.FAILURE

J F M A M J J A S O N D J F M A M J J A S O N D J F M A M J J A S O N D J F M A M J
↑1970   ↑1971   ↑1972   ↑1973

FIGURE 6.8 An automated summarization program developed by researchers at Stanford University examines an ARAMIS database (containing laboratory-test results, symptoms, and physical findings) and summarizes the data in terms of higher-level events such as renal failure, urinary-tract infection (UTI), and glomerulonephritis (a kidney disease). (*Source:* Adapted with permission from Downs, S. *A program for automated summarization of on-line medical records.* Knowledge Systems Laboratory, Stanford University, Report KSL-86-44, 1986, p. 6.)

such questions as they flip back and forth in the chart searching for facts to support or refute one in a series of evolving hypotheses. Having the record in computer-stored form does not eliminate the work of searching for a particular fact, but it can allow the user to see data in a highly structured form (for example, in flowsheets) that makes it easier to find needed information. More important, some programs can do much of the searching, and can present data relevant to particular medical problems. For example, COSTAR produces specialized flowsheets for hypertension, hematology, endocrinology, and other problem areas (Figure 6.10). On a more sophisticated level, a computer could produce lists of abnormalities that are not attributable to known problems or indicate drug side effects that could explain recent changes, such as an elevation in liver enzymes. By searching and subsetting data according to the context of a particular medical problem, the program can speed the assimilation of

```
ABNORMAL FINDINGS SUMMARY for : TEST,EDWARD 9999999-7 Age =68 Sex =M Race =W
============================================================================

The computer has identified, and tried to account for, all of the
patient's abnormal findings. The 'conclusions' are coarse approximations
intended as an aid in your analysis of the patient.
_____


HEMATOLOGIC PROBLEMS

  hemolysis pres, Probable
     +++      HGB SERUM FREE......=    41 h         On 02 APR 73
     --       HAPTOGLOBIN.........=   105           On 03 APR 73
     ++       RETIC COUNT.........=   2.7 h         On 12 AUG 77
     ++       LDH (SMA)...........=   305 h         On 05 JUN 78
     ++       MACROCYTES..........= few             On 14 DEC 81

  leukocytosis, Probable
     +++      BANDS...............=    10 h         On 01 JAN 87
     +++      WBC.................=    12 h         On 01 JAN 87

ENDO/METABOLIC PROBLEMS

  hyperthyroidism, Probable
     ---      T4 INDEX''..........=   6.6           On 31 JAN 83
     +++      CERVICAL THY CT.....= thyroid nodule hot On 11 JAN 87

  hypocalcemia, Definite
     +++++    CALCIUM.............=    5 L          On 02 MAR 88

  hypokalemia, Definite
     +++++    POTASSIUM...........=   2.5 l         On 01 JAN 88

  hyponatremia, Definite
     +++++    SODIUM..............=   131 l         On 01 JAN 88

  hyperphosphatemi, Definite
     +++++    PHOS................=    5 h          On 02 MAR 88

  hypercholesterolemia, Definite
     +++++    CHOLESTEROL.........=   335 h         On 02 MAR 88

GASTROINTESTINAL PROBLEMS

  cholelithiasis, Definite but contradictory evidence, ? Bad data,
     -----    SURGICAL HX.........= cholecystectomy On 01 JAN 87
     +++++    CHOLECYSTOGRAM......= cholelithiasis  On 07 JAN 87
     +++++    GALLBLADDER ULTRASOU= cholelithiasis  On 07 JAN 87

  pancreatitis, Possible
     ++       AMYLASE.............=   146 h         On 11 DEC 81

  hepatomegaly, Definite
     +++++    ABDOMEN CT SCAN.....= hepatomegaly    On 07 JAN 87
     +++++    LIVER ULTRASOUND....= hepatomegaly    On 11 JAN 87
_____

TEST,EDWARD 9999999-7        Printed 10 AUG 88 12:10AM    ABNORMAL FINDINGS SU
                                  1
```

FIGURE 6.9 The Patient Summary, produced by the Regenstrief Institute's Medical Gopher System, is intended to aid physicians in evaluating their patients. The summary identifies abnormal findings in a patient's computer-based medical record and presents the abnormalities according to their common possible causes. (*Source:* Courtesy of Regenstrief Institute.)

```
                                                                              PAGE 4

   EXAMPLE,CASE    (M)   57 YRS                                       UN1 DEMO-017


                        --  HEMATOLOGY FLOWCHART  --

   DATE     I HCT I WBC I RBC I HGB I MCV I MCH I MCHCI PLT I PT   I ESR I RET I DIFFERENTIAL
            I     I     I     I     I     I     I     I     I      I     I     I WBC COUNT
   ================================================================================================
   3/18/83 I 44.4I     I     I     I     I     I     I     I      I     I     I
   ------------------------------------------------------------------------------------------
   5/7/83  I       I#321 I     I     I     I     I     I     I      I     I     I
   ------------------------------------------------------------------------------------------
   3/18/83 I       I#9400I     I     I     I     I     I     I      I     I     I
   ------------------------------------------------------------------------------------------
   9/10/82 I#47.8I     I 15.2I     I     I     I     I     I      I     I     I
   ------------------------------------------------------------------------------------------
   10/3/81 I#49  I     I 15.8I     I     I     I     I     I      I     I     I
   ------------------------------------------------------------------------------------------


                        --  ENDOCRINE/METABOLIC FLOWCHART  --

   DATE     I GLU       I CHOL     I TRIG     I THYR     I T3R      I FT4I     I TSH
   ================================================================================================
   10/3/81 I 110       I 293      I          I          I          I          I
           I (NON-FAST)I          I          I          I          I          I
   ------------------------------------------------------------------------------------------


                        --  ELECTROLYTES/RENAL FLOWCHART  --

   DATE     I NA   I K   I CL  I CO2 I BUN I CRE  I CAL  I PHOS I MG  I URIC I FE  I IBC
   ================================================================================================
   3/17/83 I      I     I     I     I#28  I      I      I      I     I      I     I
   ------------------------------------------------------------------------------------------
   9/10/82 I      I#3.4 I     I     I     I      I      I      I     I      I     I
   ------------------------------------------------------------------------------------------
   10/3/81 I      I 3.9 I     I     I 18  I      I      I      I     I      I     I
   ------------------------------------------------------------------------------------------


                        --  URINALYSIS  FLOWCHART  --

   DATE     I URINALYSIS
   ================================================================================================
   10/3/81 I - ML 10/3/81
   ------------------------------------------------------------------------------------------
```

FIGURE 6.10 Specialty flowsheets from the COSTAR system provide a chronological display of laboratory-test results and clinical observations. Each section is designed to record information related to a specific problem area. (*Source:* Courtesy of Massachusetts General Hospital.)

patient data and the evolution of diagnostic hypotheses (Figures 6.8 and 6.9). Ultimately, a computer system may be smart enough to infer the kinds of information needed by the physician strictly from context.

Graphical Displays

In many cases, humans can assimilate graphical information much faster than they can assimilate textual or numeric equivalents. Graphical presentations of medical records can be grouped into three classes:

1. *Presentation graphics.* These are the typical line or bar graphs found in published case reports that show clearly the temporal relationships among clinical events and the correlations among variables. The daily ICU reports from HELP take this approach (Figure 6.11). We discuss HELP, a hospital information system, in Chapter 7.

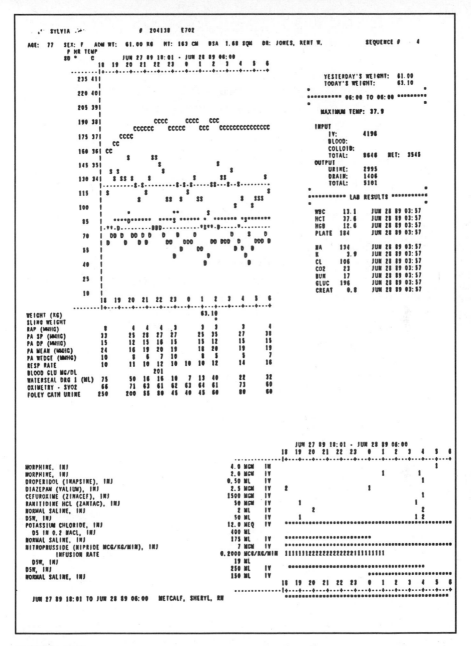

FIGURE 6.11 The HELP system daily report for patients in the intensive-care unit at Latter Day Saints Hospital. The complex display shows time-oriented data. In the upper-left corner, S and D refer to systolic and diastolic blood-pressure measurements; C is the patient's temperature in degrees centigrade. The upper-right corner shows cumulative input and output measurements over a 24-hour period, as well as recent laboratory-test results. The middle section shows a time-oriented flowsheet; the lower portion shows the drug treatment the patient has received. (*Source:* HELP System, LDS Hospital.)

2. *Diagrammatic reports.* These combine diagrams with numbers or traditional graphs. A good example is the reports generated by the Cedars-Sinai Medical Center Surgical ICU system (Figure 6.12).
3. *Continuous curves and pictures.* ECG strips, radiographic images, and even photographs of patients can be stored electronically and displayed on VDTs. Computer displays of ECGs and pressure tracings are common in ICU systems. More elaborate picture-processing radiology systems display digitized radiographs [Schneider and Dwyer, 1988] (see Chapter 11). As moderately priced devices for storing and manipulating pictures and curves become available, these display techniques will be employed increasingly in medical-record systems.

Narrative Reports

Computer-stored medical-record systems often provide facilities for producing specialized reports, such as for exercise stress tests or spirometry (evaluation of the air capacity of the lungs). In this case, physicians usually complete a structured input form (partially multiple choice, partially text; Figure 6.13), from which the computer can generate flowing text narrative automatically (Figure 6.14). Dedicated ECG and spirometry computer systems mix graphics and text in attractive specialized reports.

Computers also can use two word-processing techniques to manufacture reports:
1. *Predefined,* or *canned, notes.* These are common phrases and paragraphs that can be inserted into dictated or written narrative with a few keystrokes. This technique is used commonly in radiology-reporting systems to summarize normal examinations and common abnormal patterns. It also could be used to generate most test-interpretation narrative reports, such as those from electroencephalograms, spirometry, and surgical pathology examinations.

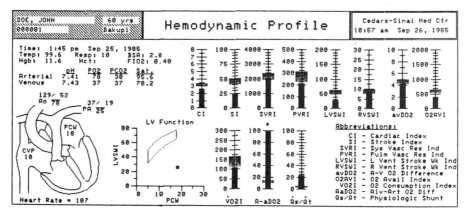

FIGURE 6.12 Cedars-Sinai Medical Center's surgical intensive-care cardiac-status display uses a number of graphical cues to present cardiac and respiratory measurements. (*Source:* Courtesy of M. Michael Shabot, M.D., Cedars-Sinai Medical Center Surgical Intensive Care Unit.)

```
                    DUKE MEDICAL CENTER                    X90001
              CAD HISTORY AND PHYSICAL FORM                84 yo wh female
                                                           10/22/84
I. HISTORY
```

A. Reason(s) for Catheterization (indicate primary *one* by P):
- (P) chest pain
- ( ) CHF
- ( ) acute evolving MI
- ( ) asymptomatic previous MI
- ( ) post-MI angina
- ( ) arrhythmia
- ( ) POS ETT
- ( ) POS RNA
- ( ) cardiac arrest
- ( ) prior cardiac surgery
- ( ) prior PTCA
- ( ) protocol
- ( ) other _____

B. Cardiovascular Risk Factors:

Hypertension .... Y (N)   Cerebrovascular disease .... Y (N)
Diabetes .... Y (N)   Smoking (> ½ pk/day in last 5 years) ... Y (N)
Peripheral vascular disease ...... Y N   Family history (age < 60) of CAD ...... (Y) N
Hyperlipidemia .... Y (N)

C. Chest Pain

Date of onset (ischemic symptoms): |0 / 15/ 82

Has the patient ever had chest discomfort felt to represent angina: (Y) N

Chest Discomfort not due to acute MI in last 6 weeks: (Y) N

IF YES: Occurs: Spontaneously or at rest .... (Y) N
                   Reproducibly with exertion/stress ...... Y (N)
                   During sleep .... (Y) N

        Relief by: Rest (≤ 10 mins) .... (Y) N
                    Nitroglycerin (≤ 10 mins) .... Y N

Type of chest discomfort (your "gestalt"):   Typical ( ),   Atypical (✓),   Not Anginal ( )

Frequency:
  If chronic Sx (> 6 weeks), average no. of episodes per week 3-5
  If new onset (≤ 6 weeks) or changing frequency, _____ episodes in the past _____ day(s)/week(s)
  If continuous, check here _____

NYHA Class (for exertional discomfort):
  ( ) I – no Sx with ordinary activity   ( ) III – Sx with ordinary activity
  ( ) II – Sx with moderate exertion   (✓) IV – Sx at rest and with any exertion

Course over last 6 weeks: Improving ( ),   Stable ( ),   Progressing (✓)

ECG documented variant angina: Y (N)

D. Hospitalizations:

Duke CCU admission to R/O MI (unstable angina) *this* hospital admission: Y N
Number of *other* CCU admissions to R/O MI in last 6 months _____

Documented MI *this* hospital admission: Y N
Prior hospitalization for *documented* MI: Y N ; If Yes, dates: _____

Prior Catheterization: Y N ; If Yes, number of prior catheterizations: _____

Most recent catheterization results:

Date: ___ / ___ / ___

# Diseased vessels: _____					
		Coronary Arteries			
EF: _____	L. Main	( ) Normal	( ) Insignificant	( ) Subtotal	( ) Total
	LAD	( ) Normal	( ) Insignificant	( ) Subtotal	( ) Total
	LCX	( ) Normal	( ) Insignificant	( ) Subtotal	( ) Total
MR Grade: _____	RCA	( ) Normal	( ) Insignificant	( ) Subtotal	( ) Total
		Grafts (specify distal anastomosis)			
# Grafts placed: _____	1. _____	( ) Normal	( ) Insignificant	( ) Subtotal	( ) Total
# Grafts patent: _____	2. _____	( ) Normal	( ) Insignificant	( ) Subtotal	( ) Total
	3. _____	( ) Normal	( ) Insignificant	( ) Subtotal	( ) Total
	4. _____	( ) Normal	( ) Insignificant	( ) Subtotal	( ) Total

FIGURE 6.13 The Duke University Medical Center history and physical form for patients with coronary-artery disease (produced by TMR). TMR uses these data to generate narrative reports, such as that shown in Figure 6.14. Some questions can be answered by multiple-choice selections; others require free-text input. (*Source:* Courtesy of Duke University Medical Center.)

```
CARDIAC CATH LAB                                        X90001
DUKE UNIVERSITY MEDICAL CENTER                          N71
                                                     10/22/84
CAD CARDIAC CATHETERIZATION

                                            CINE NO.: 123456


CLINICAL HISTORY:

   BETTY ROSS is an 84-year-old white female from DURHAM, NC who was
evaluated for chest pain.
   The patient has experienced symptoms since 10/15/82 and has had chest
discomfort in the last six weeks. The chest discomfort is considered to be
atypical angina, and occurs at rest and during sleep. It does not occur with
exertion. It is relieved by rest (<= 10 mins). The pain is chronic, with an
average of 3–5 episodes per week and is considered to be NYHA Class IV. The
course over the last six weeks has been progressive. The pain is not
considered to be preinfarctional angina. There is no history of congestive
heart failure. There have been no prior hospitalizations for documented MIs.
   Medications include: none.
```

FIGURE 6.14 A narrative report produced automatically by TMR from data collected on the form shown in Figure 6.13. (*Source:* Courtesy of Duke University Medical Center.)

2. *Mail merge.* Many word-processing systems provide a means of reproducing a standard letter or report, which is then tailored to specific individuals. The text script consists of variable and fixed components; the user produces a final report for a patient by inserting into the variable parts the patient-specific information. An example is a patient appointment reminder; the variable components of the shell are the patient's name and address, the date and time of the appointment, and the physician whom the patient is scheduled to see. Figure 6.15 shows a more sophisticated application—informing dialysis patients of their recent laboratory-test results and suggested therapy changes.

6.3.3 Query and Surveillance Systems

The query and surveillance capabilities of computer-stored records have no counterpart in manual systems. Medical personnel and administrators can use these capabilities to generate alerts about important clinical events, to retrieve a patient's selected medical or administrative characteristics, and to summarize information statistically. **Query** is the retrieval and aggregation of data about groups of similar patients. **Surveillance** is the detection and flagging of patient conditions that need medical attention.

Although these functions are quite different, their internal logic is similar. In both, the central procedure is to examine a patient's medical record and, if the record meets prespecified criteria, to generate an appropriate output. Query generally addresses a large subset or all of a patient population; the output is a tabular report of selected raw data on all the patient records retrieved, or a statistical summary of the values

```
                    THE NEPHROLOGY SERVICE
                      DURHAM VA HOSPITAL
                   ERWIN RD. & FULTON ST.
                      DURHAM, NC 27705
                          04/03/85


Ms. Margaret Bloom
12 Byte St.
Durham, NC 27705


Dear Ms. Bloom:

  The following are the results of the blood work from 03/25/85.

   NA:   139          K:    5.3      CL:   100      CO2:
   CA:   9.7          PO4:  6.4      BUN:   79      CREAT:  14.3
   GLUC:              TP:            ALB:           U AC:
   TBIL:              ALKP: 124      LDH:           SGOT:
   HCT:   23      FERRITIN:          HAA:           HAA AB:


Increase basaljel by 1 tablet or tablespoon per dose.

                                     Sincerely yours,




                             Steve Cox, PA
                             for William Stead, M.D.


Copy to: Samuel Barnes, M.D.
```

FIGURE 6.15 Letter to a patient reporting results of tests performed by the Duke University nephrology service (produced by TMR). The report also describes changes to the treatment regimen. (*Source:* Courtesy of Duke University Medical Center.)

contained in the records. Surveillance generally addresses only those patients under active care; its output is an alert or **reminder message** such as the message shown in Figure 6.16.

Query and surveillance systems can be used for clinical care and research, retrospective studies, and administration:

Clinical care. Computer reminders have increased substantially physicians' use of preventive care in eligible patients. Surveillance systems can identify patients who are due for periodic screening examinations such as immunizations, breast examinations, and cervical PAP tests, and can remind physicians to perform these procedures during the next visit. For example, physicians given computer reminders quadrupled the use of certain vaccines in eligible patients, compared to those who did not receive reminders [McDonald et al., 1984]. When physicians use an online surveillance system directly, as they do with HELP (Chapter 7), to order tests or treatments, there is an

23–Aug–85 "ENTRY__CTL: C06"

Please return to Regenstrief Institute, do not chart.

TIDBITS FROM THE COMPUTER

These suggestions are based on incomplete data;
your judgment shoud take precedence.

GOLD, M.   AGE: 60   SEX: F   RACE: B   PHONE: 000-0000
Scheduled to BARTON APTS on 27-AUG-85 at 02:00 PM (2)

GAVISCON LIQ, prescribed on 01-JUL-85, is high in sodium and may interfere with blood pressure control.

Patient's last occult blood test was dated 05-APR-84. It is time for his/her yearly screen.

Consider immunizing patient with pneumovax because age (60) places patient at high risk for pneumococcal pneumonia. Do not give if patient has ever been immunized.

Consider getting annual chest x-ray to follow up cardiopulmonary symptoms of CHEST PAIN identified in Problem list on 15-JUN-85.

There is no mammogram on record for this patient. The HIP study (R:2083) showed that, in patients between the ages of 50 and 70, mammography and physical exam reduced the breast cancer death rate by 1/2. The Canadian Medical Association and the Canadian Gynecological Society recommend breast physical exam every year and mammogram every 1 to 3 years. R:2408, R:2386

FIGURE 6.16 The Regenstrief Medical Record System produces a reminder report prior to a patient's visit. The CARE reminder report contains recommendations to the physician about the preventive procedures that should be performed, the problems that should be evaluated, and the drug therapies that are contraindicated and thus should be avoided or altered. (*Source:* Courtesy of Regenstrief Institute.)

even greater potential for improving the cost-effectiveness and quality of patient care. Query systems are particularly useful for conducting ad hoc searches—for example, to identify and contact patients receiving a drug that is recalled from the market. These systems also can facilitate the completion of quality-assurance activities, such as accreditation-required drug reviews. They can identify candidate patients for retrospective audits, and can gather much of the data required to complete such audits.

Clinical research. Query systems can be used to identify patients who meet minimum entrance requirements for prospective clinical trials (see Chapter 16). For example, an investigator could identify all patients seen in a medical clinic who were male, were over 50 years of age, and were taking antihypertension medication. Surveillance facilities can support the execution of a study by tracking patients through their visits, and by following the steps of a clinical trial as described in the study protocol to ensure that treatments are given and measurements obtained when required.

Retrospective studies. Randomized prospective studies are now the gold standard for clinical investigations, but retrospective studies of existing data have contributed to medical progress. Retrospective studies can obtain answers at a small fraction of the time and cost of comparable prospective studies. (We discuss the relative advantages and disadvantages of retrospective studies in Chapter 16.) Medical-record systems can provide many of the data required for a retrospective study. They can, for example, identify study cases and comparable control cases, and can perform the statistical analyses needed to compare the two groups [McDonald and Tierney, 1986b].

Computer-stored records do not eliminate all the work of completing epidemiologic studies; chart reviews and patient interviews may still be necessary. If more information can be retrieved from the record, however, these time-consuming tasks generally may be conducted less frequently and less intensively. Computer-stored records are likely to be most complete and accurate with respect to drugs administered, laboratory-test results, and visit diagnoses, especially if the first two types of data are entered directly from automated pharmacy and laboratory systems. Consequently, computer-stored records are most likely to contribute to research on a physician's practice patterns, the efficacy of tests and treatments, and the toxicity of drugs.

Administration. As we shall discuss in Chapter 19, fixed-cost reimbursement for specific diseases (DRGs or capitation payments) and competitive bidding for health-care contracts provide incentives for administrators to consider clinical as well as cost information in deciding what services to market, to whom, and at what price. In addition, administrators must be able to monitor physicians' use of resources for various classes of patients, and to provide appropriate feedback for physicians whose behavior is far from the norm. Medical query systems can provide information about the relationships among diagnosis, indices of severity of illness, and resource consumption. Thus, query systems are important tools for administrators attempting to make informed decisions in the increasingly cost-sensitive world of health care.

Query and Surveillance Languages

Medical query and surveillance languages are similar in many respects to query languages of general-purpose database-management systems (DBMSs; see Chapter 4). Like most formal computer languages, they have facilities for assigning values to variables, for controlling flow from one statement to the next, and for applying standard logical (AND, OR) and comparison ($<$, $>$, $=$) operators. In addition, they permit the selection and transformation of a series of repeated measurements by means of operations such as first, last, maximum, minimum, trend, number of elements found, amount of change, interval between observations, and so on. A physician can use these kinds of operators to determine the average of the serum glucose measurements observed in the first year after a patient begins insulin treatment, or to find the maximum serum potassium after initiation of potassium-supplementation therapy. Finally, the languages also provide a means to specify what message should be sent to whom when a patient's record meets the search criteria.

The HELP system; MQL, which runs under COSTAR; and CARE, which runs under RMRS, are the oldest and best-known medical query and surveillance systems. (For a more complete discussion of these systems, see Adams' article, listed in the Suggested Readings.) Examples of queries written in each of the languages are given in Figure 6.17. In each example, the computer has been instructed to retrieve records in which the patient's most recent serum-potassium result was critically low.

A fictional *HELP* sector

BLOCK #9.3
SECTOR 300 SERUM POTASSIUM===MEQ/L IS BELOW CRITICAL LEVEL
OWNER: CHEM. TEST   SECURITY: AAA   PRIORITY: 0
ALWAYS SEND DESTINATION LIST: TO CALLING PROGRAM, TO PATIENT RECORD
    TO INFA FOR DEBUGGING--SECTOR STATUS
FINAL EVALUATIONS
A VAL: A
SECTOR LOGIC
  A SEARCH: [FC] CHEM LABS, [N] ELECTROLYTES, [ADJ]POTASSIUM===MEQ
  B EXISTS: IF NOT A THEN EXIT FALSE
  C ARITH: IF A GE 2.9 THEN EXIT FALSE

A fictional *MQL* example

```
 10   /Alarm for low potassium
 20   FOR EACH PATIENT
 30   WHEN DIVISION = TEST
 40   WHEN CODE = POTASSIUM
 50   SET [LASTDATE] ="" ""
 60   DO LAST
 70   WHEN [LASTDATE] IS NOT NIL
 80   SET DATE = [LASTDATE]
 90   WHEN VALUE <3.0
100   LIST OF "SERUM POTASSIUM OF",VALUE," MEQ/L IS BELOW CRITICAL LEVEL
      ON", DATE, UNIT NUMBER, DATE, VALUE
110   STORE ALARMFILE: UNIT NUMBER, DATE, VALUE
200   /Subquery to find date of last potassium measure
210   DEFINE LAST
220   FOR EACH DATE
230   SET [LASTDATE] = DATE
```

A fictional *CARE* example

BLOCK CHEMS
CARE SET C09
! Screen for dangerously low potassium.
IF LAST "K+" IS LT LOWCRIT THEN Serum potassium "K+"{VALUE} mEq is
  below critical level. R:566
END OF BLOCK CHEMS
R"566 THE ROLE OF SERUM POTASSIUM IN CARDIAC FUNCTION
    GREEN S.A., GLUE B.F
    REVS. ELEM. PHYSIOL. 21, 188-237 (1952)

FIGURE 6.17 Examples of query statements from the HELP, COSTAR, and Regenstrief systems. In each example, the statements instruct the computer to retrieve records in which the patient's most recent serum-potassium result was critically low. (*Source:* Reprinted, with permission, from Adams, J. B. Three surveillance and query languages for medical care. *M.D. Computing,* 3(1):11–19, 1986, Springer-Verlag New York.)

MQL and CARE are similar in that both permit query or surveillance functions with one command syntax and both were originally designed for use in outpatient care and are batch-oriented. HELP is designed purely for surveillance; it employs a companion program for queries and was originally used only in inpatient settings. In HELP, alerts can be *event-driven*; the entry of an abnormal laboratory result or a prescription of a drug potentially dangerous to the patient can initiate the reminder logic.

Opportunities and Pitfalls

Given the success of epidemiologic studies using only hundreds of paper charts, we are optimistic that automatic access to tens of thousands of electronic charts will produce new clinical insights. A computer record does not in itself, however, create a research utopia, in which a push of the button produces a scientific article; serious practical and methodological problems exist.

First, a researcher cannot obtain accurate information from a medical-record system without intimate knowledge of what its content is, and of how the information was obtained, encoded, and stored. If you wish to identify all patients taking phenytoin (a drug used to treat some forms of epilepsy), you might need to know that phenytoin is stored under three codes corresponding to the tablet, the suspension, and the injectable forms of the drug. If your goal is to find the prevalence of routine urinalysis among adult patients, it is necessary to know how most urinalysis results are obtained and recorded. The computer may receive reports for all those tests analyzed by the laboratory, but few of those performed by physicians in their offices, because the doctors may note the results of the latter in their visit reports only.

There may be important delays in data receipt. A case-abstracting system may create a 2- to 3-month delay between patient discharge and entry of the discharge diagnoses in the computer. As we emphasized in Chapter 2, a general rule is that computer-stored records are never complete. If data capture depends on the cooperation of health-care professionals in completing special forms, then the forms almost surely will be less than complete. Thus, users of a query system must understand the limitations of the data-collection procedures before they write queries to answer particular questions.

6.4 Examples of Automated Ambulatory Medical-Record Systems

An automated medical record is a key feature of both a hospital information system and an automated ambulatory medical-record system (AAMRS)—both support patient-care and administrative functions. In an outpatient setting, however, many of the functions performed by a hospital information system—for example, dietary service planning and intensive-care monitoring—are unnecessary.

Most AAMRSs contain modules for maintaining medical records, managing financial and administrative information, and generating reports. Although many of the general issues of medical-record systems apply in both hospital and outpatient settings, we shall illustrate the features of medical-record systems by describing four ambulatory-care systems: COSTAR, the Regenstrief Medical Record System (RMRS), The Medical Record (TMR), and Summary Time Oriented Record (STOR). These systems have fairly long histories, and people have written about them extensively. Blum's 1984 book (listed in the Suggested Readings) contains chapters describing in greater detail these and other AAMRSs. In Chapter 7, we shall investigate the broader functions of (inpatient) hospital information systems.

6.4.1 COSTAR

COSTAR was developed in the late 1960s by Barnett and his colleagues at the Laboratory of Computer Science at Massachusetts General Hospital. Originally designed to support the operation of the Harvard Community Health Plan (HCHP), the system later was revised for use by other ambulatory-care practices. The developers expanded its functional capabilities (to allow billing, for example), and removed many of the features designed specifically for HCHP. In 1978, the version called COSTAR 5 was made available to any organization that wanted to use or market the product. Today, a practice that wants to install COSTAR can implement the public-domain version or one of the many enhanced commercial versions. The total number of COSTAR users is unknown; however, a 1986 survey of users obtained information from more than 110 separate installations [Barnett et al., 1979; Campbell, 1986].

Two design goals of COSTAR 5 were (1) to facilitate patient care by improving the availability and organization of the medical record, and (2) to support the function of an ambulatory-care practice by providing administrative, managerial, and financial support functions. To meet these goals, system developers chose a modular design, thus allowing each user organization to tailor the system to meet its administrative and clinical needs and its financial constraints, and permitting phased installation of the system. The basic COSTAR 5 system includes modules for (1) system security and data integrity; (2) patient registration, (3) appointment scheduling, (4) billing and financial reporting, (5) collection and storage of medical records, and (6) management reporting. Only the security and registration modules and a minimal medical record are required; the extended medical-record functions and the other modules are optional.

COSTAR can operate as a fully automated medical-record system. Once entered, all medical data are available online; thus, the need for a paper medical record is eliminated. Prior to a scheduled patient visit, the system prints out a summary medical record for review by the physician, as well as a blank encounter form that is used to capture administrative and medical data from the visit. The encounter form contains no preprinted patient-specific information.

During the course of patient visits, physicians collect medical data and complete the encounter forms. They check off relevant diagnoses, signs, and symptoms from coded lists of problems and indicate the status of problems—a major problem is indicated with an "M," an inactive problem with an "I," and so on. They can add comments at the bottom of the forms or dictate notes that will be processed separately. After a visit, clerical personnel enter the data from the form into the computer system.

The medical-record module produces three standard output reports in addition to the encounter (input) form:

- *The encounter report* summarizes a single patient visit, including diagnoses, results of the physical examination and of laboratory tests, and medication orders (see Figure 6.5)
- *The status report* summarizes the patient's current medical status, including a record of preventive measures; allergies; major and minor problems; family, social, and past medical histories; recent laboratory-test results; and current medications (see Figure 6.7)
- *Specialty flowcharts* summarize the temporal course of diseases or clinical findings by displaying a chronological listing of clinical observations and laboratory-test results (see Figure 6.10)

The management-reporting module produces a variety of standard reports (for example, the number of visits by patient, by provider, or by specialty service). Practices can easily program the system to produce other periodic reports. In addition, COSTAR supports a medical query language (MQL) that can be used to perform arbitrarily complex searches of the database on an ad hoc basis.

6.4.2 The Regenstrief Medical Record System

The Regenstrief Medical Record System (RMRS) was developed by McDonald and his colleagues at the Indiana University Medical Center. It has been in operation at Wishard Memorial Hospital since 1974. In 1988, it maintained medical histories for over 250,000 patients—more than 9 years of data for at least 50,000 patients [McDonald et al., 1983; McDonald et al., 1988]. It contains almost 25 million separate patient observations, all of which are encoded and fully retrievable. RMRS is part of a larger administrative support system that handles appointment scheduling and charge capture. The unique feature of the medical-record component is a reminder system that actively reviews patient data and produces reminder notes for the physician based on 1400 encoded protocol rules. An evaluation study of the initial version of the system demonstrated that the reminders significantly improved the behavior of physicians in remembering to order laboratory tests when appropriate, and in prescribing or modifying medication plans [McDonald et al., 1984].

RMRS schedules all appointments and produces three documents prior to the patient's visit:

1. *The quality-assurance report* contains recommendations to the physician about the preventive procedures that should be performed, the problems that should be evaluated, and the drug therapies that are contraindicated (see Figure 6.16). The report is discarded after the visit.
2. *The flowsheet summary* is a time-ordered summary of the clinical database (see Figure 6.6).
3. *The patient encounter form* is a patient-specific form used to capture medical data during the visit (see Figure 6.4). The contents of the form (problem list, active prescriptions, commonly ordered tests, and flowsheet observations to collect) are determined by the system based on patient data and physician-specified rules.

After a visit, the physician writes the progress report, updates the problem list, and orders laboratory tests and drugs, all on the encounter form. A data-entry clerk then enters the flowsheet observations into the clinical database. RMRS also accepts history and progress-note information in coded format; however, due to the high cost of data entry, in practice little of this information is entered. Instead, a copy of the encounter form is filed in the paper record. Thus, RMRS supplements rather than replaces the traditional record. Laboratory-test results and drug-administration information are obtained directly from the Regenstrief clinical laboratory and pharmacy systems.

CARE, a medical query language, is used to query the medical-record files and to produce quality-assurance reports. A set of CARE statements defines the search criteria (see Figure 6.17). The output of a retrieval is a set of patient records that meet the criteria. For a quality-assurance run, the output is a set of relevant reminder messages.

6.4.3 The Medical Record

The Medical Record (TMR) was developed by Stead and Hammond at Duke University starting in 1975. An original design goal was to eliminate the paper medical record. Thus, system developers emphasized the capture and storage of patient-care data, although TMR also provides appointment-scheduling and billing capabilities [Stead et al., 1983; Stead and Hammond, 1988]. By 1989, the system was used at over 25 sites in the United States and Canada. The Duke University nephrology clinic uses one version of TMR. Since 1981, all patients seen by the service have been tracked using the computer record; no other patient records are kept. The system maintains for each patient a complete list of diagnoses and procedures, and a time-oriented record of subjective and physical findings, laboratory data, medications, and procedures.

Prior to a patient's visit to the nephrology clinic, TMR reviews the patient's medical record and generates a patient-specific encounter form that summarizes recent clinical findings and treatments (see Figure 6.3). The physician uses this form to review the patient's record and to collect new data. Although physicians may record information on this form for later entry by clerical personnel, they are encouraged to enter their prescriptions directly, thus taking advantage of the system's ability to warn against drug allergies and drug interactions, and to calculate correct doses.

Physicians may view the complete patient record on a VDT. TMR can display data in one of three orientations: problem, time, or encounter. Doctors can view sequential values of a finding or test either numerically or graphically. The system also can generate a narrative text report (see Figure 6.14) from data entered in a multiple-choice form, such as the form for patients with coronary-artery disease shown in Figure 6.13.

6.4.4 Summary Time Oriented Record

Summary Time Oriented Record (STOR) was developed by Whiting-O'Keefe and his associates at the University of California, San Francisco (UCSF) [Whiting-O'Keefe et al., 1988]. In 1985, 6 years after beginning work on the pilot system, the developers began to implement STOR throughout inpatient and outpatient locations as UCSF. By 1988, STOR contained 60,000 outpatient medical records, supported 22 clinic locations with 200,000 outpatient visits per year, and responded to 2000 online queries per day. An evaluation study demonstrated that STOR communicated more information to clinical users than did the traditional paper medical record [Whiting-O'Keefe et al., 1985].

STOR provides two areas of clinical service: (1) the computer-based storage and retrieval of ambulatory medical records, and (2) the online display of inpatient and outpatient clinical information in response to user queries. To provide these functions, STOR creates a common inpatient and outpatient database that contains patient information gathered via a LAN from seven ancillary and departmental computer systems in the hospital. The real-time reports available through STOR include flowsheets, graphs and charts, problem and therapy lists, and registration data. In addition, reverse chronological displays of clinical laboratory data, operative notes, pathology reports, radiology reports, discharge diagnoses and medications, and electrocardiogram reports are available at any time at any STOR terminal.

Before each clinic visit, STOR updates its database through the LAN, prints a patient-specific encounter form, and orders retrieval of the paper medical record when clinic-defined criteria are met (STOR replaces the traditional paper record in about 75 percent of outpatient visits). The encounter form is a compact, multipart summary of patient information that includes a flowsheet of problems, therapies, and specified laboratory-test results; clinic notes (when available); information from ancillary systems; additional (untrended) problem, therapy, and laboratory data; and optional charts and graphs (Figures 6.1 and 6.2). The format and content of this document is determined by clinic-, diagnosis-, and patient-specific criteria. During the examination, the physician uses this form to update the problem and therapy lists, to record new data observations, and to record a progress note. Clinic clerks then enter the information into the computer. All clinics enter their problems and therapies, but retain the option either to enter progress notes or to keep copies of the notes in a local file.

STOR's problem list is unusually flexible in that it is an arbitrary depth hierarchy of coded or uncoded items—items may be problems, diagnoses, disease manifestations, or simply headings. Each item can be associated with one or more data values (coded or uncoded) that have been observed at different points in time. Items may be combined to define more complex items—for example, EXPECTED PREGNANCY WEIGHT is defined as a function of INITIAL PREGNANCY WEIGHT and WEEKS PREGNANT.

6.5 The Future of Automated Medical-Record Systems

To date, the health-care field has invested most of its computer dollars in administrative systems—for example, systems that schedule appointments, register patients, or generate bills. Computer-stored medical-record systems are used in relatively few institutions. It is easy to understand why: Billing systems are simpler, require fewer data, and are less expensive than are systems designed to manage clinical information as well. Two trends will work to make computer-based medical-record systems more cost-effective: (1) the decreasing cost of hardware, and (2) the tendency of health-care units to aggregate into large outpatient clinics, health-maintenance organizations, and proprietary hospital chains. Large institutions are better able to invest in expensive computer systems and can benefit from economies of scale in the management of great numbers of clinical and administrative data. Within a decade, we expect the use of computer-stored medical records to be universal in both hospital and office-practice settings.

Several technical problems must be solved, however, before health-care professionals will embrace these systems enthusiastically. Of most importance, we must determine how best to enter physician-collected data into the system. Also, we must develop powerful, yet intuitive, mechanisms for retrieving and viewing information (the user interface). As we mentioned before, new tools such as mouse pointing devices, touch screens, voice-input devices, and menus will facilitate data entry. In addition, intelligent terminals, high-resolution display monitors, and graphical interfaces will enable health-care workers to interact with the computer system more naturally.

We have stressed the importance of an integrated medical record that combines data from multiple sources. Comprehensive, integrated systems will minimize the problems of data capture and data entry and will provide a broader scope of data for use with automated decision aids. Ensuring continuity of care between outpatient encounters and hospital visits will remain problematic, however. Advances in network technology and the establishment of standard formats and procedures for data exchange will make it simple to transfer medical records among sites electronically. The development of wallet-sized card medical records (a plastic card much like a credit card that magnetically stores digitally coded information and that is carried by the patient between health-care visits) could provide a simple means for communicating information among independent health-care providers.

The use of computer technology to aid directly in physician decision making gradually will become more common (see Chapter 15). The ONCOCIN system developed by researchers at Stanford University is being used experimentally in the therapeutic management of cancer patients receiving certain forms of chemotherapy. Physicians directly enter the data collected during a visit from the physical examination and laboratory tests (for example, white-blood-cell count). The system then uses its encoded knowledge of chemotherapy protocols to evaluate data from the patient's current and past visits and to suggest appropriate doses and schedules for drug administration. The ultimate success of ONCOCIN and of other sophisticated decision-support systems will rely heavily on these systems' ability to integrate smoothly with the medical record, so that physicians can obtain the data necessary for decision making without having to enter all the data themselves.

We believe that a microcomputer-based medical workstation linked to a hospital information system eventually will serve as a comprehensive information resource for health-care professionals. (See the McDonald and Tierney article, listed in the Suggested Readings, for a discussion of one such microcomputer system.) The computer can provide access to patient data and to general medical information, such as recommended drug doses, common drug side effects, laboratory-test sensitivities, and disease definitions and related findings. It also can aid physicians in decisions associated with order writing; for example, it can detect drug–drug, drug–test, and drug–diagnosis interactions. Someday, physicians may be able to access data for a specific patient, summarize the collective experience with similar patients in the institution or even in numerous locations, consult knowledge bases of expert opinions, and search the medical literature. Thus, physicians of the future could find all the information they need linked in one seamless web, available at any time through their medical-record workstations.

Suggested Readings

Adams, J. B. Three surveillance and query languages for medical care. *M.D. Computing*, 3:11, 1986.

> *This article reviews the tasks of medical surveillance and query systems, then compares and contrasts the designs and capabilities of the HELP system, MQL, and CARE.*

Barnett, G. O. The application of computer-based medical-record systems in ambulatory practice. *New England Journal of Medicine*, 310:1643, 1984.

> *This article compares the characteristics of manual and automated ambulatory medical-record systems, discusses implementation issues, and predicts future developments in technology.*

Blum, B. I. (ed). *Information Systems for Patient Care*. New York: Springer-Verlag, 1984.

> *Most of the papers in this collection were published originally in the Proceedings of the Symposium on Computer Applications in Medical Care (SCAMC 1977–1982). The book contains chapters on COSTAR, RMRS, TMR, and other ambulatory-care systems, as well as chapters that describe the HELP and PROMIS hospital information systems.*

McDonald, C. J. (ed). Computer-stored medical record systems. *M.D. Computing*, 5(5):1–62, 1988.

> *This issue of* M.D. Computing *contains invited papers on the STOR, HELP, RMRS, and TMR systems. The objective of the issue is to describe the design goals, functions, and internal structure of these established, large-scale computer-based medical-record systems.*

McDonald, C. J. *Action-Oriented Decisions in Ambulatory Medicine*. Chicago: Year Book Medical Publishers, 1981.

> *This book summarizes a 5-year project to define medical decision rules for outpatient practice. The body of the text is a casebook of defensible practices in ambulatory medicine, as reflected in the detailed medical logic (CARE rules) used by the Regenstrief Medical Record System.*

McDonald, C. J. and Tierney, W. M. The medical gopher: A microcomputer system to help find, organize and decide about patient data. *The Western Journal of Medicine*, 145:823, 1986.

> *McDonald and Tierney describe research conducted at the Regenstrief Institute for Health Care in developing a microcomputer-based medical workstation that can help physicians to organize, review, and record medical information.*

Pryor, T. A., et al. The HELP system. *Journal of Medical Systems*, 7:87, 1983.

> *This article summarizes the HELP system's objectives and describes HELP's use in clinical decision making.*

Weed, L. L. *Medical Records, Medical Education and Patient Care: The Problem-Oriented Record as a Basic Tool.* Chicago: Year Book Medical Publishers, 1969.
   In this book, Weed presents his plan for collecting and structuring patient data to produce a problem-oriented medical record.

Questions for Discussion

1. What do we mean when we speak of the *scope* of an information system? What problems arise when the scope of the medical record exceeds the scope of control of the organization maintaining the record?
2. Discuss three ways in which a computer system could facilitate information transfer between hospitals and ambulatory-care facilities, thus enhancing continuity of care for previously hospitalized patients who have been discharged and are now being followed by their primary physicians.
3. Describe and contrast the characteristics of records of a hospital stay and of an outpatient visit—note differences in the number of data collected, the level of detail of recording, the intensity of monitoring, and the number and variety of health-care professionals collecting and recording the data. Describe three ways in which the design of ambulatory-care medical-record systems and inpatient-care medical-record systems should reflect these differences.
4. Among the key issues for designing a computer-based medical-record system are what information should be captured and how it should be entered into the system.
   a. Physicians may enter data directly or may record data on a paper worksheet (encounter form) for later transcription by a data-entry worker. What are the advantages and disadvantages of each method?
   b. Discuss the advantages and disadvantages of entry of free text, of entry of fully coded information, and of an intermediate or compromise method.
5. Consider the task of creating a summary report for the time-series data stored in a computer-based medical-record system. Clinical laboratories traditionally provide summary test results in flowsheet format, thus highlighting clinically important changes over time. A medical-record system that contains information for patients with chronic disease must present serial clinical observations, history information, and medications, as well as laboratory-test results. Suggest a suitable format for presenting the information collected during 10 ambulatory-care patient visits.
6. Someday, a person may carry a plastic card on which is stored her complete medical record. Such a card could be read by a scanner, and the information could thus be made available to a computer in, for example, a pharmacy or clinic. How do you think increased use of computers in medicine, and increased networking of those machines, will influence the traditional strict confidentiality maintained between health-care provider and patient?

7

Hospital Information Systems

Gio Wiederhold and Leslie E. Perreault

After reading this chapter, you should know the answers to these questions:

- What are the economic factors that make hospital information systems important?
- What are a hospital's primary requirements for information?
- What are the clinical and administrative functions provided by a hospital information system?
- What are the difficulties that arise from the lack of integration of information within a hospital?
- What are the relative advantages and disadvantages of *central, modular,* and *distributed* hospital information systems?
- How does a hospital information system's design depend on the functional goals of the system developers?
- What are the significant barriers slowing the acceptance of medical information systems? What are the factors that will encourage future development of these systems?

7.1 Information Management in Hospitals

In a hospital, health-care personnel constantly make decisions, both while caring for patients and while managing and running the institution. Physicians evaluate their patients' conditions and decide on appropriate treatments. Nurses assess patient status, plan patient care, and administer treatments. Administrators determine staffing levels, manage inventories of drugs and supplies, and set charges for services. The governing boards of hospitals make decisions about investing in new facilities and eliminating underutilized resources.

The purpose of a **hospital information system (HIS)** is to manage the information that health professionals need to perform their jobs effectively and efficiently. Many of the functions of an HIS are analogous to those of the automated ambulatory medical-record systems we discussed in Chapter 6. HISs and ambulatory medical-record systems both facilitate communication, integrate information, and coordinate action among multiple health-care professionals; in some cases, they also aid in patient monitoring. In addition, they assist in the organization and storage of information, and they perform some record-keeping functions. In fact, all the features of an ambulatory medical-record system also are provided by a computer-based HIS. The degree to which specific features are emphasized, however, differs.

An HIS generally is more comprehensive than an ambulatory medical-record system, and the functions it supports are more complex. These differences arise because hospitals and outpatient facilities provide different types of health care. For example, hospitalized patients usually receive continuous care over a course of days, rather than occasional care over a period of years. Furthermore, hospital personnel must attend to the needs of many inpatients; an HIS can help the staff to coordinate housekeeping and room services, to plan meals in accordance with dietary requirements and restrictions, to track the administration of medications, and to provide other such routine services that outpatients do not receive professionally. The complexity of a hospital's functions places great demands on an HIS to organize and manage the large number of data collected for each patient and to provide health-care workers with timely access to accurate and up-to-date information.

7.1.1 Information Requirements

From a clinical perspective, the most important function of an HIS is to provide communication among the many health-care workers who cooperate in caring for patients, and to organize and present patient-specific data so that the staff can more easily interpret and use those data in decision making. From an administrative perspective, the most pressing information needs are those related to the daily operation and management of the hospital—bills must be generated accurately and rapidly, employees and vendors must be paid, supplies must be ordered, and so on. In addition, administrators need information to make short- and long-term planning decisions.

We can classify a hospital's informational needs in three broad categories: support for daily operations, support for planning, and documentation.

- *Operational requirements.* Health-care workers require detailed and up-to-date factual information to perform the daily tasks that keep a hospital running—the bread-and-butter tasks of the institution. Examples of queries for operational information are: Where is patient John Dinkelman? What drugs is he receiving? When is he scheduled to be released? Who will pay his bill? An HIS can support these operational requirements for information by organizing data for prompt and easy access.
- *Planning requirements.* Hospital personnel also require information to make short- and long-term decisions about patient care and hospital management. An HIS should help health professionals to answer queries such as these: Will surgical treatment lead to a better prognosis for this patient than will medical treatment? How many free beds will be available for new patients this weekend? Is the inventory of codeine adequate, or should additional supplies be ordered? What are the financial and medical implications of closing the maternity ward? Often, the data necessary for planning are generated by many sources. An HIS can help planners by aggregating, analyzing, and summarizing the information relevant to decision making.
- *Documentation requirements.* The need to maintain records for future reference or analysis makes up the third category of informational requirements. Some requirements are internally imposed. For example, a complete record of each patient's health status and treatments is necessary to ensure continuity of care across multiple providers and over time. External requirements create a large demand for data collection and record keeping in hospitals. As we discussed in Chapter 2, the medical record is a legal document. If necessary, the courts can refer to the record to determine whether a patient received proper care. Insurance companies require itemized billing statements, and medical records substantiate the charges submitted to them. Hospital-accreditation boards have specific requirements concerning the content and quality of medical records. Furthermore, to qualify for participation in the Medicare and Medicaid programs, hospitals must follow accepted procedures for auditing the medical staff, monitor the quality of patient care, and be able to show that they meet the safety requirements for infectious-disease management, building, and equipment.

The importance of appropriate clinical decision making is obvious—we devoted all of Chapter 3 to explaining methods to help clinicians select diagnostic tests, interpret test results, and choose treatments for their patients. The decisions made by administrators and managers are no less important. Their choices concerning the acquisition and use of hospital resources affect both the quality of care that patients receive and the financial health of the institution. Administrators can use current and historical data when scheduling nurses, staff physicians, and emergency-room staff; when ordering drugs, blood, and other perishable supplies; when scheduling the use of hospital beds, surgical suites, and medical equipment; and when deciding whether to add or eliminate services.

Scheduling in the hospital is complicated because the patient load and resource utilization can vary rapidly through the course of the day simply due to chance; also, both variables are subject to periodic variations according to time of day, day of the week, season of the year, and so on. In the longer run, changes in local economic conditions and in the composition of the population can profoundly affect hospital-utilization patterns. The effective management of a hospital requires that sufficient resources be on hand to meet ordinary fluctuations in demand. At the same time, resources must not remain unnecessarily idle. If hospital planners can analyze the data to detect trends in resource utilization and can make predictions about demand, they can expand or contract hospital services to an appropriate level.

In the past, waste and inefficiency caused by poor operating procedures and inappropriate choices simply were translated into higher health-care costs. In the 1980s, however, a switch by the government to fixed reimbursement based on diagnosis-related groups (DRGs), rather than on costs or charges, placed increasing pressure on hospitals to analyze and control their costs (see Chapter 19). Inefficient institutions lose money and go out of business. Hospital administrators must collect and analyze many data to monitor resource utilization, to determine the costs of providing care, to estimate the productivity of health-care personnel, and to monitor the quality of the care provided.

7.1.2 The Cost of Information

In a 1966 study of three New York hospitals, researchers found that information handling to satisfy requirements such as those discussed above accounted for approximately 25 percent of the hospitals' total operating costs [Jydstrup and Gross, 1966]. On average, workers in administrative departments spent about three-fourths of their time handling information; workers in nursing units spent about one-fourth of their time on these tasks (Table 7.1). Over 20 years later, the basic conclusions of the study still hold true: Information management in hospitals is a costly activity. The collection, storage, retrieval, analysis, and dissemination of clinical and administrative information necessary to support a hospital's daily operations, to meet external and internal requirements for documentation, and to support short-term and strategic planning are important and time-consuming aspects of the jobs of hospital workers.

Because of the level of spending attributable to information management, it is a concern of hospital administrators, patients, third-party payers, and, ultimately, all members of society. Health-care costs have grown rapidly over the last 2 decades, from an expenditure level of $42 billion in 1965 to more than $458 billion in 1986—nearly 11 percent of the gross national product, or $1835 for each person in the United States. Increasing concern about this large and growing commitment in resources led to many changes in the health-care industry during the 1980s. Hospital costs, which account for approximately 40 percent of national health-care expenditures, have been the primary target of programs to contain health-care spending (see Chapter 19).

7.1.3 The Functions of a Hospital Information System

A carefully designed computer-based system can increase the productivity and effectiveness of health professionals, and potentially can provide a means to decrease a hospital's labor costs. Friedman and Martin proposed a functional model for an HIS

TABLE 7.1 Time Spent on Information Handling by Type of Employees (Rochester General Hospital)

Department and Type of Employee	Percentage of Employee's Available Useful Time Spent on Information Handling
Nursing:	
One medical-surgical unit:	
Head nurse and assistant head nurse	64
Registered nurses	36
Practical nurses	22
Nursing aides	9
Ward clerks	85
Total (except students)	34
All units—North- and Westside	28
Operating, labor, and delivery rooms	14
Central supply and I.V. service	6
Emergency department	28
Nursing offices	40
Total[a]	25
Administrative departments:	
Accounting, etc.[b]	95
Other—administrative office, admitting, telephone, purchasing, personnel, health office, etc.	66
Total	73
Radiology (Diagnostic, Therapeutic, Isotopic):	
Radiologists[c]	35
Technicians	28
Others—secretaries, clerks, orderlies	70
Total	42
Laboratories:	
Bacteriology (including prorated part of clerical)	17
Hematology	20
Chemistry	30
Pathology	37
Total (including photography)	28
Other:	
Medical records	95
Interns and residents	30
Dietary (10 dieticians—35%; 75 other—3%)	7
Physical medicine (1 director—50%; 3 clerks—80%; 11 other—5%)	22
Outpatient department	35
Pharmacy	26
EKG, BMR, EEG[d]	36
Social service	45
Maintenance (chief and assistant—36%; 42 others, including secretaries—4%)	6
Housekeeping ⎫ Laundry ⎭	<3
Total Hospital (958 equivalent full-time employees)	26

[a]Except students, whose information handling cost is zero by definition.
[b]Almost entirely information handling.
[c]Not on payroll.
[d]EKG = electrocardiogram, BMR = basal metabolic rate, EEG = electroencephalogram.
Source: Reprinted with permission from Jydstrup, R. A. and Gross, M. J. Cost of information handling in hospitals. *Health Services Research,* 1(3):242, 1966. Copyright by the Hospital Research and Educational Trust, 840 North Lake Shore Drive, Chicago, Illinois, 60611.

that consists of components that perform six distinct functions: (1) core applications, (2) business and financial functions, (3) communications and networking, (4) departmental management, (5) medical documentation, and (6) medical support [Friedman and Martin, 1987].

Core systems perform the basic centralized functions of hospital operation, such as patient scheduling, admission, and discharge. Maintenance of the hospital census usually is one of the first tasks to be considered for automation; the majority of hospitals today use a computer to store patient-identification information and other critical demographic data that are acquired during the patient-registration process. The census is maintained by the **admission–discharge–transfer (ADT)** component of an HIS, which updates the census whenever a patient is admitted to the hospital, discharged from the hospital, or transferred to a new bed. Before computers were used, the census often was posted on a board in a central location to facilitate access by all staff members. Using a computer-based system, health-care workers can examine and update the centralized patient database from remote locations via terminals.

Census data serve as a reference base for the financial programs that perform billing functions. When an HIS is extended to the pharmacy, laboratory, and other ancillary departments, the core system can provide a common reference base for use by these systems as well. Without access to this centralized database, these subsystems would have to maintain duplicate patient records. In addition, the transmission of ADT data can trigger other activities, such as automatic retrieval of medical records from archival storage when patients are admitted, notification of hospital housekeeping when a bed becomes free, and application of predictive functions to estimate future bed availability in times of high occupancy.

Business and financial systems assist with traditional financial functions, such as managing the payroll and accounts receivable. The majority of these data-processing tasks are well structured, labor-intensive, and repetitious—ideal applications for computers. Furthermore, the basic financial tasks of a hospital's business office do not differ substantially from those of such offices in other industries. Data-processing techniques developed to meet the needs of general industry were adapted easily for use in hospitals. For these reasons, it is not surprising that financial functions typically were the first to be automated; most hospitals now use some type of computer system to support their financial applications. In the future, more sophisticated systems will provide tools to help financial managers make investment decisions, manage costs, set charges, and respond to bids from third-party payers.

Communications and networking systems allow the integration of all components of an HIS. In the hospital, the ward is the hub of clinical activity. It is at the bedside that health professionals assess patients' health status and order drugs, laboratory tests, diagnostic radiology tests, and other procedures. An HIS can facilitate communication between the ward and the ancillary departments that provide these services. The departments most commonly served by an HIS are the pharmacy, the radiology department, and the clinical laboratories. An HIS also might provide communication links with the dietary service, operating room, social services, physical therapy, or housekeeping.

In a manual system, physicians write orders for drugs and laboratory tests. A nurse or a ward clerk then fills out an order slip, which is physically transported to the appropriate destination. Automated **order entry** and **results reporting** are two important functions provided by a computer-based HIS. Health professionals can use the HIS to communicate with ancillary departments electronically, eliminating the easily misplaced paper slips and thus minimizing delays in conveying orders. The information then is available online, where it is accessible to health professionals who wish to review a patient's drug profile or previous laboratory-test results.

Departmental-management systems support the informational needs of individual departments within the hospital—for example, the laboratory, pharmacy, and radiology departments. Often, they are installed as standalone systems designed to perform circumscribed tasks, and they are unable to communicate directly with other computers. If, however, the departmental systems are integrated with the rest of an HIS (either through shared computers or via communications networks), they can use data collected in other parts of the hospital as inputs for their own internal functions. For example, order data, entered on the wards, can be used to create specimen-collection lists in the clinical laboratory, to control inventory in the pharmacy, and to schedule the use of computed-tomography (CT) and X-ray equipment in the radiology department. We shall discuss computer-based information systems to support laboratories, pharmacies, and radiology departments in Chapters 9, 10, and 11.

Medical-documentation systems perform the functions of the standard medical record in collecting, organizing, storing, and presenting the clinical information used to manage the care of individual patients (see Chapters 2 and 6). In an HIS that supports automated order entry and results reporting, the medical-documentation component stores the order and result data. These data represent an important subset of a patient's clinical record. A comprehensive medical record, however, also includes a variety of data that staff have collected by questioning and observing the patient. Some HISs also support the management of these data. For example, they help nurses to chart vital signs, to maintain medication-administration records, and to record other diagnostic and therapeutic information.

Medical-documentation systems also can assist in hospitalwide activities, such as infection control, discharge planning, quality assurance, and utilization review. **Quality assurance (QA)** is a critical concern of hospitals, of hospital-accreditation boards, and of the government and other third-party payers—all are concerned that patients receive high-quality health care. Medical-documentation systems assist in the collection and preliminary analysis of data that help hospital administrators to assess patient outcomes, quality of workers' performance, and compliance to hospital policies and standard procedures. Once administrators have defined computable performance indicators (for example, mortality, morbidity, or the incidence of medication errors), the HIS can monitor and report performance on these measures. Administrators then can use this information to identify potential problems and to evaluate the effectiveness of existing hospital policies.

During **utilization review,** patient data are analyzed to detect inappropriate use of resources. The classification of hospitalizations by DRG can aid in QA by identifying unusual cases (cases in which costs or length of stay are significantly different from the average), which hospital administrators or external agencies then can scrutinize. Before the advent of DRG-based reimbursement, hospital administrators were required to conduct periodic reviews of the length of hospitalizations to detect unusually long stays, and hence excessive charges to the reimbursing agencies. Under the new system of fixed reimbursement per hospitalization, utilization reviews are needed to help identify abnormally *short* stays and omitted services, thus ensuring that patients do not receive inadequate care because of the financial pressure placed on the hospitals to reduce costs.

Medical-support systems directly assist clinical personnel in data interpretation and decision making. Once the clinical components of an HIS are well developed, clinical-support systems can use the information stored there to monitor patients and to issue alerts, to make diagnostic suggestions, and to provide limited therapy advice. For example, a useful adjunct to an order-entry system is a program that helps physicians to calculate patient-specific drug-dosing regimens. Decision support was a major motivation in the development of the HELP system (see Section 7.3.2 and Chapter 15); the direct assistance this system provides in monitoring and interpreting patient information encourages complete and timely recording of the data [Warner, 1979]. We shall describe other examples of decision-support systems in Chapter 15. Such services are not yet common features of HISs, however.

7.1.4 Integration of Hospital Information

Clinical and administrative personnel have distinct areas of responsibility and perform many of their functions separately. Thus, it is not surprising that clinical and administrative data traditionally have been managed separately—administrative data in business offices and clinical data in medical-records departments. When computers are used, the hospital's information processing often is performed on separate computers. These computers may also be managed separately, thereby avoiding conflicts about priorities in services and investment.

The lack of integration of data from diverse sources creates a host of problems. If clinical and administrative data are stored on separate systems, then data of mutual interest must be copied either from the source documents into both systems or from one system to the other. It is not unusual for the output generated by one computer system to be manually entered into another independent computer system. In addition to the expense of redundant data entry and data maintenance incurred by this approach, the consistency of information tends to be poor because data may be updated in one place and not in the other, or information may be copied incorrectly. Inconsistencies in the databases can result in lost charges, inappropriate patient management, and inappropriate resource-allocation decisions. For example, during an emergency, a blood specimen may be sent directly to the laboratory. No charge is entered via the order-entry system, however, and the test is not listed on the patient's discharge bill.

Clearly, the administrative and clinical functions of an HIS are related in many ways. A complete and accurate medical record is crucial not only for clinical practice, but also for billing, quality-assurance activities, and longer-term resource planning. Conversely, the hospital census maintained by the ADT system is useful not only to the administrators who monitor occupancy rates, but also to the clinicians and nurses who must know where to find their patients. In general, much more information flows from the clinical to the administrative side than moves in the opposite direction.

The integration of data from myriad sources in the hospital produces a rich database for decision making. If these data collectively are accessible to application programs, extremely sophisticated applications are possible. Infection-control programs provide a clear example of the advantages of integrating clinical and administrative data. Infection surveillance is required to alert the hospital to the possibility of a hospital-based epidemic, an event of concern both to clinical health professionals and to administrators concerned with quality assurance.

An infection-control program might monitor current infection rates and compare them with the rates that have been recorded in the past, possibly adjusting for differences in the patient population. If the system detects a significant discrepancy, hospital-census data could be used to identify patients who might have been in contact with the infected patients, and staff work schedules could be used to identify health workers who might carry the infection. The final product of such an infection-monitoring system would be a set of infection notices to hospital personnel and to areas that are likely sources of the infection, as well as a listing of patients who might have been exposed to the infection, and thus should be tested for the presence of the organism.

Although freestanding systems still are common in hospitals, we envision an increasingly integrated approach to the design of an HIS in which the communication component is essential. The objectives of high-quality and cost-effective health care cannot be satisfied if multiple computer systems operate in isolation. The integration and sharing of data in common databases eliminates redundancy and produces a synergistic effect; sophisticated applications (such as the infection-control program) are easier to implement when data are shared globally than when independent systems have access to only a subset of the data collected within the hospital. An integrated HIS does not require that all services be provided by a single, large computer—such an approach, however, is not unusual.

7.2 Alternative Architectures
for Hospital Information Systems

In this section, we shall describe three alternative models for an integrated HIS: the central, modular, and distributed models. In theory, each of these architectures provides the same range of functions; from a user's point of view, the differences among the systems may not be obvious. From the perspective of the computing personnel who design, develop, and maintain the systems, however, the differences are striking. The choice of architecture affects the choice of hardware and the design of software for storing, accessing, and transmitting data. Each of the three architectures has advantages and disadvantages. During the 1960s and 1970s, the relative merits of the central and modular approaches were the subject of much controversy. To a large extent, this debate predated the availability of powerful microcomputers and the development of network technologies. In general, we have seen an evolutionary trend in the development of HISs from central, to modular, to distributed systems.

7.2.1 Central Systems

The earliest HISs were designed according to the theory that a single, comprehensive, or **central system** (often called a *total* or *holistic* system) could best meet a hospital's information needs. Advocates of the central approach emphasized the importance of initially identifying all a hospital's information needs and of designing a single, unified framework to meet these needs. A system should not evolve through a patchwork of solutions to problems in individual application areas. The natural implementation of this theory is a system in which a single, large computer performs all information processing and manages all the data files using application-independent file-management programs. Users obtain information via general-purpose terminals (Figure 7.1).

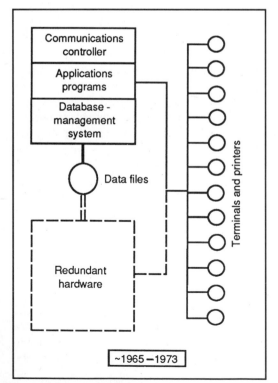

FIGURE 7.1 The earliest hospital information systems were central systems. In this model a large, central computer serves the information needs of the entire hospital. Users access the computer from video display terminals via general interface programs.

Central systems integrate and communicate information well because they provide users with a general method to access information simply and rapidly. On the other hand, large systems are expensive to implement and operate. Large initial investments are necessary, first by the vendor, to develop and test a sufficiently complete product, and then by the hospital, to bring the entire system into operation. Central systems are difficult to install because many areas of a hospital are affected simultaneously, and backup is particularly costly because of the expense of purchasing redundant hardware to be used when the primary computer is unavailable. An insidious problem is that, by the time a vendor has developed a comprehensive system that supports all the functions a hospital might want, technological obsolescence will have crept in. Central systems are not easily modified to accommodate previously unrecognized or changing needs. Furthermore, they often poorly serve individual users who compete with all other users within the hospital for the computer's resources.

The biggest limitation of central systems is the latter's inability to accommodate the diverse needs of individual application areas. There is a tradeoff between the uniformity (and relative simplicity) of a general system and the nonuniformity and greater power of custom-designed systems that solve specific problems. Generality—a characteristic that enhances communication and data integration—can be a drawback in a hospitalwide system because of the complexity and heterogeneity of the information-management tasks.

Central HISs implemented on time-shared mainframe computers accessed by video display terminals (VDTs) on the wards were developed in the late 1960s, and were installed in the early 1970s. Many of the major computer manufacturers (among others, Burroughs, Control Data Corporation, International Business Machines, Honeywell, and National Cash Register) invested in providing systems for hospitals. In general, these companies met with limited success. Many of them subsequently withdrew from the market, wholly or in part because their systems failed to achieve sufficient acceptance to become profitable. Each of the systems had certain strengths, but many failed to support adequately the complex activities on the wards, or required such a degree of custom-tailoring that they could not be transferred to other institutions. Logistical problems of slow response times and poor user interfaces also inhibited acceptance of many early HISs.

Of the early medically oriented HISs, the Technicon Medical Information System (TMIS; see Section 7.3.1) was the most successful and the most widely distributed. TMIS is one of the strongest examples of what we should expect from a large, centrally operated HIS. Now a mature system, it can provide a large number of services reliably and still is marketed today. TMIS typically runs on a duplex installation of IBM-compatible mainframes. One computer is used for tasks that involve direct interaction with users. The other is used for batch-oriented tasks, such as billing and report generation; it also can provide backup when the primary computer requires maintenance or fails unexpectedly. Depending on the size of the central machine, a TMIS center can support several hospitals to a total equivalent of a few thousand beds. Because of this high capacity, one computer installation can serve multiple hospitals in an area. The hospitals are connected via high-speed (50,000-baud) dedicated telephone lines to the central computer. Within a hospital, a switching station connects the telephone lines to an onsite network that leads to stations on all the wards. Each ward station has at least one VDT and one printer for accessing and displaying information.

7.2.2 Modular Systems

By the 1970s, modular HISs began to emerge. Decreases in the price of powerful hardware and improvements in software made it feasible for individual departments within a hospital to own and operate their own computers. In a **modular system,** one or a few machines are dedicated to the hospitals. Distinct software application modules carry out specific tasks (Figure 7.2), and a common framework, which is specified initially, defines the interfaces that will allow data to be shared among the modules. Major tasks may be performed by freestanding systems. Thus, a hospital can acquire hardware and software modules incrementally and can tailor the HIS to meet its information needs and financial constraints by "plugging in" appropriate modules as desired.

The modular approach solves many of the problems of central systems. Although individual modules are constrained to function with the predefined interfaces, they

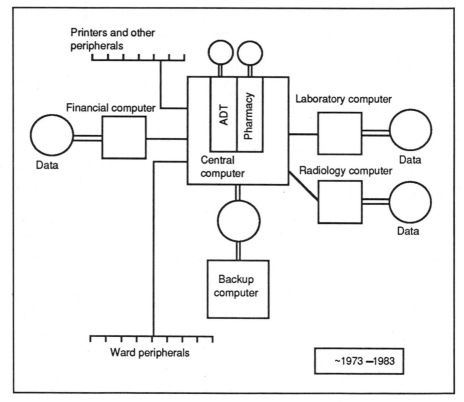

FIGURE 7.2 In modular systems, much information processing is performed locally on dedicated machines that communicate with a central machine via direct interfaces. [ADT = admission–discharge–transfer.]

do not have to conform to the general standards of the overall system, so they can be designed to accommodate the special needs of specific areas. For example, the processing capabilities and file structures suitable for managing the data acquired from a patient-monitoring system in the intensive-care unit (analog and digital signals acquired in real time) differ from the features that are appropriate for a system that reports radiology results (text storage and text processing). Furthermore, modification of modules, although laborious using any approach, is simpler because of the smaller scope of the system. As long as the interfaces are undisturbed, subsystems can be modified or replaced without the remainder of the HIS being disrupted.

Modular systems also are more responsive to local users because much processing can be performed locally on the departmental machines. The central machine with shared data files can be smaller, because it does not handle all processing. The price for this greater flexibility is increased difficulty in integrating data and allowing communication among modules. In reality, installing a subsystem never is as easy as simply plugging in the connections.

The IBM Patient Care System (PCS) exemplifies the modular approach. It provides a framework for comprehensive HIS services and is designed on the premise that a standard medical record and standard interfaces for medical-transaction programs permit the development of relatively independent modules, which together provide a powerful HIS. In PCS, the medical records are viewed as a database that unites all the functions in the hospital and also provides a long-term record of the patient's stay. PCS is built on top of a general database, communication, and transaction-management system. The desired hospital applications are placed within this framework. Hospitals typically purchase PCS through a vendor, who provides a number of basic applications with the system. The hospital data-processing staff can append their own custom-developed applications.

The most ambitious project based on the modular approach is the Distributed Hospital Computer Program (DHCP) for the Veterans Administration (VA) hospitals. The system has a common database and a database system (FileMan), which was written to be both hardware-independent and operating-system-independent. A small number of support centers in the VA develop the software modules in cooperation with user groups. The CORE—the first set of applications to be developed and installed—consists of modules for patient registration, ADT, outpatient scheduling, laboratory, outpatient pharmacy, and inpatient pharmacy. Modules to support other clinical departments (such as radiology, dietetics, surgery, nursing, and mental health) and administrative functions (such as financial and procurement applications) have been developed subsequently. During 1984 and 1985, the Veterans Administration installed DHCP in 169 of its approximately 300 hospitals and clinics. The software is in the public domain; it is now being used in private hospitals and other government facilities [Munnecke and Kuhn, 1989].

7.2.3 Distributed Systems

By the 1980s, HISs based on the new network communications technology were being developed. In a **distributed system,** an HIS consists of a federation of independent computers that have been tailored for specific application areas. The computers operate autonomously and share data (and, sometimes, programs and other resources, such as printers) by exchanging information over a local-area network (LAN; see Chapter 4) using a standard protocol for communication (Figure 7.3).

The advantages of a distributed system are that individual departments have a great deal of flexibility in choosing the hardware and software that optimally suits their needs. Smaller ancillary departments that previously could not justify a major computer acquisition because of insufficient workload now can purchase microcomputers and participate in the computer-based information system. Health-care providers in nursing units (or even at the bedside), physicians in their offices, and managers in the administrative offices can access and analyze data locally using microcomputers. Some computers may handle resources that are shared by all users—for example, the ADT information, the active medical records, the index to archived medical records, and the mail exchanged electronically between individual users. Several LANs

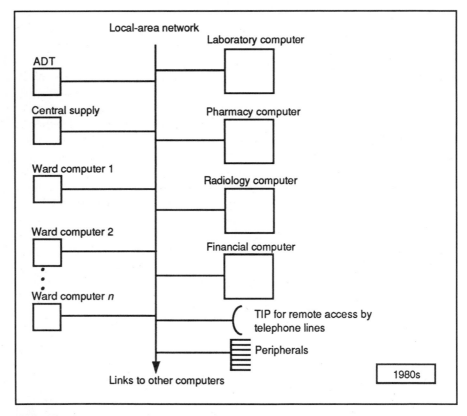

FIGURE 7.3 Network technology enables users to perform all information processing locally. Independent machines share data over the network by passing messages according to a communication protocol. A terminal-interface processor (TIP) is a utility communications computer that is used to attach video display terminals and other communications devices to the local-area network. [ADT = admission–discharge–transfer.]

can be linked together by gateway computers (see Chapter 4). Thus, networks can provide for communication outside the hospital as well as within it—for example, by linking the HIS with the information systems serving affiliated outpatient facilities, nursing homes, and outside laboratories.

The distribution of information processing and responsibility for data among diverse systems makes the tasks of data integration and communication even more difficult. The development of industrywide standard network protocols has eased the technical problems of electronic communication. Still, there are many obstacles to overcome in managing and controlling access to a patient database that is fragmented over multiple computers, each with its own file structure and method of file management. Furthermore, when no global structure is imposed on a hospital system, individual departments may encode data values in ways that are incompatible with the definitions chosen by other areas of the hospital. The promise of sharing among independent departments and even independent institutions increases the importance of defining data standards. Once the health profession agrees on minimum data sets to collect and devises standard coding schemes for medical data, staff at diverse institutions will have easier access to the data they need and will be able to interpret these data correctly. Investigators have developed one such standard for the exchange of laboratory information and are working to define standards for other types of clinical data as well [McDonald and Hammond, 1989].

In the early 1980s, researchers at the University of California, San Francisco (UCSF) Hospital successfully implemented a LAN to support communication among several of the hospital's standalone systems. Using technology developed at the Johns Hopkins University, they were able to connect minicomputers serving patient registration, medical records, radiology, the clinical laboratory, and the outpatient pharmacy. In the traditional sense, each of the four computers is incompatible with the other three: The computers were made by different manufacturers and run different operating systems [Simborg, 1984].

The University of Michigan Hospital in Ann Arbor, Michigan adopted a hybrid strategy to meet its information needs. The hospital emphasizes the central model of HIS architecture and operates a mainframe computer to perform core HIS functions. In early 1986, however, a LAN was installed to allow communication among all the clinical laboratories within the facility and to allow physicians to obtain laboratory-test results directly from the laboratory information system (LIS). At the time of installation, more than 95 percent of all the peripheral devices in the laboratories were connected to the network, rather than hardwired to the LIS computer. One month later, a second clinical host computer, which supported the radiology information system, was added to the LAN, thus allowing physicians to access radiology reports directly. Although the mainframe HIS initially was not connected to the LAN, the hospital later adopted the strategy of installing *universal workstations* that can access both the mainframe computer and the clinical hosts via the LAN [Friedman and Dieterle, 1987].

Commercial systems based on the distributed model are beginning to appear. Examples include the products of Simborg Systems Corporation and the Protouch System of Second Foundation, Inc.

7.3 A Comparison of Three Hospital Information Systems

We saw in the previous section how changes in hardware and software technology have played a role in shaping the evolution of HISs. The nature of a computer system also is highly dependent on the functional goals of its developers. Requirements analysis (problem definition) is the first step of the system-development process (see Chapter 5). Decisions at this earliest phase set the stage for the design and implementation choices that follow. Thus, the final form of the system depends greatly on which problems the developers aim to solve. We shall illustrate this point by describing the goals and designs of three of the best-known information systems developed during the 1970s: TMIS, HELP, and PROMIS. Table 7.2 shows the relative emphases of the three systems on information management, physician guidance, and clinical research. The Office of Technology Assessment report, cited in the Suggested Readings, includes more detailed descriptions and comparisons of TMIS, PROMIS, and COSTAR (see also Chapter 6).

7.3.1 The Technicon Medical Information System (TMIS)

TMIS is among the oldest and most successful of the comprehensive HISs. System development began in 1965 as a collaborative project between Lockheed and El Camino Hospital, a community hospital in Mountain View, California. Technicon (now TDS Healthcare Systems Corporation) bought the system from Lockheed in 1971 and continued to develop and market it. By 1987, TMIS had been installed in more than 85 institutions. The El Camino installation of the system probably has been more thoroughly evaluated than has any other HIS.

TMIS stresses the information-management and communication aspects of a hospital's informational needs. It was designed to allow physicians or nurses to enter orders directly into the system using menu-driven selection screens. Other screens allow health professionals to review and change existing orders and to review the results of the completed tests—for example, laboratory-test results and text reports of radiologic studies. The clinical information contained in the medical record can be organized in a variety of formats, and the system can summarize patient-care plans,

TABLE 7.2 The Designs of the TMIS, HELP, and PROMIS Systems Reflect the Functional Goals of The Developers*

System	Function		
	Information Management	Physician Guidance	Clinical-Research Support
TMIS	+++	0	0
HELP	+++	++	+
PROMIS	++	+++	0

*The symbols "+++" indicate that the function is emphasized strongly in the system; "0" indicates no emphasis on that function.

drug-distribution plans, and the like. Figure 7.4 shows an architectural overview of TMIS and indicates the information flow within the system.

Although TMIS was designed to allow physicians to enter their orders directly, the designers explicitly tried to avoid the appearance of directing the physician's decisions with respect to diagnostic or therapy planning for patient care. In addition, there was no intent to use the patient data for longer-term purposes, such as surveillance or clinical research; in the initial version of the system, the patient record was not available after the patient was discharged from the hospital.

7.3.2 The HELP System

The University of Utah's HELP system, on the other hand, was designed to meet not only the clinical needs, but also the teaching and research needs of hospital personnel [Pryor et al., 1983b]. Administrative functions were added later. Developed by Warner and colleagues at the Latter Day Saints (LDS) Hospital—a teaching hospital in Salt Lake City, Utah—HELP was viewed primarily as an information-management

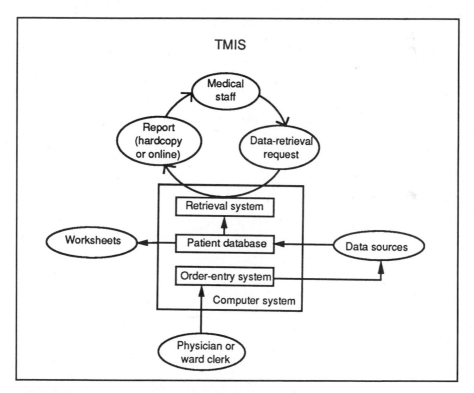

FIGURE 7.4 Physicians and nurses use TMIS to enter orders, which then are automatically communicated to the various data sources (for example, laboratories, radiology department, and pharmacy). Staff also may use a data-retrieval program to review the results of the tests they have ordered.

vehicle within the hospital setting. However, HELP provides decision support in the form of *knowledge frames,* which are modules of specialized decision logic that permit the computer to react to data as the latter are entered into patients' files, and thus to generate patient-specific warnings, alerts, diagnostic suggestions, and limited management advice (Figure 7.5). HELP protocols also can be written to evaluate the patient database at set periodic intervals—for example, to check whether a patient who is receiving a potassium-wasting diuretic has had his serum-potassium level measured during a prespecified time period.

Expert collaborators define the search criteria of the HELP frames using a HELP Frame Language that was designed to be easily understood by clinicians (see Chapters 6 and 15). Researchers can analyze the clinical and administrative database by writing HELP protocols to identify study populations with particular characteristics and to retrieve variables of interest. HELP's research subsystem is interfaced with statistical programs that can analyze the differences among study populations; the results then can be used in clinical research, in administrative audits, or as the basis for the creation of additional HELP frames to assist in patient management.

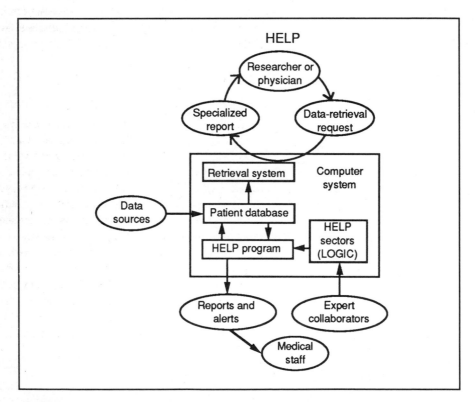

FIGURE 7.5 In HELP, the typical functions of a hospital information system are augmented by HELP frames that encode decision logic. When data in the patient database satisfy the preconditions of a frame, the program generates an advisory report or warning.

7.3.3 The Problem-Oriented Medical Information System (PROMIS)

The Problem-Oriented Medical Information System (PROMIS), implemented on a few wards at the Medical Center Hospital of Vermont by Weed and colleagues at the University of Vermont during the early 1970s, explicitly emphasized physician guidance [Fischer et al., 1980]. Whereas HELP reacted to patient data and generated a variety of online or paper guidance reports, PROMIS was designed to be used routinely by the physician in lieu of all paper record keeping. Physicians used a computer terminal not only to order tests and drugs, but also to record and review medical histories, data collected during physical examinations, progress notes, and the like. PROMIS actively *guided* the interaction, taking steps to ensure that the data entered were complete and were entered according to conventions that would allow the physician's logic to be apparent. Support of clinical research was not the goal of the system; rather, this HIS was designed to replace all paper records and to enhance uniformity and quality of care (Figure 7.6).

PROMIS implemented Weed's vision of the problem-oriented medical record, a record in which all diagnostic and therapeutic actions are tied to an underlying patient problem. This philosophy was expressed in a collection of strictly defined logic pathways for data collection and problem solving. At each point in a computer session, a user was presented with a set of related choices. When the user selected an item, the information was recorded in the medical record; the program's logic then determined which screen of related choices was presented next.

Of the three systems, PROMIS clearly had the most sophisticated user interface and the greatest capacity to structure and organize medical information. Yet, in part because of the dogmatic and inflexible nature of the system, PROMIS was not well accepted by its physician users and is not used in any major hospital today. The concept of the problem-oriented record, however, influenced the design of all subsequent medical-record systems and provides an important base for tracking clinical problems and for summarizing patients' medical histories.

7.4 Hospital Information Systems: Present and Future

Hospitals currently use a variety of strategies to meet their information needs. They may use locally developed and maintained programs running on hospital-owned or leased computers, they may purchase vendor-supplied and vendor-supported computer systems, or they may contract with outside service organizations. In 1985, at least 200 vendors supplied information systems or services to hospitals [Grams and Peck, 1986]. A handful of companies (American Express, Baxter Healthcare Corporation, GTE, HBO, Meditech, Shared Medical Systems [SMS], and TDS Healthcare Systems Corporation) control a large part of the market; most provide comprehensive administrative services and some support for nursing and medical care.

Many of the biggest companies sell both hardware and software. A number of other vendors provide services to hospitals from remote locations. These companies

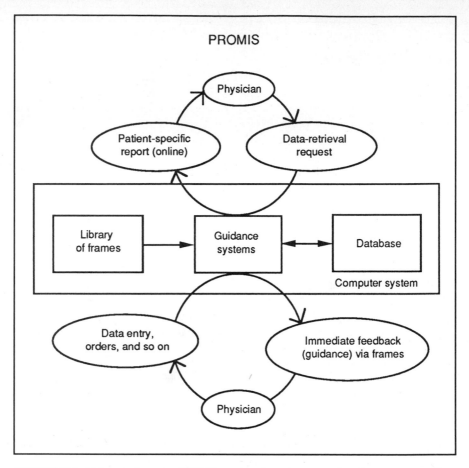

FIGURE 7.6 All interaction with PROMIS occurs through a central guidance system. The system updates and retrieves patient information from the database using a special library of *frames* that encode the guidance logic. Each frame fills one computer terminal screen; the physician can select options by touching the touch-screen display. The order of frames to be displayed is determined by the options that the physician has selected on earlier screens. Both data retrieval and data entry follow this same interactive scheme.

permit users in the hospital to access the vendor's computer to obtain selected information; these linkages, however, primarily support financial functions and rarely fulfill clinical requirements. For example, SMS's Information Systems Center provides remote online processing of administrative and financial data. Alternatively, customers may purchase or lease turnkey systems, or they may choose a hybrid solution of in-house clinical systems combined with remote financial services. Some vendors now provide a *remote computing option* in which a hospital's information systems reside on a remote, vendor-operated computer.

The choice of offerings for HISs is still varied, but a definite trend—due primarily to reduced hardware costs—is to move more functions into the hospital. Use of large, shared systems, operating from remote locations, is declining, and most companies no longer provide hospital services from centralized locations. Rather, they sell turnkey systems or control the operation of vendor-supplied inhouse systems.

Total expenditures on medical information systems in the United States were estimated to be $4.5 billion in 1987, and were projected to reach $7 billion by 1990 [Kennedy et al., 1987]. Hospitals accounted for the majority of the expenditures—nearly $4 billion. On average, hospitals spent about 3.7 percent of their total budget on information systems in 1987 [Packer, 1987a]. This figure is expected to increase as more hospitals move to inhouse data processing and purchase commercial systems. Furthermore, many of the systems in operation today now are obsolete and are expected to be replaced by newer systems.

Most hospitals with 100 beds or more use computers to handle some of their information-processing needs, but the majority currently limit their use of computers to functions related to billing and patient accounting. Results from the 1985 National Survey of Hospital Data Processing [Grams and Peck, 1986] show that, although approximately 80 percent of hospitals used a computer to assist in financial data processing and roughly 70 percent used one to help with admissions and patient registration, only about one-quarter of hospitals had a system that allowed personnel on the wards to access the computer interactively and thus to enter orders and to review test results. The proportions of hospitals that currently use a laboratory, pharmacy, or radiology system were about 25, 30, and 10 percent, respectively [Grams and Peck, 1986]. The rough estimates are probably reliable, but little weight should be placed on the exact figures reported—questionnaires were sent to over 7000 hospitals registered with the American Hospital Association, but only 22 percent responded. A 1987 survey conducted by Shared Data Research (SDR) obtained data from over 3700 hospitals. Of these, 96 percent had an automated financial system [Packer, 1988], and about 30 percent had a laboratory information system [Packer, 1987b]. The actual percentages for all hospitals are undoubtedly lower.

The capabilities of the typical HIS lag far behind those of the most sophisticated HISs in use today. Why does this disparity exist? In Chapter 5, we discussed many of the difficulties inherent in designing and implementing computer systems that are accepted by users and that function well in health-care settings. HIS developers now understand hospitals' information needs better than they did 20 years ago; however, hospitals still find that vendor systems are inflexible and do not completely satisfy their needs. Insufficient technical support for both end users and inhouse data-processing personnel is a common problem. Furthermore, lack of expertise within health-care institutions hinders both the identification of problem areas suitable for computers and the design of appropriate solutions—and, of course, a poor fit between problem and solution causes poor user acceptance of the system.

In addition to technical and logistical obstacles to success, there are economic barriers. An HIS is expensive to purchase and maintain. Although HISs seem to increase the productivity of workers, there has been no clear demonstration that a comprehensive HIS can reduce costs; without accompanying changes in the organizational and managerial structure of the hospital, many of the benefits of an HIS cannot be realized. For example, reorganization of nursing tasks is required for nurses to translate time savings scattered throughout a shift into usable blocks of productive time [Gall, 1976].

Despite these barriers to the adoption of HISs, we expect hospitals to continue to expand their information systems in response to demands from health-care personnel for help in meeting growing information-processing requirements. Hospitals are becoming increasingly sophisticated purchasers of information services, and some hospitals are creating a high-level management position, the chief information officer (CIO), who is charged with planning and overseeing information services in an institution. There is a growing recognition that information is the basis for every decision made in the hospital and that the integration of data collected throughout the institution is critical if a hospital is to function effectively in today's competitive health-care environment. The cost of an HIS is not expected to be offset by increased revenues or lowered direct costs; rather, it represents a necessary expense of doing business.

Both medical and administrative requirements drive the development of HISs. Although these two types of requirements may be at times different, hospital administrative data are meaningless without the medical component, and consistent collection of medical data requires administrative support. Although clinicians will continue to demand technology that assists directly in patient care—for example, magnetic-resonance imaging (MRI) technology, CT scanners (see Chapter 11), and many of the patient-monitoring devices found in the intensive-care unit (see Chapter 12)—we expect the strongest pressures to acquire and expand computing functions to come from administrators and managers, primarily as a response to changes in information requirements related to cost-containment policies.

Demands for data integration and better capability to access and analyze information are producing the following trends in HIS development:

- *Local-area communication networks* are becoming increasingly common in hospitals. Whereas only 5 percent of hospitals were using LAN technology in 1985, about 25 percent of hospitals had installed at least one LAN by 1986 [Packer, 1987c]. Many of the technical limitations apparent even a few years ago have been overcome, and network technology now is a viable means for hospitals to integrate their information services while preserving many of the advantages of standalone and microcomputer-based systems. Hospitals that report the highest level of satisfaction with their LANs invested the most time in planning prior to installation; their preparation included carefully determining the appropriate number of workstations, standardizing new hardware and software, training users, and planning for maintenance and growth.
- *Workstations and personal computers* continue to increase in importance in hospitals—a companion trend to the growth of LANs. Local processing provides faster response time. Furthermore, the selection of user-friendly software available for use on PCs is wider than that available for use on larger computers. Thus, hospital personnel using PCs that are linked into a LAN will have greater access to data and greater flexibility in analyzing and using data for decision support. For example, hospital managers often must rely on printed reports to obtain the information they need for decision making; typically, reports are generated on a

monthly or quarterly basis and their formats are relatively inflexible. Current database query languages are inadequate to allow managers to query a complex hospital database directly; computer programmers must formulate queries for information. The installation of management workstations can greatly improve access to information. Managers can extract relevant subsets of data from the HIS, use spreadsheet software to assess the effects of hypothetical changes, and display and summarize the results using graphical-presentation and word-processing programs.

- *Bedside terminals* allow physicians and nurses to record data as they collect the data from the patient, rather than first jotting down notes and later transcribing the notes. These **point-of-care systems** potentially can increase the productivity of nurses by reducing the amount of paperwork, can provide more accurate and timely access to the detailed clinical information for better cost-management and quality-assurance activities, and even can improve the quality of care—for example, by reducing the number of medication-administration errors. By 1989, however, the use of bedside terminals was still uncommon, although there were already at least five vendors in the marketplace. The cost and space requirements of current bedside terminals have inhibited general acceptance of this approach.

- *Linkages between hospitals and physicians* are becoming more common as hospitals install LANs and physicians automate their offices. Physicians will be able to access hospital information from on the ward, from their offices, and even from their homes. The majority of hospital patients are admitted by independent practitioners; hospitals view hospital–physician linkage as a means to attract physicians and thus patients. The growth of health-maintenance organizations (HMOs) and the tendency of nonhospital facilities (such as nursing homes, outpatient surgical centers, and emergency-care clinics) to affiliate with multihospital systems also will increase the demand for linkages for communication among hospital and nonhospital providers.

The HIS technology adopted will continue to differ by type of institution. Large hospitals, which typically support specialized functions for tertiary-care activities, have unique demands; these centers often have complex financial arrangements with schools, with other hospitals in their areas, and with governmental institutions. To accommodate their special needs, many of these hospitals will have to develop and maintain their own systems; they will not be able to rely heavily on vendors or on contributions from other, similar hospitals. Community hospitals and moderately sized institutions will have to depend heavily on vendors of packaged systems, although more hospitals are purchasing their own hardware and software. Membership in a hospital organization can help these institutions to acquire services at a reasonable rate and also to obtain advice on making appropriate decisions on investments in information technology. It is in this arena that standardization will show its greatest benefits. Smaller institutions will depend largely on turnkey systems provided by vendors and modified only nominally, if at all. Because the simple billing, order-entry, and reporting functions are now mature, those will be the primary functions available to the small hospitals. Medical records will not be a major part of the services provided for these institutions, except as needed to document reimbursement requests.

The interaction of administrative and clinical demands, with increasing techno-logical capabilities, will continue to push the development of HISs. Because of the pressure of cost containment, however, hospitals do not have the same freedom to experiment and the same breadth of research activity that they enjoyed until the early 1980s. We expect that, in most instances, hospitals will focus on short-term practical demands and will adopt the results of long-term scientific developments from leading institutions only when the new technologies become commercially available.

Suggested Readings

Cook, M. and McDowell, W. Changing to an automated information system. *American Journal of Nursing,* 75:46, 1975.

This article describes how nurses at the El Camino Hospital use the Technicon Medical Information System to perform information-management tasks related to patient care. The authors also recount the history of the system's installation—the problems that were en-countered and the steps that were taken to implement the HIS successfully.

Fischer, P. J., et al. User reaction to PROMIS: Issues related to acceptability of medical innovations. In O'Neill, J. T. (ed), *Proceedings of the Fourth Annual Symposium on Computer Applications in Medical Care.* Washington, D.C.: IEEE, 1980, pages 1722–1730.

The authors summarize the objectives of the PROMIS system and present the results of a study to evaluate the system's acceptability to physicians, nurses, and ancillary person-nel in the pharmacy, laboratory, and radiology departments at the Medical Center Hospital of Vermont.

Friedman, B. A. and Martin, J. B. Hospital information systems: The physician's role. *Journal of the American Medical Association,* 257:1792, 1987.

This short commentary proposes a model for the future organization and development of hospital information systems. It emphasizes the need for physicians to participate actively in strategic policy making and in the development of such systems.

Kennedy, O. G., et al. Computers and software: Special report. *Hospitals,* (Au-gust 5):61, 1987.

This report provides an industry perspective on the current status of information systems in hospitals. Short articles by many different authors address topics such as the emergence of integrated information systems, financial systems to assist in cost management, point-of-care systems, and software tools for hospital marketing.

Lindberg, D. A. B. *The Growth of Medical Information Systems in the United States.* Lexington, MA: Lexington Books, 1979.

This book describes the evolution of medical information systems (MISs) in the United States. The author discusses the evaluation of MISs, characterizes barriers to the development and diffusion of MISs, and describes how federal research support and health-care reim-bursement policies affect the adoption of MIS technology.

Office of Technology Assessment. *Policy Implications of Medical Information Systems.* Washington, D.C.: U.S. Government Printing Office, 1977.

The Office of Technology Assessment conducted this study on the policy implications of computer-based medical information systems in response to increasing concern over the costs and quality of health care. The report describes the TMIS, PROMIS, and COSTAR systems, discusses the potential benefits and limitations of the systems, considers factors that influence the adoption of information systems in health settings, and evaluates policy alternatives for the federal government with regard to such systems.

Pryor, T. A., et al. The HELP system. *Journal of Medical Systems,* 7:87, 1983.
This article recounts the history of the HELP system from that system's beginnings in the late 1950s through its use in the early 1980s. It explains the design objectives that shaped HELP's development and the system's decision-support, research, and administrative capabilities.

Simborg, D. W., et al. Local area networks and the hospital. *Computers and Biomedical Research,* 16:247, 1983.
The authors examine the informational needs of a hospital and argue that distributed systems are well suited to meet these needs. They explain the basic features of local-area communication networks that can support a distributed HIS.

Wiederhold, G. Hospital information systems. In Webster, J. G. (ed), *Encyclopedia of Medical Devices and Instrumentation,* vol 3. New York: John Wiley & Sons, 1988.
This article provides an encyclopedic list of the functions of an HIS, discusses interactions among these functions, and describes the growth in functionality of HISs over time.

Questions for Discussion

1. Briefly explain the differences among a hospital's operational, planning, and documentary requirements for information. Give two examples in each category.
2. Describe three situations in which the separation of clinical and administrative information could lead to inadequate patient care, loss of revenue, or inappropriate administrative decisions.
3. Describe the key concepts underlying the design of central, modular, and distributed HISs. What are the advantages and disadvantages of each architecture?
4. Assume that you are the CIO for a large teaching hospital. You have been charged with the task of implementing an HIS. You have identified three leading vendors, each offering a system with a different architecture—central, modular, and distributed. Describe the pros and cons of each of the three systems as you discuss each of the following issues:
   a. The growth of the hospital, which includes adding a new patient-care wing.
   b. The introduction of an all-digital radiology department.
   c. The addition of a new program to track outbreaks of infection among patients.
   d. A decision to provide HIS information to physicians for outpatient care (for example, hospital discharge summaries and profiles of current medications).
5. How do you think that bedside terminals will affect the quality of physician–patient and nurse–patient interactions? Explain both the benefits and the drawbacks you perceive.

8

Nursing Information Systems

Judy Ozbolt, Ivo L. Abraham, and Samuel Schultz II

After reading this chapter, you should know the answers to these questions:

- How does nursing care complement and differ from medical care?
- What are the primary tasks of clinical nursing practice and of nursing administration?
- What is a nursing taxonomy? Why has the lack of agreement on a taxonomy hindered the development of nursing information systems?
- What are the factors that have constrained the development of computer-based nursing systems to aid in clinical practice?
- How have changes in health-care financing affected the nursing profession?

8.1 Nursing as a Professional Health-Care Discipline

Throughout human experience, societies have made some provision for caring for the sick and injured. Modern nursing, however, began with Florence Nightingale. Nightingale established that effective nursing was not merely the intuitive, nurturant action natural to any woman, as the popular belief of her day held; rather, nursing consisted of the knowledgeable, considered application of specific skills—knowledge and skills that had to be learned. According to Nightingale, to be a nurse is to "have charge of somebody's health" [Nightingale, 1860]. She continued, "[Nursing] ought to signify the proper use of fresh air, light, warmth, cleanliness, quiet, and the proper selection and administration of diet—all at the least expense of vital power to the patient." For Nightingale, then, nursing was characterized by nurturance, but a nurturance vested with authority and guided by knowledge.

These basic concepts are still central to nursing. Over the years, many nurses have elaborated on the nature of their professional practice. One of the most influential such writers is Virginia Henderson. In 1955, Henderson offered a description of nursing that has been adopted by the International Council of Nurses, and by many nursing organizations, agencies, and schools worldwide:

> Nursing is primarily assisting the individual (sick or well) in the performance of those activities contributing to health, or [to] its recovery (or to a peaceful death) that he would perform unaided if he had the necessary strength, will, or knowledge. It is likewise the unique contribution of nursing to help the individual to be independent of such assistance as soon as possible. [Henderson, 1960]

Thus, nurses provide the care that people are unable to provide for themselves because those people are debilitated or because the care requires specialized knowledge and skills. Nurses help people, whenever possible, to increase their ability to care for themselves.

Nursing has become highly sophisticated since Nightingale's day. As nursing has become more complex and sophisticated, it has become more dependent on knowledge and information. Furthermore, as health-care technology has evolved, the amount of knowledge and information potentially available to nurses has expanded dramatically. In this chapter, we shall see how computer-based **nursing information systems (NISs)** can improve nurses' ability to access this information and to use it productively. It would be impossible to review all existing systems; therefore, we shall focus on a number of professional, scientific, and technical issues pertaining to the development of NISs. We shall identify important problems, discuss possible solutions, and examine the ways in which system developers have attempted to solve these problems.

As we discussed in Chapters 6 and 7, hospital information systems (HISs) and computer-based medical-records systems promise to increase the productivity of nurses by reducing paperwork, performing record-keeping functions, making information more accessible, and facilitating communication of information. Nurses typically are the primary users of HISs; features such as the order entry, results reporting, and automated charting of many HISs are used most often by nurses performing the documentation and communication aspects of their jobs. Thus, NISs and HISs are integrally related. In addition, NISs have specialized components to help with the unique tasks of nursing. For example, NISs help nurses to determine nursing diagnoses, to formulate and implement care plans, and to evaluate the care provided; they help nursing administrators to run nursing departments, to manage staff and nonpersonnel resources, and to perform quality-of-care audits. Thus, the use of NISs can result in improvements in the quality and consistency of nursing care. Furthermore, the nursing data collected and stored in nursing databases will promote research and education in nursing science.

8.1.1 Clinical Practice

Nursing often contributes to *cure,* but its special focus, authority, and responsibility are *care,* and it is toward the end of effective care that the nursing profession develops and directs its knowledge and technology. Nursing's mission, then, is complementary to but different from medicine's. Rather than focusing on the prevention, diagnosis, and treatment of disease, nurses focus on how people respond to and cope with issues of health and illness and on people's ability to care for themselves in the interests of their health. Figure 8.1 illustrates the similarities between the medical- and nursing-care processes in the context of information flow within a hospital.

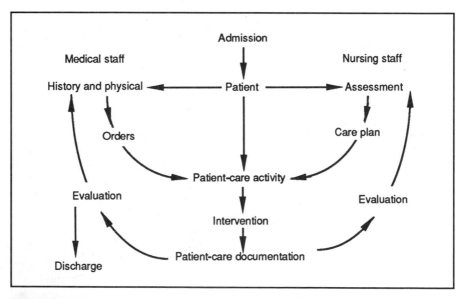

FIGURE 8.1 The medical-care and nursing-care processes are complementary, but different. Physicians obtain medical histories, conduct physical examinations, and order medical treatments; nurses assess patients' needs, plan patient care, administer treatments, educate, and provide emotional support. (*Source:* Courtesy of Ralph A. Korpman, M.D., Professor, Loma Linda University School of Medicine, and President and Chairman, Health Data Sciences Corporation. Reprinted with permission from Korpman, R. A. Patient care information systems: Looking to the future. Part 4. The changing role of computers in nursing. *Software in Healthcare,* Oct/Nov:58–64, 1984.)

To provide appropriate care, nurses must determine the nature of the care required and must assess the ability of the client[1] to care for himself. Nursing action, therefore, is preceded by a diagnostic process. Indeed, the American Nurses' Association (ANA) has defined nursing as "the diagnosis and treatment of human responses to actual or potential health problems" [American Nurses' Association, 1980]. The focus is phenomena such as "the impact of illness-effects upon the self and family and related self-care needs."

For nursing, the process of diagnosis consists of looking not for patterns of signs and symptoms that point to a particular disease state, but rather for indicators of how the person responds to an actual or potential health problem, and of the person's ability to provide independently for her own care. Nursing treatment then includes a wide range of actions, from providing emotional support to a client anticipating surgery, to giving a bed bath to an immobilized person, to helping a chronically ill person plan and implement health-promoting changes in lifestyle, to counseling an emotionally disturbed person, to carrying out complex treatment regimens, to operating sophisticated electronic monitoring devices and interpreting readings. The common characteristic of all such nursing actions is that they are part of a deliberative process in which the nurse assesses the patient, diagnoses that patient's capacities and deficiencies in coping with health problems or providing self-care, and formulates and executes a **nursing care plan** to maintain and enhance the patient's capacities and to compensate for and, if possible, to overcome the patient's deficiencies. The nurse analyzes each client situation in the light of professional knowledge to arrive at appropriate decisions for care (Figure 8.2).

The provision of computer-based support for the nursing process is complicated by two factors: (1) the fledgling state of nursing science, and (2) the complexity of the process itself. Unlike medicine, nursing has no generally accepted taxonomies of nursing diagnoses, nursing objectives, or nursing interventions. Lacking a taxonomy of diagnoses, nurses have been unable either to identify the data that would be critical indicators of each diagnosis, or to trace logical pathways from data to diagnoses. These deficiencies obviously impede development of decision-support systems for nursing diagnosis. Most clinical settings have "assessment guides" for data collection, but the purpose and function of each datum are undefined. Consequently, irrelevant data may be collected, and potentially useful data may be ignored. Furthermore, the leap from data to diagnoses is not logical but intuitive. Such assessment guides are therefore not a sufficient basis for developing computer-based systems that can use the data intelligently.

With the growing pressure to control costs while maintaining the quality of care, however, it is increasingly important for nurses to avoid missed diagnoses, which have the potential for causing complications and prolonging hospitalization, and to substantiate the diagnoses they do make, to justify expenditure of resources. Thus, a task of information processing that forms the foundation of nursing's professional

---

[1]Many nurses prefer to refer to the people for whom they care as *clients,* rather than using the more restrictive term *patient.* We shall use *client* and *patient* interchangeably throughout this chapter.

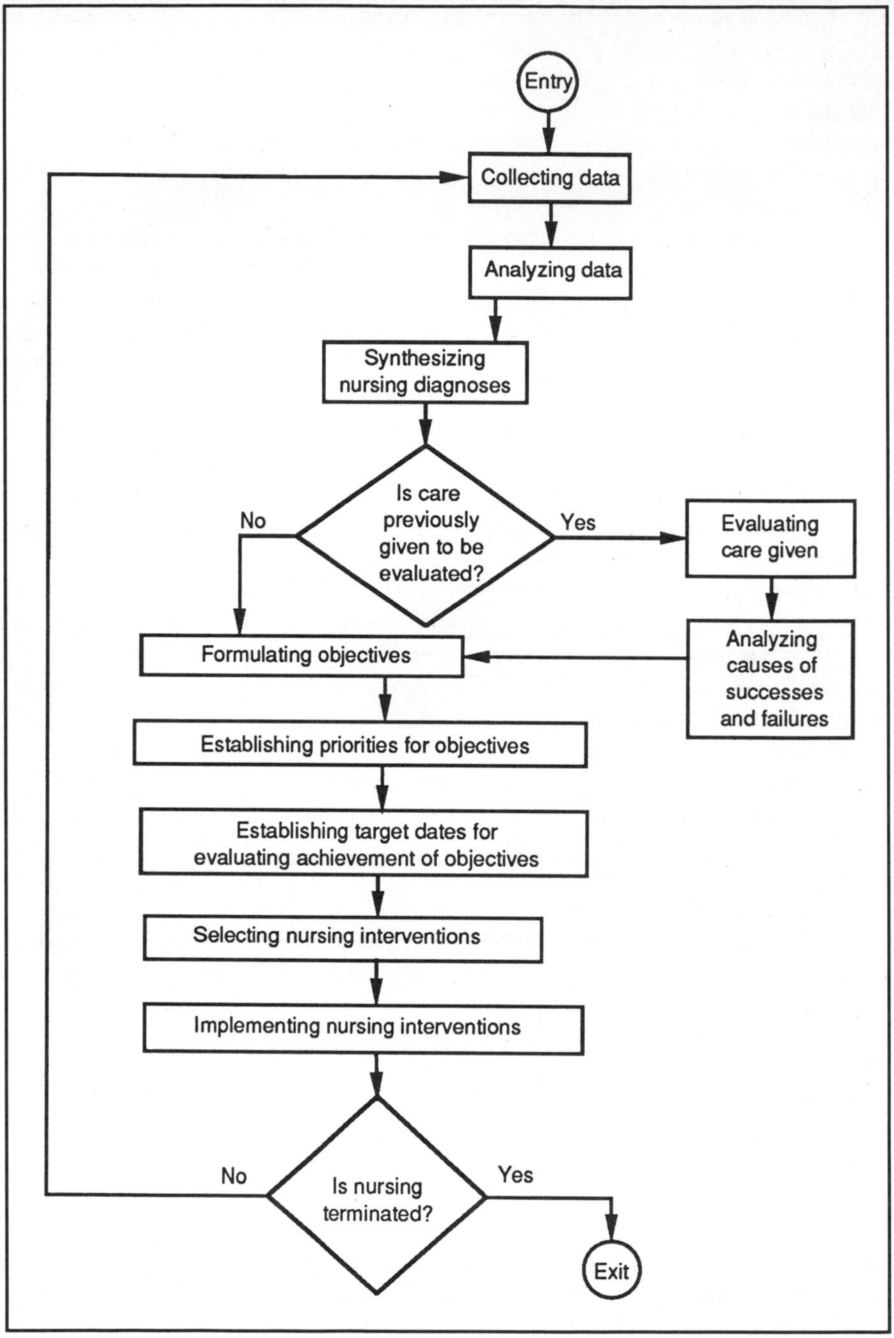

FIGURE 8.2 The provision of nursing care is an iterative process that consists of steps to collect and analyze data, to plan and implement interventions, and to evaluate the results of interventions. (*Source:* Adapted with permission from Ozbolt, J. G., et al. A proposed expert system for nursing practice. *Journal of Medical Systems,* 9:57–68, 1985.)

service and economic justification—deriving nursing diagnoses from client data—remains largely undefined. The developers of decision-support systems have had to make ad hoc decisions about terminology, data, and logical links.

Subsequent steps of the nursing process are similarly problematic. Once a diagnosis is established, nurses set objectives for the client behaviors or conditions to be achieved. In the absence of any standard taxonomy, objectives are idiosyncratic. To the degree that the objectives are individually tailored to the client, this lack of standardization can be an advantage. Unless objectives are stated in observable, measurable terms, however, it is difficult to evaluate whether they have been achieved, and busy nurses may not always state objectives clearly. Furthermore, idiosyncratic statements of objectives make it difficult to compare the effectiveness of particular interventions across clients: How can nurses determine the frequency of success of an intervention for clients who have a common problem if the objective is stated differently for each client? As in the case of diagnoses, the lack of a taxonomy of objectives hinders the development of computer systems that can document nursing objectives, much less support decision making.

Nursing interventions themselves vary in the specificity and the standardization of their definitions. Some interventions, particularly those involving routine physical care, are spelled out in detailed procedure manuals. Teaching plans and guidelines also may be available for commonly occurring learning needs of clients—for example, nurses often teach clients about upcoming surgical procedures to prepare their clients physically and emotionally for surgery. On the other hand, many nursing interventions, especially those involving emotional care, are idiosyncratic to the particular nurse–client dyad—for example, the act of listening supportively as the client talks about anxieties and concerns (see Figure 2.4). In the best cases, these differences make for sensitive, individualized care. They also, however, make it difficult to identify what the best nurses are doing to be effective, so that their behavior can be replicated by other nurses, and can be tracked and supported by computer-based systems.

Thus, although the nursing care of each client is planned, implemented, and evaluated by means of a deliberative process, nurses are handicapped in carrying out this process by the lack of a standard taxonomy of data, diagnoses, objectives, interventions, and outcomes, and by the absence of explicit rules for decision making at each stage of care and for moving from one stage to the next. As a result, nursing-care planning often is unsystematic and intuitive; statements of diagnoses, objectives, and interventions usually are so varied as to make comparisons difficult; and nurses receive little if any feedback on the effectiveness of care. We shall discuss attempts to formulate nursing taxonomies and the implications for clinical systems later in this chapter.

Other problems of information management in clinical-practice environments arise not from nursing's stage of development, but rather from the complexity of the situations with which nurses must deal. To provide for the total care needs of their clients, nurses must not only have a thorough knowledge of their clients and of these clients' needs for nursing care, but also must consider, interpret to the clients, and help to implement the plan of medical care and related services such as pharmacy, laboratory, radiology, physical therapy, and so on. Except in intensive-care settings, where one-on-one staffing is common, nurses must manage all this information not just for one client but for many, and must coordinate and schedule not only their own efforts on behalf of their clients but also those of the other members of the health-care team. Because of their unique role in providing 24-hour care, nurses often act as advocates and intermediaries for clients, alerting other team members to changes in the client's condition, or to conflicts in or problems with care plans. The necessity of keeping their own records and of communicating with other professionals results in nurses' spending up to 40 percent of their time on paperwork [Richart, 1976; Jydstrup and Gross, 1966]. Concern about nursing productivity has spurred the development and implementation of computer systems to make documentation and communication faster and easier.

Clearly, the responsibilities of nurses for information management are complex and time consuming. Furthermore, the amount of information confronting nurses who must make decisions about the care of individual patients, and must coordinate the care of many patients in concert with the entire health-care team, far exceeds the limits of human capacities for information processing [Abraham, 1986; Edwards, 1968]. Nurses must select the data to which they will attend in reaching any decision, but lack any systematic method for doing this. Because humans inherently are conservative decision makers [Edwards, 1968], nurses may wait to make a decision until they collect more information than is necessary, thereby delaying needed treatment and risking negative consequences for the client. Conversely, because humans can remember and apply only a limited number of data in making any decision, nurses may forget key points and make less than ideal decisions. Information systems, therefore, can assist nurses in data selection, acquisition, and management, as well as in making inferences based on these data.

In the clinical setting, data required to make accurate decisions are not always available; nurses must then rely on hunches and guesses. Considering the complexity of the clinical situation and the limits of human information processing, the wonder is that nurses so often do make decisions that are beneficial to their clients. It is not surprising, however, that the nursing literature contains many discussions of job stress, anxiety, guilt, and burnout.

8.1.2 Nursing Administration

Information management also is a problem for nurse administrators. Major administrative responsibilities include determining the need for nursing resources in a particular setting; scheduling personnel in accordance with the clients' needs for care and with the abilities, needs, preferences, and constraints of individual nurses; and generating reports of clients' needs, and of the quantity, quality, and cost of the services provided.

Organizing and administering nursing services is complex. Nurse administrators must have a thorough knowledge of the clinical problems and the nursing challenges occurring on the units they manage. They must identify the knowledge, skills, time, and resources necessary to provide high-quality, cost-effective nursing for each of their clients, and they must plan how to provide those human and material resources to all their clients, 24 hours per day, 7 days per week. Nurse administrators in hospitals must consider the different levels of education, knowledge, skill, and experience of their personnel, as well as the constraints on the personnel's availability, and they must match those variables to the needs of clients to provide necessary services three shifts per day, every day. Nurse administrators in community settings must ensure that services are responsive to community needs, that care provided to individuals and families is sensitive and appropriate, and that caseloads and workloads are reasonable, equitable, and productive. In all settings, nurse administrators must project needs for nursing services, conduct budget and personnel planning, and develop reports of services rendered, quality of care, and costs.

To determine the need for nursing services, administrators must assess the physical, emotional, and social conditions of the clients on their units and determine what kinds of care those clients require, what the clients can do for themselves, and what nurses must do for the clients. Ideally, administrators could compile this information from the care plans of individual patients. As we discussed, however, care plans are likely to vary in organization, terminology, and content. Needed information may be disguised in a variety of formats and presentations, or may be missing altogether. To attempt to retrieve this information manually would be laborious, time consuming, and possibly futile. Consequently, administrators have relied on other, less optimal methods to determine the need for nursing services.

Prior to 1960, most hospitals assigned a fixed number of nurses to each unit. Scheduling was the responsibility of the head nurse, and usually the same number of nurses was scheduled to work every day. In 1960, Connor established that this fixed model was inefficient, because workloads vary widely from day to day even on the same unit [Connor, 1960]. Furthermore, workloads across units vary independently of one another, so that a heavy workload on unit A today does not imply that unit B also is experiencing a heavy workload today. These findings were substantiated by a number of other investigators during the 1960s and 1970s. As a result, hospitals have resorted to a variety of methods to assign nurses to units on the basis of the workload anticipated for the assigned shift. Most of those methods involve applying a formula to a checklist to determine the number of hours of nursing time required to meet client needs; the checklist includes the kinds of problems clients present and the kinds of assistance clients require.

This approach has been criticized because the estimates of required nursing time on which these formulae are based represent the *average* times nurses spent in the past to care for patients with certain needs. It is not known whether those average times represent the optimum for either productivity or quality of care. It would be desirable to have clinical-practice data linking patient needs or problems (nursing diagnoses) with objectives, interventions, and outcomes of care. It then would be possible to determine which interventions are most effective and efficient, and to use the times required for productive, high-quality care in computing the nursing hours needed on a unit. Until such information is available, however, and until computer systems are developed to manage it, nurse administrators must depend on indirect, somewhat imprecise estimates of the needs for nursing services.

Whatever method is used to arrive at needs for nursing services, the next step is to schedule personnel to meet those needs. A number of factors make scheduling a complex task. First, the education and experience of nursing personnel vary widely. The roster may include nursing assistants, licensed practical nurses, and registered nurses with diplomas, associate degrees, bachelor's degrees, master's degrees, and occasionally doctoral degrees; from these people, the administrator must select the correct mix to meet nursing needs. Second, the staff cannot be assigned arbitrarily to any shift or any day they might be needed. Rarely are enough nurses willing to be assigned permanently to the evening and night shifts or to weekends, and humane considerations, safety concerns, and often collective-bargaining agreements limit the frequency with which nurses can be required to rotate shifts or to work weekends and holidays. Third, nurses are likely to have preferences and special requests for shift assignments and days off. Fourth, flexibility is needed to deal with unanticipated absences by nurses and unexpectedly light or heavy workloads. Nurses, however, often are reluctant to be assigned temporarily to a unit other than the one where they usually work; when they are assigned to another unit, their lack of familiarity with clients and the setting can result in a lower quality of care. To attain the necessary flexibility, hospitals may rely on "float pools" of nurses employed by the hospital to work part-time, or on agencies that supply temporary staff. This approach, however, does not resolve concerns about the effects of lack of familiarity with the unit on the quality of care.

Scheduling, then, requires that the nurse administrator consider simultaneously an array of requirements and constraints, and resolve them in a way that meets client needs and ensures nurse satisfaction. Traditionally, this laborious task has consumed a significant portion of the nurse administrator's time. Scheduling systems can optimize the scheduling process and can link the process to other resource-management applications that help nursing managers to allocate their resources rationally and cost effectively. The resultant time savings will allow managers to focus on other, less tedious and more creative activities.

It also is important to recover the cost associated with nursing care. If nursing care plans and records were sufficiently detailed, standardized, and complete, it would be relatively simple to look at each client's nursing-care requirements and to charge accordingly. In the absence of such plans and records, administrators must find other means to justify differential charges for nursing care. Some hospitals, such as St. Luke's Hospital and Medical Center in Phoenix, Arizona, and Stanford University Hospital, in California, are using various checklist methods to classify and charge patients according to the level of nursing care required [Walker, 1982]. Like other aspects of nursing, accounting for costs and revenues clearly stands to benefit from improvements in information management.

Costs and revenues, of course, are only one side of the nursing equation. The other side is the quality of the services provided. Since Donabedian's classic work in the mid-1960s, people have recognized that the quality of health services can be measured along any of three dimensions: structure (or resources), process, and outcomes [Donabedian, 1966]. Most quality-assurance programs in nursing have focused on the first two dimensions.

Structure is relatively simple to measure. The evaluator looks at the number of nursing personnel, the personnel's qualifications and experience, the working conditions, the material resources for providing care, and similar variables.

Process is somewhat more difficult to measure. The evaluator reviews written records to determine whether each of a sample of clients had an appropriate nursing assessment and care plan, whether timely and reasonable interventions were carried out in response to identified needs and problems, and whether the results of care were recorded. Because of the nonstandard, free-form narrative structure of most written nursing records, retrieving, coding, and analyzing these data are time-consuming and expensive tasks. Furthermore, even if the records show that the care provided appears reasonable and appropriate, there has been insufficient nursing research linking interventions and outcomes to permit a judgment of whether the most effective processes were used. Thus, measures of structure and process allow nurses to evaluate the degree to which the elements necessary for good care are present, but they do not provide information about the effectiveness of care.

Evaluation of *outcomes* of nursing care rarely is included in nursing quality-assurance programs. Nurses have shied away from the use of outcomes in part because of concern that any outcome is not solely due to nursing, but rather is influenced by many factors, from the client's own resilience to the care provided by other members of the health-care team. Other researchers, however, have recognized that certain outcomes are strongly influenced by nursing, and that, although it is impossible to predict with certainty the outcome for any individual, clients who receive better nursing care will, on the average, have better outcomes than will clients with similar problems who receive lower-quality nursing care [Horn and Swain, 1978]. Ideally, evaluations of the quality of nursing care would look at all three dimensions—structure, process, and outcomes—so that nurses could determine how variations in one dimension affected the other dimensions. Once again, however, the lack of standardized taxonomies and of systematic methods of recording make it impossible to use clinical records to compare diagnoses, objectives, interventions, and outcomes across groups of clients.

For the present, then, nurse administrators charged with evaluating the quality of care use slow, costly, manual methods to retrieve narrative information about the structure and process of care, and can only hope that what they consider to be positive structures and processes will lead to positive outcomes. Quality-assurance programs, like other procedures for which nurse administrators are responsible, can benefit greatly from improvements in information management.

8.1.3 Nursing Research and Development

Nursing research in clinical settings is hampered by the same problems of information management that plague nursing practice, administration, and education. Clinical nursing records are so unstandardized, disorganized, incomplete, and difficult to retrieve as to be virtually useless as a resource for research. Nurse researchers must develop their own operational definitions of variables and collect research data separately from clinical data. This is true even when the research problem and the clinical problem overlap, as in a test of the effectiveness of nursing interventions.

Standardizing the taxonomies and organization of clinical nursing records and providing for ready retrieval of data would offer important advantages for the development of nursing knowledge. Instead of being separate from practice, research could be done routinely in day-to-day nursing practice, vastly increasing the potential for building new knowledge. Clinical records could provide the data for studies to measure the incidence of particular nursing diagnoses, the relationships among phenomena, and the relative effectiveness of alternative nursing interventions to resolve problems. Clinical practice would raise questions for research, and research would be directly applicable to practice.

8.2 A Historical Perspective: Development of Computer Systems for Nursing

Computer applications are increasingly popular in all the nursing settings we have discussed. In clinical practice, NISs—independently or as components of total HISs—assist nurses in planning and documenting care. Although these systems offer no direct support to decision making, they organize clinical data more systematically than do traditional paper-based systems, and thus significantly reduce the time nurses spend processing information. In nursing administration, computer-based systems help to classify clients according to the level of care needed, and to project staffing requirements. Increasingly sophisticated systems are being developed to relieve nurse administrators of the burdens of scheduling. Advances are being made in cost and revenue accounting. Computer-based NISs also include mechanisms for assessing the quality of nursing care. In nursing education, computer-aided instruction (CAI) is being developed to teach the nursing process (including the specific cognitive, decision-making tasks) and to provide clinical simulations for practice in decision making with immediate feedback at no risk to clients. In nursing research, a variety of statistical programs facilitates analysis of complex, multivariate data sets. The problem of providing standardized, reliable clinical data for research, however, has not yet been resolved.

The development of viable computer applications in nursing is a relatively recent phenomenon. Prior to 1980, there were few real computer systems designed by or for nursing. The neophyte nature of nursing informatics was reflected in the scant literature of the period; most of the literature of the 1960s and 1970s consisted of commentaries on how to educate nurses about computing or how to implement computers in various nursing settings. We shall discuss a few notable exceptions from this period, but 1980 marked the beginning of a new era of research in computer applications for nursing.

During the last decade, a growing number of nurses discussed the effective use and design of NISs. Their interest was evidenced by the organization of periodic conferences devoted to nursing informatics, the increasing number of nursing submissions to the annual Symposium on Computer Applications in Medical Care (SCAMC), the inauguration in 1983 of *Computers in Nursing* (the first journal devoted entirely to the field), and the publication of the first textbook on the subject (the book by

Ball and Hannah that is listed in the Suggested Readings), which was quickly followed by other texts. Today, we see new developments and applications in all areas of the profession and a greatly foreshortened window between development and application in nursing, as computing becomes a basic tool to be applied across the professional panorama.

8.2.1 Systems for Clinical Practice

The history of clinical practice applications of computers in nursing mimics the overall history of computers in nursing. There were a few isolated bursts of activity in the early 1970s; until recently, however, few comprehensive and professionally satisfactory systems had been developed. Most systems that have been developed have taken a limited clinical view of nursing or have supported administrative functions more directly than they have clinical nursing care.

Reasons for such a slow development include
- The view that the existence of a satisfactory comprehensive HIS must precede the development of a nursing system
- The lack of agreement about and complete development of taxonomies in nursing
- The lack of computer resources in nursing
- The difficulty of attempting to develop isolated clinical applications in a profession dedicated to caring for patients' total health needs
- The lack of acceptable online environments within which to implement such tools

Early Prototypes of Clinical Nursing Systems

Among the earliest computer applications for nursing were programs to facilitate nursing diagnosis. Lagina, using a FORTRAN program, demonstrated the successful application of a Bayesian approach (see Chapters 3 and 15) to assessing the anxiety of awaiting surgery [Lagina, 1971]. Recognizing that a similar approach could be extended to other cognitive tasks of the nursing process, Ozbolt and Edwards carried out a systems analysis of the nursing process, wrote a program to diagnose the functional status of the skin and appendages, and described how their methods could be applied to diagnosis in other functional areas as well as to setting objectives, choosing interventions, and evaluating care [Goodwin and Edwards, 1975]. Nursing-care systems based on these prototypes could be implemented today in a number of computer-based nursing environments. At the time these programs were written, however, no comprehensive information systems offering this level of decision support were operational or even under development. Lacking opportunities for implementation, these early prototypes had little immediate influence.

Nursing in Hospital Information Systems

The Technicon Medical Information System (TMIS; see Chapter 7) was the first commercially usable system to include nursing-care subsystems. Technicon's implementation of a wide variety of care-planning and patient-outcome matrices represented a new height in applications development for nursing [Cook and Mayers, 1981]. Critics of the system, however, contend that, although the system allows rapid collection of patient data and execution of tasks such as order confirmation, there exists little linkage between patient data and care plans in the system. This lack probably reflects the state of the art of nursing theories and taxonomies in the early 1970s, when the system was developed.

Whereas the Technicon system has used a superficial, unsophisticated approach to the nursing process, other systems such as COSTAR (see Chapter 6) and PROMIS (see Chapter 7) have virtually ignored that process. Although these systems offer features such as the automated **Kardex** and the problem-oriented record to make nurses' work easier, they reflect no mature understanding of nursing's primary professional responsibility—the provision of appropriate, effective care via the nursing process.

More specific nursing applications have been developed outside the context of comprehensive information systems. These include many small systems for advising nurses regarding medications, pediatric assessment, health-risk appraisal, and so on [Johnson and Razenberger, 1981]. However, because nurses often have lacked access to microcomputers or to hospital mainframes, systems such as these rarely have been implemented.

The middle to late 1980s saw the development of more sophisticated clinical nursing systems within comprehensive information systems. The HELP system (see Chapter 7) incorporated modules for advising nurses in emergency and intensive-care situations; research and development were underway to support other aspects of nursing. ULTICARE, another recently developed system, basically serves as a shell that can incorporate modules for nursing assessment, diagnosis and inference, care planning, care monitoring, and care implementation.

Community-Health Nursing Systems

Traditionally, public-health facilities collected little systematic information on the services they provided. However, federal regulation enacted in the mid-1960s (for example, Medicaid, Medicare, and family-planning programs) required documentation to justify continued funding. Computer-based information systems have been essential for the collection and analysis of data both to plan and control organizational activity and to evaluate the benefits and costs of programs. Thus, federal support facilitated the development of a number of nursing systems in community-health settings.

Brown and colleagues' pacesetting work in the development of a patient-care information system (PCIS) for community-health nursing in the Indian Health Service benefited from early support for such systems by the Division of Nursing of the Bureau of Health Manpower, Department of Health, Education, and Welfare [Brown et al., 1971]. PCIS was developed in the 1960s to support community-health nurses working on the Papago Indian reservation in southwestern Arizona. Due to the mobility of the population and other factors, medical information tended to become fragmented among the records of multiple clinics, public health offices, and other institutions. PCIS stored medical, socioeconomic, and environmental information on each member of the tribe in a central database. Nurses could retrieve summary reports of patients' recent clinical visits, chronic problems, medications, and other medical data. The system also printed monthly appointment lists, generated summaries of nursing activities (for example, a breakdown of nursing hours by federal program), and provided community information on request (for example, a listing of children who had not been immunized).

Eight other projects, started in the 1960s and 1970s, have led to several successful implementations [Saba, 1982; Saba, 1983]:

1. The Patient Progress Methodology by the Division of Nursing of the Department of Health and Human Services
2. The Rockland County Project
3. The Systematic Nursing Assessment Project
4. The Philadelphia Community Nursing Services System
5. The New Jersey Home Health Management Information System
6. The Florida Health and Rehabilitation Services Nursing System
7. The Burlington/PROMIS Project
8. The Omaha Visiting Nurses' Association System (VNA).

Although some of the community-health nursing systems were primitive in their use of computer resources, their number and variety suggest that computer applications for nursing have developed more readily outside the hospital setting. This difference may be due in part to nursing's relative autonomy in community settings where applications do not need to compete for priority with other potential uses of computing resources, as they do in a complex hospital setting.

8.2.2 Systems for Nursing Administration

Early work in the organization and administration of nursing services via computer was done by Freund and Mauksch [Freund and Mauksch, 1975]. This important research, supported by the federal government, was among the first projects to provide nursing staffing advice on the basis of clients' needs for care. It led to the development of many later systems and computer staffing models. Early commercial systems for nurse staffing include the CSF system [Gabbert et al., 1975] and the Medicus system, which were modeled on the PASS system; PASS was one of the first systems for allocating and scheduling nursing staff [Jelinek et al., 1973]. Finlayson described an early implementation of the Medicus system, including its apparent ease of use, power, and flexibility [Finlayson, 1976]. It is interesting to note that, in spite of the wide availability of systems for computing nurse staffing needs, there continues to be great dissatisfaction in many areas with most nurse-staffing methodologies.

Critics maintain that, despite the computational precision of the computer-based systems and the time-and-motion studies on which the algorithms are founded, these systems at best project the *average* time required for the *usual care* of a patient with specific problems. Leaving aside questions of how to assess the reliability of the checklist data fed into these systems, in most cases there is no basis in research for determining whether the usual care is necessary, sufficient, or appropriate for achieving desired patient outcomes. Furthermore, patient-classification systems for determining staffing needs are expensive to purchase, maintain, and use; the data required to project staffing needs must be gathered and entered at frequent intervals—in some cases, once per shift. Yet no researcher has demonstrated that these systems provide an estimate of staffing needs more accurate than is the assessment made by the head nurse.

8.2.3 Systems for Nursing Education

Nursing education perhaps has been the area where the development of computer applications has been most dramatic and prolific. Much of the work on CAI in nursing began in the early 1970s, paralleling research in medical CAI (see Chapter 17). Although nursing-specific CAI was poorly represented at most centers, several sterling examples of effective computer-based instruction were successfully developed, tested, and implemented. Two seminal works are those of Bitzer and Bailey.

Bitzer's project extended research conducted at the University of Illinois on the PLATO project (see Chapter 17) [Bitzer and Boudreaux, 1969]. The system presented nursing students with simulated patients and problem situations, questions, and textual and pictorial information, and asked them to collect data, to perform experiments, and to answer questions (Figure 8.3). The program then judged the students' performances in managing cases. The use of CAI allowed students to control the rate and direction of their learning, and encouraged the development of critical thinking and problem solving. Thus, Bitzer applied all the creativity of the prescient PLATO technology to nursing. Further, her research to test the effectiveness of CAI methodology served as a model for later researchers, demonstrating better test scores and more rapid assimilation than was obtained by nursing students who had conventional instruction.

Bailey's MR. MARSHALL, which included such concepts as continuity of patient care, represented one of the first patient simulations to be incorporated into a nursing curriculum [Bailey et al., 1972]. The program provides students the opportunity to plan and manage the care of a patient, with immediate feedback on the consequences of their decisions.

SYPH and GASTRO, by Donabedian and Schultz, were two of the first case-finding simulations for community-health nursing [Donabedian, 1976]. Students were presented with the description of a situation that involved an outbreak of illness, either syphilis or food poisoning. Each scenario was followed by a set of questions designed to test understanding of key concepts and to stimulate interest in the subject matter. The computer provided immediate feedback as the student answered each question, including explanations of why an answer was correct or incorrect.

Until 1980, development of CAI for nursing was limited. Tymchyshyn, who also worked on the PLATO project, gives a good reason for this observation: the lack of sufficient rewards for nursing faculty members to invest the considerable time and work necessary to design and program CAI [Tymchyshyn, 1982]. This problem was partially overcome in the 1980s by the advent of good authoring software (for example, PILOT [Zucconi, 1986], NEMAS [Grobe, 1983]), of inexpensive microcomputers, and of publishers interested in providing support. Any recent issue of *Computers in Nursing* will demonstrate clearly the proliferation of CAI in nursing.

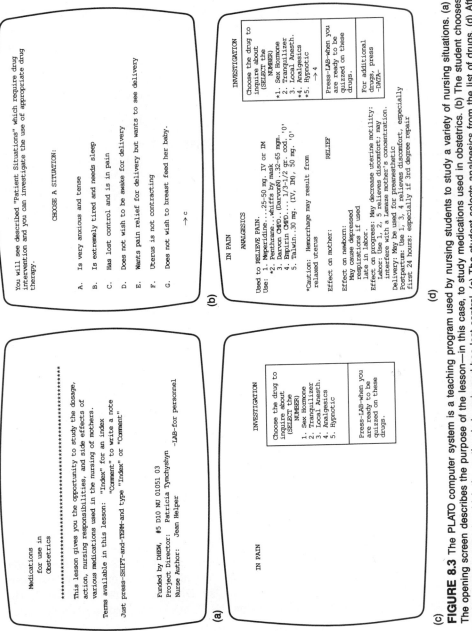

FIGURE 8.3 The PLATO computer system is a teaching program used by nursing students to study a variety of nursing situations. (a) The opening screen describes the purpose of the lesson—in this case, to study medications used in obstetrics. (b) The student chooses to explore the situation in which the mother is in pain and has lost control. (c) The student selects analgesics from the list of drugs. (d) After investigating the use of analgesics in obstetrics, the student can opt to be quizzed on the information, or can select another drug. (*Source: Courtesy of Pat Tymchyshyn, R.N., Ph.D. In Tymchyshyn, P. An evaluation of the adoption of an innovation: CAI with PLATO into a nursing program, Ph.D. thesis, College of Education, University of Illinois, Champaign-Urbana, 1982.*)

8.3 Fundamental Issues for Nursing Information Systems

The primary functions of an NIS are to assist nurses in record keeping and in decision support. In clinical practice, these functions translate to assistance in planning, implementing, documenting, and evaluating patient care. Fundamental to each of these tasks is a method for characterizing patient status, categorizing patient conditions (the nursing diagnoses), and creating patient-care plans. In nursing administration, NISs assist in scheduling nursing staff, managing resources, and assessing the quality of the care that is provided.

It should be clear from the discussion of nurses' clinical and administrative duties in Section 8.1 that the lack of a standardized terminology and a framework for viewing problems complicates all aspects of nurses' tasks. As we discussed in Chapter 2, the lack of a standard language is particularly detrimental to computer-based systems. If NISs are to be more than electronic filing cabinets, calculators, and pneumatic tubes for transmitting information, nurses and systems designers must create systems that *use* the information put into them, that *transform* raw data into more useful forms, and that *propose* clinical inferences for the nurse's consideration. For such systems to become possible, nurses must define the content of each step of the nursing process in clear and consistent language, and must tell how the elements fit together within each step and between steps. That is, they must develop a taxonomic structure for nursing, or perhaps several taxonomies that can be evaluated for their relative usefulness.

8.3.1 Taxonomies of Nursing Phenomena

Perhaps because nurses view their concern as the whole person and their responsibility as providing all the care that is needed that is not provided by anyone else, they have found it difficult to articulate and agree on more specific definitions of nursing. There is general agreement that nursing care is delivered via a problem-solving process that includes collecting data, formulating diagnoses, setting objectives, choosing and implementing interventions, and evaluating outcomes. But what data are to be collected? What is the nature of nursing diagnoses and objectives? What are effective nursing interventions? What outcomes are to be evaluated, and how? Taxonomies for these elements of the nursing process have yet to be fully developed and accepted.

Historically, nursing diagnoses have been the most common topic for discussion. Even the term *nursing diagnosis* was controversial as recently as the early 1970s, until it became clear to nurses and other health-care professionals that it referred not to nurses making a medical diagnosis but to nurses identifying problems (or resources) that were the particular focus of nursing practice. One factor in establishing the legitimacy of nursing diagnoses was the formation in 1973 of the National Conference Group for Classification of Nursing Diagnoses—now called the North American Nursing Diagnosis Association (NANDA)—which endeavored to generate and classify nursing diagnoses.

To generate diagnoses, NANDA researchers have worked inductively, first eliciting statements of problems nurses say they confront in their practices, and then searching for general organizing principles. The diagnoses they derive contain three elements: a statement of the problem itself, a statement of etiology in the form of a list of possible causes, and a list of defining characteristics (observable behaviors, signs, and symptoms) indicating that the problem is present. NANDA has generated a partial list of nearly 100 nursing diagnoses (see Figure 8.4), but some researchers have questioned the internal consistency of the diagnoses [Roy, 1982] and the centrality of the diagnostic labels to nursing concerns [Kritek, 1984].

Having generated a set of nursing diagnoses, the group subsequently faced the problem of organizing the diagnoses in a conceptual framework. One possible conceptual framework takes "unitary person" [Rogers, 1970] as the focus of nursing, derives categories from this framework, and fits the diagnostic labels into the categories, making some modifications both in the categories and in the labels to achieve a better fit [Kritek, 1984]. A problem with this approach is that it requires looking at unitary person as an integral and indivisible whole, whereas nurses are accustomed to dealing with diagnoses that describe some aspect of the person. Later versions of the structure of nursing diagnoses included nine patterns of unitary persons related to nine categories of alterations in human responses (Table 8.1). The pattern of *exchanging,* for example, was structured to include alteration in nutrition, elimination, oxygenation, circulation, and physical integrity. Current activities in the development of a structure of diagnoses include reviewing how nurses actually record clinical phenomena, so that the terminology of newly created labels can be useful to practicing nurses [Kritek, 1984].

While NANDA has been working inductively to generate nursing diagnoses and then classifying them in a general framework, independent researchers have been attempting to generate nursing taxonomies deductively. In 1972, Ozbolt and Edwards began designing a prototype computer program to aid the nursing process [Goodwin and Edwards, 1975]. This team perceived that the first task in such an undertaking was to define the nature of the problems addressed by the nursing process. Useful direction was provided by McCain's approach to the systematic assessment of patients [McCain, 1965]. McCain described nursing's primary goal as assisting clients and their families to attain and maintain optimal functional abilities, and she developed a guide to data collection that would provide information about functional abilities. Working within this rudimentary conceptual framework, Ozbolt and Edwards decided that the problems addressed by the nursing process, or nursing diagnoses, logically should deal with alterations in function. Nursing diagnoses, then, would describe areas of optimal functioning (*eufunctions*) or of problematic functioning (*dysfunctions*). Thirteen areas of functioning were included in McCain's assessment guide (for example, respiratory status, circulatory status, nutritional status, emotional status).

Selecting one of these areas—state of skin and appendages—Ozbolt and Edwards first listed all the functions of the skin, hair, and nails, then catalogued the data that would indicate whether each function was currently in a state of dysfunction or eufunction. Finally, they wrote a program that requested patient data, analyzed them, and

Approved Nursing Diagnostic Categories (1988)

Activity Intolerance
Activity Intolerance, Potential
Adjustment, Impaired
Airway Clearance, Ineffective
Anxiety
Aspiration, Potential for
Body Image Disturbance
Body Temperature, Potential Altered
Breastfeeding, Ineffective
Breathing Pattern, Ineffective
Communication, Impaired Verbal
Constipation
Constipation, Colonic
Constipation, Perceived
Decisional Conflict (Specify)
Decreased Cardiac Output
Defensive Coping
Denial, Ineffective
Diarrhea
Disuse Syndrome, Potential for
Diversional Activity Deficit
Dysreflexia
Family Coping: Compromised, Ineffective
Family Coping: Disabling, Ineffective
Family Coping: Potential for Growth
Family Processes, Altered
Fatigue
Fear
Fluid Volume Deficit
Fluid Volume Deficit, Potential
Fluid Volume Excess
Gas Exchange, Impaired
Grieving, Anticipatory
Grieving, Dysfunctional
Growth and Development, Altered
Health Maintenance, Altered
Health Seeking Behaviors (Specify)
Home Maintenance Management,
  Impaired
Hopelessness
Hyperthermia
Hypothermia
Incontinence, Bowel
Incontinence, Functional
Incontinence, Reflex
Incontinence, Stress
Incontinence, Total
Incontinence, Urge
Individual Coping, Ineffective
Infection, Potential for
Injury, Potential for
Knowledge Deficit (Specify)
Noncompliance (Specify)
Nutrition: Less than Body Requirements,
  Altered

Nutrition: More than Body Re-
  quirements, Altered
Nutrition: Potential for More than Body
  Requirements, Altered
Oral Mucous Membrane, Altered
Pain
Pain, Chronic
Parental Role Conflict
Parenting, Altered
Parenting, Potential Altered
Personal Identity Disturbance
Physical Mobility, Impaired
Poisoning, Potential for
Post-Trauma Response
Powerlessness
Rape-Trauma Syndrome
Rape-Trauma Syndrome: Compound
  Reaction
Rape-Trauma Syndrome: Silent Reaction
Role Performance, Altered
Self Care Deficit
  Bathing/Hygiene
  Feeding
  Dressing/Grooming
  Toileting
Self Esteem, Chronic Low
Self Esteem, Situational Low
Self Esteem Disturbance
Sensory/Perceptual Alterations (Specify)
  (visual, auditory, kinesthetic, gustatory,
  tactile, olfactory)
Sexual Dysfunction
Sexuality Patterns, Altered
Skin Integrity, Impaired
Skin Integrity, Potential Impaired
Sleep Pattern Disturbance
Social Interaction, Impaired
Social Isolation
Spiritual Distress
Suffocation, Potential for
Swallowing, Impaired
Thermoregulation, Ineffective
Thought Processes, Altered
Tissue Integrity, Impaired
Tissue Perfusion, Altered (Specify Type)
  (renal, cerebral, cardiopulmonary,
  gastrointestinal, peripheral)
Trauma, Potential for
Unilateral Neglect
Urinary Elimination, Altered
Urinary Retention
Violence, Potential for: Self-directed or
  Directed at Others

FIGURE 8.4 The nursing diagnoses accepted by the North American Nursing Diagnosis Association include physiological, functional, behavioral, and psychological classifications. (*Source:* Courtesy of North American Nursing Diagnosis Association, St. Louis, MO.)

TABLE 8.1 One Proposed Structure for Nursing Diagnoses

Patterns of Unitary Persons	Alterations in Human Responses (Normless)
Exchanging	Nutrition, elimination, [oxygenation], [circulation], [physical integrity]
Communicating	[Communication]
Relating	[Role]
Valuing	Spiritual [state]
Choosing	Coping, [participating]
Moving	Activity, rest, [recreation], [activities of daily living], [self-care]
Perceiving	Self-concept, sensory perceptual
Knowing	Knowledge, [learning], thought processes
Feeling	Comfort, [emotional integrity]

Source: Reproduced by permission from: Kritek, P. B. Report of the group work on taxonomies. In Kim, M. J., et al. (eds), *Classification of Nursing Diagnoses: Proceedings of the Fifth National Conference*, St. Louis, MO, 1984, The C. V. Mosby Co.

printed out nursing diagnoses with a summary of the data supporting each diagnosis (Figure 8.5). Although the program was clumsy and slow by today's standards, its development entailed the deduction of nursing diagnoses that were consistent with a conceptual framework and with one another, the identification of data necessary and sufficient to make the diagnoses, and the specification of logic linking data to diagnoses. The project was thus a step toward a coherent, internally consistent taxonomy of nursing diagnoses.

In subsequent work, Ozbolt organized diagnoses in a self-care conceptual framework by the degree to which self-care requisites were met and by the degree to which clients were able to continue meeting them. The valid and reliable measures developed during the Horn–Swain quality-of-care project [Horn and Swain, 1978] provided data items to determine the diagnoses. The foundation for an alternative nursing taxonomy was thus constructed. Furthermore, extrapolating from Orem's framework of self-care [Orem, 1980], and extending it to other stages of the nursing process, made it possible to enlarge the taxonomy to include objectives (requisites will be met; the client will become able to meet the requisites independently), interventions (actions to supplement and foster self-care), and outcomes (conceptually the same as diagnoses and objectives, differing perhaps in degree).

Ozbolt and other researchers implemented this taxonomy in developing prototype computer programs to aid nurse decision making at each step of the nursing process [Ozbolt, 1982; Ozbolt et al., 1984]. The taxonomy has been useful and practical for this purpose. Still, it has not been widely adopted. By contrast, the diagnoses developed by NANDA, for all their problems of internal consistency and incompleteness, have the endorsement of the hundreds of nurses nationwide who have worked to develop them. Will they prove useful? Will some other taxonomy prove most useful for nursing? Or will a variety of taxonomies be developed and used in different settings?

The function of the skin and mucous membranes
in preventing the entry of microorganisms is
impaired by:

> Presence of pathogens
> One
>> incision(s)
>>> not more than 20 cm in length or diameter
> Drainage with odor suggesting infection

Location:

> Abdomen

FIGURE 8.5 Ozbolt and Edwards' program for determining the state of skin and appendages requested patient data, analyzed them, and printed out nursing diagnoses with a summary of the data supporting each diagnosis.

8.3.2 Computer-Aided Planning and Documenting of Care

Despite lack of widespread agreement on a classification scheme for patient diagnoses, the developers of NISs have adopted standard vocabularies so that computers can assist in patient care. In most clinical settings today, nurses use locally generated sets of diagnostic statements to refer to common problems, and supplement these as needed with their own idiosyncratic diagnoses of less common conditions. The same approach has been applied to interventions, and, if they are recorded, to outcomes. Thus, nurses are able to record nursing assessments in automated nursing-history notes, and diagnoses in the automated Kardex.

The description of a patient's condition is not only a summary but also a point of departure. It serves as the foundation for the planning of nursing interventions and their implementation. Information systems are indispensable in this phase of the clinical process; they can aid in the development and execution of a treatment plan. In fact, an NIS that provides no aid in this phase is of limited value.

Generation of treatment objectives and actual treatment activities can take several forms. One extreme is to present nurses with quasiprescriptive actions to take (or a list of "things to do"), with no room for additions, specifications, or changes. Such a system is undesirable, as it would reduce nurses to automatons and ignore their professional expertise. The other, even less useful, extreme is to generate a list of all possible nursing interventions, with minimal advice about which ones are appropriate, which ones have higher priority, and so on. Nurses would just check off their selections, retaining all decision making.

Clearly, the solution lies somewhere in the middle. Standardized care plans undoubtedly are useful. First, they save time in terms of compilation and writeup. Second, and more important, they provide consistency over time, and reduce the probability of errors. The danger in the use of standardized care plans is that the plans are linked to problems considered in isolation from one another. An understanding of the whole person and of the interrelationship of problems and resources may require minor or major modifications in the standard care plan or sophisticated decision making about the timing of its implementation. Consequently, nurses must have the opportunity to add to or to change the standard care plans.

Currently available NISs offer standardized care plans for a limited number of nursing problems and allow the nurse to modify them according to the patient's needs. In the future, NISs may select and combine elements of standard care plans to generate a plan tailored to the individual patient's array of problems and resources. Such systems still would need to permit modification by the nurse, to allow for the diversity of human interaction that is central to nursing.

The nursing component of the Technicon system, used at the El Camino Hospital in Mountain View, California and at the NIH Clinical Center, among other sites, offers a rudimentary level of decision support to nurses (see Section 7.3.1). After the medical diagnosis, orders, and nursing-assessment data have been entered, the system helps to generate a nursing-care plan by proposing certain nursing actions, which the nurse can modify or augment. The proposals generated by the system, however, concern only routine nursing care associated with the medical diagnosis and orders. The system offers little more than a blank slate on which to write; to individualize the care plan and to make use of the rich nursing database, nurses must rely on their own intellectual processes.

The Technicon system employs a *deterministic* approach to propose routine nursing care associated with certain medical conditions—if a given set of data is entered (thus indicating the presence of a particular medical condition), a corresponding intervention is recommended in the nursing-care plan. This intervention will be generated if and only if all of the prespecified conditions have been met. More recent work on other systems takes into account the continuous nature of many nursing phenomena; decisions are triggered when certain data exceed a threshold [Ozbolt, 1982; Ozbolt et al., 1984]. For example, preoperative anxiety is normal, but when it exceeds the level judged by the nurse to be normal, intervention is indicated to reduce it. This work has extended the applicability of deterministic paradigms to clinical NISs. Still, clinical phenomena are modeled as discrete events, even if acknowledged to be of a continuous nature.

Some projects are underway to develop NISs that apply probabilistic and heuristic approaches (see Chapter 15), rather than deterministic approaches. These projects, however, are still in the experimental stages. The need to work in this new direction emerges from the nature of inference in nursing. First, clinical inference in nursing does not end with the identification and classification of a disease. It entails the continuous and sustained assessment of the patient over time until the initial problems have disappeared or have been otherwise managed. Second, the domains of clinical inference in nursing are multiple (physical, psychological, and social). Each domain must be assessed independently, and these assessments must be integrated into a coherent, multidimensional assessment. Finally, parameters in nursing practice seldom have discrete values (for example, normal versus abnormal); rather, the values lie on a continuum.

Abraham and colleagues proposed a multivariate mathematical algorithm for diagnostic information systems, which is designed to assess the status of continuous temporal processes with multiple dimensions [Abraham et al., 1984a; Abraham et al., 1984b]. The algorithm presumes that a patient's clinical condition can be expressed, at any point in time, as a vector that describes the patient's status along several functional domains. The patient's clinical-condition vector can be compared at any time with two other vectors that define the upper and lower limits of normalcy in a population—the boundaries of the *population criterion interval*. Clinical inference, then, consists of determining whether the clinical-condition vector falls within or outside the population criterion interval. If it falls within, normalcy is inferred, and the decision, therefore, is that there is no need for nursing action. Conversely, a locus outside the interval indicates a clinical nursing problem and implies the need for nursing interventions. Assessments such as these can be performed for the client's overall status, as well as for specific functional domains.

8.3.3 Evaluating Care

The linkage in an NIS of nursing-assessment data and nursing orders and objectives offers the possibility of using computer-based methods to evaluate the quality of the nursing care process. Two tasks constitute the evaluation procedure: (1) the evaluation of the patient's condition, and (2) the evaluation of the nursing care rendered. An NIS should permit both.

Evaluating the patient's conditions essentially consists of measuring change. Performing a nursing assessment at the beginning of the clinical process and again at the end is one possible approach. The appropriateness of this method can be questioned, however, on the grounds that assessment—total and partial—is a continuous activity. Information systems should therefore accommodate multiple time points.

Allowing nurses to set multiple time points might be preferred over determining time points a priori. In the latter case, it is likely that an information system's prompts for patient evaluation data would not coincide with clinically critical moments of evaluation. The vector algorithm proposed by Abraham and colleagues (see Section 8.3.2) addresses this problem. The clinical-condition vector summarizes the patient's state at a particular point in time. In other words, the clinical-condition vector is a time-specific indicator of the patient's status, and as such is a parameter for evaluation. Significant alterations over the previous time point indicate change—improvements or deteriorations in the patient's condition. Such changes can be recorded for the patient's overall condition, and for functional domains.

Evaluation often occurs in a recursive fashion as well. The need for information may prompt the nurse to return to data acquired at an earlier point in the clinical process, and to update the patient information base with new or more detailed information. Clinical updating is an important procedure in nursing inference, because it maximizes accuracy, detail, and sophistication.

As professionals, nurses need to monitor the quality of the care they provide, a function in which computer-based assistance might prove useful. More commonly known as quality assurance, the monitoring of care and services is an evaluative endeavor that concerns the client, nursing staff, and hospital at large. One avenue for performing quality assurance is to build into the NIS subroutines for auditing the nursing-care plans and documentation of care. This has been the most frequent approach in both paper- and computer-based systems. Some people have questioned, however, whether documentation accurately reflects the care actually provided, and whether the care that is considered appropriate is in fact the most effective. Computer-aided systems can promote accuracy of documentation by increasing the speed and ease with which this activity is performed. They can facilitate evaluation of the effectiveness of care by analyzing correlations among diagnoses, objectives, interventions, and outcomes to determine the degree to which the care provided led to achievement of objectives. Self-correcting mechanisms then can be applied to the standardized care plans to promote the most effective care.

A final aspect in the evaluation of the quality of nursing care is receiving increasing attention as hospitals attempt to determine the costs of nursing care. Nursing administrators must determine the costs (as well as the effectiveness) of providing different levels of nursing care, so that they can allocate their resources optimally, choosing the types of care that provide the greatest benefits to patients, relative to costs.

8.4 Current Nursing Information Systems

In this section, we shall illustrate progress and problems in developing NISs by discussing a few systems in the areas of nursing practice, administration, and education.

8.4.1 Systems for Nursing Practice

Perhaps most representative of clinical information systems for nursing is TMIS, the Technicon system (see Section 7.3.1). It reflects the state of the art of nursing with respect to process and outcome specifications, measurement, and documentation circa 1970. It provides extremely rapid confirmation of physicians' orders, medications, and so on, and rapid switching of computer screens to produce care plans quickly and conveniently. There appears to be, however, little or no connection between the data collected by nurses and the care plans produced by the system. Essentially, the system lacks nursing knowledge, operating only at a gross paper-replacement level rather than using knowledge of the nursing process.

IBM's Patient Care System (PCS; see Section 7.2.2) goes a step beyond the Technicon system in relating nursing diagnoses to the care plan. In this system, care plans consist of (1) nursing diagnoses, (2) factors related to the nursing diagnoses, (3) patient goals, (4) outcome criteria, and (5) nursing measures and assessments. Like Technicon, PCS uses standardized nursing care plans. To use the system, the nurse selects the nursing diagnosis or problem that most nearly corresponds to the client's condition, calls up the standard care plan, and modifies the plan according to the patient's needs. The system is said to reduce the time nurses spend doing paperwork while encouraging them to maintain comprehensive up-to-date care plans [Light, 1983]. Like Technicon, however, the PCS provides no assistance in deriving diagnoses from clinical data, and little or no other support for nurse decision making. We clearly have a long way to go before we develop systems that use nursing data to advise nurses on the care of patients.

The COMMES (Creighton On-Line Multiple Medical Expert System) prototype is a notable example of a system designed to assist with nursing decision making [Ryan, 1985]; COMMES has been under development at Creighton University in Omaha, Nebraska since the mid-1970s. One part of the system, the Nursing Protocol Consultant (NPC), provides patient-specific information to guide nurses in developing patient-care plans. In response to specific requests for information, NPC identifies critical nursing goals and itemizes nursing interventions to achieve these goals. To provide this assistance, NPC interacts with the Generalist Knowledge Base, which encodes in a hierarchy of goals and subgoals the knowledge that a generalist nurse must use to provide safe, comprehensive care. A comparison of COMMES-generated nursing protocols with protocols produced by qualified nursing consultants revealed that the computer's protocols were comparable to those written by educators and clinicians. On the basis of the results of the evaluation, COMMES is being implemented in a clinical setting [Cuddigan et al., 1987].

The ULTICARE system, developed by Health Data Sciences and implemented at William Beaumont Hospital in Royal Oak, Michigan, is an ambitious system that potentially could change nursing practice. Essentially, it provides a shell environment within which to embed nursing knowledge regarding assessment, inference and diagnosis, care planning, and care documentation. Users can custom-tailor ULTICARE to a degree not possible with other clinical nursing systems. The system's greatest advantage is that it allows the evaluation of nurses' clinical inference processes. Thus, it provides an environment for intelligent processing of nursing information and integration of decision support and consultation for clinical nursing practice.

8.4.2 Systems for Nursing Administration

The style of administrative systems was, to a great extent, fixed by the mid-1970s, with the release of systems such as Medicus (now NPAQ). NPAQ still is commercially successful; many nurse administrators depend on it for staffing and scheduling.

NPAQ uses a patient-classification instrument and a quality-monitoring system as its sources of data. Other systems, such as GRASP,[2] also are dependent on quality-of-care measures, whether based on the outcomes or on the process of care. The inherent unreliability of current quality-measurement systems is well documented, however, and calls into question the usefulness of most such systems [Schultz II, 1978]. The computer-based tools of today probably often simply legitimate "squeaky-wheel" staffing more than they predict true workload and thus needs. Further,

---

[2]GRASP was developed in the late 1960s as PETO. Later, the system was refined extensively. It is now marketed by the First Consulting Group in Long Beach, California.

patient-acuity measures, another critical index of staffing needs, also suffer from un-reliability and the continuing flux in modalities of patient care driven by diagnosis-related groups (DRGs; see Chapter 19) and other financing directives. Although there are many anecdotal accounts of successes, few tools are tested thoroughly or are sub-jected to close scrutiny while in use with today's complex mixes of skills, patients, and care. A step in the right direction is provided under COSTAR (see Section 6.4.1), in which CASH (Commission on Administrative Services for Hospitals) and PIRS (Patient Information Review System) provide quality-assurance audits as part of the total system.

8.4.3 Systems for Nursing Education

The availability of affordable microcomputers has facilitated the introduction of com-puters into nursing schools. It is now common to see microcomputers in schools of nursing, and some schools have built impressive computer laboratories for educa-tional (and research) applications. Publishing houses joined in the movement to use microcomputers for nursing education; there now are commercially available soft-ware programs to teach fundamental aspects of nursing, to simulate nursing care prob-lems, and to test nursing skills and knowledge.

A CAI system with great potential for nursing is the Nursing Education Modular Authoring System (NEMAS), developed by Grobe and associates at the University of Texas at Austin [Grobe, 1983]. NEMAS helps nursing instructors to write patient simulations that will teach specific cognitive skills in the nursing process. Grobe's analysis of the cognitive tasks inherent in the nursing process is one of the few explications of this critical aspect of nursing. Key skills of clinical judgment that heretofore had been scarcely articulated can now, thanks to NEMAS, be taught ex-plicitly. Furthermore, instructors who use the authoring system do not need to have specific prior knowledge of Grobe's cognitive analysis. They enter client informa-tion in response to prompts, and NEMAS structures the learning activity to teach the cognitive skills of the selected step of the nursing process.

Other applications that have attracted publishing houses are software programs for testing nursing competency. Most of them are electronic compilations of the books that prepare students for the nursing licensure examination, although there are a few more generic testing programs. More recently, test-authoring programs have appeared on the market.

8.5 A Look to the Future

The changes in computing technology that are shaping the development of HISs af-fect the ways and the extent to which nurses use computers in their work. As the primary users of HISs, nurses will benefit from the assimilation of local-area net-works in hospitals, the installation of bedside terminals, and the development of user-friendly software running on microcomputers; progress in these areas will simplify and streamline many of nurses' information-management tasks. More fundamental advances will come through the development of specialized NISs—information systems to support nursing decision making and the professional aspects of nursing practice, rather than just the clerical aspects.

The development of standard nursing plans is an important first step toward improving the consistency and efficiency of the nursing care process. Deterministic approaches, however, ignore the richness of the patient information that could be used in patient-care planning. In the future, research in the application of artificial-intelligence techniques to NISs may produce usable clinical systems to assist in *patient-specific* planning and evaluation of nursing care. If they are to be truly useful, these systems must not merely emulate what nurses do, but rather must complement the nursing process. For example, they may calculate complex interrelationships among multiple data to propose nursing diagnoses that would be apparent only to the most expert nurses. Such systems might assist even experts to compose a complex care plan quickly and easily.

These and other developments in NISs will be driven by pressures to control the costs of health care. Undoubtedly, one of the most important changes in health-care financing in recent years was the introduction of prospective reimbursement based on DRGs. With it came an increasing awareness among health-care administrators of nurses as a focus of resource utilization. Nursing administrators now face great pressure to reduce staffing levels and to allocate resources optimally. At the same time, nursing treatment is growing more intensive; as clients' lengths of stay shorten, and as nurse-to-client ratios decrease, nurses have more work to do and more goals to achieve in less time. Furthermore, outpatient surgery and other nonhospital forms of care are becoming more common, thus increasing the importance of continuity of care between hospital, outpatient facilities, and home.

External pressures are forcing nurses to describe more explicitly the nature of their work, and to justify the costs of that work. Thus, the changing health-care environment has led to a growing interest among nurses and hospital administrators in defining standard nursing taxonomies, developing uniform treatment procedures, and studying ways to make the nursing staffing more responsive to the level of patient needs in the hospital. Computer-based tools have a great potential to help with nursing tasks. First, however, we need to develop a deeper understanding of what is entailed in nursing care. Perhaps, ironically enough, by forcing nurses to explain the nature of their practice, the next generation of computer systems will help them to realize more fully Nightingale's view of the profession as artful but deliberate, as nurturant but knowledgeable—as the considered application of specialized skills to bring about better health for nursing's clients.

Suggested Readings

Ball, M. J. and Hannah, K. J. *Using Computers in Nursing.* Reston, VA: Reston Publishing Company, 1984.

The first text devoted to computer applications in nursing, this book provides a basic introduction to computer hardware and software, and covers topics such as the use of com-

puters in primary and continuing education, in research, and in hospital- and community-based practice settings.

Ball, M. J., et al. (eds). *Nursing Informatics.* New York: Springer-Verlag, 1988.
More than 30 collaborators worked together to create this volume, which summarizes the current state of nursing informatics and the discipline's relation to patient care. The first section of the book delineates the field of nursing informatics; it defines new roles for nurses and discusses the challenges of integrating nursing and computing. The second section describes computer applications in four functional areas of nursing: clinical practice, administration, research, and education.

Gordon, M. Practice-based data set for a nursing information system. *Journal of Medical Systems,* 9:43, 1985.
This article proposes 17 categories of data for inclusion in a standard nursing data set. The categories include patient-identification, demographic, care-provider–identification, and care-provision information. Definitions and rationales for inclusion also are presented.

Korpman, R. A. Patient care information systems: Looking to the future. Part 4. The changing role of computers in nursing. *Software in Healthcare,* (October/November):58, 1984.
The fourth in a series on patient-care information systems, this article focuses on the potential benefits to be derived from the automation of the nursing-care process. The paper contrasts nursing assessment, care planning, Kardex and patient-schedule maintenance, and charting and continuing patient assessment under manual and computer-based systems.

Ozbolt, J. G., et al. A proposed expert system for nursing practice. *Journal of Medical Systems,* 9:57, 1985.
The authors first describe the nursing process and discuss the nature of nursing knowledge, then outline an approach to constructing an expert system designed to help nurses in determining nursing diagnoses and formulating individualized care plans.

Ryan, S. A. An expert system for nursing practice. *Journal of Medical Systems,* 9:29, 1985.
This article on COMMES describes the operation of the Nursing Diagnosis Consultant and the structure of the Generalist Knowledge Base.

Werley, H. H. and Grier, M. R. (eds). *Nursing Information Systems.* New York: Springer-Verlag, 1981.
This volume grew from research presented at the first Research Conference on Nursing Information Systems in 1977. It includes discussion of tasks such as identifying data for nursing practice, implementing these data in computer-based systems, and evaluating NISs. Although, at the time of the conference, few computer-based NISs existed, the participants and their research helped to build foundations for future work in nursing informatics.

Zielstorff, R. (ed). *Computers in Nursing.* Wakefield, MA: Nursing Resources, 1980.
This collection of articles provides an introductory-level overview of what computers are, how they are used in nursing, and what some of the impediments are to their more widespread adoption.

Zielstorff, R. D., McHugh, M. L., and Clinton, J. *Computer Design Criteria for Systems that Support the Nursing Process.* Kansas City, MO: American Nurses' Association, 1988.
This document, written for both practicing nurses and computer-system vendors, describes criteria for the success of computer applications that support and document the nursing process. The monograph reviews many factors related to the design, selection, and use of automated systems for nursing practice.

Questions for Discussion

1. For which aspects of health care does nursing have primary responsibility? How is nursing's domain of responsibility different from and complementary to medicine's?

2. Consider the differing and complementary domains of nursing and medicine and the different methods for delivering services in the two professions. Describe the extent of nursing's responsibility for documentation and communication, and explain the importance of these tasks. What improvements do existing computer-based systems offer over nonautomated systems for these nursing tasks of documentation and communication?

3. What factors have hindered the development of clinical decision-support systems for nursing? Briefly describe two prototype systems, and explain how these systems addressed each of the problems you have described.

4. Describe how researchers have applied inductive and deductive approaches to develop taxonomies of nursing diagnoses. What are the strengths and weaknesses of each approach? Describe the taxonomies yielded in each case.

5. What are the strengths and limitations of standardized nursing care plans as elements of computer-based care-planning systems? How might future systems use artificial-intelligence techniques to overcome some of the limitations you mentioned?

6. What are the advantages and limitations of staffing systems that classify patients according to level of need for nursing services? What kinds of systems are needed to permit analyses of nursing costs and effectiveness and of quality of care?

7. Describe three computer-based systems that have been used in nursing education. How might the growing use of CAI change the way nursing is taught? More fundamentally, how might increasing use of automated systems, including those that use artificial-intelligence techniques, change nursing practice, and what changes in nursing education would be necessary?

8. Traditionally, physicians have been slow to accept the use of computers in medical practice—especially the use of decision-support systems. Do you think that developers will face the same problems with nursing systems? Explain your answer.

9

Laboratory Information Systems

Jack W. Smith, Jr. and John R. Svirbely

After reading this chapter, you should know the answers to these questions:

- What are the most common divisions of the clinical laboratory, and what are their functions?
- What are the reasons for using computer-based information systems in the clinical laboratory?
- What tasks make up the extralaboratory and intralaboratory cycles of information processing?
- What functions are provided by the current generation of commercial laboratory information systems?
- How will laboratory information systems of the future help physicians and other health-care professionals in test ordering and interpretation?

9.1 Handling Information in the Clinical Laboratories

Laboratory-test results are an important source of information for health-care professionals. Physicians may order tests to assist in the diagnosis of disease, to guide the treatment of known disorders, or to screen patients for inapparent disease. The primary functions of the clinical laboratories are to acquire, validate, interpret, and communicate the information derived from analyzing patient specimens. The quality of laboratory services depends not only on the accuracy and precision of the test results, but also on the timeliness of test completion and the availability of the results.

For over 2 decades, the number of tests performed in clinical laboratories has increased at an average annual rate of 10 to 15 percent (Figure 9.1). Clinical laboratories in large community and teaching hospitals routinely perform several million tests each year [Miller et al., 1980]. Computers were introduced into clinical laboratories during the late 1950s to help laboratory personnel meet this rapidly growing demand for testing. The implementation of DRG-based reimbursement for Medicare-insured hospital patients forced clinical laboratories to become more efficient, thus producing additional incentives to use computers. While the laboratory workload has been increasing in recent years, the number of technical personnel has actually been decreasing (Table 9.1). Today, computers are widely distributed and are well integrated into the clinical laboratory.

Laboratory information systems (LISs) support fundamental functions in both data processing and laboratory management. Not only have computers become integrated into the instruments that process the specimens, but also they help to analyze the primary data, to store and distribute test results, to monitor testing quality, to document laboratory procedures, and to provide information used by managers in controlling inventory, monitoring workflow, and assessing laboratory productivity.

9.1.1 Organization of the Clinical Laboratory

To meet the demands of medical practice, clinical laboratories perform many kinds of tests, some of which must be available 24 hours per day. Although we often speak of the clinical laboratory, it is more realistic to refer to various specialized laboratories: clinical chemistry, hematology, microbiology, surgical pathology, blood bank, and so on. Each laboratory handles different types of specimens, and uses different analytical techniques.

* The *clinical chemistry* laboratory performs chemical analyses on specimens such as plasma, serum, whole blood, urine, and cerebrospinal fluid. Typically, a *reagent* is mixed with a sample specimen, causing a chemical reaction. The intensity of the reaction is proportional to the chemistry being measured; the test result is determined by matching the observed change to a standard set of changes (Figure 9.2). Common tests measure the concentrations of electrolytes (for example, sodium, potassium, and calcium), blood gases (for example, oxygen and carbon dioxide), enzymes, lipids, carbohydrates, proteins, physiologic waste products, hormones, drugs, and poisons. In many medical situations, these chemical determinations are crucial for the management of critically ill patients; thus, a significant proportion of chemistry tests are performed as emergency (stat) procedures.

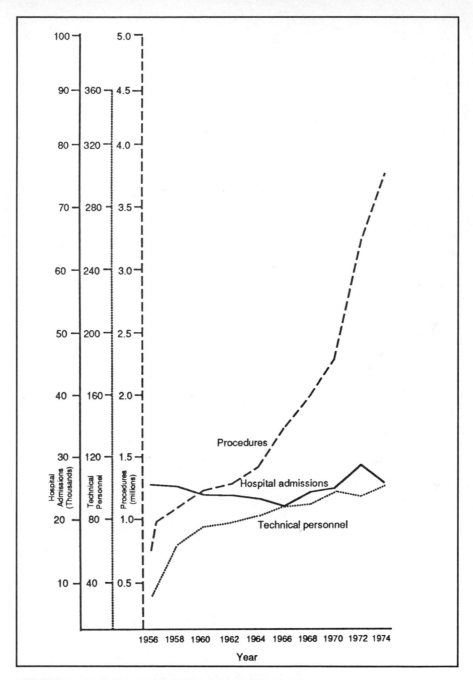

FIGURE 9.1 Between 1956 and 1974, the number of laboratory tests performed at the Ohio State University Hospitals rose much faster than did either the number of patients or the number of laboratory staff. (*Source:* Reprinted with permission from Speicher, C. D. and Smith, J. W., Jr. *Choosing Effective Laboratory Tests.* Philadelphia: W. B. Saunders, 1983, p. 4.)

TABLE 9.1 Increased Efficiency in Clinical Laboratories in Response to DRG-Based Reimbursement

Year	FTEs[a]	CAP[b] Work Units
1985	294	20,850,000
1986	289	20,938,093
1987	275	23,178,000
1988	265	23,788,992

[a]FTE = full-time equivalent.
[b]CAP = College of American Pathologists; see Section 9.3.7.
Source: Ohio State University Hospitals.

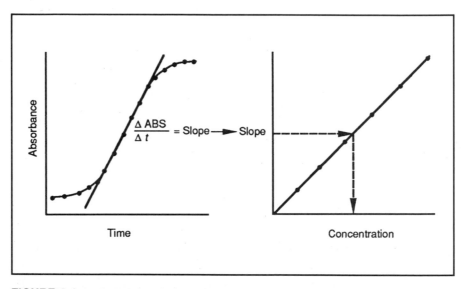

FIGURE 9.2 In clinical chemistry testing, specific reagents are added to a patient specimen to produce a chemical reaction that causes a detectable change (in color, for example). The underlying premise is that the measured intensity of the reaction is proportional to the amount of substance being measured. By comparing the observed reaction to similar reactions produced by standardized samples of known concentrations, the computer can extrapolate the level of the chemical compound in the patient's specimen.

- The *hematology* laboratory performs tests to characterize the cellular elements of the blood—the red and white blood cells, and the platelets. One of the most commonly performed blood assays is the complete blood count (CBC), a panel of tests that determines the numbers, sizes, and hemoglobin content of the cells. Blood also may be examined under a microscope to determine the *differential counts* of red blood cells at various stages of development.
- The *clinical microbiology* laboratory identifies the infectious agents (bacteria, fungi, parasites, viruses) present in patient specimens. Specimens may be examined under a microscope, cultured in isolation, or subjected to biochemical analysis. In some

cases, the laboratory performs tests to determine the sensitivity of the organisms to various antibiotic compounds; this information is used by physicians to prescribe effective therapeutic regimens.

- The *cytology* laboratory examines specimens for malignant cells. The most commonly performed tests are screening examinations, such as the Pap smear to screen patients for cervical tumors or sputum smears to screen for lung tumors.
- The *immunology* laboratory measures antigens and antibodies in body fluids to diagnose infectious disease and immunological disorders.
- The *surgical pathology* laboratory examines all specimens removed during surgery to diagnose the type and extent of the diseases present. Although sometimes only gross (direct visual) examination of the material needs to be performed, typically very thin sections are cut from the tissue and are examined microscopically. Specialized laboratories may conduct additional studies using techniques such as immunological staining or electron microscopy.
- The *blood bank* is responsible for storing and distributing blood products. In addition, it tests donor and recipient bloods to ensure that the blood types are compatible and that only biologically safe products are released for transfusion.

The optimum organization of the laboratory is determined by the type and size of the medical installation, the location of the laboratory, and the kinds of tests the laboratory performs. Typically, large clinical laboratories are organized into two or more divisions, each specialized to perform tests in a particular medical domain (microbiology, hematology, and so on). Because emergency tests require special handling procedures, laboratory divisions may be further subdivided by expected turnaround time (routine versus stat). In smaller laboratories, clear-cut divisions may not exist, and many kinds of tests may be performed in the same area.

9.1.2 Information Flow in the Clinical Laboratory

The clinical laboratory, like all ancillary-care departments, responds to external demands for services. The order for a test, usually written by a patient's attending physician, is the first in a series of steps in the testing process, which includes specimen collection, test performance, and report generation. We can distinguish two cycles in the testing process—one that takes place outside the laboratory and another that functions within the laboratory (Figure 9.3). In the **extralaboratory cycle,** specimens and test requests are delivered to the laboratory, and test results are communicated to requesting physicians. The **intralaboratory cycle**—the analysis cycle—consists of steps to label each specimen with a unique accession number, to divide the specimen into aliquots (small portions), to deliver the aliquots to the appropriate workstations, to perform the tests, and to prepare the report of test results.

Laboratory managers carefully monitor the testing process to measure the volume and distribution of test orders, the productivity of laboratory workers, and the testing turnaround time and error rate. They use parameters such as these to help in scheduling personnel, controlling inventory, purchasing equipment, and estimating the budget. In addition, these process measures are used to evaluate the quality of laboratory services and to understand how existing procedures can be improved.

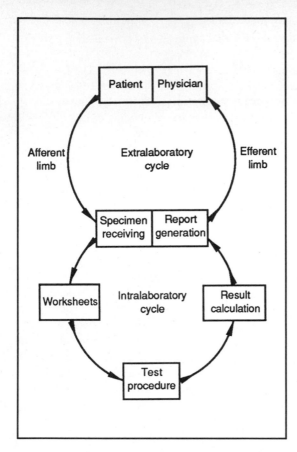

FIGURE 9.3 The testing process comprises two cycles. In the extralaboratory cycle, specimens and test requests are delivered to the laboratory, and final test results are returned to requesting physicians. Within the laboratory, technologists analyze specimens and prepare reports of test results.

9.2 Historical Development of Laboratory Information Systems

Until the late 1950s, most laboratory tests were performed individually by hand. The same technologists who analyzed the specimens also did much of the associated paperwork. These clerical duties accounted for 15 to 30 percent of laboratory personnel's work time [Peacock et al., 1965; Flynn et al., 1968]. The manual systems functioned adequately while the workload was low and the timeliness of the results was not crucial, but as the volume of work increased and as physicians demanded results with greater urgency, the quality of laboratory services deteriorated. By the late 1950s, laboratories were overburdened. Tests were ordered but never completed, specimens were misidentified, erroneous results were generated, and reports were misplaced. Laboratory managers hoped that the introduction of automated analytical instruments would solve these problems. The clinical laboratory was a natural application area for computers; computers could perform the high volume of repetitive tests rapidly and accurately.

In 1957, Skeggs described an automated analyzer for performing chemistry tests continuously. This process was first implemented as Technicon Instruments' Auto Analyzer, which could perform the majority of the tests requested in the clinical chemistry laboratory; the analyzer sequentially sampled the specimen, added reagent, and measured the intensity of the chemical reaction. With the continued introduction of other automated analyzers in the early 1960s, laboratories were able to perform rapidly panels of analytical tests on a single specimen.

Automated laboratory instruments greatly improved the ability of the clinical laboratories to perform the tests inhouse. However, they generated large numbers of data; consequently, they overwhelmed the data-interpretation processes within the laboratory. In some respects, automation of test performance aggravated laboratories' information-handling problems. Hence, the development of LISs; computers were used to acquire data from laboratory instruments, to manipulate and store the information, and to generate reports of test results.

Initially, the output from instruments had to be entered manually into LISs. The first attempts at data acquisition used offline input via mark-sense cards (forms that are marked with a pencil and scanned optically) or punched cards and some human coding of instrument outputs. Later, instruments produced output on a machine-readable medium that could be fed into a computer. Finally, direct instrument-to-computer interfaces were used for data input, with the earliest success being achieved with the Auto Analyzer, the IL flame photometer, and the Coulter blood-cell analyzer. Currently, many automated instruments come equipped with preprocessors that convert the analog data generated by the instruments into digital format, and transmit the digital data in real time to the LIS without human intervention. Removal of the transcription step eliminates human errors and time delays associated with data collection and data entry.

In 1970, Du Pont introduced the first computer-controlled laboratory instrument, the Automated Clinical Analyzer (ACA). A hardwired computer, which was incorporated into the instrument, controlled the ACA's functions, calculated results from raw data, and reported the final results. Since then, the trend has been toward highly automated, intelligent, standalone instrument systems. Reductions in the size and price of processors hastened the incorporation of computers into laboratory instruments. Currently, numerous instruments use microprocessors to control many phases of operation. For example, the computer of the Sequential Multiple Analysis Computer (SMAC) system assists in all phases of testing. It automatically calibrates each testing channel, identifies samples, calculates data, reports results, and assists in troubleshooting.

Computers were first used in laboratories for administrative and managerial support in the mid-1960s. Not only were clerical functions performed automatically, but also computers interfaced directly with laboratory instruments. Even the earliest, and relatively unsophisticated, computer systems produced tangible benefits, including

- Decreased turnaround time from test request to reported result
- Increased accuracy of test results and marked reductions in the numbers of transcription errors and misplaced results
- Improved quality control and better monitoring of equipment

- More efficient storage and more timely retrieval of data used in research and teaching
- Increased productivity per laboratory worker
- Greater availability of information used for administrative and managerial purposes

9.3 Fundamental Functions of Laboratory Information Systems

The benefits of today's LISs derive from these systems' ability to facilitate information flow both within the laboratory and between the laboratory and the health-care personnel who use the laboratory's services. Currently, LISs are used primarily for data collection, record keeping, and process control, although more sophisticated patient-care applications are possible and some interpretive systems are being developed.

9.3.1 Test Ordering and Results Reporting

Historically, the communication of orders and results between the laboratories and the patient wards has been a source of errors and delays. Before LISs were developed, health-care personnel relied on handwritten test-order forms to request tests and to receive results (Figure 9.4). These paper slips sometimes were misplaced and were vulnerable to transcription errors and misinterpretation of handwritten results. More urgent results often were conveyed verbally over the telephone, a potential source of misunderstanding and incomplete data transfer. Pneumatic tubes and other transmission devices were used to minimize errors and delays in communication, particularly to key areas, such as the emergency room and intensive-care unit. The use of computers greatly improved the ability of laboratories to deliver results rapidly and accurately by allowing remote printing of information via devices located on the wards. If an LIS supported automated order entry and results reporting, paper order slips could be eliminated entirely, and legible results became available without delay to all authorized health professionals who had access to the patient's online records.

9.3.2 Patient and Specimen Identification

Currently, the most problematic step in the testing process is the identification of patients and specimens. LISs assist in the identification process by producing specimen-collection lists by room number and by preprinting specimen labels. No completely reliable, generally accepted, and cost-effective system for identification exists, however. Many blood banks use bar-coded labels to identify blood products, but despite their potential for reducing identification errors, bar-coded patient-identification wristbands and specimen labels are not widely used. In many laboratories, specimen-collection personnel still must either read patients' identification bracelets or ask patients for names and birthdates.

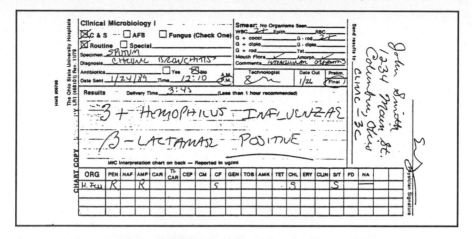

FIGURE 9.4 In manual laboratory information systems, health-care personnel order laboratory tests by filling out paper order slips, such as this request for a sputum culture. The laboratory performs the requested tests, writes the results on the slip, and returns a copy of the form for inclusion in the patient's chart. Cumulatively, these handwritten slips supply a large amount of information, typically without accompanying interpretation. Furthermore, they are subject to problems of illegibility. (*Source:* Ohio State University Hospitals.)

9.3.3 Data Processing and Record Keeping

Central to LIS functions are the clerical tasks associated with the testing process. LISs tabulate test requests and prepare specimen-collection lists. Once specimens are received, they are assigned unique accession numbers, which are logged into the system. Computer-generated worklists then help technicians to prepare specimens for analysis at individual workstations. Typically, these worklists also include any special-handling instructions or precautions to be used while the test is being performed. LISs also maintain tracking logs that allow laboratory personnel to determine when and by whom each step of the testing process was performed.

9.3.4 Data Acquisition

Clinical laboratories perform two general categories of tests: (1) tests that measure numeric quantities, such as concentration or counts; and (2) tests that require visualization and interpretation, such as the classification of biopsied tissues or the identification of cultured organisms. In either case, test results must be entered into the LIS and displayed in a format that is meaningful to the health-care professionals caring for patients. The characteristics of the data determine the mechanisms used by the LIS for data acquisition and report generation.

Most chemistry and hematology tests are performed by automated instruments and produce numeric results. An online interface converts voltages measured by the instrument to digital values that can be processed by a computer (analog-to-digital conversion; see Chapter 4). The computer then evaluates the raw digital data to determine the final numeric result (Figure 9.5). Results must be associated with individual specimens; typically, a technician enters into the computer an ordered list of accession numbers and loads the specimens into the instrument in exactly the same order. Thus, there is a one-to-one correspondence between specimen numbers and results.

In the earliest LISs, the central laboratory computer performed all analysis of the raw data. Today, dedicated computers contained in the instruments themselves process raw data, check the consistency of results, associate results with individual specimens, and transmit numeric results in real time via a direct hardware connection to the LIS. The LIS may acquire and integrate information from multiple instruments, store the results online, and produce reports of laboratory-test results (Figure 9.6).

The development of LISs to support microbiology and pathology laboratories has proceeded more slowly than did development of comparable systems for the chemistry and hematology laboratories. Some of the difficulties derive from the nature of the testing process in these departments. First, many of the steps in processing specimens are not automated; technologists must view specimens directly, interpret findings, and summarize their conclusions. Second, the testing process may vary depending on preliminary results—for example, if initial microbiology-culture results identify an infectious organism, additional tests may be performed to determine the organism's sensitivity to different types of antibiotics. Third, a variable, and sometimes long,

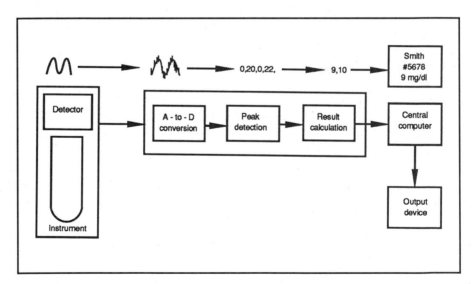

FIGURE 9.5 Automated testing instruments produce a continuous stream of data as each specimen is tested in turn. The computer converts the analog data to digital form, smooths the curve, and detects the peaks associated with individual specimens. The measured values then are interpreted as medically meaningful values (see Figure 9.2), and results are matched with specimens. Initially, the intermediate processing steps were performed by the central LIS computer, but now they are performed within the instruments themselves.

period of time may be required to process a specimen completely; some microbiology cultures are grown for weeks or even months. These characteristics of the testing process make data entry problematic and necessitate a flexible system for report generation.

```
OHIO STATE U HOSP                    CUMULATIVE REPORT            1028 01/24/89   PG  1
CARL SPEICHER MD LAB DIR NS: U9W        ROOM: 0969 2    H#:
                                 DOB: 07/20/1964  SEX: F   R#:
DR:                                   OS                 NAME:

          **************************** H E M A T O L O G Y *************************
   TEST:    RBC     HEMOGLOBN HEMATOCRT     MCV        MCH        MCHC      RDW
   LO-HI: 4.2-5.4    12-16     37-47      82-99      27-31      32-36    11.5-14.5
   UNITS: MIL/CMM    GM/DL       %          FL         PG        GM/DL       %

R01/18/89                 8.2    *   23.4   *
   1140HR
R01/19/89                 6.3    *   18.4   *
   1530HR
R01/20/89                 8.6    *   24.8   *
   0235HR
R01/20/89                 8.8    *   25.1   *
   1040HR
\R01/24/89    3.29   *   10.9   *   31.1   *    94       33.1   *   35.1      17.8
\  0835HR

          ************ E L E C T R O N I C   D I F F E R E N T I A L ***********
   TEST:   WBC
   LO-HI:   5-10
   UNITS: THOU/CMM

\R01/24/89    7.3
\  0835HR

          ***************** R O U T I N E   C H E M I S T R Y ****************
   TEST:           UREA    GLUCOSE    CREAT     SODIUM   POTASSIUM  CHLORIDE
   LO-HI:          5-24    65-115    .7-1.3    136-146    3.7-5.3   101-111
   UNITS:          MG/DL   MG/DL     MG/DL      MM/L       MM/L      MM/L

C01/18/89 R01/18/89    16            1.5   *    135   *    3.6   *    109
  07??HR    1140HR
C01/19/89 R01/19/89    14            1.6   *    139        4.0        111
  07??HR    1530HR
C01/20/89 R01/20/89    16            1.6   *    140        3.3   *    109
  07??HR    1040HR
\C01/24/89 R01/24/89   33   *   86   1.7   *    138        3.3   *    103
\  07??HR    0830HR


   TEST:          CO2 CONT
   LO-HI:          21-31
   UNITS:          MM/L

C01/18/89 R01/18/89    21
  07??HR    1140HR
C01/19/89 R01/19/89    24
  07??HR    1530HR
C01/20/89 R01/20/89    25
  07??HR    1040HR




                                                                          PG  1
```

FIGURE 9.6 This cumulative laboratory report displays the results of the hematology and chemistry tests that have been completed during the patient's hospitalization. (*Source:* Ohio State University Hospitals.)

In addition, the use of nonstandardized nomenclature in free-text reports limits the ability of the computer to perform analyses based on content. This problem was partially resolved in pathology laboratories by the development of standardized coding schemes such as SNOP and SNOMED in the late 1960s (see Chapter 2). (Although microbiology has a more constrained vocabulary than does pathology, its terminology causes similar problems.) The use of coding schemes allowed gross summarization of results by diagnosis and made possible selective retrieval of reports by result. Some LISs have extended coding to include common comments; however, the most frequently used approach is to generate free-text reports using a word processor and to encode the high-level diagnosis (Figure 9.7).

Form 9425
Rev 11/83

SURGICAL PATHOLOGY

THE OHIO STATE UNIVERSITY HOSPITALS

COLUMBUS, OHIO 43210

Path. No.		Name	Hospital #		Service/Nursing Unit
84-00000		Doe, Jane	00000000	07C	MR
Age	**Sex**	**Tissue Submitted**	**Date In**	**Date Out**	**Physician**
80	F	Lesion of back	07-25-84	07-26-84	

Clinical History

T01000-M80903
Lesion of back (Th-1-3-bx)

SURGICAL PATHOLOGY REPORT

GROSS:
The specimen is received in a properly labeled container designated lesion of back and consists of a 25 x 10 mm. ellipse of skin and two additional skin fragments, the largest of which measures 15 mm. in its greatest dimension, the smaller 10 mm. in its greatest dimension. The container is designated short tie at 9:00, long tie at 12:00, additional two fragments from 9:00 margin. There is a piece of suture up to 8 mm. along one edge at one corner of the ellipse and another similar piece of suture measuring less than 3 mm. at an end along one lateral margin. The specimen has a maximum depth of about 8 mm. The central area is somewhat depressed and pearly in appearance. The entire base of the piece of skin is inked and the epithelial surface is inked at the 9:00 margin. Summary of cassettes: A, B, 9-3:00 (9:00 inked); C, 12:00; D, 6:00; E, 9:00 (re-excised margin). Stock. RG/bj

MICROSCOPIC:
The skin shows a reticular pattern of strands of basaloid cells arising from the epidermis at more than one point and extending deep into the dermis associated with a fibrovascular stroma that shows chronic inflammation. Focally the tumor has more solid "nests" of cells, also with associated fibrous stroma. Adjacent dermis shows fibrosis. The surgical margins are free of tumor. This tumor morphologically is consistent with fibroepithelioma of Pinkus which is a variant of basal cell carcinoma. It should be treated as a basal cell carcinoma.

DIAGNOSIS:

SKIN, BACK, FIBROEPITHELIOMA OF PINKUS (SEE MICROSCOPIC)

PATHOLOGIST

FIGURE 9.7 Surgical pathology reports detail pathologists' observations about a specimen and their interpretations of findings. In addition to giving a diagnosis, such a report also may include therapy recommendations. (*Source:* Ohio State University Hospitals.)

9.3.5 Report Generation

Once results have been stored online, the LIS can produce reports in a variety of formats that can help health professionals in interpreting results. Computer-generated laboratory reports typically include the normal ranges and reference values of each test, along with the measured values; in addition, they often flag abnormal values. Summaries of a patient's recent laboratory-test values often are printed in a time-oriented flowsheet. Alternatively, the values could be displayed graphically to facilitate the detection of subtle trends. More sophisticated programs can generate lists of diagnostic possibilities or can perform automatic patient-specific interpretation of tests. For example, Figure 9.8 shows an interpretive report for serum protein electrophoresis[1] that was produced by the clinical laboratory system at the Ohio State University Hospitals.

9.3.6 Quality Control

The purpose of **quality control (QC)** in the clinical laboratories is to monitor the quality of work performed. A primary concern is the correct operation of testing equipment. Chemistry laboratories routinely include aliquots of standard samples in *production-analytic runs*. By comparing the measured and expected results derived from the standard samples, laboratory personnel can determine whether instruments are operating correctly. In addition, statistical analysis of control samples analyzed over time can help to define the accuracy and precision of test results, and can distinguish trends in patient data from problems with instruments or reagents (Figure 9.9).

Another common quality-control check is the *absolute-limit check,* in which someone reviews all test results outside certain limits to verify the accuracy of the value. For example, laboratories may routinely confirm results that are more than two standard deviations away from the mean. *Delta checks* identify instances in which the current result differs significantly from the same patient's previous test result. If the difference exceeds a specified threshold, laboratory technicians will look for an explanation. If they can find no reasonable medical reason for the disparity, they will investigate other possible causes, such as sample mixup, contamination, and reagent errors.

Laboratories are inspected and certified by the Joint Commission for the Accreditation of Health Organizations (JCAHO) and by the College of American Pathologists. In addition, blood banks are certified by the American Association of Blood Banks, and any laboratory that uses radioactive tracers in testing must comply with Nuclear Regulatory Commission regulations. An important criterion for accreditation is documented adherence to strict quality-control protocols. For example, all the equipment

---

[1]Electrophoresis is a technique used to analyze the composition of mixtures in solutions. When a protein mixture is exposed to an electromagnetic field, it separates into its constituent proteins, primarily because the different particles carry different charges, and thus travel at different rates through the medium in which they are dispersed.

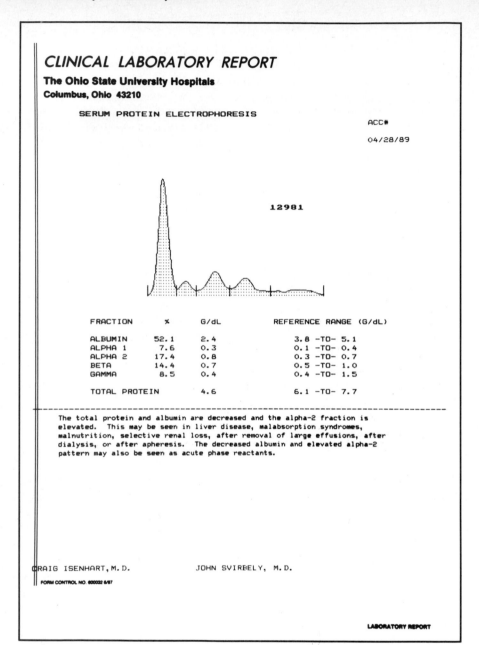

CLINICAL LABORATORY REPORT

The Ohio State University Hospitals
Columbus, Ohio 43210

SERUM PROTEIN ELECTROPHORESIS

ACC#

04/28/89

12981

FRACTION	%	G/dL	REFERENCE RANGE (G/dL)
ALBUMIN	52.1	2.4	3.8 -TO- 5.1
ALPHA 1	7.6	0.3	0.1 -TO- 0.4
ALPHA 2	17.4	0.8	0.3 -TO- 0.7
BETA	14.4	0.7	0.5 -TO- 1.0
GAMMA	8.5	0.4	0.4 -TO- 1.5
TOTAL PROTEIN		4.6	6.1 -TO- 7.7

The total protein and albumin are decreased and the alpha-2 fraction is elevated. This may be seen in liver disease, malabsorption syndromes, malnutrition, selective renal loss, after removal of large effusions, after dialysis, or after apheresis. The decreased albumin and elevated alpha-2 pattern may also be seen as acute phase reactants.

CRAIG ISENHART, M.D.   JOHN SVIRBELY, M.D.

FORM CONTROL NO. 800032 6/97

LABORATORY REPORT

FIGURE 9.8 This interpretive report displays the results of electrophoresis of a patient's serum proteins. The upper plot shows the relative densities of the separated protein fractions; these percentages and the total protein are used to calculate the amount of each fraction. Possible causes for the observed pattern of changes are also presented. (*Source:* Report courtesy of Dr. John Lott, The Ohio State University Hospitals.)

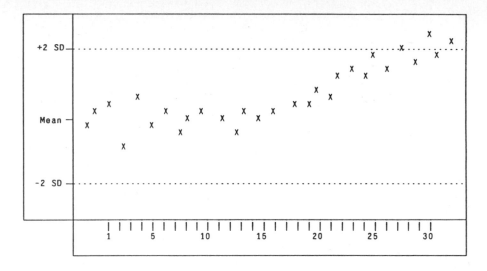

FIGURE 9.9 Laboratories routinely test standard control samples. The results are plotted over time and the plots are examined to detect patterns (dispersion, shift, trends) that indicate problems with the instruments or with the quality of reagents. [SD = standard deviation.] (*Source:* Reprinted with permission from Smith, J. W., Jr. and Svirbely, J. R. Laboratory information systems. *M.D. Computing,* 5(1):38, ©1988, Springer-Verlag New York.)

and most of the utilities (such as water and electricity) in the laboratory must be monitored and periodically maintained. Reagents must be assayed to verify that they have been properly prepared and labeled. Laboratories must maintain detailed records of all specimens that they receive and all tests that they perform. Blood banks must keep records of all blood products transfused and must report all recipients' adverse reactions. LISs can perform many of the record-keeping tasks associated with QC activities.

9.3.7 Managerial Reporting

LISs can perform various data-collection and data-analysis tasks that help laboratory managers to evaluate current laboratory procedures and to suggest changes that will improve the laboratory's efficiency. The LIS can collect and analyze information on test requests, including data such as specimen-receipt time and test-completion time. Reports of the laboratory workload by time help managers to identify periods of peak and slack load—information useful for scheduling personnel and for identifying problems with laboratory workflow, such as excessive turnaround times (Figure 9.10).

An LIS also can produce reports that help laboratory managers to evaluate departmental productivity. A commonly accepted measure of laboratory workload is a standard created by the College of American Pathologists (CAP). On the basis of time–motion studies, CAP determined the average amount of time required to perform

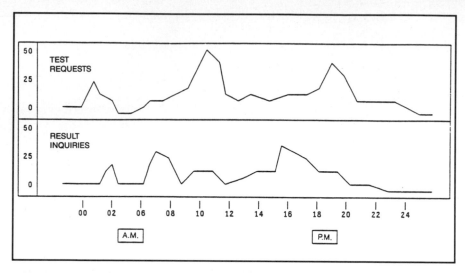

FIGURE 9.10 An analysis of the numbers of test requests and result inquiries during a 24-hour period may expose patterns in the demand for laboratory services. Managers can use this information when making decisions about personnel scheduling. (*Source:* Reprinted with permission from Smith, J. W., Jr. and Svirbely, J. R. Laboratory information systems. *M.D. Computing,* 5(1):38, ©1988, Springer-Verlag New York.)

various test procedures within the laboratory. The labor required to perform each test is expressed in CAP units; each CAP unit represents 1 minute of clerical or technician time. The LIS can determine the total number of CAP units performed at a given workstation by multiplying the number of procedures performed by the procedures' corresponding CAP unit values. The administrator can determine the productivity of the laboratory by comparing the number of personnel hours committed to a project with the number of CAP units of production.

Inventory control, another duty of laboratory managers, poses a significant problem in certain laboratories. It is especially critical in the blood bank, where an LIS can keep records of the current inventory of blood products, the sources, and the expiration dates. Similarly, microbiology and other laboratories often maintain large inventories of frozen organisms or cells. An LIS can greatly simplify the record-keeping tasks associated with inventory management.

9.4 Contemporary Laboratory Information Systems

The clinical laboratories in a growing number of hospitals use some form of computer-based information system. Relatively few, however, have integrated all laboratory divisions under a single LIS. Fewer still have integrated the LIS with the HIS, although the development and implementation of local-area networks (LANs) is changing this situation rapidly. Although some institutions—particularly large hospitals—have chosen to develop custom inhouse systems, most clinical laboratories use vendor-supplied turnkey systems. In 1987, there were at least 40 vendors of commercial LISs [Hatchell and Winsten, 1987]. We shall discuss two vendors' systems to illustrate typical features of such products.

9.4.1 The Citation Systems

In 1987, Citation Computer Systems was one of the largest vendors of LISs, controlling nearly 20 percent of the market. Citation markets a family of LAN-based, menu-driven systems designed to support the fundamental information-management tasks of the clinical laboratories. We shall describe these systems briefly to illustrate the functions of the current generation of commercial LISs.

The basic Citation system supports real-time data acquisition from automated testing instruments; record keeping; and report generation for chemistry, hematology, and urinalysis tests. It automatically generates specimen-collection lists, instrument-loading lists, and other documents used to track specimens and to control workflow. Citation also collects data for and creates a variety of reports used by laboratory administrators and managers, including reports on CAP unit workload statistics, QC, reagent inventory control, billing, costs, and revenues. In addition, Citation provides subsystems to support microbiology laboratories, blood banks, anatomical and surgical pathology services, and business offices.

- *The MicroBiology subsystem* allows users to define tables of specimen types, procedures, organisms, antimicrobial drugs, and susceptibility panels (used in testing the relative sensitivity of isolated organisms to panels of antimicrobials). It uses this information, along with stored patient data, to produce the patient-specific worksheets that guide technologists in performing tests and recording results, and to generate reports of preliminary, interim, and final test results. The system also calculates epidemiology statistics that can help laboratory personnel to identify outbreaks of hospital-acquired infection. For example, for particular organisms of interest, it can monitor the number of positive test cultures by location of patients within the hospital.
- *The Blood Bank subsystem* can support health-care facilities that perform both transfusion and donor functions. It maintains online databases of information about patients, donors, and individual units of blood and blood components. Prior to distribution of blood products for transfusion, the system evaluates patient and unit information and prints out a warning if it detects an incompatibility in blood type or cross-type. The system also assists in controlling inventory, by recording the status and disposition of each unit of blood and by automatically producing lists of critical inventory—those units that are about to reach their expiration dates. Blood-bank personnel can query the system directly to identify units that are available for cross-matching for a specific patient, and, if no compatible units are on hand, to locate appropriate donors.
- *The Surgical and Anatomical Pathology subsystem* helps to streamline workflow in the pathology department and permits the tracking of specimens from receipt through final report. An optional feature of the system is the automatic SNOMED

encoder. The encoder scans the text of pathology reports, identifies pathology words that are associated with SNOMED codes, and produces a list of the codes and their meanings. A pathologist then verifies the appropriateness of the codes and appends them to the tissue report. The SNOMED codes also are used to index the findings within the database of pathology reports.

- *The Business Manager subsystem* can be used by independent laboratories and other laboratories that have a significant business component to manage accounts receivable and to assist in billing insurance companies, private patients, physicians, and clinics. In addition, it produces a variety of financial-management reports, such as reports of revenue by physician, by patient type, and by procedure.

9.4.2 PathNet

The PathNet information system is marketed by Cerner Corporation. Although a relative newcomer to the laboratory marketplace (it was founded in 1979), Cerner has expanded rapidly to become one of the major laboratory-software vendors. The reasons for this performance include the company's use of current communication and networking technologies, and its emphasis on management decision support.

PathNet runs on VAX minicomputers manufactured by the Digital Equipment Corporation. Because of the complexity of the software, the system requires a relatively large CPU to ensure rapid response time. PathNet provides a variety of component subsystems. The wide selection of system options allows individual buyers to choose the configuration of services that best matches the laboratories' operational needs.

- *The Core subsystems* handle essential functions, such as order entry, results inquiry, and maintenance of basic patient data files.
- *The General Laboratory subsystems* support basic laboratory functions, such as printing of labels, generation of specimen-collection lists, assignment of accession numbers, generation of worklists, and entry of test results. These systems are particularly suited for highly automated laboratories, such as hematology and chemistry.
- *The Microbiology and Blood Bank subsystems* support information management for those clinical laboratories performing tests that require complex textual interpretations, that have variable and unpredictable turnaround times, or that frequently need additional testing.
- *The Anatomical Pathology subsystems* support the functions of pathology laboratories that process anatomical tissue. These subsystems share the general features of the Microbiology and Blood Bank subsystems, but also support the laboratories' need to handle more unpredictable terminology, to produce longer reports, and to store archived information for longer periods of time. Software packages are available in three levels of complexity (simple, intermediate, and advanced), which allows a hospital to choose a system that closely matches the complexity of its information requirements.
- *The Management subsystems* assist laboratory managers in the effective control of inventory, personnel, and other essential resources. In addition, managers can

use the Cerner Command Language (CCL) to produce ad hoc reports with which they can monitor laboratory costs and utilization of resources.

- *The Commercial subsystems* handle business-related aspects of laboratory practice, such as billing and maintenance of accounts receivable, market analyses, and evaluation of profitability. Additional subsystems facilitate equipment maintenance and data communications.
- *The Common subsystems*—such as those for report generation, infection control, workload recording, and quality control—provide functions that are shared by multiple PathNet subsystems. These functions improve laboratory responsiveness in the extralaboratory communication cycle, and facilitate the solution of intralaboratory technical and management problems.

9.5 Expert Systems in the Clinical Laboratories

In the previous section, we described commercial LISs that support the operational and managerial activities of a clinical laboratory. Computer-based tools have also been developed to support the professional functions of the physicians and technologists who work in these settings. For example, an essential task of anatomical pathologists is the examination of tissue specimens to diagnose the type and extent of the diseases present. Likewise, blood banks and other specialized laboratories need to provide both test results and interpretations of the significance of those results. In this section, we shall describe two systems designed to support data interpretation and diagnosis in the clinical laboratories. Chapter 15 is devoted to a more complete discussion of computer-based decision-support systems.

9.5.1 Pathfinder/Intellipath

During the mid-1980s, researchers at the Stanford University School of Medicine and the University of Southern California School of Medicine developed an expert system called Pathfinder, which was designed to assist surgical pathologists in interpreting the findings noted on microscopic examination of lymph-node tissue [Heckerman et al., 1989]. The Pathfinder project explored automated approaches to hypothetico-deductive reasoning (Chapter 2), using probability theory to assess belief in the likelihood of alternative diagnoses and decision theory to guide the questioning process. Intellipath, a commercial spinoff of the Pathfinder project, is one of the first computer systems designed to assist primarily with the clinical, rather than with the clerical and administrative, functions of the laboratory. It integrates an expert reasoning system for pathology diagnosis with a videodisc library of histological slides. The result is a powerful educational tool that can assist pathologists in learning and teaching about pathology diagnosis. Development of the lymph-node pathology knowledge base and videodisc library has been completed; by 1989, the system was being used in over 100 pathology practices in North America. In addition, experts in different pathology subspecialties are cooperating to build knowledge-base modules for other tissue areas. Eventually, Intellipath's developers intend to provide modules that support diagnosis of pathology in tissue sections from all 40 organ systems of the human body.

Intellipath has the ability to form a differential diagnosis of plausible diseases based on the histological features that have been entered into the system. It uses the subjective probabilities of experts to infer the probability that each disease is responsible for the evidence that has been reported (see Chapters 3 and 15), and orders the diseases by the relative likelihood that each is present. As the pathologist enters new findings, the differential is updated to reflect the new information. At any point in a diagnostic session, the user can ask the system to indicate the features that will best help to distinguish among diagnoses.

Pathologists can recall images from the slide library to view cases that illustrate diseases and histological features. The system also provides definitions of diseases and features, explanations of the relevance of laboratory tests, and important references from the medical literature. In addition, Intellipath can automatically generate pathology reports that include histologic findings, diagnosis, SNOP code, and relevant references; it also provides a database system for archiving and retrieving case reports.

9.5.2 RED

As we have described in previous sections, many LISs support inventory control, donor recruitment, and other clerical tasks in blood banks. Researchers have paid little attention, however, to applying computer processing to the problem-solving tasks of technologists. One of the primary concerns of the blood bank is to identify red-cell antibodies in the serum of prospective transfusion recipients, so as to prevent transfusions that could result in adverse reactions; these transfusion reactions range from fever and anemia to acute renal failure. Over 300 red-cell antigens, in addition to the ABO antigens, have been identified. Prior knowledge of the identity of the antibodies permits the selection of blood units in which the red cells lack the corresponding antigens.

Investigators in the Ohio State University Pathology Department have been developing an expert system, RED, that helps technologists in the blood bank to interpret the information derived from antibody-identification tests [Smith et al., 1985]. Interpretation of the data is complicated, especially when multiple antibodies are present. In many respects, the problem-solving approach is similar to the hypothetico-deductive approach used by physicians in making diagnoses (see Chapter 2). RED uses knowledge gained from expert technologists to classify antibodies in four categories: present, likely present, possibly present, and absent. Eventually, this module may be incorporated into a more comprehensive system that determines ABO blood groups, interprets the results of screening tests for red-cell antibodies, chooses potentially compatible units of red cells based on information about transfusion recipients and inventoried units, and evaluates the results of cross-match testing.

9.6 The Future of Laboratory Information Systems

A significant proportion of health-care expenditures is spent for laboratory testing. Thus, attempts to contain costs have had a profound effect on the practice of laboratory medicine. Whereas in the past laboratories generated revenue for hospitals and passed on increased costs to patients, current reimbursement schemes have produced a situation in which less money is available for the laboratory, despite rising costs and increasing demand. Undoubtedly, continuation of these economic pressures will shape the scope of future computer-based LISs. There are at least three ways in which LISs can help to reduce costs, while still maintaining the quality of services.

First, labor costs represent a significant proportion of the laboratory budget. LISs have proved to be cost-effective in performing many of the clerical functions associated with the clinical laboratories and thereby increasing the productivity of laboratory workers. We can expect that more hospitals will implement LISs to provide these functions, and that LIS vendors will continue to enhance their products with administrative and managerial functions that will further streamline the testing process.

Recently, hospital laboratories have begun to experiment with alternative marketing arrangements; for example, many larger laboratories have started to perform outside work to keep expensive instruments busy during nights and other traditionally slack times. Some smaller hospitals have contracted their laboratory operations and now send out all nonemergency laboratory work. Other laboratories are experimenting with joint ventures with laboratories at competing hospitals, or with reference laboratories. Arrangements such as these will stimulate an even greater need for information systems to perform record-keeping functions and for communications networks that facilitate rapid and accurate transmission of information.

Second, computer-based information management can reduce laboratory-test costs by minimizing the number of tests performed. More extensive networking of LISs, regional databanks, and long-term storage can decrease the number of duplicate tests by making results available to all who need them; for example, hospitals will have access to preadmission tests performed by community physicians, and community physicians will be able to review the results of tests performed during hospitalizations.

Third, LISs can contribute to the decentralization of the clinical laboratories, thereby reducing transportation time and costs. In the past, laboratories were centralized because large automated analyzers were expensive and required highly trained operators. Newer instruments can perform measurements on smaller samples, at lower cost. These instruments employ built-in microcomputers that control operation and provide digital outputs of fully processed data for direct display or for transmission to other computers.

The availability of instruments such as these will encourage the geographical dispersion of laboratory testing, especially where there is a high demand for testing and a need for rapid turnaround. Another development that will contribute to distribution of chemical analyses is the availability of implantable biosensors (such as an automatic infusion pump; see Chapter 12). These instruments will provide continuous real-time biochemical information about patients, thus eliminating the need to collect specimens and to wait for test results. As more data become available and data collection becomes more widely distributed, there will be greater need for LISs to collect, store, and manage the information so that it is accessible to those who need it.

In addition to improving the cost-effectiveness of laboratories, future LISs will be capable of assisting physicians in both the ordering and interpretation of laboratory tests. The volume of laboratory testing exceeds the capacity of humans to assimilate the information provided, especially in areas such as the intensive-care units, where patients are monitored closely. Furthermore, the knowledge required to interpret the information effectively is substantial and is increasing rapidly. A computer-based system could reduce the risk of clinicians ordering tests inappropriately and of their misinterpreting laboratory data when caring for patients.

Typically, laboratory-test results are displayed with their normal ranges and reference values; abnormal results are highlighted to attract attention. As LISs become integrated into HISs, and therefore have access to nonlaboratory data, they will be able to provide more direct interpretive assistance. For example, an LIS might analyze patients' past test results to provide patient-specific normal values for each test. Or the system might help health professionals to interpret patients' patterns of laboratory values, perhaps in combination with relevant clinical information. Automated surveillance, such as that performed by the HELP (Chapter 7) and RMRS (Chapter 6) systems, can aid the laboratory-testing process by reminding health professionals to take appropriate action when certain clinical situations occur, or by recommending additional studies.

Decision-support systems have been developed to provide more sophisticated assistance for physicians in test ordering and interpretation. Investigators have tried a variety of problem-solving strategies, including the use of Bayes' theorem, decision-analytic techniques, and sequential branching algorithms (see Chapter 3). During the 1980s, researchers began to explore artificial-intelligence approaches to laboratory-support systems. The EXPERT language has been used to construct decision-support systems for serum-protein analysis and for interpretation of various enzyme tests [Weiss et al., 1981; Smith, 1984]. These interpretation modules are commercially available as part of a serum-protein electrophoresis instrument produced by Helena Laboratories. In the future, we expect that knowledge-based decision-support systems will be increasingly incorporated into LISs.

The LIS of the future will be a distributed computer network in which microcomputers in instruments communicate with more powerful processors that collate data, generate reports, perform data correlation, and execute medical interpretive functions. As an integral part of a broader-based HIS, the expanded LIS will share laboratory data with computer systems performing other patient-care applications, and will collect data from a variety of sources to perform detailed interpretive functions.

Suggested Readings

Aller, R. D. and Elevitch, F. R. Symposium on computers in the clinical laboratory. *Clinics in Laboratory Medicine,* 3(1):1, 1983.

> *This collection of papers discusses a variety of issues related to the use of computers in the laboratory, including justifications for acquiring a computer-based information system and applications of LISs in laboratory management.*

Benson, E. S. and Rubin, M. *Logic and Economics of Clinical Laboratory Use.* New York: Elsevier, 1978.

> *This conference proceedings contains papers that address issues of laboratory economics, test selection for decision analysis, data interpretation, and resource utilization.*

Bronzino, J. D. *Computer Applications for Patient Care.* Menlo Park, CA: Addison-Wesley, 1982.

> *This book discusses a variety of medical applications for computers, including patient monitoring, medical imaging, and ECG interpretation. It contains one chapter on the use of computers in the clinical laboratory, which describes the functions of the hematology and clinical chemistry laboratories, explains the pattern of information flow in the laboratory, and identifies instrument- and management-level issues in the use of computers.*

Elevitch, F. R. and Aller, R. D. *The ABCs of LIS: Computerizing Your Laboratory Information System.* Chicago: American Society of Clinical Pathologists Press, 1986.

> *This book is an excellent source for people who have the responsibility for selecting an LIS for a hospital laboratory.*

Gates, S. C. and Becker, J. *Laboratory Automation Using the IBM PC.* Englewood Cliffs, NJ: Prentice-Hall, 1989.

> *This "how to" book demonstrates hardware and software aspects of laboratory automation by teaching the reader how to attach a scientific instrument to a personal computer, how to control the instrument, and how to collect and analyze data. It includes discussions of analog-to-digital and digital-to-analog converters, noise-reduction techniques, and techniques for data analysis. A floppy disk containing all the computer programs listed in the book also is provided.*

Henry, J. B. *Clinical Diagnosis and Management by Laboratory Methods,* 17th ed. Philadelphia: W. B. Saunders, 1984.

> *This book is one of the standard textbooks on laboratory medicine; it is recommended for people who are unfamiliar with laboratory practice. In addition to an explanation of laboratory information processing, it describes each major laboratory division, and discusses laboratory management and quality assurance.*

Lundberg, G. D. *Using the Clinical Laboratory in Medical Decision-Making.* Chicago: American Society of Clinical Pathologists, 1983.

> *Through examples of selected clinical situations, this book shows how the laboratory can assist clinicians in their problem-solving strategies. Flow diagrams of decision-making processes are of particular interest.*

Spackman, K. A. and Connelly, D. P. Knowledge-based systems in laboratory medicine and pathology. *Archives of Pathology and Laboratory Medicine,* 111:116, 1987.

> *The authors introduce the fundamental concepts of knowledge-based systems and review applications and research in the domains of laboratory medicine and pathology.*

Speicher, C. D. and Smith, J. W., Jr. *Choosing Effective Laboratory Tests.* Philadelphia: W. B. Saunders, 1983.
> *This book addresses the efficient use of laboratory resources. The first part of the book
> describes the application of artificial-intelligence and cognitive-science approaches to
> medical problem solving. These approaches are then applied to selected clinical problems
> and to laboratory-test findings to illustrate their practical uses.*

Questions for Discussion

1. The microbiology laboratory notifies you that a specimen cannot be accessioned
   into its standalone computer. The problem is that the patient's hospital identification number, which is supposed to be unique to that patient, has apparently been
   assigned to another patient. You note the following facts: (1) the patient whose
   specimen has been received is on the obstetric ward, and (2) the first name and
   age of the patient whose specimen has been received are the same as those of
   the other patient with the same number. What are some possible explanations for
   this situation? What would you need to do to verify whether your hypotheses are
   correct? How could communication between the central HIS and the LIS help
   to minimize such problems?
2. You would like to place terminals in the intensive-care units of your hospital to
   increase the speed of reporting results. You are concerned about people using these
   terminals to gain improper access to data in the system, particularly to the records
   of prominent persons. How would you secure your system?
3. As reflected in the daily delta-check report, a patient shows a change in an enzyme activity value from 50 units to 560 units over a 24-hour period. This level
   of activity is seen only in serious diseases, but your review of the patient's chart
   indicates that this man has been admitted for minor eye surgery and is in excellent
   physical health. What would you do to find the cause of the discrepancy? Why
   would you need to find it? How would your problem-solving approach differ if
   you knew that enzyme results were entered manually into the LIS, rather than
   via a direct instrument–computer interface?
4. You use your LIS computer to monitor patterns of test ordering and test-result
   inquiry; the results are shown in Figure 9.10. You know that (1) doctors round
   on (visit) their patients from 8 to 10 A.M., and from 4 to 6 P.M; (2) nurses work
   on shifts from 7 A.M. to 3 P.M., from 3 P.M. to 11 P.M., and from 11 P.M. to 7 A.M.;
   and (3) the bars in town close at 2 A.M. What are your explanations for the times
   of heavy usage? How would this information help you to schedule personnel for
   the laboratory?
5. Your hematology laboratory does a test profile (a series of tests) to detect a red-
   blood-cell disorder. The tests included are total iron determination, a white-blood-
   cell count, and plasma folate level; the unit values (where 1 unit is the amount
   of work an ideal technologist can perform in 1 minute) are 16, 8, and 24 respectively. Twenty of these profiles are done per day by one technologist working Mon-
   day through Friday. Calculate the workload per year for this test profile and the

productivity (workload divided by the number of hours worked) of the technologists, assuming that the technologist works a 40-hour week, 50 weeks per year. Based on your result and the definition of the unit value, what staffing recommendation would you make?

6. The blood bank has just been notified that there is a person in the emergency room who is bleeding massively from a ruptured aorta. In addition, there is an ambulance coming with two persons who have been involved in a major automobile accident. Most of the currently available blood is in a peripheral-storage refrigerator for use in the two open-heart surgeries now in progress. The local Red Cross has no blood reserves, but its personnel will start checking with other hospitals in the state for available blood. Would a computer-based inventory system be of use in such a situation? What information would the system need to provide? (Do not forget that whole blood has a short shelf-life and must be transfused within 30 days of collection.)

7. The chief of the medical staff asks for a monthly log of the laboratory use for each physician admitting to the hospital. After meeting with her, you realize that she would like to be able to see not only which physicians are ordering the most laboratory tests, but also how the physicians compare in ordering tests when confronted with patients with the same diagnosis. What information would you want to include in such a report? How could you use an interface between the LIS and the HIS? Could workload recording in conjunction with these data be used to control testing costs?

10

Pharmacy Systems

Stuart M. Speedie and Alan B. McKay

After reading this chapter, you should know the answers to these questions:

- What are the eight steps of the drug-use control process?
- What are the four major areas of pharmacy practice? What are the primary functions of each area?
- What roles have computer systems played in the evolution of pharmacy practice from a product- to a patient-oriented profession?
- What characteristics of pharmacy information make many pharmacy tasks particularly well suited for implementation in computer-based systems?
- How do clinical pharmacists use computers to design patient-specific drug regimens?
- What resources do pharmacists use to collect and disseminate information about drugs and drug effects?

10.1 Overview of Pharmacy Practice

Pharmacy systems manage medical information related to drugs and to the use of drugs in patient care. Due to the nature of the tasks performed and of the information requirements, the pharmacy was one of the earliest patient-care services to benefit from the development of medical information science and from the introduction of computers into health-care settings. Today, computer-based information systems are an integral part of the practice of pharmacy, both in hospitals and in the community. In this chapter, we shall review the background of pharmacy services, discuss how pharmacy functions lend themselves to the application of principles from medical computer science, and explore possible future developments in computer-based pharmacy information systems.

Pharmacy for many years was viewed as a product-oriented profession concerned with the collection, extraction, and preparation of medicinal agents to create the finished dosage forms suitable for human consumption. Assumption of these drug-preparation functions by drug manufacturers gradually has shifted the role of the pharmacist; modern pharmacy practice comprises a predominantly patient-oriented, distributive set of functions that is characterized collectively as drug-use control. **Drug-use control** has been defined as "the sum total of knowledge, understanding, judgments, procedures, skills, controls, and ethics that assures optimal safety and efficacy in the distribution and use of medication" [Brodie, 1966, p. 39].

Ideally, control of the use of drugs implies surveillance from the moment the substance enters the health-care system until the time that that substance is eliminated from the body or is destroyed. The steps of the drug-use process are as follows (see also Figure 10.1):

1. *Diagnose:* Identify the patient's problem
2. *Determine drug history:* Ascertain the patient's history of drug prescriptions, drug allergies, and prior adverse reactions
3. *Prescribe:* Determine a drug therapy that treats the patient's problem effectively and that is not contraindicated by the patient's drug-prescription history
4. *Select product:* Choose a specific drug product that satisfies the prescription
5. *Dispense:* Distribute the drug
6. *Counsel:* Educate and counsel the patient concerning the drug's proper use, risks, and potential side effects
7. *Administer:* Administer the drug to the patient
8. *Monitor:* Observe the patient receiving drug therapy for evidence of drug effectiveness and for signs of adverse reaction

In addition, pharmacy personnel provide advice and instruction to other health professionals regarding drug-related therapy. The basis for this advice is the science of **pharmacology**—the study of the properties, uses, and actions of drugs. Notice that pharmacists, physicians, nurses, other health-care staff, and patients cooperate to complete the steps of the drug-use process and to ensure that drug therapies are beneficial, rather than detrimental, to the patients' health. The practice of pharmacy encompasses a large number of health-care–related functions performed in a variety of settings. The four major areas of pharmacy service are (1) inpatient pharmacy

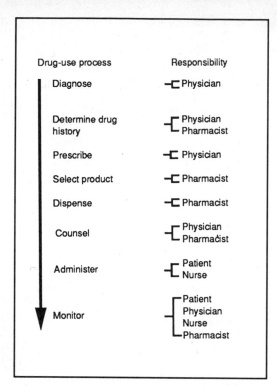

FIGURE 10.1 Once the physician forms an initial diagnosis, pharmacists, nurses, and patients participate in the remaining steps of the drug-use process, from the selection of appropriate drug therapies to the administration of drugs and the monitoring of patients.

services, (2) community (outpatient) pharmacy services, (3) clinical pharmacy services, and (4) drug-information services.

10.1.1 Inpatient Pharmacy Services

Most physicians' first encounter with pharmacy services occurs in a hospital. The inpatient or hospital pharmacy service has the fundamental task of providing (dispensing) drug products in response to physicians' orders for drug therapy. This dispensing role can be summarized as "getting the right drug to the right patient at the right time." On receiving an order, the pharmacist verifies it for accuracy and evaluates it in the context of what is known about the patient's current drug therapy. A significant component of this activity involves examining the patient's medication history and clinical data to identify potential drug–drug and drug–food interactions, allergies, and other drug sensitivities that may adversely affect the patient. When pharmacists detect problems, they consult with the patient's physicians to determine the most appropriate course of action. Once a prescription has been approved, a drug that meets the patient's treatment requirements without conflicting with the patient's other needs is retrieved from the pharmacy's inventory (in the case of capsules, tablets, and so on) or is formulated (in the case of intravenous solutions). The order as dispensed is recorded in the patient's **medication profile,** and the drug is delivered to the nursing station for administration to the patient.

There are two distinct approaches to the drug-distribution function. In the older approach, still used in many hospitals, the pharmacy dispenses multiple doses of a drug for a particular patient. The drug is delivered in a labeled container to the nursing station to be used for the patient's entire course of therapy. This traditional approach minimizes record keeping by the pharmacy, but has several potential problems, including waste of drugs, inappropriate administration of therapy, and illegal diversion of drugs.

With **unit-dose dispensing,** each drug is packaged, labeled, and distributed to nursing stations in its unit of use—a single pill or injection. The pharmacy distributes to each nursing station a cart that contains the medications for the current administration period, typically a single day (Figure 10.2). This approach significantly decreases the amount of wasted drugs and provides better control over the patient's drug therapy because orders can be discontinued instantly. On the other hand, record keeping within the pharmacy is increased; the patient's medication profile must be recalled and updated each time that a new unit of a drug is dispensed. With a computer-based system to maintain the medication-administration records and to print the labels, however, the additional burden is slight and is more than offset by the benefits.

In support of and related to the dispensing function, the inpatient pharmacy performs a number of other tasks. These responsibilities include acquisition of drug products, provision of information for billing, and maintenance of certain legally required

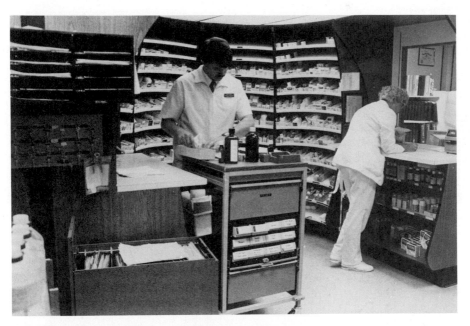

FIGURE 10.2 In pharmacies that use the unit-dose method of drug dispensing, pharmacists package and label individual doses of drugs and deliver them to nursing stations in carts that contain medications for the current drug-administration period. (*Source:* Photograph courtesy of Ken Heinen ©1989.)

records, such as those related to dispensing and administering narcotics. The hospital pharmacy, in conjunction with the pharmacy and therapeutics committee, also compiles and manages the use of the **drug formulary**, a document that specifies which drugs are to be kept in the pharmacy's inventory, and that details any restrictions on the use of these drugs.

Finally, the hospital pharmacy may provide a variety of special services to physicians and patients. For example, it often collects and evaluates published information about drugs, and disseminates this information through educational programs or on request. The hospital pharmacy also may perform more complex tasks related to drug therapy, such as calculation of optimum drug doses for specific patients and consultation with patients' physicians regarding therapeutic decisions.

10.1.2 Community (Outpatient) Pharmacy Services

The community pharmacy has essentially the same functions as does the inpatient pharmacy, but must perform its tasks in a more open and complex environment in which it has much less control over the drug-use process (Figure 10.3). Unlike hospitalized patients, patients in the community choose which pharmacy to patronize. Multiple physicians may be treating a patient for different medical conditions; each may be ignorant of the drug therapies prescribed by the others. Furthermore, out-

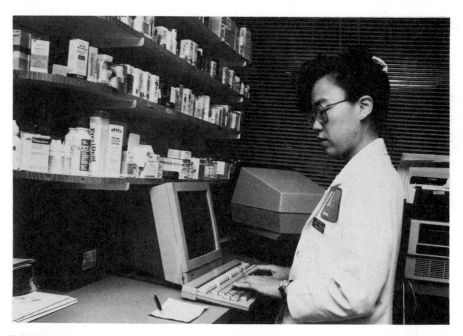

FIGURE 10.3 Like hospital pharmacists, community pharmacists dispense drugs on the orders of physicians. In addition, they evaluate drug therapies with respect to drug interactions and contraindications, and they educate and counsel clientele about potential drug side effects and interactions.

patients often are taking chronic (long-term) medication. In the inpatient setting, the number of patients is limited to the number of beds (fewer than 500 beds in about 95 percent of hospitals); in contrast, a typical community pharmacy provides drug therapy to 3000 to 5000 clients at any one time.

The primary responsibility of community pharmacies, like that of hospital pharmacies, is the dispensing of drugs on the orders of physicians. In performing this task, the pharmacist conducts professional evaluations of drug therapies with respect to drug interactions and contraindications. Most community pharmacies now maintain medication profiles for their patrons. In addition, community pharmacists educate and counsel clientele. They are among the most accessible of health professionals, and they enjoy a high degree of public trust. This puts them in an ideal position to teach consumers about potential drug side effects and interactions. Furthermore, they often are asked about general health concerns, and thus serve as an entry point into the health-care system.

A community pharmacy also faces a significantly greater number of tasks associated with the financial aspects of a business than does a hospital pharmacy. These include ordering products, managing inventory, billing medical-insurance companies, maintaining client charge accounts, tracking product sales, and preparing financial summaries.

10.1.3 Clinical Pharmacy Services

Clinical pharmacy is a relatively new area of pharmacy practice. It focuses more on assessing patients' drug therapies than on the traditional dispensing roles. Clinical pharmacists work closely with physicians to determine the optimal drug therapies for patients, and often assist in monitoring the effects of such therapies. In carrying out this task, they not only provide physicians with information about drug effects, contraindications, and appropriate dosing regimens, but also evaluate patients' medical histories and review laboratory-test results and other clinical data to detect and prevent therapeutic problems. In some settings, such as nursing homes, clinical pharmacists provide legally mandated reviews of patients' drug therapies.

10.1.4 Drug-Information Services

The evaluation and dissemination of comprehensive drug information to the institution's staff and patients has been identified as an important aspect of pharmaceutical services [Brown and Smith, 1986]. The mechanism often used to accomplish this task is the drug-information service.

The basic function of pharmacy personnel working in the drug-information service is to answer drug-related questions posed by the hospital staff (primarily physicians and nurses). In addition, pharmacists participate in the activities of the pharmacy and therapeutics committees by evaluating new drugs, developing drug-use policies, and maintaining drug formularies. They disseminate drug and poison information by publishing drug newsletters and developing drug-related educational programs for staff and patients. In support of these educational activities, pharmacists conduct drug-utilization reviews to determine areas of educational need; for example, they identify drugs that are being used inappropriately and implement programs to increase health professionals' understanding of these drugs.

10.2 Historical Perspective—The Evolution of Pharmacy and Drug-Information Systems

Computer systems were first introduced to hospital pharmacies in the mid-1960s as an extension of the record-keeping functions of larger hospital computer systems. Their initial tasks were to monitor the flow of drug products into the pharmacy and to permit accurate and timely patient billing. Other traditional pharmacy functions were added gradually. By 1975, approximately 7 percent of all hospitals had some form of computer service in the pharmacy. The proportion increased gradually to about 9 percent by the end of the 1970s [Gouveia et al., 1986]. A smaller number of pharmacies also began to use computers for isolated patient-care activities, such as calculating drug regimens, screening for drug allergies and previous adverse reactions, and identifying duplicate drug orders.

With the increasing availability of powerful mini- and microcomputers in the late 1970s and early 1980s, smaller hospitals began to install their own computer systems, which functioned as standalone systems or were linked electronically to a central hospital computer (see Chapter 7). The major improvements in communications capabilities brought about by local-area networks (LANs) provided the means for pharmacy computer systems to share information and to communicate electronically with other hospital computer systems. The same trends caused a similar movement within the pharmacy away from the use of single computers toward multiple, networked microcomputers sharing a common database. By 1987, over 50 percent of hospitals had implemented some form of computer system [Stolar, 1988]. Roughly 75 percent of hospitals with automated pharmacies used commercially available software; the other 25 percent developed their own inhouse systems [Packer, 1986].

Use of computers in community pharmacies lagged behind that in hospital pharmacies because of the high initial and maintenance costs and the need for links to larger mainframe systems. Most of the community pharmacy systems introduced in the early 1970s were *online systems*; pharmacies purchased processing time or services from private computer vendors or computer service bureaus and accessed the systems via telephone lines. Often, the only functions provided by such systems were the preparation of prescription labels and the automatic calculation of prices.

Although early estimates of computer use are sketchy, probably no more than 7 percent of all community pharmacies were using computer technology directly (either online or standalone), and a total of roughly 18 percent were using some form of computer-based service (for example, computer billing or insurance-claim submission). In the late 1970s, declining hardware costs, expanding computer communication networks, and improved pharmacy-system software prompted large numbers of pharmacies to acquire computer systems. By 1987, approximately 80 to 90 percent of community pharmacies used some form of computer service or planned to acquire a system within the next 2 years [Banaham, 1987; Burton et al., 1986].

Today, pharmacy systems are among the most widely used computer systems in medical care. Because they provide a range of business, operational, and clinical functions that greatly improve the efficiency and cost-effectiveness of pharmacy practice, they have become a fundamental tool for the practice of pharmacy in many hospital and community pharmacies.

10.3 Fundamental Concepts for Pharmacy Systems

Pharmacies, like all health-care–related practices, face a growing need to manage large amounts of medical information. Likewise, they confront contradictory pressures to provide high-quality service at low cost. The implementation of computer-based solutions to information-management problems has been a significant boon to the practice of pharmacy in all four pharmacy settings.

First, maintenance of complete, accurate, and up-to-date records concerning all aspects of drug therapy is requisite for high-quality patient care. Furthermore, these records must exist in forms suitable for a number of purposes, from professional evaluations to ensure optimal drug therapy to routine billing. The maintenance of such records is a major burden for all types of pharmacy services. The use of a computer system to maintain pharmacy records has all the advantages of computer-based medical-record systems over paper record systems (see Chapter 6), including greater accuracy and more timely access to information, as well as the ability to organize and display information in a variety of formats, to aid directly in evaluating drug orders and monitoring patients, and to submit claims to insurance companies.

Second, cost-control strategies in the pharmacy focus on maximizing the efficiency of pharmacy personnel and on controlling tightly the acquisition, storage, and distribution of drugs. Pharmacy information systems can help staff to achieve these goals. They relieve pharmacy workers of many time-consuming clerical and record-keeping tasks, thus increasing worker productivity. They also can support departmental decision making by helping managers to collect and analyze pharmacy costs, worker-productivity measures, and drug-utilization information.

Drug-information services is the third area in which computers provide significant benefits to pharmacy practice. The dramatic increase in the amount of information available concerning drugs and their effects requires that personnel in drug-information services regularly consult and review a wide variety of references. To acquire and disseminate such information efficiently, the service must have a method for quickly searching and reviewing the drug-related literature.

10.3.1 Functions of a Pharmacy Information System

Evaluations of existing hospital pharmacy computer systems clearly show that the use of computers is an effective means of controlling the drug-use process in the hospital. Pharmacy computers increase the accuracy and efficiency of drug distribution and perform routine medication monitoring and screening for drug interactions.

The following are examples of drug-use control and distribution functions that are aided by computer systems:

- *Online order entry.* In the most advanced pharmacy systems, health-care personnel enter physicians' orders for drug therapy directly via terminals located on the hospital wards. These orders are transmitted instantly to the pharmacy for processing and dispensing. The entire process of creating, transferring, and reading paper orders is thus eliminated. In less advanced systems, paper orders are generated and delivered to the pharmacy, where pharmacy personnel enter them into the stand-alone system.

- *Pharmacist review.* After an order has been entered into the system, it is held for professional review by a pharmacist. Pharmacists may consult patients' medication profiles to detect potential problems (such as duplicate orders or drug interactions), or the computer may screen automatically for such problems by reviewing the information contained in its databases. In the latter case, the system may present warning messages to pharmacists via terminals when appropriate. Pharmacists then use their professional judgment to determine the best action to take.

- *Medication-profile update.* Once an order has been approved, the system automatically updates the patient's medication profile to reflect the new order. Thus, the database always contains the latest information about the patient's drug therapies, as known to the pharmacy.

- *Printed labels.* Medication-profile information can be used to print labels with the patient's identification and location, and with instructions for administration. Automatic generation of labels is a practical necessity for unit-dose distribution systems because of the frequency of dispensing.

- *Drug-dispensing reports.* Most pharmacy computer systems automatically generate dispensing reports that instruct technicians to assemble drug orders for distribution to nursing stations. Computer-generated dispensing reports are particularly useful in hospitals that use the unit-dose approach to distribution, because the reports are easily updated to reflect last-minute changes.

- *Medication-administration reports.* The medication-profile database permits timely generation of custom-tailored medication-administration recording forms for use by nursing personnel. These forms provide detailed instructions about which medications are to be administered to which patients at what times; thus, they significantly improve control over the drug-use process.

- *Inventory maintenance and automatic drug reorder.* Inventory figures can be adjusted continually to reflect the quantities of drugs dispensed from the pharmacy. The availability of up-to-date inventory information facilitates automatic reordering of drugs and allows pharmacy managers to analyze drug utilization by item and by company.

- *Drug-use review reports.* The medication-profile database can be used to identify and track problems related to suboptimal drug therapy. Such problems include the prescription of excessive or subtherapeutic doses, the administration of therapies for too long or too short a period, the use of expensive drugs when less costly ones are available, and the failure to monitor the patient adequately during the course of therapy. Once problems have been identified, pharmacists can design and implement educational programs aimed at physicians, nurses, and other pharmacists.

- *Controlled-drug reports.* Information from the medication-profile and drug-inventory databases is used to generate product- and patient-specific reports concerning the utilization of federally controlled drugs, such as opiates and other narcotics. These reports facilitate accurate control and accountability, which are mandated by law.

Almost all modern hospital pharmacy information systems perform at least this set of basic functions. In addition, many systems provide features to support business and managerial functions. For example, they may generate bills for patients or third-party payers and maintain the pharmacy payroll. Pharmacy information systems also can collect statistics on pharmacy productivity, sales volume, prescription activity, and drug usage—information that managers need to run the pharmacy efficiently. Some systems also include software to support clinical pharmacy functions, such as drug-dose calculation and patient-specific therapy monitoring. We shall describe these clinical functions in Section 10.3.2.

In most respects, the functions of community pharmacy systems in distributing drugs, evaluating drug therapies, and managing the pharmacy parallel the functions of hospital systems. They are differentiated by the nature of community pharmacy practice, which requires systems that can handle larger numbers of patients, but with much lower frequencies of transactions per patient and much less available patient information. In addition, systems that support community practices must perform a larger number of fiscal functions, including billing third-party payers and maintaining charge accounts.

Community pharmacists view the computer as a means of freeing themselves from time-consuming clerical drug-distribution activities by taking advantage of computer-generated labels, prescription numbers, and patient receipts, as well as of rapid retrieval of prescription-pricing and inventory data. Activities that formerly occupied a large proportion of the pharmacist's work routine now can be performed rapidly and efficiently by a computer. Many systems allow pharmacies to update their drug-pricing and drug–drug interaction databases via a telephone line connection to a centrally maintained database. Newer systems facilitate direct submission of claims to Medicaid and other insurance agencies using a similar mechanism. Some systems even provide computer interfaces to automated drug-dispensing cells, thus eliminating the need for pharmacists to count and package pills manually.

10.3.2 Drug-Related Decision Support

The newest developments in pharmacy information systems are applications that assist physicians and pharmacists directly in the drug-use process. Pharmacy systems play an important role in the provision of safe and effective therapy by maintaining accessible, legible, and up-to-date medication records. Some systems have been implemented that can evaluate computer-stored records to screen automatically for drug–drug interactions. More sophisticated systems can verify that appropriate monitoring tests are being ordered and can detect clinically significant changes in laboratory-test results that may be related to drug use. In addition, computers now are used to custom-tailor drug regimens for patients receiving powerful drugs with a narrow therapeutic range (a small margin between the minimum effective dose and the maximum nontoxic dose; see Figure 10.4) and to choose the ingredients of intravenous solutions for patients receiving all their fluids and nutrients intravenously.

Prior to the 1970s, physicians performed most clinical drug dosing by prescribing standard doses of drugs and adjusting dosing regimens intuitively based on patients' clinical responses. Such empirically derived dosing guidelines were designed to provide safe and effective therapy for most patients in a population. Dosing guidelines worked well for most drugs, but the effects of some drugs were extremely sensitive to interpatient variability; the use of standard doses produced unacceptably high rates of drug-related morbidity and mortality. The introduction of laboratory techniques for determining drug-concentration levels in the blood and the development

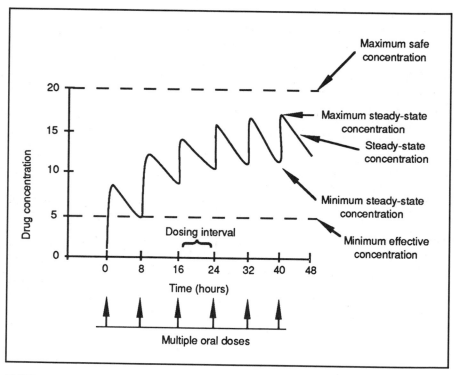

FIGURE 10.4 Drug-concentration levels in the blood rise as orally administered drugs are absorbed into the body, and fall as the drug spreads to other body tissues, then is biotransformed and eliminated from the body. In drugs with a narrow therapeutic range (drugs with only a small margin between the minimum effective level and the maximum safe level), dosing intervals and amounts must be calculated carefully to ensure that drug levels stay within that range. Too low a level is subtherapeutic; too high a level can cause side effects and, in some cases, death. (*Source:* Reproduced by permission from *Bedside Clinical Pharmacokinetics, Revised Edition,* by Carl Peck, published by Applied Therapeutics, Inc., Vancouver, Washington, ©1989.)

of **pharmacokinetic models** for interpreting the clinical significance of these levels allowed researchers to devise a new approach to dosing based on measured drug concentrations [Peck, 1989].

Researchers have developed pharmacokinetic models that represent the drug levels over time as a function of the amount and timing of drug doses; the route of administration; drug-specific **pharmacokinetic parameters** (for example, drug-elimination half-life, and the rate of clearance from the body); patient factors (for example, age, gender, and ideal body weight); and concurrent therapies and disease factors that influence the drug's effects (for example, congestive heart failure, pneumonia, smoking behavior, and concurrent use of phenobarbital are some of the factors that influence the effects of theophylline, a bronchodilator often used to treat bronchospasm in bronchial asthma and emphysema). Health professionals use pharmacokinetic models to forecast future drug levels, and, thus, to design optimal therapeutic regimens.

In the early 1970s, Jelliffe and colleagues reported one of the first systems designed to assist physicians in developing dosing regimens for digitalis [Jelliffe et al., 1972]. (Digitalis is used to treat congestive heart failure and certain cardiac arrhythmias. Excessively high serum digitalis levels can produce life-threatening arrhythmias.) A few years later, Sheiner and his associates described *Bayesian forecasting models* that adjust the parameters of the pharmacokinetic model based on the results of drug-level tests. The model is tailored to an individual patient and, therefore, produces a better fit between measured and predicted drug levels [Sheiner, 1975]. Today, programs are available that permit rapid calculation of drug concentrations using complex pharmacokinetic equations; these calculations assist clinicians in predicting the efficacy of drug therapy and enhance the role of clinical pharmacists in providing pharmacokinetic consultations.

Recently, computers also have been used to determine the formulation of solutions for patients receiving intravenous feeding—partial or total parenteral nutrition (TPN; see Figure 10.5) [Moliver and Coates, 1987]. Physicians and pharmacists must consider a variety of factors, both singly and in combination, when formulating solutions. These factors include the patient's fluid and caloric requirements, dextrose (sugar) and lipid (fat) levels, and electrolyte balance (potassium, sodium, calcium, and so on). Prescription of TPN is particularly complicated for neonates and other pediatric patients, because these young patients often have high nutritional and caloric requirements, but need severe fluid restriction. Without the help of computers, pharmacists and pediatricians may spend hours calculating and verifying prescriptions that satisfy the multiple constraints.

10.3.3 Characteristics of Pharmacy Information

Pharmacy information systems possess many of the same characteristics as do the hospital information systems (HISs) we discussed in Chapter 7; in fact, we can consider pharmacy systems (and other departmental systems) to be components of more comprehensive HISs. For example, the drug-order data maintained in pharmacy medication-history records and used in drug-use control and dispensing applications are information typically contained in the medical-record portions of an HIS.

```
                    MONTREAL CHILDREN'S HOSPITAL
                    PRESCRIPTION FOR PARENTERAL NUTRITION        (89/07/19 11:22)
RX DATE: 89/07/17
                                                                  RX:      2064
                                                                  HOSP:

Name:                              Sex:          M
Born: 89/04/03                     Wt:           3.970 kg
Ward: 9D                           Day of TPN:   35
Input 89/07/17 08:43               Physician:
                                   Solution:     SPECIAL
Effective thru 89/07/18            Route:        CENTRAL

Total daily fluid:       131.08 ml/kg =   520 ml
Formula:                   0.00 ml/kg =     0 ml
Other Non-TPN Fluid:      55.67 ml/kg =   221 ml
TPN fluid without lipids: 57.91 ml/kg =   230 ml
                                                  9.6 ml/hr  ( 24.0 hrs) =
                                                  9   ml/hr  ( 10   hrs)
                                                  10  ml/hr  ( 14.0 hrs)
Osmolarity: 1730 mosm/L

              ENERGY                                  I.V. LIPIDS

I.V. Lipids:               146 kJ/kg        20% emulsion
I.V. Dextrose:             297 kJ/kg        3.5 g/kg
P.O.                         0 kJ/kg        69.5 ml
TOTAL:                     444 kJ/kg        2.9 ml/hr (24.0 hrs) =
I.V. Protein:               31 kJ/kg        2   ml/hr (  2   hrs)
TOTAL (incl. prot.)        475 kJ/kg        3   ml/hr ( 22.0 hrs)
Energy/nit. ratio:        1242 kJ/g nitrogen
                    METALS, VITAMINS AND HEPARIN
Trace metals #2: <20 kg (1ml/kg)            3.97 ml = 17.27 ml/L
Multivitamins: MVI PEDIATRIC (0–11 yrs)     5.00 ml = 21.75 ml/L
Heparin: 1 unit/ml TPN fluid minus lipids   230 units
```

	/kg PO	/kg IV	/kg IV + PO	Total IV	per litre	Qty (ml)
Dextrose (mmol)	—	71.04	—	282.03	1226.8	112.81
Protein (g)	0.00	2.28	2.28	9.04	39.3	90.35
Sodium (mmol)	0.00	3.00	3.00	11.91	51.8	1.96
Potassium (mmol)	0.00	2.00	2.00	7.94	34.5	1.95 KCL–
Phosphate (mmol)	0.00	0.71	0.71	2.83	12.3	1.35 KPHOS
Calcium (mmol)	0.00	0.68	0.68	2.70	11.7	11.83
Magnesium (mmol)	0.00	0.34	0.34	1.34	5.8	0.67

```
Sterile H20 to volume:                                                0.00

TOTAL:                                                              229.89

****IF  TPN  IS  INTERRUPTED,  HANG  D10W  TO  PREVENT  HYPOGLYCEMIA****
Pharmacist: _____     Physician: _____
```

FIGURE 10.5 At the Montreal Children's Hospital, physicians use an interactive computer program to prescribe solutions for intravenous feeding (total parenteral nutrition, or TPN). Final prescriptions, such as this one, are printed automatically in the pharmacy. (*Source:* Courtesy of Montreal Children's Hospital.)

The unique components of pharmacy systems relate to facts about drugs and drug effects; this information base is essential to the practice of pharmacy. For example, clinical information, such as common side effects and drug interactions, is relevant to the drug-information services and is used in patient-specific therapy-monitoring programs. Drug-specific pharmacokinetic parameters, such as the mean drug-elimination rate, may be encoded in dose-calculation programs, and detailed information about specific drug products (for example, shelf life) is used by inventory-management applications.

Many pharmacy functions are well suited to implementation on computers because much drug information is easy to define. An advantage of pharmacy systems is that the information with which they deal generally is straightforward. Drug names, for example, are easier to encode than are disease states. As a result, collections of pharmacy-related information are more easily organized, managed, and controlled than are data from other types of medical information systems, for which the vocabulary is not as precise. Pharmacy also has an established and precise record-keeping function, primarily a result of legal requirements that dictate which elements of information must be captured and that designate the time periods for retention of those elements. In addition, the basic functions of pharmacy practice are well-defined processes with definite inputs, and they constitute a stepwise progression of activities that results in a definable product. Established software methodologies related to information management, such as the design of databases and other data-processing techniques, are thus directly applicable to the tasks encountered in pharmacy practice.

More problematic is the development of pharmacy applications that directly support decision making regarding drug therapies. Therapeutic goals and the criteria for success in meeting these goals are less easily defined and encoded than are lists of interacting drugs. In Chapter 15, we shall discuss research in knowledge representation and in the development of reasoning mechanisms to perform medical problem-solving tasks such as these.

10.4 Modern Systems to Support Pharmacy Practice

Over the past 20 years, researchers have developed a number of computer systems for pharmacy practice in the areas of inpatient, community, clinical, and drug-information services. In institutional settings, the pharmacy, like the business office and the clinical laboratory, is one of the areas most likely to have computer systems in place and functioning as part of its operation.

10.4.1 Pharmacy Information Systems

A 1986 survey of 4370 hospitals, conducted by Shared Data Research (SDR), identified 49 companies that offer pharmacy applications to hospitals [Packer, 1986]. Of these, nine companies controlled 60 percent of the market. These nine vendors provided software that ran on a variety of machines, from personal computers to mainframes. Their systems supported most of the functions discussed in Section 10.3.1, including online order entry, maintenance of medication-administration records, automatic generation of refill-dispensing reports, order crediting and debiting, label generation, performance of drug compatibility checks, and duplicate-order checking. Some of the systems also supported patient-care functions, such as allergy screening and drug-dose calculation; research functions, such as the creation and maintenance of historical databases; and financial-management functions, such as cost accounting.

10.4.2 Clinical Pharmacy Systems

The most exciting systems from a clinical perspective are those that directly help pharmacists and physicians to prescribe drugs and to monitor patients receiving drug therapies. A number of research groups and, more recently, companies have developed software to assist health professionals in calculating and adjusting drug doses of dangerous drugs, such as digoxin, gentamicin, theophylline, heparin, and warfarin. These systems employ pharmacokinetic models to forecast drug levels based on patient characteristics and drug-administration information. One of the most recent systems is PK Monitor, which was developed by researchers at the Stanford University Medical Center as part of the MENTOR therapeutic monitoring program [Lenert et al., 1988]. PK Monitor uses information about the amount and timing of doses and the levels of the drug detected in a patient's blood to monitor the use of digoxin and to provide dosing recommendations for physicians.

Researchers at the Montreal Children's Hospital have developed a decision-support system to assist in prescribing TPN for pediatric patients of all ages and weights, including premature neonates [Moliver and Coates, 1987]. The system interactively guides physicians through the prescription process and uses encoded rules to custom-tailor its recommendations based on the patient's age, weight, length of therapy, and previous prescriptions. During the process, it performs safety checks to identify and flag high doses and other out-of-range values. Physicians can override most of these limits, but some actions are never permitted. For example, physicians are never allowed to prescribe concentrations of calcium, phosphate, and magnesium that exceed the levels at which these elements might precipitate out of solution. Completed orders are stored in the database, where they are accessible from terminals that are connected to the HIS. In addition, orders are transmitted to the pharmacy, where they are printed (Figure 10.5). Pharmacists can direct the TPN system to calculate additional information needed to fill orders, including the absolute ingredient totals, ingredient totals for individual bottles, and the cumulative volume levels after each ingredient is added.

The automation of TPN ordering has reduced delays in the transmission of orders to the pharmacy, and has saved the hospital pharmacy about 25 minutes per prescription by eliminating the need for pharmacists to calculate and verify prescriptions manually, to locate physicians to supply missing and illegible information, and to type bottle labels. In addition, an online help facility outlines the system's criteria for recommending values and for generating safety warnings—an educational tool for health professionals in training.

The MEDIPHOR system, developed by researchers at Stanford University School of Medicine in the early 1970s, was one of the first computer systems to use a pharmacy's medication records to provide online drug-interaction surveillance [Tatro et al., 1975]. As pharmacy personnel enter new prescription orders into the pharmacy system, MEDIPHOR updates patients' drug profiles, then uses information stored in its drug-interaction database to determine whether the new drugs interact with drugs that have been ordered previously. When it identifies a potential interaction, the system produces a drug-interaction report to alert pharmacists and health-care professionals caring for the patient to the potential danger. Each report contains information about the pharmacological effect and mechanism, speed of onset, and the severity of the interaction (Figure 10.6). In addition, MEDIPHOR produces prescription labels and patient-specific drug profiles for the pharmacy and serves as an online resource for the retrieval of drug-interaction information. Since mid-1973, MEDIPHOR has been used at Stanford University Medical Center to evaluate the prescriptions of all inpatients receiving medication. It also is available commercially.

The MENTOR system, developed by researchers at Stanford University and the University of Maryland, is designed to monitor the drug therapies of hospitalized patients, thereby reducing the incidence of adverse drug reactions [Speedie et al., 1988]. MENTOR combines the wealth of clinical information collected and stored by modern HISs (Chapter 7) with the reasoning power of expert systems (Chapter 15). The system's evaluation process can be triggered by a variety of *events,* including orders for drugs, laboratory tests, and surgical procedures. MENTOR determines the set of events of interest for any particular patient, based on the patient's current drug therapy, laboratory-test results, pending laboratory-test orders, and scheduled surgical procedures. During each patient-monitoring cycle, MENTOR builds a profile of events, which determines the types of monitoring to be performed, as well as the timing and type of future evaluation. The system generates appropriate advisory messages to physicians and other health-care professionals when it detects problems related to the drug therapy (Figure 10.7).

The HELP system developed at the LDS Hospital in Salt Lake City is a comprehensive medical-information system that uses a different approach than MENTOR to support a variety of pharmaceutical services (see Chapter 7). In addition to warning physicians of potential drug–drug interactions and adverse side effects, it also identifies abnormal chemistry levels, concurrent diseases, and other patient conditions (for example, impaired renal function) that should be considered when particular drugs are prescribed (see Figure 15.10). Recently, HELP was extended to monitor the use of prophylactic antibiotics [Evans, 1987]. By integrating the surgical-scheduling programs with the hospital information system, HELP is able to identify patients who should receive prophylactic antibiotics within 2 hours before surgery and patients who are receiving unnecessary antibiotics (48 hours postoperative and no evidence of infection). A preliminary evaluation showed that use of the monitoring system significantly lowered the overall rate of hospital-acquired infection and saved thousands of dollars by reducing the unnecessary use of antibiotics.

10.4.3 Drug-Information Services

Bibliographic-retrieval systems are the primary computer-based information systems used by drug-information services. They are used to access bibliographic databases of indexed literature citations and abstracts, medical information bases containing machine-readable forms of entire journal articles and books, and medical knowledge bases (organized collections of distilled and validated factual information). These systems facilitate the provision of drug-information services by allowing rapid access to the large body of drug-related medical literature. In the following paragraphs, we

STANFORD UNIVERSITY MEDICAL CENTER ● DIVISION OF CLINICAL PHARMACOLOGY

DRUG INTERACTION REPORT #782   4-MAY-89 9:47:45

JANE DOE   01-234-567 0 123   NICU

REASON FOR REPORT: A potentially interacting drug combination has been prescribed for this patient. Pharmacist/nurse: Place report in progress notes.

INTERACTING DRUGS:

THEO-DUR (THEOPHYLLINE) with ERYTHROMYCIN

ONSET: Delayed   SEVERITY: Moderate   CLINICAL SIGNIFICANCE: Established
----

EFFECTS: Pharmacologic effects of THEO-DUR may be increased. Elevated theophylline plasma levels with toxicity characterized by nausea, vomiting, cardiovascular instability, and seizures may occur. The effectiveness of ERYTHROMYCIN may also be decreased. (see discussion.)

MECHANISM: The hepatic metabolism of THEO-DUR may be inhibited by ERYTHROMYCIN.

MANAGEMENT: May need a 15% to 40% lower dose of THEO-DUR during concurrent administration of ERYTHROMYCIN. Monitor theophylline plasma levels and the patient for symptoms of theophylline toxicity; adjust the dose accordingly. May also need a higher dose of ERYTHROMYCIN.

DISCUSSION: Controlled studies involving normal subjects or patients with pulmonary disease have shown that a 5 to 10 day course of erythromycin decreases theophylline metabolic clearance by 15% to 40%, and prolongs the elimination half-life by as much as 60% (3-8,10,11). Theophylline toxicity due to this interaction has been reported (1,4,12). Others have failed to observe this interaction, usually when erythromycin is administered for 5 days or less or in smokers (2,7-9,13). One study suggests that the magnitude of the effects of this interaction may depend on the dose of theophylline (14).   Based on current data, consider that in some patients, particularly nonsmokers with theophylline levels in the upper the therapeutic range, toxicity may occur when a course of five or more days of erythromycin is added to the therapeutic regimen.   Dyphylline (a less potent, renally excreted theophylline derivative), probably does not interact.

Theophylline has also been reported to decrease erythromycin concentration (10, 15). In one study, erythromycin serum levels were more than 30% lower in the presence of theophylline (15).   The mechanism and significance of this finding remains to be established.

REFERENCES: 1. Kozak PP et al: J Allergy Clin Immunol 60:149(1977). 2. Pfeifer HJ et al: Clin Pharmacol Ther 26:36(1979). 3. Zarowitz BJM et al: Clin Pharmacol Ther 29:601(1981). 4. LaForce CF et al: J Pediatr 99:153(1981). 5. Renton KW et al: Clin Pharmacol Ther 30:422(1981). 6. Prince RA et al: J Allergy Clin Immunol 68:427(1981). 7. May DC et al: J Clin Pharmacol 22:125(1982). 8. Richer C et al: Clin Pharmacol Ther 31:579(1982). 9. Maddux MS et al: Chest 81:563(1982). 10. Iliopoulou A et al: Br J Clin Pharmacol 14:495(1982). 11. Reisz G et al: Am Rev Respir Dis 127:581(1983). 12. Parish RA et al: Pediatr 72:828(1983). 13. Hildebrandt R et al: Eur J Clin Pharmacol 26:485(1984). 14. Vercelloni M et al: J Int Med Res 14:131(1986). 15. Paulsen O et al: Eur J Clin Pharmacol 32:493(1987). 16. Rieder MJ et al: J Asthma 25:195(1988). <review>

FIGURE 10.6 This MEDIPHOR drug-interaction report describes a potential interaction between theophylline and erythromycin. Each report indicates the severity of the interaction and the rapidity of onset, describes the effects and the mechanism of the interaction, and provides references to substantiate its contents. (*Source:* Courtesy of Terrence Blaschke, M.D., Division of Clinical Pharmacology, Stanford University.)

MENTORx
Advisory

Doe, Matthew
E2A-4

ADVISORY Inappropriate Antibiotic Therapy
CONDITION *9:40 A.M. March 2, 1989*

RECOMMENDED
ACTION

• **Review Microbiology Susceptibility Result**

• **Revise Antibiotic Therapy**

WHY • Blood cultures ordered on March 1 revealed **facultative**
Gram-Negative Rods, possibly Klebsiella

• Susceptibility result for the first set of cultures is available

• Blood isolate is not sensitive to currently administered
antibiotic--**erythromycin**

*This report is based on information available to the
Hospital Pharmacy and Laboratories at 9:30 A.M.*

*MENTOR advisories are intended as background to help inform the judgments of
physicians and clinical pharmacists. Any use of this information is the responsibility of
the individual physician or pharmacist.*

FIGURE 10.7 The MENTOR system issues this advisory message to indicate inappropriate antibiotic therapy. The organism detected through laboratory testing is not susceptible to the drug that the patient is taking. (*Source:* Courtesy of Terrence Blaschke, M.D., Division of Clinical Pharmacology, Stanford University.)

briefly discuss systems that provide access to drug information; we shall examine bibliographic-retrieval systems in greater depth in Chapter 14.

The MEDLINE system of the National Library of Medicine (NLM) provides access to the world's largest, most comprehensive, and most up-to-date selection of citations and references from the medical literature. The database consists of both English and foreign-language references and abstracts from over 3000 journals and other publications. Because it contains practically all the published literature on drugs and their effects, MEDLINE is an invaluable resource for drug-information specialists. In addition to MEDLINE, the NLM maintains a variety of other databases, some relevant to pharmacy. These include TOXLINE, Registry of Toxic Effects of Chemical Substances (RTECS), and Toxicology Data Bank (TDB).

There are a number of other bibliographic databases that contain pharmacological information.

1. *International Pharmaceutical Abstracts (IPA)*. Produced by the American Society of Hospital Pharmacists, the IPA database covers more than 600 worldwide publications from 1970 to the present.

2. *Excerpta Medica*. The Excerpta Medica database provides comprehensive coverage of the pharmaceuticals literature and is used to produce two drug-related bibliographies: Drug Literature Index and Adverse Reactions Titles.

3. *BIOSIS Previews*. Produced by BioScience Information Service, BIOSIS Previews is the online database of *Biological Abstracts* (journal abstracts) and *Biological Abstracts/RRM* (abstracts of reports, reviews, and meetings). It contains citations from publications in the life sciences, including journals, books, government reports, and conference proceedings.

4. *Pharmaceutical News Index (PNI)*. PNI is produced by Data Courier. Its database contains references to literature on finances, government regulatory activities, and health-care legislation related to pharmaceuticals, cosmetics, medical devices, and other health fields.

Several commercial services provide access to the full text of selected journals and textbooks. The American Society for Hospital Pharmacists sells a full-text medical-literature information base that relates specifically to drugs and drug therapy. It consists of a comprehensively indexed series of published drug evaluations. Such full-text information bases are particularly helpful to pharmacy personnel because they can provide immediate access to all entries within the information base on a particular drug or drug class. The COLLEAGUE system, discussed in Chapter 14, also allows full-text retrieval. This general medical system contains a significant number of articles related to drug therapy.

In addition to indexing the published literature, knowledge bases can store expert summaries of the articles and related conclusions. When users consult such a knowledge base, they do not retrieve or locate references; rather, they retrieve factual information and valuations, which an expert has written based on clinical knowledge and the current literature. Micromedex's DRUGDEX database is an example of such a knowledge-based system. It contains over 6000 referenced monographs of drug information and answers to specific patient-care questions about drugs and drug therapies. The information in the database is contributed by experts in a variety of fields and is updated on a quarterly basis. Drug monographs are organized as a series of indexed paragraphs, each of which can be accessed individually. Figure 10.8 shows typical computer screens from the microcomputer-based DRUGDEX system. Menus on each screen allow users to move from topic to topic within the database. The DRUGDEX database is available in three formats: the traditional microfiche, magnetic tape for use with mainframe computers, and CD-ROM for use with microcomputers.

10.5 A Look at the Future of Pharmacy Systems

Pharmacy practice is in the midst of redefinition and transformation. Rapid advances in medical and pharmacological knowledge and in the number, sophistication, and power of drugs create a growing need for tighter drug control and make it increasingly difficult for physicians and nurses to understand the many drugs they use in caring for patients. Recently, some pharmacists and pharmacologists have begun to call for expansion of the professional role of pharmacists to embrace greater responsibility in patient care and in the medication-use process.

At the same time, changes in health-care financing and delivery place pressure on health institutions, including pharmacies, to minimize costs while maintaining high-quality patient care. The implementation of computer-based information systems that perform many of the data-processing and record-keeping functions that occupied pharmacists previously will hasten this shift from a product- to a patient-oriented profession.

In the future, it is likely that computer systems will assume many of the dispensing and distribution functions of the pharmacy as well. The technology now is available to automate much of the drug-use process, from the time a therapeutic decision is made until the drug is administered to the patient; someday, the computer routinely will screen orders for potential adverse interactions, flag complicated or unusual therapies for review by pharmacists, count out tablets and capsules automatically, and package them for delivery to patients.

The use of bar codes in the pharmacy will remove the last major technological obstacle to automated drug dispensing by computer-controlled dispensing machines. Ubiquitous in supermarkets, bar-code technology already is used in some hospitals for tracking blood supplies, medical records, and X-ray film jackets. Pharmacy robots are used in Japan, and prototypes are being tested in the United States. Other potential uses of bar-code technology in the pharmacy are automated monitoring of inventory levels and computer-assisted tracking of drug-product expiration and disposal. Bar codes even can reduce drug-administration errors—health professionals can verify that the correct drug is given to the correct patient by scanning both the bar-coded patient-identification bracelet and the bar-coded drug label prior to administering a drug.

The availability of high-density storage technology will rapidly reduce the size and cost of pharmacy computer systems. A single WORM (write once, read many [times]) optical disc has the capacity to store all the information collected and used by a community pharmacy during 5 years of operation. This higher storage capacity will also allow information bases, such as the DRUGDEX database, to be incorporated into pharmacy information systems.

Advances in networking and communications technology also affect pharmacy practice. The automation of the drug order-entry process will allow quicker and more accurate filling of orders, but also provides the opportunity to give immediate feedback to physicians about their orders. For example, if a physician enters an order for a drug and a potential drug–drug interaction is detected, she can be instantly warned of the problem, rather than receiving a report hours later—and perhaps hours too late. In addition, pharmacies will not be restricted to local databases, but will have access to national databases of information about drug prices, drugs approved for reimbursement by specific third-party payers, and criteria for optimal drug use. The Health Care Financing Administration (HCFA) is developing a system for processing drug-prescription claims under the Medicare Catastrophic Coverage Act of 1988. The system will perform real-time processing of claims, while simultaneously evaluating the prescriptions for potential problems, such as drug–drug interactions. Participating pharmacies will be directly connected to HCFA via telephone lines, thus allowing them to obtain immediate decisions about prescriptions.

This same communications technology will also promote increased professional communication via pharmacy computer systems. For example, the University of Maryland School of Pharmacy recently initiated the PCRx project, a telecommunications-mediated conferencing system for pharmacists in the state of Maryland. Any

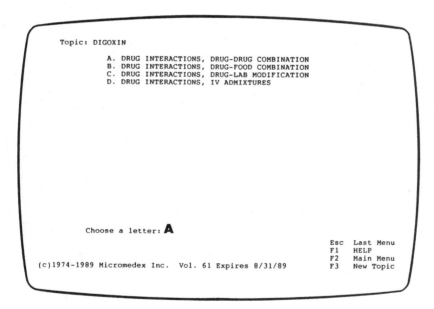

(a)

FIGURE 10.8 Users can obtain drug-specific information from Micromedex's microcomputer-based DRUGDEX system. A physician who wishes to learn about potential interactions between digoxin and acebutolol can navigate through the system rapidly by (a) selecting the DRUG–DRUG COMBINATION option from the list of drug interactions for digoxin, and (b) choosing ACEBUTOLOL from the list of interacting drugs. (c) The drug-evaluation monograph provides detailed descriptions of each drug interaction. An overview of the drug and its effects, dosing information, summary of clinical applications, and pertinent references also are available. (*Source:* Gelman CR & Rumack BH (eds): DRUGDEX® Information System. Micromedex, Inc., Denver, Colorado [Edition expires 8/31/89].)

```
     Topic: DIGOXIN

                   A. ACEBUTOLOL
                   B. ALPRAZOLAM
                   C. AMILORIDE
                   D. AMIODARONE
                   E. AMPHOTERICIN B
                   F. ANTACIDS
                   G. ASPIRIN
                   H. ATROPINE
                   I. BEPRIDIL
                   J. CALCIUM
                   K. CARBAMAZEPINE
                   L. CHOLESTYRAMINE
                   M. CIMETIDINE
                   N. CISAPRIDE
                   O. COLESTIPOL
                   P. CYTOTOXIC AGENTS
                   Q. DIAZEPAM
                   R. DILTIAZEM




             Choose a letter: A                        Esc   Last Menu
                                                       F1    HELP
                            * PgDn MORE *              F2    Main Menu
     (c)1974-1989 Micromedex Inc.  Vol. 61 Expires 8/31/89    F3    New Topic
```

(b)

```
                    DRUG EVALUATION MONOGRAPHS
                                                    A.Overview
     Topic: DIGOXIN                                 B.Dose Info
       3.5 DRUG INTERACTIONS                        C.Kinetics
         3.5.1 DRUG-DRUG COMBINATIONS             ➞D.Cautions
           A.  ACEBUTOLOL                           E.Clin Appl
             1.  No significant interaction was reported during      F.Mfg Info
                 concomitant therapy with acebutolol and digoxin (Tech   G.Reference
                 Info, 1985).                       H.Author
           B.  ALPRAZOLAM
             1.  Concomitant administration of aprazolam (1.5 mg/day)
                 and digoxin was reported to result in no change in
                 digoxin clearance or other kinetic variables of     ↑   Up 1 Line
                 digoxin; in addition, creatinine clearance was not   ↓   Dn 1 Line
                 affected significantly during concomitant alprazolam
                 administration (Ochs et al, 1985).  Based upon these  PgUp Up 1 Page
                 data, it appears that therapeutic alprazolam doses   PgDn Dn 1 Page
                 should have no effect on digoxin serum concentrations.
                 However, more studies are needed to evaluate the effect  Esc  Last Menu
                 of higher alprazolam doses and in more seriously-ill  F1   HELP
                 patients.                           F2   Main Menu
             2.  For More Information :              F3   New Topic
                 See Drug Consult reference:  "ALPRAZOLAM-DIGOXIN     F4   Print
                 INTERACTION"                        F5   DC ref
           C.  AMILORIDE

     (c)1974-89 Micromedex Inc.      More data follows   Vol. 61 Expires 8/31/89
```

(c)

FIGURE 10.8 *Continued.*

pharmacist in the state may register to participate. The system allows users to sign up for and participate in a variety of topical conferences by dialing a local telephone number to connect to the University's system. From their personal computers, participants can scan the list of messages posted under the conference topic and can add their own comments.

The implementation of point-of-care systems using bedside terminals to collect critical information, such as vital signs and drug-administration data, will produce more comprehensive medical databases and will facilitate sophisticated, patient-specific drug-therapy monitoring. It will be possible, for instance, to determine exactly which drugs the patient has taken and when they were administered. Detailed and accurate drug-administration and vital-sign information is crucial for evaluating therapeutic regimens, monitoring the effects of drug therapies, and detecting adverse drug reactions.

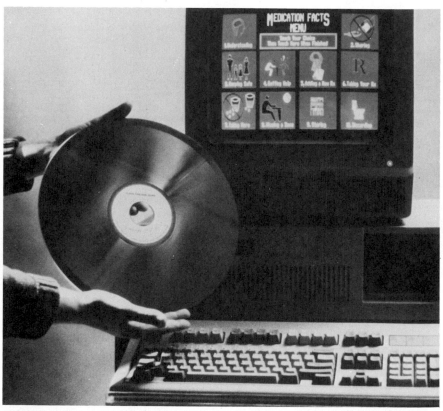

FIGURE 10.9 A project under development by the United States Pharmacopeia uses a computer-based educational program and videodisc technology to teach patients about the drugs they are using. The interactive system explains how each drug works, how it should be taken, and what the side effects are. These explanations are illustrated with video segments that explain potential side effects and provide instructions for drug use. (*Source:* Photograph by B. Conatha.)

Online access to detailed clinical data and the application of artificial-intelligence (AI) techniques to drug-therapy monitoring will improve significantly the ability of such monitoring systems to detect and make recommendations concerning potential problems with drug therapy. In addition, the continuing development of pharmacology knowledge bases will have a major influence on drug-information services. The integration of such knowledge-based systems and HISs will provide online access to current drug information by pharmacy and other health-care personnel. Someday, health professionals even may obtain expert therapy-planning advice from clinical-consultation systems.

The integration of videodisc technology with computers will soon change the ways in which patients can learn about the drugs they are taking. A recent example of this approach to patient education is a project under development by the United States Pharmacopeia. The patient identifies the drug she is taking, and the interactive system explains how the drug works, how it should be taken, and what the side effects are (Figure 10.9). The explanations are heavily illustrated with video segments that visually illustrate potential side effects and instructions for drug use. Someday, systems of this type will be routinely available in pharmacies for use by clients.

In summary, the future holds increased automation of pharmacy practice. The use of computer-based systems to perform drug-distribution, record-keeping, and routine monitoring functions will simplify many time-consuming tasks, and thus will allow pharmacists to emphasize the patient-care aspects of their practices—assisting in drug-therapy decision making and monitoring and providing drug information to health-care personnel and patients. Computer-based information systems will better equip pharmacy services in both the inpatient and community settings to provide high-quality patient care in the face of growing pressure to control health-care costs.

Suggested Readings

Brodie, D. C. and Smith, W. E. Implications of the new technology for pharmacy education and practice. *American Journal of Pharmaceutical Education,* 49(3):282, 1985.

> *The authors present descriptive vignettes that summarize important technological changes, describe the problems created by these changes, and discuss the implications of the new technologies for pharmacy education and practice.*

Fassett, W. E. and Christensen, D. B. *Computer Applications in Pharmacy.* Philadelphia: Lea & Febiger, 1986.

> *This textbook provides a basic introduction to the computer hardware and software used in hospital and community pharmacies. Individual chapters are devoted to drug-therapy monitoring, drug-use review, drug information services, and clinical pharmacokinetics. The article concludes with a list of unanswered questions relevant to the future of the profession.*

Gouveia, W. A., Neal, T., and Nold, E. G. *1986 Report: Hospital Pharmacy Computer Systems.* Bethesda, MD: American Society of Hospital Pharmacists, 1986.

> *This report from the American Society of Hospital Pharmacists presents the 1986 results of a periodic survey of computer use in hospital pharmacies. The report covers not only*

the hardware and software systems used, but also the pharmacy applications provided by each system.

Helper, C. D. Unresolved issues in the future of pharmacy. *American Journal of Hospital Pharmacy,* 45:1071, 1988.

> *This article discusses the technological, economic, and societal forces that are shaping the future of pharmacy practice. It explores unresolved issues in pharmacy and describes alternative ways to redefine pharmacy practice.*

Peck, C. C. *Bedside Clinical Pharmacokinetics,* rev. ed. Vancouver, WA: Applied Therapeutics, Inc., 1989.

> *This manual provides an understandable introduction to pharmacokinetic concepts and to techniques for individualizing drug therapy. It provides an overview of the time course of drugs in the body, outlines major factors that influence drug effects, and explains techniques for using pharmacokinetic models to produce patient-specific drug therapies.*

Tatro, D. S., et al. Online drug interaction surveillance. *American Journal of Hospital Pharmacy,* 32:417, 1975.

> *The authors describe the goals, design, and implementation of MEDIPHOR, a computer-based system that evaluates drug orders and alerts health-care personnel when it detects interacting drug combinations.*

Questions for Discussion

1. Pharmacy-system implementation has been possible in part because pharmacy practice deals with large numbers of well-defined data and tasks, which has allowed adaptation of existing hardware and software. Compare and contrast the types of data managed by pharmacy information systems with those handled by computer-based medical record systems.

2. A major factor in the successful implementation of a computer system is the degree to which users accept the system. Why might pharmacy systems be accepted more easily than are other medical computer systems?

3. Delegation of routine and time-consuming tasks to a computer allows pharmacists to concentrate on the clinical aspects of the practice. Do you think that eventually other health-care professionals will spend more time in direct patient-care activities? Or might the trend toward increasing use of computers have the opposite effect, such that people become experts more in running computer programs than in dealing with patients? In your discussion, keep in mind the pressures that are speeding adoption of medical computer systems.

4. Modern computer networks support direct communication among computer systems in multiple locations. Currently, however, many of the systems that we discuss in this book operate independently. What are the implications for pharmacists and other health-care professionals of the establishment of direct connections between physicians' office computer systems and pharmacies' computer systems?

5. Almost all pharmacy information systems in community pharmacies contain only information on the prescriptions filled at a single geographic location. What

implications does this have for a pharmacist's ability to counsel patients concerning drug therapies? A nationwide system of drug profiles has been proposed as a part of the new Medicare program. How would giving pharmacists access to patients' global profiles change that ability to provide counseling?

6. Most patients today receive the majority of information about drug therapies directly from their physicians and pharmacists. Describe three new technologies that have been developed to provide information to health professionals about drugs and drug effects. How could such systems be adapted to provide information to the general public? In what ways would the adapted systems differ from the systems described in this chapter? In what ways will these new approaches to providing information affect pharmacists and physicians?

11

Radiology Systems

Robert A. Greenes and James F. Brinkley

After reading this chapter, you should know the answers to these questions:

- What information-management tasks are supported by computer-based radiology information systems?
- How are medical images, such as X-ray films, computed-tomography scans, and ultrasound images, generated?
- What factors account for the relative lack of success of computer-based systems for radiologic-image interpretation?
- What are the important human-engineering issues that shape the design of image-interpretation workstations?
- What are the functions of a picture-archiving and communication system?
- What are the technical problems that must be solved before all-digital radiology departments become feasible?

11.1 Information Processing Within a Radiology Department

The primary function of a radiology department is the acquisition and analysis of medical images. Through imaging, health-care personnel obtain information that can help them to establish diagnoses, to plan therapy, and to follow the courses of diseases or therapies. Diagnostic studies in the radiology department are provided at the request of referring clinicians, who then use the information for decision making. The radiology department produces the images, and the radiologist provides the primary analysis and interpretation of the radiologic findings. Thus, radiologists play a direct role in clinical problem solving and in diagnostic-workup planning.

The activities of the radiology department can be divided into four categories: image generation, image analysis, image management, and information management. Each of these tasks is amenable to the use of computers. In fact, radiology is one branch of medicine in which even the basic data can be produced by computers and stored directly in computer memory.

11.1.1 Image Generation

Medical image generation is the process of producing the images that health professionals use to visualize the internal structure and functions of the body indirectly. A variety of **imaging modalities** (such as film-based X-ray imaging, computed tomography, and ultrasound imaging) are available. In many cases, the use of computers to create and manipulate digital images has been indispensable in the image-generation process.

Film-based **radiography** is the primary modality used in radiology departments today. A typical X-ray image is produced by projecting an X-ray beam—one form of **ionizing radiation**—from an X-ray source through a patient's body and onto an X-ray–sensitive film. Because an X-ray beam is differentially absorbed by the various body tissues, the X-rays produce shadows on the radiographic film. The resultant *shadowgraph* is a superposition of all the structures traversed by each beam (Figure 11.1). **Digital radiography** applies the same techniques, but the images are digitized, and these data are recorded in computer memory rather than on film.

The most dramatic application of computers to image generation is **computed tomography (CT)**. CT scanners also use X rays to generate images. However, instead of depicting a directly measurable parameter (the absorption of X-ray beams as they pass through the body), CT mathematically reconstructs an image from X-ray–attenuation values that have been measured from multiple angles. As a result, it is possible to view cross-sectional "slices" through the body, rather than two-dimensional projections of superimposed structures (Figure 11.2). Thus, CT images provide a precise mapping of the internal structures of the body in three-dimensional space, a function not provided by standard X-ray images. They also greatly improve contrast resolution.

Another common imaging modality is **ultrasound imaging** (echosonography). Ultrasonography uses pulses of high-frequency sound waves, rather than ionizing radiation, to image body structures. As each sound wave encounters tissue interfaces in

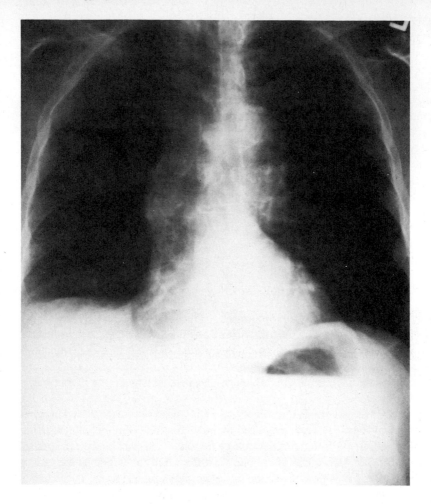

FIGURE 11.1 A standard chest X-ray image. (*Source:* Courtesy of Dr. William Shuman, Department of Radiology, University of Washington, Seattle.)

a patient's body, a portion of the wave is reflected and a portion continues. The time required for the echo to return is proportional to the distance into the body at which it is reflected; the amplitude (intensity) of a returning echo depends on the acoustical properties of the tissues encountered and is represented in the image as brightness. The system constructs two-dimensional images by displaying the echoes from pulses of multiple adjacent one-dimensional paths (Figure 11.3). Such images can be stored in digital memory or recorded on videotape, then displayed as television (raster-display) images.

The desire to obtain clinical information about physiologic function as well as about anatomical structure led to the development of other imaging modalities. In **nuclear-medicine imaging,** a radioactive isotope is chemically attached to a biologically active compound, then injected into the peripheral circulation. The compound

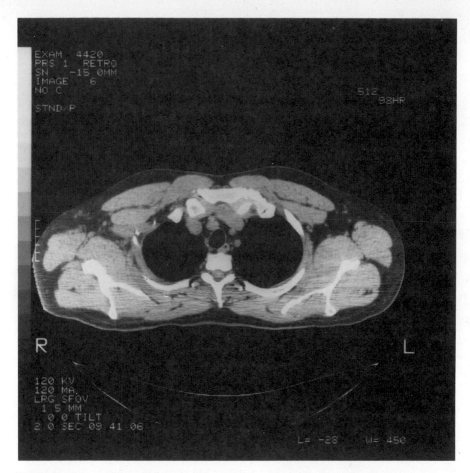

EXAM 4420
PRS 1 RETRO
SN -15 0MM
IMAGE 6
NO C
512
93HR
STND/P

R
L

120 KV
120 MA
LRG SFOV
1 5 MM
0 0 TILT
2 0 SEC 09 41 06
L= -28   W= 450

FIGURE 11.2 A computed-tomography (CT) image of the thorax of a patient. The gray-level settings have been optimized for the display of bone. (*Source:* Courtesy of Dr. William Shuman, Department of Radiology, University of Washington, Seattle.)

collects in the specific body compartments or organs (such as the thyroid or liver) where it is stored or processed by the body. The isotope emits radiation locally and the radiation is measured using a special detector. The resultant nuclear-medicine image depicts the level of radioactivity that was measured at each point (Figure 11.4). Because the counts are inherently digital, computers have been used to record them. Multiple images also can be processed to obtain dynamic information, such as the rate of arrival or of disappearance of isotope at particular body sites. Newer nuclear-medicine techniques use methods similar to CT for reconstructing images from projections.

An exciting recent development in medical imaging is **magnetic resonance imaging (MRI)**. All atomic nuclei within the body have a net magnetic moment, which means that they act like tiny magnets. When a patient is placed in an intense magnetic field, these nuclei line up in the direction of the field, spinning about the axis of

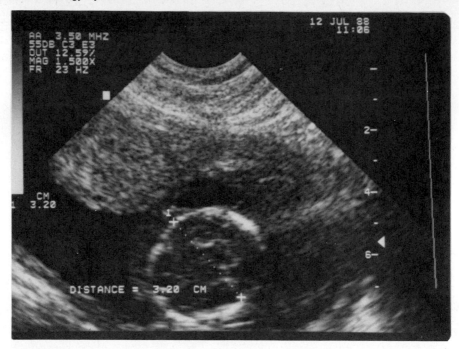

AA 3.50 MHZ
55DB C3 E3
OUT 12.59%
MAG 1.500X
FR 23 HZ

12 JUL 88
11:06

CM
3.20

2—

4—

6—

DISTANCE = 3.20 CM

FIGURE 11.3 An ultrasound image of a fetal head. The electronic calipers show a head diameter, which is useful for assessing fetal growth. (*Source:* Courtesy of Dr. William Shuman, Department of Radiology, University of Washington, Seattle.)

the field with a frequency dependent on the type of nucleus and on the strength of the magnetic field. If a radio pulse of the same frequency is applied at right angles to the stationary magnetic field, those nuclei with rotation frequency equal to that of the radio-frequency pulse will resonate with the pulse and absorb energy. The higher energy state causes the nuclei to change their orientation with respect to the fixed magnetic field. When the radio-frequency pulse is removed, the nuclei return to their original aligned state, emitting a detectable radio-frequency signal as they do so. The intensity and duration of this signal are dependent on several parameters related to the density and type of nuclei. Such differences can be measured, and these values can be used to generate images that depict biological differences among tissues (Figure 11.5).

One reason for the excitement about MRI is its potential to perform noninvasive *chemical* analyses of regions of the body. Different atoms respond differently to the application of the radio-frequency waves. Hence, they can be identified and imaged by the MR scanner. One of the easiest atoms to visualize by MRI—the hydrogen atom—is also among the most common in the body. Thus, it is possible to observe metabolism and to characterize tissues, perhaps in some cases differentiating normal versus cancerous tissue. MRI technology is currently an active area of research; many clinical applications are being developed.

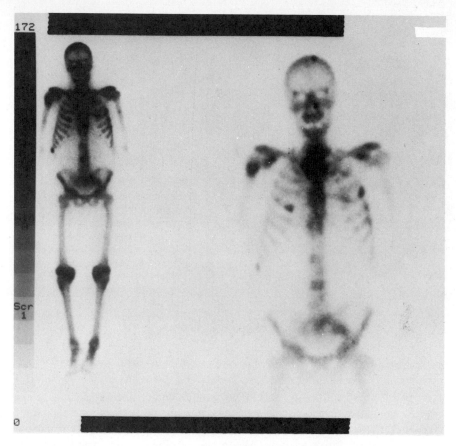

FIGURE 11.4 Whole body nuclear-medicine scan (two views) of a patient with metastatic prostate cancer. Small dark areas in the ribs, spine, and upper arm are bone metastases. (*Source*: Courtesy of Dr. Michael M. Graham, Division of Nuclear Medicine, University of Washington, Seattle.)

11.1.2 Image Analysis

Once images have been generated, they must be analyzed. Traditionally, image analysis has been the primary role of radiologists, who use their clinical knowledge, their perceptual abilities, and information about specific patients to interpret medical images. Radiologic examinations usually are requested for four basic reasons: visualization, quantitation, localization, and screening.

Physicians often request an imaging procedure to rule in (confirm) or to rule out specific disease hypotheses. The images are used to *visualize* body structure or function, and thus to determine whether the features of the disease are present. The growing trend toward digital imaging means that radiology personnel can use computers to manipulate the images to allow better visualization of disease processes. For example, technologists can adjust the gray scale of a CT image to display the regions of

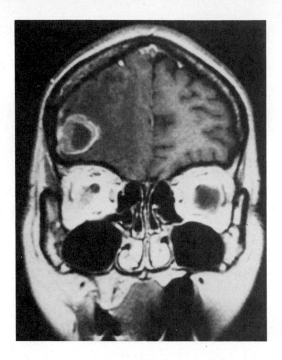

FIGURE 11.5 Coronal magnetic resonance imaging (MRI) section through the forebrain. The bright rounded area on the patient's right side (as viewed from the front) is a tumor surrounded by edema. The edema has compressed the surrounding brain tissue (compare with the left side). (*Source:* Courtesy of Dr. Gary Stimac, North Shore Magnetic Imaging Center, Boston.)

interest optimally. In addition, many of the image-enhancement procedures developed for the National Aeronautics and Space Administration (NASA) space program have been or will be used for this purpose. For example, digital filtering techniques can be applied to remove signal noise, to enhance edges, and otherwise to sharpen blurry images. Image enhancement for improved visualization currently is the principal use of the computer for image analysis. As three-dimensional–image data become increasingly available, particularly via MRI, the computer also will be used to display imaging data in ways that promote more effective viewing. For example, the computer might display only portions of an image, such that organs obscured by overlying structures can be visualized.

Computers also can be used to *quantify* measurable parameters, such as the volume of the heart or the size of a fetus. In most contemporary systems, these parameters are measured on the instrument's display screen using electronic calipers or on photographs using mechanical calipers. Light-pen systems, in which a technician points to areas on the screen, and thus enters coordinates, also have been developed. Typically, the computer records the measurements and performs calculations. Because these types of measurements are tedious for radiologists to perform, they also are subject to error. Automatic measurement of quantifiable parameters could improve both the consistency of measurements and the productivity of radiologists.

Often, radiologists use measurements from two-dimensional images to estimate organ volumes, by assuming that the organ has a simple mathematical shape, such as a cylinder or an ellipsoid. These calculations are not accurate, however, because organs are not easily described in terms of simple shapes. The availability of three-dimensional image data will make it possible to calculate volumes more accurately, but the number of parameters will become too large for manual measurement. In these cases, automatic or semiautomatic measurement will be a necessity.

For certain purposes, such as surgery or radiation therapy, precise *localization* of a lesion (an injury or pathological change) is the primary reason for a study. Localization is crucial for **interventional radiological procedures,** such as needle-aspiration biopsies and drainage of abscesses. Radiologists analyze medical images to ascertain precisely the best site for approaching a lesion and to determine the angle and depth of approach. Three-dimensional image data are invaluable for localization because a lesion's location usually must be related to external landmarks on the body (as, *3 centimeters above the umbilicus*). Such data also are useful in radiation-therapy planning, where oncologists must determine the volume of the treatment zone precisely.

Because the careful interpretation of radiologic images is time consuming, it is costly for trained radiologists to process large numbers of images. Thus, some researchers have worked to develop systems for computer-aided image interpretation. These systems might be particularly useful in settings in which X-ray examinations are commonly used for *screening* purposes—for example, preoperative chest examinations or periodic mammograms. In screening settings, the likelihood of true-positive findings is inherently relatively low, and manual reading remains tedious and time consuming. The goal of an automated image-analysis system in these settings is to flag abnormal and questionable images for later interpretation by a radiologist. This notion of automated screening has been applied successfully to the interpretation of ECG recordings, as described in Chapter 12.

11.1.3 Image Management

One of the major burdens of the radiology department is the storage and retrieval of the images themselves. Currently, most medical images are recorded and stored on film. Even images such as CT and MRI scans, which are inherently digital, are typically transferred to film once the technologist has optimized them for viewing. Radiologists then place the filmed images on illuminated light boxes, where the films can be analyzed in batches and can be compared easily with previous and related studies. Occasionally, as in the case of ultrasound studies, the images are transferred to videotape for later review and interpretation.

Radiology personnel prepare a film folder for each examination (or type of examination), label it with patient-identification information, and file it with the patient's master film jacket in the film library. The staff must locate and retrieve the master jacket each time the images are needed for review. If a clinician wishes to take a film out of the department, the staff must make a duplicate film or transact a loan.

Film storage requires a large amount of space in a radiology department. Typically, departments have the capacity to store films only for those patients who have had studies within the past 6 to 12 months. Older studies, usually retained for at least 7 years, are stored in a basement or warehouse.

Digital acquisition of images offers the exciting prospect of reducing the physical space requirements, material cost, and manual labor of traditional film-handling tasks, through online digital archiving, rapid retrieval of images via querying of image databases, and high-speed transmission of images over communications networks. Development of a system with such capabilities—a **picture-archiving and communication system (PACS)**—is an active area of research in medical informatics (Figure 11.6). A number of complex problems must be solved before PACSs become practical, however, including standardization of image transmission and storage formats; development of storage-management schemes for enormous numbers of data; and design of workstations, or consoles, that are as convenient and acceptable to radiologists for the interpretation of digital images as are the illuminated light boxes used for film-based interpretation.

11.1.4 Information Management

The management of work flow in a radiology department is a complex activity that involves not only maintenance of the film library, but also scheduling of examinations, registration of patients, performance of examinations, review and analysis of studies by radiologists, transcription of dictated reports, distribution of radiology reports to referring physicians, and billing for services.

In addition, department managers must collect and analyze process-control and financial data to prepare budgets, to make informed decisions regarding appropriate staffing levels and the purchase of additional equipment, and to identify problems, such as overly large numbers of retakes of films, too many portable or stat examination requests, excessive patient waiting times, and unacceptable delays in report transcription or signature. Inventory control, quality assurance, radiation-exposure monitoring, and preventive-maintenance scheduling are other important managerial functions.

As we have noted in previous chapters, many information-intensive tasks yield readily to automation; computer-based **radiology information systems (RISs)** have been developed to handle almost the entire spectrum of information-management tasks in the radiology department. RISs have been implemented either as standalone systems or as components of larger information systems. In either case, an RIS must be integrated with other information systems within an institution to allow reconciliation of patient data, to support examination scheduling and results reporting, and to facilitate patient billing.

11.2 Historical Perspectives

X rays were first discovered in 1895 by Wilhelm Conrad Röntgen, who was awarded the 1901 Nobel prize in physics for this achievement. The discovery caused worldwide excitement, especially in the field of medicine; by 1900, there already were several medical radiological societies. Thus, the foundation was laid for a new branch of medicine devoted to imaging the structure and function of the body [Dewing, 1962].

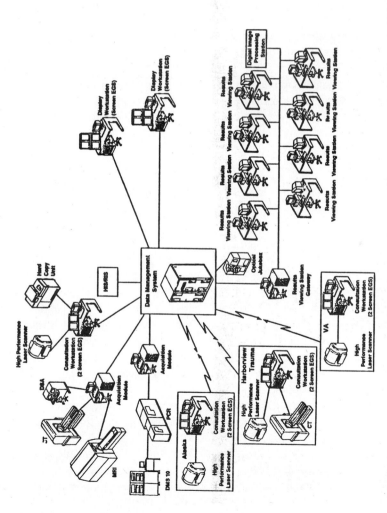

FIGURE 11.6 A picture-archiving and communication system (PACS) supports the management of digital images. A PACS integrates imaging devices, image archiving nodes (shown here as an optical jukebox), database systems, and workstations for image interpretation and review. [CT = computed tomography; DSA = digital subtraction angiography; MRI = magnetic resonance imaging; EGS = enhanced graphics system; PCR = Philips computed radiography; HIS = hospital information system; RIS = radiology information system; VA = Veterans Administration; DMS = data-management system.] (*Source:* Courtesy of Philips Medical Systems N.A., Inc.)

333

11.2.1 Development of Medical-Imaging Modalities

Both film and fluoroscopic screens were initially used for recording X-ray images, but the fluoroscopic images were too faint to be used clinically. By the 1940s, however, television and image-intensifier technology were used to produce clear real-time fluorescent images. Today, a standard procedure for many types of examinations is to combine real-time television monitoring of X-ray images with the creation of selected higher-resolution film images. Until the early 1970s, film and fluoroscopy were the only X-ray modalities available.

A challenge for early researchers was to find a solution to the problem of super-position of structures. The X-ray image at a given point represents the total attenuation due to all the overlaid structures traversed by a beam as it passes through the body; shadows cast by surrounding structures may obscure the object that the clinician wishes to visualize. **Contrast radiography**—the use of radiopaque contrast material to highlight the areas of interest—was used as early as 1902 to help deal with this problem. The first clinical experiments with **angiography**—imaging of blood vessels performed by the injection of opacifying agents into the bloodstream—were conducted in 1923.

The desire to separate superimposed structures also led to the development of a variety of tomographic techniques. In analog methods, the X-ray source and detector were moved in opposite arcs, thereby causing a thin tomographic (planar) section to remain in focus while other planes were blurred. This method, however, exposes the patient to a relatively high X-ray dose, because the blurred areas are continuously exposed. A method of axial (cross-sectional) tomography, introduced by Takahashi in 1957, avoided this problem by rotating a fan beam of X rays about the patient. The images produced by this method were blurred, however, and researchers recognized that a computer would be needed to make them clearer.

Mathematical methods for reconstructing images from projections were first developed by Radon in 1917, and later were improved by other researchers. These methods were used in the 1950s and 1960s to solve scientific problems in many fields, including radio astronomy and electron microscopy. In the late 1960s, Cormack used the techniques to reconstruct **phantoms** using X rays. Phantom reconstruction is a technique still used for machine calibration. An image is obtained of a phantom, an object with a known shape. The accuracy with which the reconstructed image matches the phantom is a measure of the accuracy of the system. This test can reveal errors in the reconstruction algorithms as well as in the hardware. In the early 1970s, Hounsfield led a team at the London-based EMI Corporation, which developed the first commercially viable CT scanner.

The development of the CT scanner dramatically improved the ability to visualize adjacent structures; for the first time, physicians were able to see inside a living human being clearly, but noninvasively. This ability led to a revolution in medicine almost as great as the one occasioned by the invention of X-ray imaging. As a result, Cormack and Hounsfield were awarded the 1979 Nobel prize in medicine.

The years following the invention of the CT scanner have seen an unprecedented proliferation of imaging techniques and modalities. Many of these modalities are variations of the basic image-reconstruction techniques used in the CT scanner. For example, computed-emission tomography produces tomographic slices from isotope radiation, and MRI produces tomograms from magnetic fields. On the other hand, ultrasonic imaging developed out of research performed by the Navy during World War II.

The expansion of medical-imaging modalities can be attributed to the convergence of many factors, including a better understanding of the physics underlying basic imaging principles, the development of improved mathematical-reconstruction techniques, and the availability of faster and less expensive computers. Continuing improvements in computer technology produced a trend toward completely digital image generation—even traditional X-ray examinations are now acquired and processed by computers. The acquisition and analysis of such digital X-ray images form the basis for a new field called **digital radiology.**

11.2.2 Automated Interpretation of Medical Images

Success in processing satellite and spacecraft images generated considerable interest in biomedical image processing, including automated image analysis for interpretation. Beginning in the 1960s, researchers devoted a large amount of work to this end, with the hope that eventually much of radiographic image analysis could be automated.

One of the first areas to receive attention was automated interpretation of chest X-ray images, because at that time most patients admitted to a hospital were subjected to routine chest X-ray examinations. (In most hospitals, such routine screening is no longer considered cost-effective, except in selected subgroups of patients.) Much of the work in automated interpretation was done at the University of California at Irvine, at Nagoya University in Japan, at the University of Southern California, and at the University of Pittsburgh. Subsequent research, however, confirmed the difficulty of performing completely automated radiographic-image interpretation. Much of the initial enthusiasm subsided, and research in this area is now less active.

Because of the relative lack of success of automated radiographic interpretation systems, much research has shifted to *enhancing* the images produced by the newer image modalities such as CT or MRI. Some researchers now believe that many of the difficulties of automated image interpretation are due to poor image quality. Thus, if the images can be improved first, then the image-interpretation task (whether performed by human or by computer) will become easier.

11.2.3 Computer-Based Information-Management Systems

The first applications of computers to radiology-information management were developed in the late 1960s. At that time, a study at the Massachusetts General Hospital (MGH) identified two major bottlenecks in the hospital's radiology department: (1) patient-examination scheduling and (2) film-library management. As a consequence of that study, the researchers designed and implemented a system to automate these two functions [Bauman et al., 1975a; Bauman et al., 1975b]. The examination-scheduling system checked for conflicting or duplicate examinations, assigned patients to examination rooms, and assisted in the registration of essential patient data.

It produced flashcards to identify patients' imaging studies, generated requests for patients' master folders in the film library, and automatically produced daily worklists for each examination area. The film-library management system demonstrated one of the first medical uses of bar-code readers and labels (Figure 11.7); bar-coded labels were used to identify film jackets and to track their locations throughout the department. In addition, the system maintained a database of film-library loan transactions.

The system was a precursor of today's RISs, and it has evolved to include a variety of other functions. A particularly important function is online transcription of radiology reports, including the capability for online editing and approval of reports by radiologists. Another feature, incorporated into the MGH system by Greenes and colleagues, was a link to a computer-based surgical-pathology accessioning system. Radiologists had automated access to confirmed pathologic diagnoses, and thus could receive automated feedback on their interpretations [Greenes et al., 1978]. Links to other hospital systems have since been incorporated.

Also in the late 1960s, several groups explored methods to allow radiologists to enter reports into computer-based systems directly, rather than dictating reports for later transcription. The most elaborate was a system developed by Margulies and later enhanced by Wheeler at Johns Hopkins University Hospital [Margulies and Wheeler, 1972]. Researchers created a set of large, graphically oriented displays on

---

EXAMINATION   FORM

Smith, Nancy   F   44 years old
111-11-11   Ambulatory
BARIUM ENEMA   23672   20-Feb-85   9:46 AM
Room: FLU 2
Physician: HEALLY, JAMES R.
History: BLEEDING

Precautions: NONE

Other Exams: NONE

A23672

FIGURE 11.7 Bar-coded patient-examination requisition forms identify the patient and provide information about the examination. (*Source:* Courtesy of R. Gilbert Jost, M.D., Mallinckrodt Institute of Radiology, Washington University Medical Center, St. Louis.)

film. The displays could be selected randomly and back-projected onto a touch-sensitive screen. Radiologists were able to compose narrative reports by touching appropriate areas of the screen to select words, phrases, and even pictures. Branching from one display to another was controlled by the choices selected by the radiologist. SIREP, a commercial version of this system, marketed by Siemens, had limited acceptance, although later reimplementations by other companies were also explored (see Figure 11.15, later in this chapter).

Bauman and colleagues at MGH also experimented with using branching hierarchical menus of displays as a means for entry of radiologic reports, but abandoned this project because the approach did not seem to fit well with the radiologists' desire for freedom of expression when creating reports [Bauman et al., 1972]. A similar menu-driven system, called CLIP, was developed by Leeming, Simon, and Bleich at Beth Israel Hospital in Boston [Leeming and Simon, 1982]. Radiologists choose from lists of statements by indicating the alphanumeric code for the desired phrase, then modify the selected statements by inserting appropriate adjectives and adverbs. The report-generation system developed in the late 1960s by Lehr and colleagues at the University of Missouri at Columbia allowed radiologists to compose reports by concatenating symbols that represented sentences or phrases. They could append additional free text to the report by typing it into the terminal. This system later added patient-registration, scheduling, and film-tracking capabilities, to become a full-function RIS known as MARS [Lehr et al., 1973]. More recently, systems that combine voice input with selection from screen-based menus have been explored [Robbins et al., 1987].

Most existing RISs facilitate the management of standard film-based images. The development of computer-based approaches to digital-image management is a relatively new area of activity, made feasible by advances in direct digital-image generation, high-bandwidth network communication, very large-volume data-storage technology, and microcomputer-based workstations. Many investigators are working to design systems for managing digital images; however, no mature systems yet exist. It is too early to predict how quickly the prototype systems described in Section 11.4.4 will evolve into fully functional systems capable of supporting entire departments. Technical advances are making the all-digital radiology department a possibility; the large costs for labor, space, and materials (especially film) associated with traditional film-based systems are making it a necessity.

11.3 Fundamental Concepts for Computer-Based Radiology Systems

A **digital image** typically is represented in a computer by a two-dimensional array of numbers (a *bit-map*; see Chapter 4). Each element of the array represents the intensity of a small square area of the picture, called a **pixel.** If we consider the image of a volume, then a three-dimensional array of numbers is required; each element of the array in this case represents a volume element, called a **voxel.**

We can store any image in a computer in this manner, either by converting it from an analog to a digital representation, or by generating it directly in digital form. Once an image is in digital form, it can be handled just like all other data. It can be transmitted over communications networks, stored compactly in databases on magnetic or optical media, and displayed on graphics monitors. In addition, the use of computers has created an entirely new realm of capabilities for image generation and analysis; images can be computed rather than measured directly. Furthermore, digital images can be manipulated for display or analysis in ways not possible with film-based images.

11.3.1 Imaging Parameters

All images can be characterized by several parameters of image quality. The most useful of these parameters are spatial resolution, contrast resolution, and temporal resolution. These parameters have been widely used to characterize traditional X-ray images; they also provide an objective means for comparing images formed by digital imaging modalities. (See Chapter 4 for a discussion of spatial and contrast resolution of bit-mapped images.)

- **Spatial resolution** is related to the sharpness of the image; it is a measure of how well the imaging modality can distinguish points on the object that are close together. For a digital image, spatial resolution is determined by the number of pixels per image area.
- **Contrast resolution** is a measure of the ability to distinguish small differences in intensity, which in turn are related to differences in measurable parameters, such as X-ray attenuation. For digital images, the number of bits per pixel determines the contrast resolution of an image.
- **Temporal resolution** is a measure of the time needed to create an image. We consider an imaging procedure to be a *real-time* application if it can generate images at a rate of at least 30 per second. At this rate, it is possible to produce unblurred images of the beating heart.

Other parameters that are specifically relevant to medical imaging are the amount of risk to the patient, the degree of invasiveness, the dosage of ionizing radiation, the degree of patient discomfort, the size (portability) of the instrument, the ability to depict physiologic function as well as anatomic structure, and the cost of the procedure.

A perfect imaging modality would produce images with high spatial, contrast, and temporal resolution; it would be low in cost, portable, free of risk, painless, and noninvasive; it would use **nonionizing radiation;** and it would depict physiologic function as well as anatomic structure. A primary reason for the proliferation of imaging modalities is that no single modality satisfies all these requirements—each is strong along one or more of the dimensions and weak along others (Table 11.1). Selection of the most appropriate modality for a particular diagnostic problem requires a tradeoff among these various dimensions.

Traditional X-ray images have high spatial resolution and medium cost. Furthermore, they can be generated in real time (fluoroscopy) and can be produced using

TABLE 11.1 Comparative Imaging Parameters for Alternative Imaging Modalities

	CT	MRI	US	NM	DSA	Digital X ray	Film X ray
Pixels per image	$(256–512)^2$	256^2	512^2	128^2	512^2	1000^2	2000^2
Bits per pixel	11–13	10	8	8	10	12	14
Spatial resolution	mod	low	mod	low	mod	high	high
Contrast resolution	high	low	low	low	mod	high	low
Radiation	mod	none	none	mod	mod	low	mod
Cost	high	high	mod	mod	mod	mod	low
Physiologic function	no	some	no	yes	no	no	no
Portability	no	no	yes	yes	no	no	yes

CT = computed tomography; MRI = magnetic resonance imaging; US = ultrasound imaging; NM = nuclear-medicine imaging; DSA = digital subtraction angiography; mod = moderate.

portable instruments. Their disadvantages are their relatively poor contrast resolution, their use of ionizing radiation, and their inability to depict physiologic function. Alternate imaging principles have been applied to increase contrast resolution, to eliminate exposure to X-ray radiation, and so on.

Improvements in one aspect, however, often are achieved at the expense of degradations in other aspects. For example, the strengths of nuclear-medicine techniques are the abilities to depict physiologic function and to improve contrast resolution by imaging only the organ in which the molecules accumulate. On the other hand, nuclear-medicine images have poor spatial resolution. Opacifying agents improve contrast resolution, but can be used only in areas where a cavity can be filled with radiopaque contrast material (for example, the heart, blood vessels, or intestinal tract). In addition, the procedure is invasive and entails some risk to patients. Ultrasound imaging, currently the modality of choice for prenatal examinations, has the advantages of low cost, noninvasive nature, small instrument size, high temporal resolution, and avoidance of ionizing radiation. Its disadvantages include relatively poor spatial resolution and an inability to image through bone or air. MRI uses nonionizing radiation to produce high-contrast images that depict physiologic function. Currently, however, it is expensive, and it provides poor temporal resolution.

11.3.2 Functional Images

The extraordinary contribution of computers to image generation is the ability to compute images that cannot be generated directly. CT scans are prime examples of such computed or **functional images.** A revolution in medical imaging has been brought about by CT's ability to portray structures without superposition and to enhance contrast resolution greatly.

Although both standard X-ray and CT images can be represented as digital images, the numbers in the pixel array represent different types of quantities. For a standard X-ray image, each pixel value is directly related to the observed intensity of the X rays striking the film. Thus, a digital X-ray image uses numbers to represent *measurable* parameters. On the other hand, the numbers (pixel values) in a CT image represent *computed* values for the X-ray attenuation within small squares of tissue along a slice through the body. These values cannot be measured directly; rather, they must be computed from a large number of measurements. Thus, a computed tomogram is a *functional image*—each pixel value is a function of other directly measurable parameters.

Figure 11.8 illustrates the basic imaging technique developed for first-generation CT scanners. The patient is placed between an X-ray–sensitive detector and an X-ray source that produces a collimated (pencillike) beam. The measured difference between the source and detector X-ray intensities represents the amount of X-ray attenuation due to the tissues traversed by the beam; this measured attenuation is a superposition, or *projection,* of the attenuations of all the individual tissue elements traversed by the beam. In the simplest reconstruction method, called **back-projection,** the measured intensity is distributed uniformly over all the pixels traversed by the beam. For example, if the measured attenuation is 20, and 10 pixels were traversed, then the CT number of each of the 10 pixels is incremented by 2 units.

The attenuation measured from a single projection is not sufficient to reconstruct an image. The same back-projection computation, however, can be applied to the attenuations measured from multiple projections. The source and detector are translated and rotated about the patient, and the X-ray attenuation is measured along each path. Because each pixel is traversed by multiple projection paths, its computed attenuation is the sum of the contributions from each path. This sum provides a reasonable first approximation of the X-ray attenuation of the individual pixel. The image is further refined using a mathematical edge-enhancement technique called **convolution.** In effect, convolution removes shadows that result from the back-projection, thus sharpening the blurry image.

This basic method of reconstruction from projections also has been applied to other modalities, including MRI, ultrasound-transmission tomography, and variants of nuclear-medicine imaging called positron–emission tomography (PET) and single-photon–emission computed tomography (SPECT).

11.3.3 Image Analysis

Many researchers have attempted to build systems that analyze medical images automatically, both because automated interpretation has medical utility and because medical images raise provocative theoretical issues related to perception. To date, a complete solution to the problem has eluded researchers; no practical systems for automatic image interpretation currently exist.

Image analysis requires visual **pattern recognition**—a perceptual process for which humans are particularly well adapted. Computers, on the other hand, perform notoriously poorly on perceptual tasks, such as vision and speech understanding. It still is a matter of debate whether computers, at least in their present form, ever will be able to duplicate human pattern-recognition abilities. Some researchers believe that a solution to image-analysis problems lies in a deeper understanding of human intelligence.

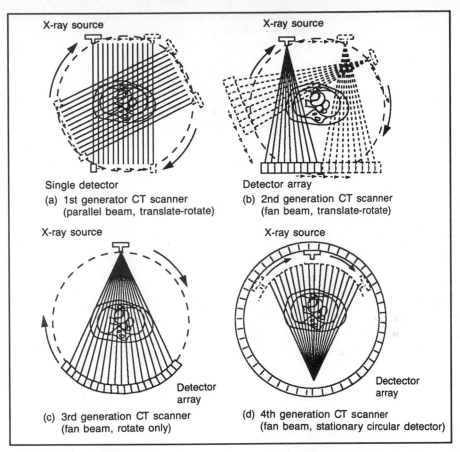

FIGURE 11.8 (a) First-generation CT scanners use a pencil beam defined by a well-collimated X-ray source and a single detector, which translate-rotate through 180 degrees in about 300 seconds. (b) Second-generation scanners use a small linear array of detectors to speed up data acquisition to about 20 seconds using fan-beam geometry. (c) Third-generation systems use a large array of detectors (usually circular), and the source and detector array can rotate through 360 degrees in less than 5 seconds. (d) Fourth-generation systems use a fixed circular array of many detectors and an X-ray source inside (or outside) of the detector ring that can rotate 360 degrees in less than 5 seconds. (*Source:* Courtesy of Dr. Richard A. Robb, Mayo Clinic. Adapted with permission from Robb, R. A. X-ray computed tomography: An engineering synthesis of multiscientific principles. *CRC Critical Reviews in Biomedical Engineering,* 7(4):265–334, 1982. Copyright CRC Press, Inc., Boca Raton, FL.)

Although completely automated interpretation is unlikely to be developed soon, systems that offer partially automated interpretation are available. These systems typically solve subtasks of the overall interpretation task. Often, they interact with the user (the radiologist or technician); users guide the computer using their intelligence and expertise, whereas the computer performs the computational and repetitive tasks. Because many image-interpretation tasks are tedious for humans to perform, even limited help from the computer is desirable.

Pattern recognition and image analysis can be divided into four subtasks: (1) global processing, (2) segmentation, (3) feature detection, and (4) classification. These subtasks are analogous to operations that scientists believe the human brain performs as it processes sensory input.

Global processing involves computations on the entire image, without regard to specific local content. The purpose is to enhance an image for human visualization or for further analysis by the computer. Global processing is the most active and most successful area of image-analysis research, because it applies well-understood physical-imaging principles developed by the aerospace industry to enhance images from outer space. Increasingly, these techniques are being applied to medical-image analysis.

One common example of global processing is *gray-scale windowing* of CT images. The CT scanner generates CT numbers in the range of −1000 to +1000 (−3000 to +4000 on newer-generation equipment). Humans, however, cannot distinguish more than about 100 shades of gray. To appreciate the full precision available with a CT image, the operator can adjust the midpoint and range of the displayed CT values. By changing the *level* and *width* of the display, radiologists enhance their ability to perceive small changes in contrast resolution within a subregion of interest. (At the same time, they sacrifice resolution in other areas of the image.) Compare Figure 11.9 to Figure 11.2; these figures show the same digital CT image displayed with different window level and width settings.

Another example of global processing applied to CT images is *histogram equalization,* in which the statistical distribution of gray levels in the image is made uniform. Such *smoothing* of the histogram often improves the contrast resolution of images. In addition, a variety of *filtering algorithms* can be applied in image processing to remove equipment noise, to enhance edges, and to sharpen blurry images. Clayton and Parker's article on digital subtraction angiography (DSA; discussed in Section 11.4.1), cited in the Suggested Readings, describes several common filtering techniques that have been applied to improve the quality of DSA images.

During the **segmentation** phase, regions of interest are extracted from the overall image. The regions usually correspond to anatomically meaningful structures, such as organs or parts of organs. The structures may be delineated by their borders, in which case *edge-detection* techniques (such as edge-following algorithms) are used, or by their composition on the image, in which case *region-detection* techniques (such as texture analysis) are used. Neither of these types of techniques has been completely successful; regions often have discontinuous borders or nondistinctive internal composition. Furthermore, contiguous regions often overlap. These and other complications make segmentation the most difficult subtask of the medical image-analysis problem.

An analogy developed by Herbert Simon helps to illustrate the limitations of current segmentation techniques. Imagine an ant crawling around on an image. The ant is able to see only those portions of the image near where it is standing—it has no way to "stand back" and get a global picture. Thus, if it is following along some edge, it will get lost if the edge disappears, or if the edge merges into the edge of an abutting region. The computer, like the ant, can "see" only one pixel at a time.

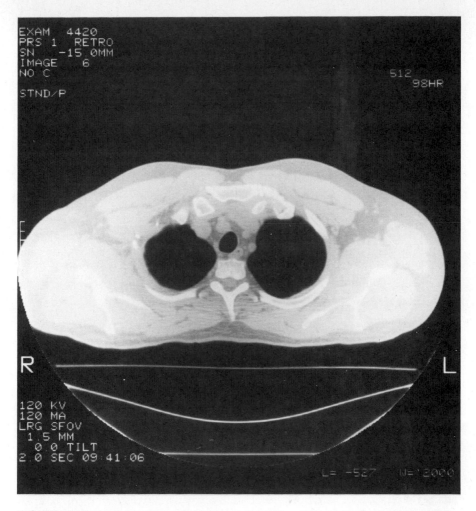

FIGURE 11.9 The same CT image as Figure 11.2 with a different window level and width, optimized to show lung tissue. (*Source:* Courtesy of Dr. William Shuman, Department of Radiology, University of Washington, Seattle.)

Because of the difficulty of the segmentation process, most systems require humans to perform segmentation manually.

Feature detection is the process of extracting useful parameters from the segmented regions. These parameters may themselves be informative—for example, the volume of the heart or the size of the fetus. They also may be used as input into an automated **classification** procedure, which determines the type of object found. For example, small round regions on chest X-ray images might be classified as tumors, depending on such features as intensity, perimeter, and area.

Mathematical models often are used to aid in the performance of image-analysis subtasks. In classical pattern-recognition applications, the subtasks of global processing, segmentation, feature detection, and classification usually are performed sequentially. People, however, appear to perform pattern-recognition iteratively. For example, radiologists can perceive faint images and can trace discontinuous borders, in part because they know for which features they are searching. Some researchers have applied artificial-intelligence (AI) techniques to imitate such interaction among subtasks. The computer is programmed with some of the higher-level anatomic knowledge that radiologists use when interpreting images. Thus, high-level organ models provide feedback to guide the lower-level process of segmentation.

11.3.4 Image Management

Most current research and development projects in PACS technology are collaborative endeavors between departments of radiology and vendors of radiologic equipment. The development of comprehensive systems that integrate image-acquisition instruments, image-archiving devices, viewing consoles for interpretation, and communications networks for transmitting imaging information is a massive undertaking that requires a thorough understanding of how radiology departments operate and how radiologists function.

Technologies for Image Archiving

Online archiving of image data for a busy radiology department requires vast amounts of storage. The number of bits that are required to store a radiologic study depends on several factors: the size of each image, the number of images in the examination, whether raw or postprocessed data are stored, and whether data-compression techniques are used.

A CT image, for example, may consist of a 256×256, 320×320, or 512×512 array of pixels. If the full dynamic range of CT numbers is saved, each pixel is represented using 11 to 13 bits. Once the radiologist or technologist has determined the optimal settings for displaying the region of interest, however, perhaps only 8 bits per pixel must be saved. A typical CT examination consists of 15 or 20 cross-sectional slices. Additional slices are required if both precontrast and postcontrast images, or other special slices, are desired. Assuming that a CT examination consists of 30 images, and assuming that the full dynamic range is retained, then $30 \times 512 \times 512 \times 13$, or approximately 100 million, bits must be saved. **Data-compression** techniques can reduce this total by a factor of three without loss of resolution, or by as much as a factor of eight, with some loss of information.

A single-view chest X-ray image consists of $2048 \times 2048 \times 14$ bits of data; therefore a typical frontal- and lateral-view examination contains about 110 million bits. A real-time ultrasound examination generates video images at 30 frames per second. Of these, a radiologist usually selects 30 to 40 frames for later analysis. Occasionally, dynamic sequences, such as those portraying a cardiac arrhythmia, are retained at the full rate of 30 images per second. Resolution per image is 512×512 pixels; about 8 bits per pixel are required to store the acoustical signal once the image has been postprocessed for optimal viewing. Nuclear-medicine images have lower resolution—typically, $128 \times 128 \times 8 = 131{,}072$ bits of data are sufficient. MRI has requirements similar to those of CT, except that data are available for a volume of the body rather than for single slices, and data on several parameters at each voxel are potentially useful.

Considering that a typical radiology department performs 250 examinations per day, and nominally assuming 25 million bits per study, then in an average day approximately 6 billion bits of data must be transmitted from the image-acquisition nodes to the image archive. Assuming 250 working days per year (ignoring weekends for simplicity), we estimate that the storage requirements per year for examination image data are on the order of 10^{12} bits. Data compression and prior selection or preprocessing of image data can reduce this number considerably.

In addition to the online maintenance of active images, an image-archiving system must provide for the storage of less current image data. Because of the large storage requirements, practical systems will use some form of hierarchical storage management, whereby the most current images are easily and rapidly accessible, and images that are less likely to be retrieved are stored in a less costly, less accessible form.

Optical-disc technology is the most promising medium for online storage of image data. Storage capacities on a single platter of 10^{10} bits are possible, and jukebox arrangements with 100 platters (optical discs) permit online access to 10^{12} bits (approximately 1 year of data in our example). Optical discs are inexpensive, on the order of $100 per platter, and should become even less costly as their use increases. Although the earliest discs could be written only once, newer discs permit optically stored data to be erased and rewritten multiple times. Magnetic storage media also are undergoing dramatic increases in capacity and decreases in price, although they are not yet competitive with the projections for optical-disc storage. It is likely that magnetic-disk storage will remain for some time as the medium of choice for intermediate storage, such as that required in distributed nodes of the image network. Various media are being considered for longer-term storage, including magnetic tape, optical discs, and laser cards.

Technologies for Image Interpretation and Review

A major task of PACS researchers is the development of monitors for viewing and interpreting digital images. The design of image-viewing consoles, suitable for interpretation of examinations by radiologists, poses a host of technical and human-engineering problems—to be acceptable, consoles must match the low cost, convenience, and flexibility of the illuminated light boxes used for interpreting film-based images.

Radiologists usually interpret the results of an examination by comparing multiple images, both from the current examination and from previous or correlative studies. Flexibility is crucial as they organize and reorganize the images to display temporal sequence, to reflect anatomic organization, and to compare preintervention versus postintervention views (such as when contrast injection is used). Furthermore, when radiologists analyze an image, their attention shifts rapidly between overview or general pattern-recognition modes of viewing and detailed inspection of specific areas. The ability to reshuffle images, to shift attention, to zoom in on a specific area, and to step back again to get an overview is essential to the interpretive and analytic processes. These effects are easy to achieve with film, but are difficult to replicate on a viewing console.

Experience with CT underscores the challenges of designing viewing consoles for image interpretation. CT is the quintessential digital imaging modality. Furthermore, viewing consoles are available to and operated by radiologists. Nonetheless, virtually all interpretation of CT scans still is done on film. The viewing console associated with a CT scanner permits the technologists to retrieve single images (slices) one at a time, to manipulate the image's gray scale for detailed inspection, and to perform limited analyses. Typically, however, it does not allow the operator to view all the images of a study concurrently, to rearrange them, or to zoom in rapidly on particular images for detailed inspection. For these reasons, the CT console is used only to determine whether patients have been properly positioned, to monitor the progress of studies, and to optimize the display before images are photographed onto sheets of film. Radiologists then interpret the film, returning to the viewing console only if they have particular questions that they cannot answer using the filmed images.

For example, the radiologist may want to use the viewing console to support general image-manipulation operations, such as gray-scale manipulation, histogram equalization, edge enhancement, image subtraction, online measurement, and other operations radiologists perform while analyzing images. The display of three-dimensional imaging data will place even greater demands on consoles to calculate and redisplay oblique slices and rotated views rapidly. In addition, some interpretation requires image-specific processing capabilities; for example, mathematical models may be used to calculate cardiac volume or fetal weight.

It is not yet clear to what extent special capabilities can or should be incorporated in the design of generic viewing consoles. Such features might more appropriately be associated with the image-acquisition device itself. This issue is particularly relevant for MRI data manipulation, because of the specialized nature of an MRI database. MRI data are inherently three-dimensional. Each point typically is associated with multiple data values, the interpretations of which are also dependent on a variety of data-acquisition and examination parameters. Considerable human engineering and experimentation will be necessary before practical image-interpretation consoles are designed.

Fortunately, a radiology department will require only a moderate number of sophisticated image-interpretation workstations. Consoles for reviewing examinations that already have been preprocessed and interpreted require significantly lower resolution, less processing and data-transmission capability, and smaller local memory— even an analog video image might be acceptable for review. Monitors for review and consultation, however, must be easily accessible, and thus must be conveniently distributed throughout an institution.

Technologies for High-Speed Image Networking

The integration of distributed viewing stations, online image databases, image-management systems, and broadband local-area networks (LANs) will allow imaging data to be shared among health professionals at remote viewing sites. Furthermore, the data can be viewed at multiple locations simultaneously. Thus, health personnel throughout an institution can have timely and convenient access to medical images.

The principal media for image transmission and networking are broadband coaxial cable and fiberoptic cable (see Chapter 4). Coaxial cable, used in the cable-television industry, supports a variety of network topologies. Coaxial networks are relatively inexpensive; they also are reliable, although they are susceptible to electrical and radio-frequency interference. Fiberoptic networks offer a high degree of reliability without interference problems, but they currently are limited with respect to the topologies that they can support and the ease with which connections can be added. A crucial consideration is that the maximum load and the rate of data transmission must be able to support the communication needs of the department.

In addition to identifying the hardware required for networking, PACS developers must agree on formats for the data to be transmitted and protocols for network communication. Standardization of network protocols using conventions such as the ISO OSI reference model (see Chapter 4) is important to ensure that a wide variety of equipment can be interfaced with the network and that the data can be recognized and interpreted correctly by all the nodes on the network. To this end, the National Equipment Manufacturers Association and the American College of Radiology have cooperated to create standard formats for image data [Lodwick, 1984].

11.4 Current Applications of Computers in Radiology

The radiology department provides examples of the most dramatic health-care computing applications to date. The use of computers in radiology has produced fundamental advances in image generation and image analysis, in addition to facilitating the communication and management of images and radiologic information.

11.4.1 Image Generation

The most striking examples of new radiology applications are the digital imaging modalities themselves. Revolutionary developments in image generation have transformed the field of radiology from a narrow, ancillary discipline into a dynamic medical specialty. Digital radiography, CT, MRI, and other computing applications provide fertile ground for both clinical and medical-computing research.

Digital Subtraction Angiography

An important use of digital radiography is **digital subtraction angiography (DSA)**—a radiologic technique for imaging blood vessels, such as the cerebral, pulmonary, and coronary arteries. A common application of DSA is the visualization of the carotid-artery bifurcation (branching) in the neck as a diagnostic test in the setting of a stroke. Pieces of atherosclerotic plaque that have accumulated in this region sometimes break off and travel through the bloodstream to the brain, where they can cause strokes— DSA is used to determine the degree of blockage at the carotid bifurcation.

The poor contrast resolution of conventional X-ray images prohibits visualization of the bifurcation directly. Thus, radiologists use angiographic techniques (they inject radiopaque contrast material into the circulatory system) to distinguish the vessels from the background. The way to visualize the carotid bifurcation while posing the least risk to the patient would be to inject the contrast through a peripheral vein, and to let it circulate to the carotid arteries. Because the contrast has to circulate through the heart and lungs before it reaches the carotid arteries, however, the resultant concentration is too low to allow adequate visualization of the area. Conventionally, radiologists have overcome this problem by inserting a catheter into an artery and threading the catheter to the carotid bifurcation, where the contrast can be injected in a high enough concentration to allow visualization. (Arterial injection carries a greater risk than does venous injection.)

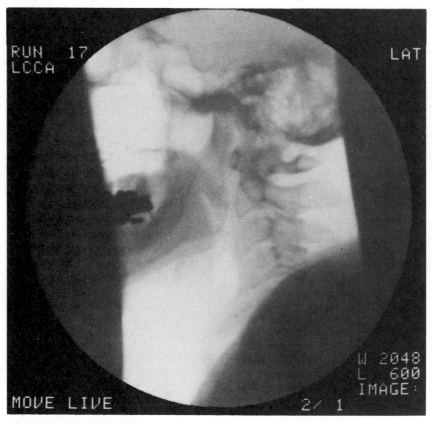

(a)

FIGURE 11.10 (a) Digital subtraction angiography (DSA) of the carotid begins with the creation of a *mask*—a fluoroscopic image that is digitized and saved in a computer. (b) Contrast material is then injected into an artery through a catheter, and a second series of contrast-enhanced X-ray images is taken and digitized. (c) In the final step, the computer subtracts the mask image from each contrast image leaving only the artery that contained the contrast material. (*Source:* Courtesy of Douglas M. Coldwell, M.D., Ph.D., and Joseph Eskridge, M.D., Department of Radiology, University of Washington, Seattle.)

The DSA technique increases visualization of low concentrations of contrast material, and therefore has been used to overcome the limitations of conventional angiography. The digital-radiography hardware is used to record a *mask* image of the vessels before contrast is injected; this mask is stored in the computer memory. Contrast is then injected and the mask image is *subtracted* from the current images in real-time. The dedicated processor performs the subtraction by simply subtracting the intensity numbers of corresponding pixels in the two images. The output images portray the *difference* between the mask image and the contrast-injected images. Ideally, the only differences between the mask image and later images are the regions where contrast material has accumulated. Thus, the output images show only the blood vessels—background tissues are subtracted out (Figure 11.10). Although the concept behind this technique is simple, DSA would be impractical without the advances in hardware that have allowed it to be performed in real time.

Initially, researchers hoped that contrast material could be injected through a peripheral vein; in practice, however, the amount of contrast material that reaches the region of interest is still not enough. Thus, although DSA is routinely employed

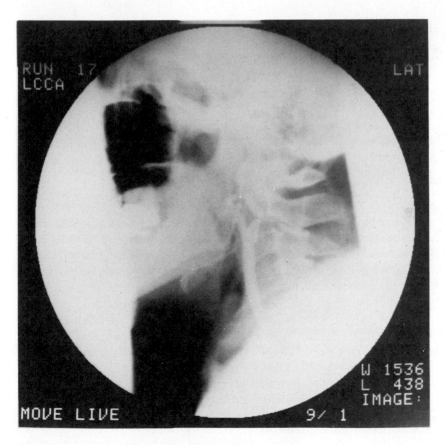

(b)

FIGURE 11.10 *Continued.*

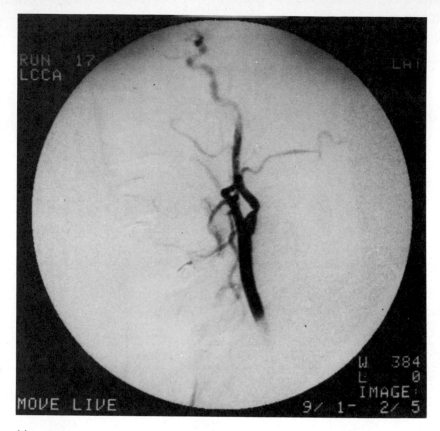

(c)

FIGURE 11.10 *Continued.*

in angiographic procedures, arterial injections continue to be used. DSA is still useful, however, because less contrast material must be injected, images are produced in real time, and the digital images can be manipulated using image-enhancement techniques.

DSA has been especially useful for imaging structures within the skull, because the overshadowing image of the skull can be subtracted out. It also has been used successfully to visualize the renal arteries, where (as in imaging of the carotid arteries) motion is minimal and high resolution is not a major factor. DSA has been used with less success for imaging other structures, such as the coronary arteries, where motion is unavoidable and resolution is more critical. If the body part moves between the creation of the mask and the creation of the new image, the subtraction technique will not work, because the area filled with contrast no longer will be the only part of the image that has changed. Image-enhancement techniques to remove motion artifacts in DSA images are a subject of active research.

Three-Dimensional Image Generation

The images produced by CT, MRI, and PET are *planar slices* through the body. It is possible to acquire parallel, closely spaced stacks of slices in order to image complete three-dimensional volumes. Current CT scanners, for example, have the ability to store collections of parallel slices, then to manipulate the data to produce images of slices with planar orientations different from those acquired originally. A drawback with conventional CT scanners is that they generally acquire data for one slice, or at most for a few slices, through the body at one time. From 2 to 6 seconds are required to complete each scan, and additional time is taken to move the patient for the next parallel scan. Therefore, patient or organ movement, which interferes with accurate reconstructions, is likely to occur. For the heart, the system can *gate* (time) the acquisition of images by coordinating with the ECG, such that each image is acquired at the same point in the cardiac cycle. Artifacts caused by other movement (such as from breathing) remain problematical.

A research group at the Mayo Clinic in Rochester, Minnesota has developed a real-time three-dimensional CT scanner [Robb, 1982]. The system achieves real-time volume imaging by partially surrounding the patient with a semicircle of 28 X-ray sources, rather than depending on the usual single source. A fluorescent screen is fixed on the side of the patient opposite to the X-ray source, and the entire source-detector assembly rotates about the patient. Each source produces a cone beam that gives rise to a two-dimensional image, which is projected onto the fluorescent screen. Images are scanned by a video camera, then are digitized and processed by special-purpose hardware. The large number of X-ray sources, plus the fact that each produces a two-dimensional projection, allows a complete three-dimensional volume image to be processed in real time.

Researchers also have produced three-dimensional ultrasound data by attaching position-locating devices to commercial two-dimensional ultrasound scanners [Brinkley et al., 1982]. Figure 11.11 shows a computer reconstruction, based on ultrasound images, of a fetus in a water bath. A series of arbitrarily oriented ultrasound scans of the fetus were acquired, then were outlined with a light pen. A custom-built position locater identified the three-dimensional position of each scan, and a computer combined the position and outline information to produce a perspective view of the fetus. Each contour in the display represents a single ultrasound slice, after that slice has been outlined and displayed in its three-dimensional relationship to all the other slices. Practical application of this type of system awaits the development of faster and more accurate three-dimensional locating devices, as well as less tedious methods for extracting the organ contours.

11.4.2 Image Analysis

Although completely automated image-analysis systems are still in the future, many partial systems have been developed. A review of the current literature reveals numerous examples of computer-assisted image interpretation. For example, computers have been used to classify lesions in lung tissue, to determine the diameters of blood vessels, to measure radiographic changes occurring in rheumatoid arthritis, to study bone morphology, to aid in the diagnosis of periodontal disease, and to assist in the design of joint prostheses.

Segmentation typically is necessary before the image can be analyzed further—for example, radiologists must determine the borders of the heart before they can

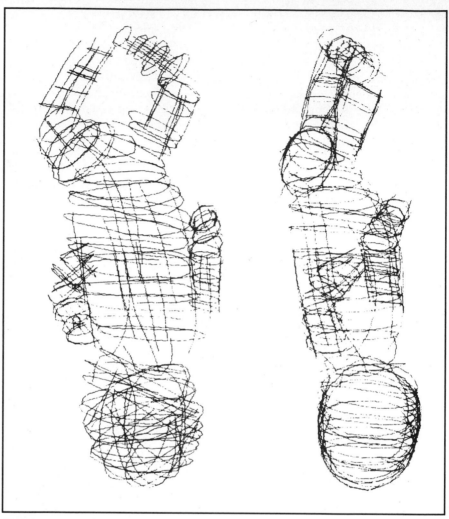

FIGURE 11.11 Each contour line in this computed ultrasound reconstruction of a fetus in a water bath represents one ultrasound slice displayed in its three-dimensional relationship to the other slices. (*Source:* Reprinted with permission from Brinkley, J. F., McCallum, W. D., Muramatsu, S. K., and Liu, D. Y. Fetal weight estimation from ultrasonic three-dimensional head and trunk reconstructions: Evaluation in vitro. *American Journal of Obstetrics and Gynecology,* 144(6):715–721, 1982.)

estimate its volume. The simplest method for finding borders is to have the human operator outline them on a video screen with a light pen or other digitizing device. Manual segmentation is the most common method used for clinical purposes, because automatic systems are still unreliable. The OBUS system employs manual segmentation to measure various fetal diameters and lengths from ultrasound scans [Greenes, 1982]. The system then uses these measurements to estimate gestational age and fetal weight, and compares the latter value to the ideal fetal weight for the estimated gestational age. A typical system for this kind of application is illustrated in Figure 11.12.

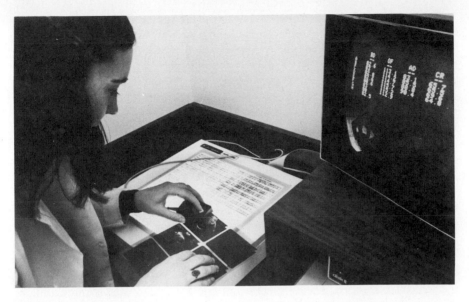

(a)

BRIGHAM & WOMEN'S HOSPITAL
    RADIOLOGY REPORT

(334–8) OBSTETRICAL ULTRASOUND   11 11 11 1
EXAM DATE: 2/21/85
M.D.: BARNES
CLINIC/FLOOR: RH2

LMP: 6/30
PREV US: 10/14   → 33.1 WKS. NOW
CLINICAL SIZE: 30 WKS.

CLINICAL INDICATION: SIZE > DATES

FINDINGS:

GENERAL: single fetus
POSITION: vertex

MEASUREMENTS & CALCULATIONS:
  BPD 77.6   OFD 100.2   AC 244.3
  GA 31.3 WKS   WT 1633 GMS (IDEAL WT 1423 GMS)

ACTIVITY: generally spontaneous; fetal heartbeat seen
MOVEMENT: diaphragm; eye
ANATOMY: neural tube normal; heart normal; GI system normal; GU system normal
AMNIOTIC VOLUME: normal
PLACENTA: normal; posterior; left
IMPRESSION: normal fetal development, consistent with LMP
FOLLOW-UP RECOMMENDED: as indicated

       James A. Smith, M.D.

(b)

FIGURE 11.12 OBUS is a microcomputer-based obstetrical reporting system. (a)
Radiologists use a graphics tablet to choose functions and to enter measurements. (b) The
system then produces summary reports of the findings. (*Source:* Reprinted with permission
from Greenes, R. A. OBUS: A microcomputer system for measurement, calculation, reporting, and retrieval of obstetric ultrasound examinations. *Radiology,* 144:879, 1982.)

This method also has been applied to estimate the volume of the left cardiac ventricle (the main pumping chamber of the heart). Although manual outlining of the ventricle is tedious, it can be used routinely to perform segmentation on ultrasound studies of one or two images. Detailed wall-motion analyses, however, require that a large number of images be outlined precisely to measure small changes in motion. In this case, the manual outlining method is unacceptably time consuming and prone to errors. Thus, researchers have attempted to develop automatic or semiautomatic border-detection techniques.

Most commercial systems for three-dimensional display of CT or MRI images use a simple thresholding technique to segment regions of interest. For example, in CT images, the voxels that represent bone and the voxels that represent soft tissues fall into different ranges of CT numbers. Therefore, it is possible to choose a threshold CT number that falls between the two ranges, and the user can instruct the computer to display only those voxels that fall in the range for bone, or only those that represent soft tissues.

This simple thresholding technique does not always work for soft tissues, because the voxel values do not fall into easily separable ranges. In these cases, edge-following methods often are used. The most common edge-following methods simply follow the organ border, searching pixel by pixel for intensity discontinuities between the organ border and the surrounding tissue. These methods have not been very successful, both because imaging limitations cause the intensity changes to disappear in certain places, and because the local intensity changes merge with spurious borders. More sophisticated systems have provided a two-dimensional tolerance region, or *plan,* within which the computer can search for the border. For example, Yachida used AI search techniques to develop an initial border on the first frame of a sequence, then used this border to guide segmentation in subsequent frames [Yachida et al., 1980].

An alternate approach is to use models to represent anatomical knowledge. This knowledge can then be used by AI programs to guide low-level image-processing subtasks, such as segmentation. For example, Shani at Rochester developed one of the few AI systems for analyzing three-dimensional medical image data. A detailed anatomic model of the kidney is used to provide search regions for finding the image of the kidney in a stack of CT slices [Shani, 1981]. Similarly, models are used to reduce the number of three-dimensional ultrasound data that must be analyzed in an ultrasound modeling system. A training set of ultrasound reconstructions is used to teach the computer the expected shape of classes of objects. This knowledge is then used to direct future analysis of ultrasound data [Brinkley, 1985].

Once the borders of an organ have been segmented on each slice, either manually or semiautomatically, the segmented two-dimensional regions can be assembled in three dimensions, as was done to produce the computer-generated illustration of a fetus in Figure 11.11. More sophisticated computer-graphics techniques may be used to show realistic perspective views of the organ (Figure 11.13). A useful application of this approach is in the design of joint prostheses. Three-dimensional reconstructions are used to identify the shape of the prosthesis precisely and to guide the creation of a mold for the fabrication of the prosthesis.

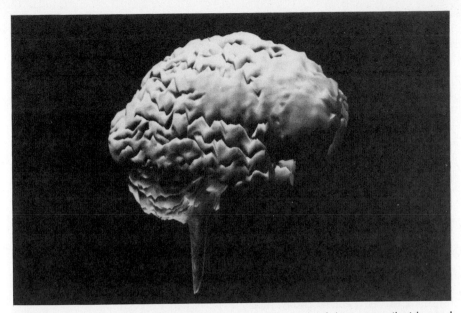

FIGURE 11.13 Three-dimensional reconstruction of the brain of the same patient imaged with MRI in Figure 11.5. The flattening effect of the tumor on the right frontal lobe is clearly seen. This image was created by hand tracing the borders of the brain structures on each of a series of coronal MRI brain sections, then displaying the surface with a graphics program developed by Jeff Prothero. (*Source:* Courtesy of John Sundsten, Jeff Prothero, and Ken Kastella, Department of Biological Structure, University of Washington, Seattle.)

11.4.3 Radiology Information Systems

With the development of new imaging techniques, the volume of and demand for radiologic studies has grown, thus stressing existing manual systems for image and information handling. At the same time, radiology departments face increasing pressures to control costs and to manage resources efficiently. Computer-based RISs rapidly are becoming necessary to schedule equipment and examination rooms for maximum usage, to assist in film-library management, to track the locations of films, and to collect and analyze the data necessary for evaluation and planning decisions. Various RISs currently exist; some are one-of-a-kind systems that have been developed within a particular institution, and others are available commercially.

Until the mid-1980s, one of the most comprehensive RISs in operation was that developed by Arenson and his associates at the Hospital of the University of Pennsylvania (HUP) [Arenson, 1984]. It was based on the system developed at MGH in the early 1970s, and expanded to support a wide range of department functions, including scheduling, patient tracking, film-library management, billing, and management reporting. Although the system now provides essentially all of the functionality outlined in Section 11.1.4, it is not commercially available.

Based on the success of the HUP implementation, a consortium of nonprofit hospitals throughout the United States (the Radiology Information System Consortium, or RISC) was organized in 1982 to design a next-generation RIS that reimplemented and enhanced the original features of the HUP system, as well as to explore and develop other radiologic applications [Arenson et al., 1982]. By 1988, RISC had almost 40 institutional members, among them many of the major teaching hospitals of the United States. The RIS specified by RISC, known as DECrad, was implemented by Digital Equipment Corporation and has been installed successfully at some member sites, as well as elsewhere.

Jost and colleagues at Mallinckrodt Institute of Radiology in St. Louis also have developed a successful comprehensive RIS [Jost et al., 1982]. One of its most interesting features is the degree to which it collects operational and process-control data. The system routinely monitors events related to patient care and provides up-to-the-minute summary statistics about the operation of the department (Figure 11.14). Thus, managers can monitor information (such as durations of patients' waits, numbers of examinations in progress, and numbers of untyped or unsigned reports) and can identify developing problems. The Missouri Automated Radiology System (MARS), developed at the University of Missouri, Columbia in the early 1970s, also has evolved into a comprehensive system, although its initial focus was on exploring methods of capturing diagnostic reports in structured rather than free-text form [Lehr et al., 1973]. MARS is available commercially from ADAC Corporation.

The report-generation process is the least developed component of RISs; transcription of dictated reports is by far the most common system for report generation. Word processors and VDTs have replaced typewriters, and computers can track the status of reports in the review and approval process. Beyond these functions, however, there has been much experimentation, but no overwhelming success. We described several of the first and best-known report-generation systems in Section 11.2.3. Similar systems employing large-screen graphical menus of words, phrases, and pictorial elements also have been made available commercially. For instance, the Xyram system is based on this approach; it was originally developed at Johns Hopkins University in the early 1970s (Figure 11.15). Except in a few circumstances, however, radiologists generally have not accepted structured forms for composing their reports; most researchers believe that unstructured dictation will be the preferred mode of report generation for the foreseeable future.

For this reason, some investigators have experimented with voice data entry for producing radiology reports. The RTAS system, for example, has been installed successfully in many radiology departments. Radiologists use a touchtone telephone to dictate reports. The voice signals are stored digitally; any authorized health professional using a standard touchtone telephone can access and play back the reports. The voice signals are never analyzed, however; the recorded messages typically are manually transcribed into a traditional reporting system to produce machine-readable reports [Jost, 1986]. The more sophisticated Kurzweil system uses a speech recognizer to generate computer-stored records directly from dictated reports. Currently, however, the choice of words is limited to a lexicon of 1000 to 5000 words. Furthermore, users must pause after pronouncing each word or phrase; the system is unable to recognize continuous speech [Robbins et al., 1987].

Radiologists have shown less resistance to using report-generation systems in domains in which the content and organization of reports are well structured. For

```
SECOND FLOOR      10:48
                  24-Apr-85
                         ARRIVAL  FILMS  DEPARTURE  MINUTES   TYPE OF
   PATIENT NAME          TIME     TAKEN  TIME       ON FLOOR  EXAM

   1   AMES, THEOPOLIS     09:09                        99    ANGIO
   2   SMITH, LUCIA E      09:20                        88    CT
   3   PEALE, FRED         09:58                        50    NEURO
   4   JACOBS, SHELLEY     10:03    10:39               45    CHEST
   5   BORDEN, HELEN       10:16    10:39               32    CHEST
   6   STARR, BEVERLY      10:19                        29    K ARTHR
   7   PAULIEN, HELEN      10:26                        22    BJ
   8   JONES, FRED         10:28                        28    BJ
   9   JOHNSON, WILLIAM    10:29    10:49               19    CHEST
  10   BARNES, HOMER DR    10:33                        15    CT
  11   MERRILL, MARGIE     10:36                        12    BJ
  12   COTTER, RUTH        10:37    10:49               11    CHEST


                                AVERAGE TIME ON FLOOR
                FOR CURRENT ROUTINE EXAMS: 27    FOR DEPARTURES: 32
                FOR CURRENT SPECIAL EXAMS: 57    FOR DEPARTURES: 66
```

(a)

```
                         REPORTING ACTIVITY


   LOCATION       REPORTS    CHARACTERS    LINES    REPTS/HR    CHARS/MIN

   2ND FLOOR        262       74962.0      2065       30.7        146.7

   5TH FLOOR        212       95334.0      2553       25.3        189.5

   8TH FLOOR        126       71766.0      1976       14.8        140.9

   QUEENY TOWER      90       32616.0      1018       10.9         65.8

   WEST PAVILION    165       74610.0      2057       19.4        146.2

   NUCLEAR MED       40       31068.0       812        4.7         61.0


                                       MOST RECENT REPORT
        TODAY'S DATE:   20-Oct-85      REQUISITION #:     D01079050
        STARTING TIME:  07:23          TRANSCRIPTIONIST:  RAB
                                       TIME TRANSCRIBED:  15:53
```

(b)

FIGURE 11.14 Two process-control displays from the radiology information system at the Mallinckrodt Institute of Radiology summarize (a) patient waiting times, and (b) transcription activity. (*Source:* Courtesy of Dr. R. Gilbert Jost, Mallinckrodt Institute of Radiology, Washington University Medical Center, St. Louis.)

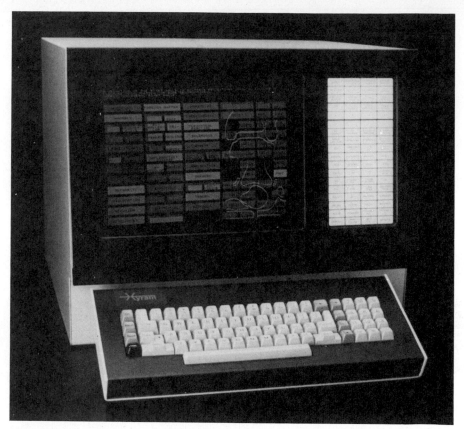

FIGURE 11.15 The Xyram system reporting terminal is a specially designed console used to input radiology reports. (*Source:* Courtesy of Xyram Corporation, New York, New York.)

example, typical obstetrical ultrasound-imaging reports identify the number, orientation, and activity of the fetuses, the site of the placenta, the amount of amniotic fluid, and the presence and normalcy of organs. Radiologists also supply specific measurements of fetal size, estimates of weight and gestational age, and an analysis of fetal growth. In the OBUS system, a graphic tablet or screen-based menu can be used to select the descriptors for composing the report rapidly (see Figure 11.12). The CLIP system, developed and used at the Beth Israel Hospital, currently produces almost 90 percent of reports for CT examinations of the head and spine at that hospital.

11.4.4 Picture-Archiving and Communication Systems

During the last decade, many researchers have worked to develop PACs that support the management of digital imaging data. Some have focused on one or two aspects of the overall PACS problem. Others have attempted to incorporate all the aspects of a PACS. The latter typically use readily available rather than state-of-the-art technologies, and initially concentrate on selected areas of the radiology department.

At the University of Kansas, Templeton and colleagues have developed a prototype system that can be used to study the image-management requirements of a PACS-supported radiology department [Templeton et al., 1988]. A high-speed LAN (initially Ethernet, but later replaced with fiberoptic cable) interconnects three types of nodes within the department: (1) image-acquisition nodes that interface with digitally formatted imaging instruments, (2) interactive-display and image-manipulation nodes, and (3) online and long-term archiving nodes.

Using this prototype system, the group investigated a hierarchical storage strategy and developed a number of projections about network capacity and archival storage requirements. Although the researchers performed a detailed cost analysis in 1982 for digital archiving and management of images in their 614-bed hospital, many of the costs have been substantially reduced since that time as a result of technological advancements [Dwyer et al., 1982]. Studies of the cost-effectiveness of PACSs need to be done based on current technology; we are not aware of any more recent studies updating the earlier estimates. As labor costs of non-PACS image archiving continue to increase, as costs of workstations, networking, and mass storage continue to decrease, and as the PACS technology becomes sufficiently robust to support full-scale implementations, the cost of a PACS probably will be justified readily.

Blaine and colleagues at the Mallinckrodt Institute of Radiology (MIR) in St. Louis have developed a PACS workbench—a set of basic tools and utilities that can be used to study PACS design and to conduct experiments related to image acquisition, transmission, archiving, and viewing [Blaine et al., 1983]. To provide demonstrations and to support research in methods of picture storage, distribution, and presentation, they have compiled a pilot database of medical images. They have also created a library of image-processing routines, carried out studies of image compression, and developed simulations to aid in network design. In addition, they are designing image-interpretation workstations, and are exploring the distribution of analog images as a low-cost way to support remote viewing and evaluation by radiologists and referring physicians of both fluoroscopic- and digital-imaging studies.

Another prototype system has been developed by Arenson and colleagues at the Hospital of the University of Pennsylvania (HUP) [Arenson et al., 1988]. A fiberoptic network, in a star configuration, is used to link digital image-acquisition devices, image-archiving nodes, and image-review stations; the central node of the network—the image manager—is connected to the department's RIS. A primary goal of the HUP project is the development of a comprehensive image database that can be used for image review and consultation throughout the institution. Images that are not already in digital format are digitized from film with a high-resolution digitizer and are stored in the database. Images can be retrieved on request by physicians communicating through the RIS, then transmitted to the requestor on particular channels of a local analog video system so that they can be viewed on standard video monitors. Clinical experience demonstrated that physicians in the medical intensive-care unit had faster access to imaging information using the prototype system than they had with the previous film-based system, and thus were able to take action more quickly when treating patients.

Development of viewing consoles for interpretation has been an active area of research at several sites, both academic and commercial. Researchers have designed workstations that can function as nodes on a network and can download sets of images onto local hard disks. The availability of large local memories allows users to perform a wide range of image-processing functions rapidly, including mathematical transformations for image analysis, enhancement for improved image display, and specialized processing for image recognition and classification. Typically, the workstations are equipped with high-resolution displays of at least 1000×1000 pixels, with 8 bits per pixel. Thus, the displays are capable of portraying fine gradations of gray, and sometimes color.

Often, multiple display monitors are used. One high-resolution monitor displays panels of miniature images, which a user can select and move with a mouse pointing device. Other monitors display selected images in full resolution, or composite displays of regions of interest segmented from several images. The systems may have zoom and roam capabilities and may produce *movie sequences,* in which the parallel slices of structural scans, or the frames of dynamic sequences, are displayed rapidly in succession. A prototype viewing station of this kind, under development by Huang and colleagues at the University of California, Los Angeles, is illustrated in Figure 11.16.

Researchers at the Mayo Clinic have developed a desktop workstation for displaying three-dimensional and four-dimensional (time-varying) images [Erickson and Robb, 1987]. The microcomputer-based system can compute and display orthogonal sections, projection images of volumes from any viewpoint, and shaded surfaces of objects of interest (Figure 11.17). In addition, radiologists can use a joystick to instruct the computer to display oblique sections of three-dimensional images. The system also can help the user to make measurements from the data and to manipulate or segment out portions of the image.

In an attempt to integrate many of the ideas presented over the past decade, the United States Army Medical Research and Development Command selected two centers, the University of Washington in Seattle and the George Washington and Georgetown Universities (working in collaboration) in Washington, D.C., as testbeds for the development and evaluation of comprehensive imaging networks. The University of Washington system will primarily use equipment provided by Philips Medical Systems; the system for George Washington and Georgetown will use equipment provided by American Telephone and Telegraph [Loop et al., 1988]. The initiation of this project, called the Digital Imaging Network/Picture Archiving and Communications System (DIN/PACS), is evidence of researchers' recognition that creating such a network will require cooperation among government, industry, and academia over a long period.

11.5 The Future: The All-Digital Radiology Department

Two major factors will continue to promote the development and acquisition of RISs: increasing demand for radiologic examinations and procedures, and growing pressure to reduce costs in radiology departments. The automation of registration and schedul-

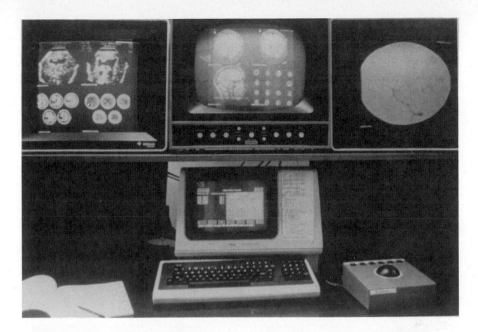

FIGURE 11.16 This image-interpretation workstation being developed by researchers at the University of California at Los Angeles has multiple display monitors. Radiologists can display single images in full resolution or can view composite displays of selected regions segmented from several images. (*Source:* Courtesy of Dr. H. K. Huang, Department of Radiological Sciences, UCLA School of Medicine, Los Angeles.)

ing functions alone justifies the implementation of RISs in busy radiology departments; patients can be moved in and out more quickly, thus increasing the capacity of the department.

The rate of adoption of PACS technology is less certain; many technical and human-engineering problems remain to be solved, and existing systems are prohibitively expensive. The importance of digital imaging for medical diagnosis and treatment continues to grow, however. Furthermore, as PACS-related technologies mature, the costs of optical storage and high-resolution monitors will fall. Eventually, the material and labor costs of film handling and storage will exceed the costs of computer-based systems, and PACSs will become an economic necessity.

Someday, PACSs will routinely connect image-acquisition devices, image-archival devices, and remote viewing stations in electronic networks. Digital images generated by X-ray, CT, MRI, nuclear medicine, and ultrasound instruments will be transmitted to digital archives and stored on optical discs. Radiologists will interpret the images using special image-interpretation workstations with extremely high-resolution monitors. For three-dimensional images, anatomical models will help to segment organs from the surrounding data. Graphics displays will be able to show two-dimensional views of the extracted organ images in different orientations. Holographic and other three-dimensional display methods also will be available for viewing the

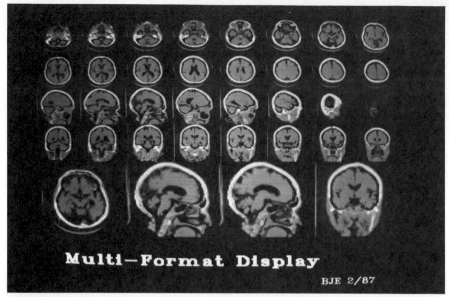

(a)

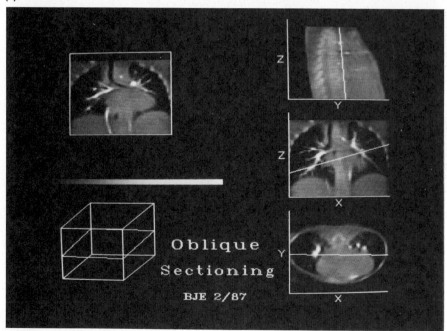

(b)

FIGURE 11.17 A desktop workstation being developed at the Mayo Graduate School of Medicine supports a variety of image-processing capabilities. For example, radiologists can view (a) multiple CT images of the head in various orientations and magnifications or (b) oblique sections through the thorax. (*Source:* With permission from Dr. Richard A. Robb, Director, Mayo Biotechnology Computer Resource, Mayo Foundation, Rochester, MN 55905.)

images. Radiologists will use knowledge-based image-analysis systems that encode clinical and anatomic knowledge to extract important features from the images for viewing and quantitation, and will use decision-support systems (see Chapter 15) to analyze the extracted features and patients' clinical data to arrive at interpretations. For example, the clinical-consultation system may suggest alternative diagnoses that the radiologist has not considered. Radiologists then will use computer-based report-generation systems to produce consultative reports.

As digital images replace analog images in the radiology department, PACSs will assume the functions of the film library. Databases of medical images, available for clinical and research purposes, will be indexed for retrieval by image, by case, by diagnosis, or by feature. The integration of RISs and PACSs will then allow coordination of all the major activities of the radiology department, from examination scheduling and patient registration; to image acquisition, storage, and retrieval; to report generation and distribution.

The radiology department in turn will be integrated with the overall HIS. Thus, health-care personnel throughout the institution will have online access to the images, as well as to radiologists' reports. Conversely, linkages between the RIS and patients' computer-based medical records will allow radiologists to access the clinical data they need to interpret images and to obtain feedback on their work.

Many parts of this scenario already are operational or are well underway at different institutions. Before the full scenario becomes a reality, however, a variety of problems must be solved. Some of the remaining problems are technical; others are financial. As investigators at the various institutions find incremental solutions, we come closer to the goal of the all-digital radiology department.

Suggested Readings

Arenson R. L. (ed). Use of computers in radiology. *The Radiology Clinics of North America*, 24(1):1–133, 1986.

This issue surveys current computer applications in radiology. It includes selections on radiology-information management (including the registration and scheduling process, the automation of film-library functions, and report-generation systems), and discusses issues related to the design of digital image networks and monitors for the display of biomedical images. In addition, one article describes the application of decision-analytic techniques to the selection of diagnostic workups.

Brody, W. R. *Digital Radiography.* New York: Raven Press, 1984.

This book gives a clear, nonmathematical explanation of the field of digital radiography. It provides understandable descriptions of basic image-processing techniques.

Greenes, R. A. OBUS: A microcomputer system for measurement, calculation, reporting, and retrieval of obstetrical ultrasound examinations. *Radiology,* 144:879, 1982.

This article describes OBUS, a microcomputer-based system that facilitates the measurement, analysis, interpretation, reporting, and retrieval of obstetrical ultrasound examinations.

Greenfield, G. B. and Hubbard, L. B. *Computers in Radiology.* New York: Churchill Livingstone, 1984.

One half of this book provides an introduction to computers; the other half discusses image generation and image analysis. Applications chapters on digital radiography, CT, and NMR are included.

Huang, H. K. Biomedical image processing. *CRC Critical Reviews in Bioengineering,* 5(3):185, 1981.

This lengthy but fairly complete survey of biomedical image processing discusses techniques for generating and analyzing medical images, and explains the application of these techniques in radiology, as well as in microscopy.

Jost, R. G., et al. A computer system to monitor radiology department activity: A management tool to improve patient care. *Radiology,* 145:347, 1982.

The authors discuss the use of a computer as a management tool to monitor activity in a radiology department. They describe a number of useful parameters that can be measured and monitored online to facilitate process and management control.

Lodwick, G. S. The ACR-NEMA standardization effort. In Jost, R. G. (ed), *Proceedings of the Eighth Conference on Computer Applications in Radiology.* St. Louis, MO: American College of Radiology, 1984.

This article describes work to develop a standard for the transmission of digital radiologic imaging data.

Parker, D. L. and Clayton, P. D. Computed tomography: The revolution in computer based medical imaging. *M.D. Computing,* 1(1):37, 1984.

This article summarizes the history of computed tomography and explains the application of back-projection and convolution algorithms to reconstruct functional images.

Parker, D. L. and Clayton, P. D. Diagnostic digital angiography: The image revolution continues. *M.D. Computing,* 1(4):48, 1984.

The authors describe the clinical applications of digital subtraction angiography (DSA), review methods for image enhancement, and discuss the technical barriers that compromise the quality of DSA images.

Schneider, R. H. and Dwyer, S. J. (eds). Medical imaging II: Image data management and display. *Proceedings of SPIE 914.* Newport Beach, CA: IEEE Computer Society, 1988.

The proceedings of a yearly conference on PACS, this collection of papers reports research in image processing and the management and display of image data.

Templeton, A. W., et al. An on-line digital image management system. *Radiology,* 152:321, 1984.

The authors describe the design considerations and tradeoffs involved in developing a PACS prototype for the digitally formatted imaging modalities.

Questions for Discussion

1. What is the general principle that underlies computed tomography (CT)? What are three advantages of CT images, as compared to conventional X-ray images?
2. Explain the general principle underlying digital subtraction angiography (DSA). What are three advantages of this method compared to older angiographic techniques?

3. Discuss three reasons why most X-ray images are currently recorded in analog form.

4. Explain what contrast, spatial, and temporal resolution are. State how each is measured.

5. Describe each of the four image-analysis steps a radiologist would apply when interpreting the chest X-ray film of a patient whom she suspects may have a lung cancer.

6. What is the segmentation step in image analysis? Why is it so difficult to perform? Give two examples of ways by which current systems avoid the problem of automatic segmentation. Give an example of how knowledge about the problem to be solved (for example, local anatomy) could be used in future systems to aid in automatic segmentation.

7. Describe the various factors that you must consider when estimating the storage requirements for image data in an all-digital radiology department. What are the major factors that could reduce the volume of data that would have to be maintained in online storage?

8. Refer to Table 11.1. How many bytes are needed to store a digitized chest X-ray image? How many bytes are needed to store a 15-panel computed-tomography study? If you have a communication line that transmits 9600 bits per second, how long will it take to transmit each of these images to the display terminals within the hospital?

9. What are the economic and technologic factors that will determine how quickly hospitals and clinics will adopt all-digital radiology departments?

12

Patient-Monitoring Systems

Reed M. Gardner

After reading this chapter,[1] you should know the answers to these questions:

- What is patient monitoring? Why is it done?
- What are the primary applications of patient-monitoring systems in the intensive-care unit?
- How do computer-based patient monitors aid health professionals in collecting, analyzing, and displaying data?
- What are the advantages of using microcomputers in bedside monitors?
- What are closed-loop and open-loop control systems?
- Why is integration of data from many sources in the hospital necessary if a computer is to assist in the majority of critical-care decisions?

---

[1]Portions of this chapter are based on Gardner, R. M., Sittig, D. F., and Budd, M. C. Computers in the intensive care unit: Match or mismatch? In Shoemaker, W. C., et al. (eds), *Textbook of Critical Care*, 2nd ed. Philadelphia: W. B. Saunders, 1989, p. 248.

12.1 What Is Patient Monitoring?

Frequent measurement of patient parameters (such as heart rate, respiratory rate, blood pressure, and blood-oxygen content) has become a central feature of the care of critically ill patients. When timely and accurate decision making are crucial for providing therapy, patient monitors frequently are used to collect and display physiological data.

We usually think of a **patient monitor** as something that watches for—and warns against—life-threatening events related to a critically ill patient. **Patient monitoring** can be rigorously defined as: "Repeated or continuous observations or measurements of the patient, his or her physiological function, and the function of life support equipment, for the purpose of guiding management decisions, including when to make therapeutic interventions, and assessment of those interventions" [Hudson, 1985, p. 630]. A patient monitor not only should alert health-care professionals to potentially life-threatening events, but also may control devices that maintain life.

In this chapter, we shall discuss the use of computers to aid health professionals in the collection, storage, interpretation, and display of physiological data. Although we shall deal primarily with patients who are in **intensive-care units (ICUs),** the general principles and techniques also are applicable to other hospitalized patients. For example, patient monitoring may be performed for diagnostic purposes in the emergency room, or for therapeutic purposes in the operating room. Techniques that just a few years ago were used only in the ICU are now used routinely on general hospital wards; some even are used by patients at home.

12.1.1 A Case Report

A case report will give you a perspective on the problems faced by the health-care team caring for a critically ill patient. A young man is injured in an automobile accident. He has multiple chest and head injuries. His condition is stabilized at the accident scene by skilled paramedics, using a microcomputer-based ECG monitor, and he is quickly transported to a trauma center. Once in the trauma center, the young man is connected via sensors to computer-based monitors that determine his heart rate, rhythm, and blood pressure. Because of the head injury, the patient has trouble breathing, so he is connected to a computer-supported ventilator. Later, he is transferred to the ICU. The results of clinical chemistry and blood-gas tests are soon transmitted from the laboratory to the ICU via electronic computer networks. The patient survives the early threats to his life and now begins the long recovery process.

Unfortunately, a few days later, the patient is beset with a problem common to multiple trauma victims—he has a major infection and develops problems with several vital organs. As a result, even more monitoring instruments are needed to acquire data and to assist with the patient's treatment; the detailed information required to care for the young man has increased dramatically. The computer provides suggestions about how to care for the specific problems, flags life-threatening situations, and organizes and reports the mass of data so the physicians can make prompt and reliable treatment decisions. Figure 12.1 is an example of a computer-generated ICU

```
                    L D S   H O S P I T A L   I C U   R O U N D S   R E P O R T
                             DATA WITHIN LAST 24 HOURS

NAME:        , STEVEN              NO.   10072      ROOM: E609                   DATE: JAN 29 14:17
DR. STINSON, JAMES B.        SEX: M   AGE:  43  HEIGHT: 178   WEIGHT:  75.40   BSA: 1.93   BEE:  1697   MOF:   0
ADMT DIAGNOSIS: FEVER UNK ORIGN, S/P KIDNEY TR   ADMIT DATE: 14 DEC 88

═══════════════════════════════════════════════════════════════════════════════════════════════════
CARDIOVASCULAR:   0                                          EXAM: _____
        -- NO CARDIAC OUTPUT DATA AVAILABLE
                    SP    DP    MP   HR  | LACT      CPK       CPK-MB      LDH-1      LDH-2
        LAST VALUES  121   68    89  113 |
        MAXIMUM      194   97   126  124 |  (    )    (    )    (    )    (    )    (    )
        MINIMUM      101   58    72   83 ·
═══════════════════════════════════════════════════════════════════════════════════════════════════
RESPIRATORY:   0
            pH    PCO2   HCO3    BE   HB  CO/MT  PO2  SO2  O2CT  %O2  AVO2  VO2   C.O.  A-a  QS/QT  PK/ PL/PP  MR/SR
29 06:21 A  7.43  27.3   18.0  -4.5 10.0  2/ 1   80   94  13.2   30                          66        0/  0/ 5  17/ 0
        SAMPLE # 74, TEMP 38.4, BREATHING STATUS : ASSIST/CONTROL
        NORMAL ARTERIAL ACID-BASE CHEMISTRY
        SEVERELY REDUCED O2 CONTENT (13.2) DUE TO ANEMIA (LOW HB)

            ------- machine settings ------- | ----------------------- patient values -----------------------
            VENT  MODE  VR   Vt   O2%  PF  IP    MAP   PK   PL  PP  m-Vt  c-Vt  s-Vt  MR   SR  TR  m-VE  s-VE  t-VE  Cth   Pc
29 14:15    B-I   A/C   16  700   30   50         32   26   5   866   731         29           21.2             34.8
29 06:05    B-I   A/C   16  700   30   50         22   20   5   830   745         19           14.2             49.7
29 14:15  5/14:16  INTERFACE: TRACH TUBE;  ALARMS CHECKED;  POSITION: SUPINE;  THERAPIST: DAVIS, TERIANNE,  CRTT
29 06:05  10/06:08  INTERFACE: TRACH TUBE;  ALARMS CHECKED;  POSITION: SEMI-FOWLER;  PATIENT CONDITION: CALM;  SUCTIONED, 3 CC,
        HEMOPTIC;  THERAPIST: TARR, TED,  RRT

    DATE    TIME   HR   VR    VT    VC    VE   MIP MEP  MVV  PK FLOW  THERAPIST               EXAM: _____
    01/29/89 07:15  109  20   600        12.0  -60                   DAVIS, TERIANNE
═══════════════════════════════════════════════════════════════════════════════════════════════════
NEURO AND PSYCH:   0
    GLASCOW  6 (08:00) VERBAL _____   EYELIDS _____   MOTOR _____   PUPILS _____   SENSORY _____

    DTR _____      BABIN. _____   ICP _____      PSYCH _____
═══════════════════════════════════════════════════════════════════════════════════════════════════
COAGULATION:   0
    PT:   14.2   (05:15   ) PTT:   50 (05:15   ) PLATELETS:   89 (05:15   ) FIBRINOGEN:   0(00:00) EXAM: _____
    FSP-CON:   0 (00:00   ) FSP-PT:   0 (00:00   ) 3P:           (00:00   )                              _____
═══════════════════════════════════════════════════════════════════════════════════════════════════
RENAL, FLUIDS, LYTES:   0
    IN   3430 CRYST  1025  COLLOID  1035  BLOOD        NG/PO  1340 | NA        (     ) K         (     ) CL        (     )
    OUT  2689 URINE   800  NGOUT     500  DRAINS   25 OTHER   1364 | CO2 21.0 (05:15) BUN    51 (05:15) CRE   4.2 (05:15)
    NET   741 WT   75.40   WT-CHG         S.G.   1.015             | AGAP   16.7        UOSM               UNA       CRCL
═══════════════════════════════════════════════════════════════════════════════════════════════════
METABOLIC --- NUTRITION:   0
    KCAL    2630  GLU 138   (05:15)  ALB   2.9 (05:15) | CA   7.7 (05:15)  FE   .0 (00:00)  TIBC   0 (00:00)
    KCAL/N2  891  UUN    .0 (00:00)  N-BAL  .0         | PO4  1.9 (05:15)  MG  1.9 (05:15)  CHOL 228 (05:15)
═══════════════════════════════════════════════════════════════════════════════════════════════════
GI, LIVER, AND PANCREAS:   0                                                              EXAM:
    HCT   29.4 (05:15)  TOTAL BILI   23.1 (05:15)  SGOT   73 (05:15)  ALKPO4  957 (05:15)  GGT    768 (05:15) _____
    GUAIAC     (    )   DIRECT BILI  17.4 (05:15)  SGPT   99 (05:15)  LDH     237 (05:15)  AMYLASE  0 (00:00) _____
═══════════════════════════════════════════════════════════════════════════════════════════════════
INFECTION:   0
    WBC  5.2(05:15 ) TEMP  40.3 (28/06:00) DIFF  26 B, 70P,  3L,  1M,  E (05:15) GRAM STAIN: SPUTUM _____ OTHER _____
═══════════════════════════════════════════════════════════════════════════════════════════════════
SKIN AND EXTREMITIES:
    PULSES _____    RASH _____   DECUBITI _____
═══════════════════════════════════════════════════════════════════════════════════════════════════
TUBES:
    VEN _____   ART _____   SG _____   NG _____   FOLEY _____   ET _____   TRACH _____   DRAIN_____

    CHEST _____   RECTAL _____   JEJUNAL _____   DIALYSIS _____   OTHER _____
═══════════════════════════════════════════════════════════════════════════════════════════════════
MEDICATIONS:

MORPHINE, INJ                        MGM  IV     20     AMPHOJEL, LIQUID                        ML    NG      30
MEPERIDINE (DEMEROL), INJ            MGM  IV    150     DIPHENHYDRAMINE (BENADRYL), INJ         MGM   IV     100
PHENYTOIN (DILANTIN), SUSPENSION     MGM  NG    300     HYDROCORTISONE NA SUCCINATE (SOLU-CORTEF)MGM, IV     200
MIDAZOLAM (VERSED), INJ              MGM  IV      5     AMIN-AID FULL STRENGTH, LIQUID          ML    NG D  1380
AMPHOTERICIN B, INJ                  MGM  IV     40     TAP WATER, LIQUID                       ML    NG      60
CEFTAZIDIME (FORTAZ), INJ            MGM  IV   1000     MAGNESIUM SULFATE 50%, INJ              GM    IV       2
SUCRALFATE (CARAFATE), TAB           MGM  NG   4000     POTASSIUM CHLORIDE, INJ                 MEQ   IV      20
FAMOTIDINE (PEPCID), INJ             MGM  IV     40     NOVOLIN REGULAR, INJ                    UNITS IV      58
                                                                                                   #087 - pg1
```

FIGURE 12.1 Rounds report used at LDS Hospital in Salt Lake City for evaluation of patients each day during teaching and decision-making rounds. The report abstracts data from diverse locations and sources, and organizes them to reflect the physiological systems of interest. Listed at the top of the report is patient-identification and patient-characterization information. Next is information about the cardiovascular system. Data for other systems follow. (*Source:* Courtesy of LDS Hospital.)

report produced by the HELP system (discussed in Chapter 7). This report summarizes 24 hours of patient data, and is used by physicians to review a patient's status during daily rounds (daily visits by physicians to their hospitalized patients).

12.1.2 Patient Monitoring in Intensive-Care Units

There are at least four categories of patients who need monitoring:
1. Patients with *unstable physiologic regulatory systems*; for example, a patient whose respiratory-control system is suppressed as a result of a drug overdose or anesthesia
2. Patients with a *suspected life-threatening condition*; for example, a patient who has findings indicating an acute myocardial infarction (heart attack)
3. Patients with a *high-risk status*; for example, a patient who has just had open-heart surgery, or a premature infant whose heart and lungs are not fully developed
4. Patients in a *critical physiological state*; for example, a patient with multiple types of trauma

Care of the critically ill patient requires prompt and accurate decisions so that life-protecting and lifesaving therapy can be appropriately applied. Because of these requirements, ICUs have become widely established in hospitals. Such units use computers almost universally for the following purposes:
1. To acquire physiological data, such as blood-pressure readings
2. To communicate data from distant laboratories to the ICU
3. To store, organize, and report data
4. To integrate and correlate data from multiple sources
5. To function as a decision-making tool that health professionals may use in the care of critically ill patients

12.2 Historical Perspective

The earliest foundations for acquiring physiological data date back to the end of the Renaissance period.[2] In 1625, Santorio, who lived in Venice at the time, published his methods for measuring body temperature with the spirit thermometer and for timing the pulse (heart) rate with a pendulum. The principle for both devices had been established by Galileo, a close friend. Galileo worked out the uniform periodicity of the pendulum by timing the period of the swinging chandelier in the Cathedral of Pisa, using his own pulse rate as a timer. The results of this early biomedical-engineering collaboration, however, were ignored. The first scientific report of the pulse rate did not appear until Sir John Floyer published "Pulse-Watch" in 1707. The first published course of fever for a patient was plotted by Ludwig Taube in 1852. With subsequent improvements in the clock and the thermometer, the temperature,

---

[2]This section has been adapted, with permission, from "Computer Monitoring in Patient Care" by D. H. Glaeser and L. J. Thomas, Jr., in the *Annual Review of Biophysics and Bioengineering*, Volume 4, ©1975 by Annual Reviews Inc.

pulse rate, and respiratory rate became the standard **vital signs.** In 1896, Scipione Riva-Rocci introduced the sphygmomanometer (blood-pressure cuff), which permitted the fourth vital sign, arterial blood pressure, to be measured. A Russian physician, Nikolai Korotkoff, applied Riva-Rocci's cuff with a stethoscope developed by the French physician Rene Laennec to allow the auscultatory measurement[3] of both systolic and diastolic arterial pressure. Harvey Cushing, a famous U.S. neurosurgeon in the early 1900s, predicted the need for and later insisted on routine arterial-pressure monitoring. Cushing also raised two questions familiar even at the turn of the century: (1) Are we collecting too many data? (2) Are the instruments used in clinical medicine too accurate? Would not approximated values be just as good? Cushing answered his own questions by stating that vital-sign measurement should be made routinely and that accuracy was important [Cushing, 1903].

Since the 1920s, the four vital signs—temperature, respiratory rate, heart rate, and arterial blood pressure—have been recorded in all patient charts. In 1903 Willem Einthoven devised the string galvanometer for measuring the ECG, for which he was awarded the 1924 Nobel prize in physiology. The ECG has become an important adjunct to the clinician's inventory of tests for both acutely and chronically ill patients. Continuous measurement of physiological variables has become a routine part of the monitoring of critically ill patients.

At the same time that advances in monitoring were made, major changes in the therapy of life-threatening disorders also were occurring. Prompt quantitative evaluation of measured physiological and biochemical variables became essential in the decision-making process as physicians applied new therapeutic interventions. For example, it is now possible—and in many cases essential—to use ventilators when a patient cannot breathe independently, cardiopulmonary bypass equipment when a patient undergoes open-heart surgery, hemodialysis when a patient's kidneys fail to function, and intravenous (IV) nutritional and electrolyte (for example, potassium and sodium) support when a patient is unable to eat or drink.

12.2.1 Development of Intensive-Care Units

To meet the increasing demands for more acute and intensive care required by patients with complex disorders, new organizational units—the ICUs—were established in hospitals beginning in the 1950s; ICUs proliferated rapidly during the late 1960s and the 1970s. The types of units include burn, coronary, general surgery, open-heart surgery, pediatric, neonatal, respiratory, and multipurpose medical–surgical units. By the mid-1980s, there were an estimated 75,000 adult, pediatric, and neonatal intensive-care beds in the United States.

The development of **transducers** and instrumentation electronics during World War II dramatically increased the number of physiological variables that could be monitored. Analog computer technology was widely available, as were oscilloscopes—

---

[3]In medicine, auscultation is the process of listening to the sounds made by structures within the body, such as by the heart or by the blood moving within the vessels.

electronic devices used to picture changes in electrical potential on a cathode-ray tube (CRT) screen. These devices were soon used in specialized cardiac-catheterization[4] laboratories, and they rapidly found their way to the bedside.

Treatment for serious cardiac arrhythmias (rhythm disturbances) and cardiac arrest (abrupt cessation of heartbeat)—major causes of death following myocardial infarctions—became possible. As a result, there was a need to monitor the ECG of patients who had suffered heart attacks, so that these episodes could be noticed and treated immediately. In 1963, Day reported that treatment in a coronary-care unit of patients who had had a myocardial infarction reduced mortality by 60 percent [Day, 1963]. As a consequence, coronary-care units—with ECG monitors—proliferated. The addition of online blood-pressure monitoring quickly followed. **Pressure transducers,** already used in the cardiac-catheterization laboratory, were easily adapted to the monitors in the ICU.

With the advent of more automated instruments, the ICU nurse could spend less time measuring the traditional vital signs and more time observing and caring for the critically ill patient. Simultaneously, a new trend emerged; some nurses moved away from the bedside to a central console where they could monitor the ECG and other vital-sign reports from many patients. Maloney pointed out that this was an inappropriate use of technology when it deprived the patient of adequate personal attention at the bedside. He also suggested that having the nurse record vital signs every few hours was "only to assure regular nurse–patient contact" [Maloney, 1968, p. 606].

As monitoring capabilities expanded, physicians and nurses soon were confronted with a bewildering number of instruments; they were threatened by **data overload.** Several investigators suggested that the digital computer might be helpful in solving the problems associated with data collection, review, and reporting.

12.2.2 Development of Computer-Based Monitoring

Teams from several cities in the United States introduced computers for physiological monitoring in the ICU, beginning with Shubin and Weil in Los Angeles [Shubin and Weil, 1966], then Warner and colleagues in Salt Lake City [Warner et al., 1968]. These investigators had several goals: (1) to increase the availability and accuracy of data, (2) to compute derived variables that could not be measured directly, (3) to increase patient-care efficacy, and (4) to allow display of the time trend of patient data. Each of these teams developed its application on a mainframe computer system, which required a large computer room and special staff to keep the system operational 24 hours per day. The computers used by these developers cost over $200,000 each in 1965! Other researchers were attacking more specific problem areas in monitoring. For example, Cox and associates in St. Louis developed algorithms to analyze

---

[4]Cardiac catheterization is a procedure whereby a tube (catheter) is passed into the heart through an artery or vein, allowing the cardiologist to measure pressure within the heart's chambers, to obtain blood samples, to inject contrast dye for radiological procedures, and so on.

the ECG for rhythm disturbances in real time [Cox et al., 1972]. The arrhythmia-monitoring system, which was installed in the coronary-care unit of Barnes Hospital in 1969, ran on an inexpensive minicomputer.

As we described in Chapters 1 and 4, the advent of integrated circuits and other advances allowed computing power per dollar to increase dramatically. As hardware became smaller, more reliable, and less expensive, and as better software tools were developed, simple analog processing gave way to digital signal processing. Monitoring applications developed by the pioneers using large central computers now became possible using dedicated machines at the bedside.

The early bedside monitors were built around *bouncing-ball* or conventional oscilloscopes and analog computer technology (Figure 12.2). As computer technology has advanced, the definition of *computer-based monitoring* has changed. The early developers spent a major part of their time deriving data from analog physiological signals. Soon the data-storage and decision-making capabilities of the computer monitoring systems came under the investigators' scrutiny. Therefore, what was considered computer-based patient monitoring in the late 1960s and early 1970s (Figure 12.3) is now built into bedside monitors and is considered simply patient monitoring. Systems with database functions, report-generation capabilities, and some decision-making capabilities are usually called **computer-based patient monitors.**

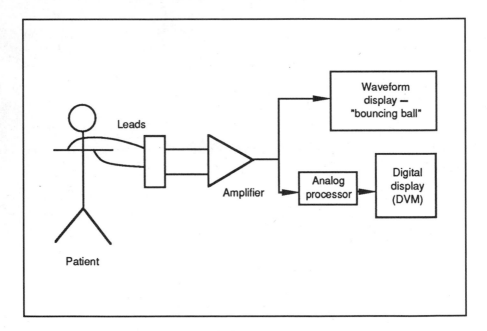

FIGURE 12.2 Block diagram of a typical analog monitor. These systems were developed in the early 1970s and are still in widespread use in hospitals today. [DVM = digital volt meter.]

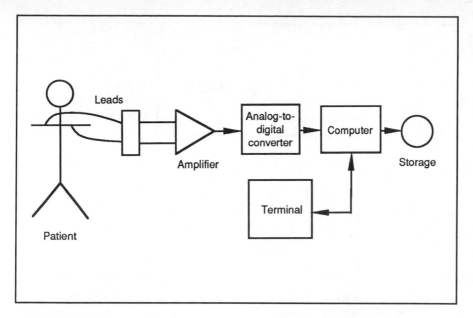

FIGURE 12.3 Analog monitor (see Figure 12.2) with a minicomputer attached. The system configuration is much like that used more than 1 decade ago by the developers of early computer-based monitoring systems.

12.3 Data Acquisition and Signal Processing

The use of microcomputers in bedside monitors has revolutionized the acquisition, display, and processing of physiological data.[5] There are few bedside monitors or ventilators marketed today that do not use at least one microcomputer. Figure 12.4 shows a block diagram of a patient connected to sensors and bedside monitors. Sensors convert biological signals (such as pressure, density, or mechanical movement) into electrical signals.

Some biological signals are already electrical, such as the currents that traverse the heart and are recorded on the ECG. Figure 12.5 shows a patient connected to ECG electrodes and an accompanying amplifier. The ECG signal derived from the electrodes at the body surface is small—only a few millivolts in amplitude. The patient is isolated from the electrical current of the monitor, and the analog ECG signal is amplified to a level sufficient for conversion to digital data using an analog-to-digital converter (ADC). Digital data then can be processed, and the results displayed (Figure 12.6).

---

[5]Portions of Sections 12.3 and 12.4 have been adapted with permission from Gardner, R. M. Computerized management of intensive care patients. *M.D. Computing,* 3(1):36–51, 1986.

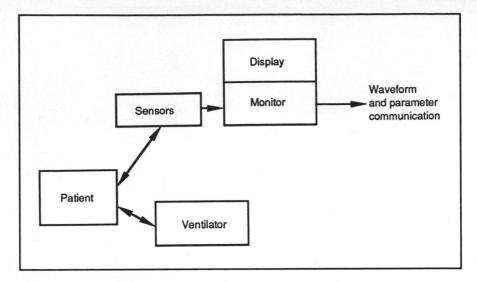

FIGURE 12.4 Block diagram of a simple bedside monitor with sensors attached to the patient. Signals are derived from the patient's physiological states and are communicated as waveforms and derived parameters to a central station display system.

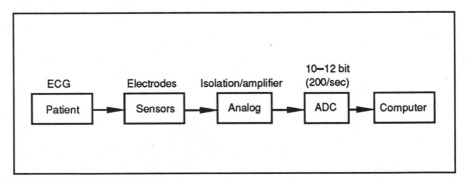

FIGURE 12.5 Front-end signal acquisition for a bedside monitor. The ECG signal is used as an example. The sensors (ECG electrodes) are attached to the patient. The resulting ECG signal is amplified by an electrically isolated analog amplifier, and is presented to an analog-to-digital converter (ADC). The signal is sampled at a rate of 200 measurements per second, with a 10- to 12-bit ADC; the resulting data are presented to the computer for pattern analysis.

As we discussed in Chapter 4, the sampling rate is an important factor that affects the correspondence between an analog signal and that signal's digital representation. Figure 12.7 shows an ECG that has been sampled at four different rates. At a rate of 500 measurements per second (part a), the digitized representation of the ECG looks like an analog recording of the ECG. All the features of the ECG, including the shape of the P wave (atrial depolarization), the amplitude of the QRS complex

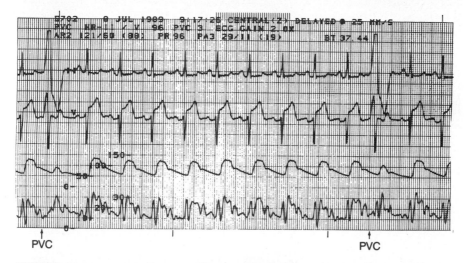

FIGURE 12.6 ECG (first [top] and second traces), arterial pressure (third trace), and pulmonary-artery pressure (fourth trace) recorded from a patient's bedside. Annotated on the recording are the bed number (E702), date (8 Jul 1989), and time (9:17:25). Also noted is regular rhythm, a heart rate from ECG (V) of 96 beats per minute, a systolic arterial pressure of 121, a diastolic pressure of 60, a mean pressure of 88 mm Hg, and a heart rate from pressure (PR) of 96. The patient is having premature ventricular contractions (PVCs) at a rate of three per minute; two PVCs can be seen in this tracing (the wide complexes noted at the beginning and near the end). The pulmonary-artery pressure is 29/11, with a mean of 19 mm Hg, and the blood temperature is 37.44° C. The self-contained monitoring system has determined the values and generated the calibrated graphical plot.

(ventricular depolarization) and the shape of the T wave (ventricular recovery) are reproduced faithfully. When the sampling rate is decreased to 100 measurements per second, however, the amplitude and shape of the QRS complex begin to distort. When only 50 observations per second are recorded, the QRS complex is grossly distorted and the other features also begin to distort. At a recording rate of only 25 measurements per second, gross signal distortion occurs, and even estimating heart rate by measuring intervals from R to R is problematic.

12.3.1 Advantages of Built-In Microcomputers

Today, the newest bedside monitors contain multiple microcomputers; they have much more computing power and memory than were available in systems used by the computer-monitoring pioneers (Figure 12.8). Bedside monitors with built-in microcomputers have the following advantages over their analog predecessors:

- The digital computer's ability to store patient waveform information such as the ECG permits sophisticated **pattern recognition** and **feature extraction.** The microcomputer uses **waveform templates** to identify abnormal waveform patterns, then classifies ECG arrhythmias. Analog computer technology allowed only a tiny

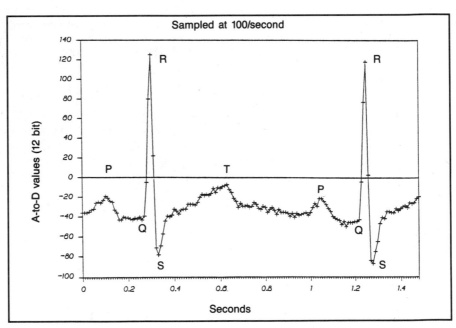

(a)

(b)

FIGURE 12.7 The sampling rate of the analog-to-digital converter determines the quality of the ECG recording. All four panels show the same ECG signal, sampled at different rates: (a) 500, (b) 100, (c) 50, and (d) 25 measurements per second. Note the degradation of the quality of the signal from (a) to (d).

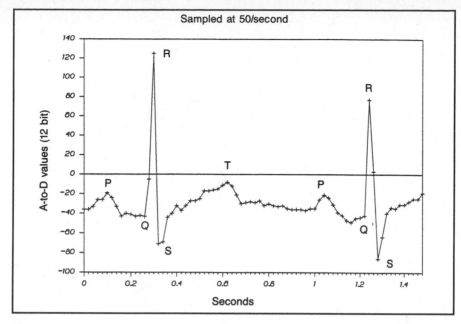

(c)

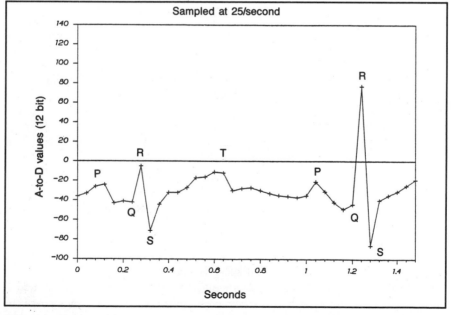

(d)

FIGURE 12.7 *Continued.*

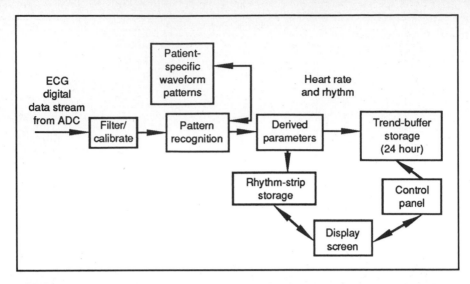

FIGURE 12.8 Block diagram of a microcomputer-based bedside monitor showing a digital data stream derived from an analog-to-digital converter (ADC), and how parameters are derived from the signal. First, the signal is calibrated, and unwanted signals are removed (such as the 60-Hz signal from the power line). Next, software pattern-recognition algorithms are applied. For ECG rhythm analysis, patient-specific waveform templates that the microcomputer-based system has learned are compared with each patient waveform. Once the signal characteristics are determined, derived parameters are generated and are stored in time-trend buffers. When arrhythmia events are detected by the pattern-recognition algorithm, the digitized signals also are transferred to a storage area for ECG recordings. Figure 12.9 shows an example of an ECG recording, or strip. The operator—usually a nurse or a physician—interacts with the monitor via a control panel and display screen.

segment of waveforms to be processed at one time, thereby permitting only a narrow view of the entire patient waveform.

- Signal quality can now be monitored and maintained. For example, the computer can watch for degradation of ECG skin-electrode contact resistance. If the contact is poor, the monitor can alert the nurse and can specify which electrode needs attention.
- The system can acquire physiological signals more efficiently by converting them to digital form early in the processing cycle. The waveform processing (for example, calibration and filtering, as described in Chapter 4) then can be done in the microcomputer. The same principle simplifies the nurse's task of setting up and operating the bedside monitor, because it eliminates the need for manual calibration.
- Transmission of digitized physiological waveform signals is easier and more reliable. Digital transmission of data is inherently noise-free. As a result, newer monitoring systems allow health-care professionals to review a patient's waveform displays and derived parameters, such as heart rate and blood pressure, at a central station as well as at the bedside in the ICU.

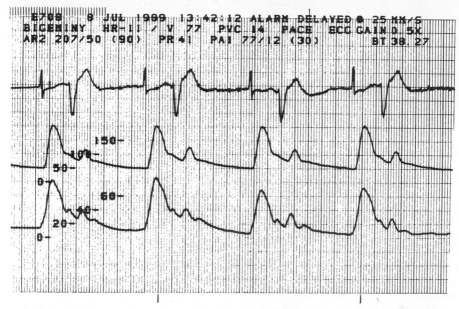

FIGURE 12.9 ECG strip showing a patient's ECG (upper trace) and arterial (middle trace) and pulmonary-artery (lower trace) pressure waveforms. The patient has a potentially life-threatening arrhythmia in which heart beats occur in pairs—a pattern called *bigeminy.* Note that, for the extra beats on the ECG pattern, the resulting pressure waveform pulsation is unusually small, indicating that the heart has not pumped much blood for that extra beat. The patient's heart rate, as determined from the ECG, is 77 beats per minute, whereas that determined from blood pressure is only 41 beats per minute. The heart is effectively beating at a very slow rate of 41 beats per minute.

- Selected data can be retained easily if they are digitized. For example, ECG strips reflecting interesting physiological sequences, such as periods of arrhythmias (Figure 12.9), can be stored in the bedside monitor for later review.
- Measured variables, such as heart rate and blood pressure, can be charted over prolonged periods to aid with detection of life-threatening trends (Figure 12.10).
- Alarms from bedside monitors are now much "smarter" and raise fewer false alarms. In the past, analog alarm systems used only high–low threshold limits and were susceptible to **signal artifacts.** Now, computer-based bedside monitors often can distinguish between artifacts and real alarm situations by using the information derived from one signal to verify that from another, and can confidently alert physicians and nurses to real alarms. For example, heart rate can be derived from either the ECG or the arterial blood pressure. If both signals indicate dangerous tachycardia (fast heart rate), the system sounds an alarm. If the two signals do not agree, the monitor can notify the health-care professional about a potential instrumentation or medical problem. The procedure is not unlike that performed by a human verifying possible problems by using redundant information from simpler bedside monitor alarms.

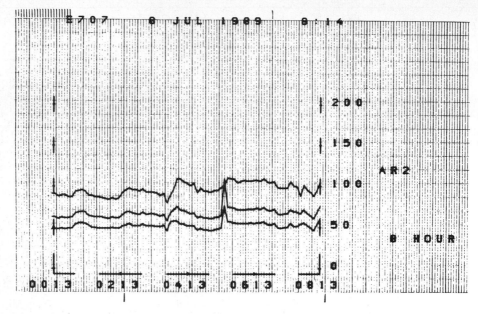

(a)

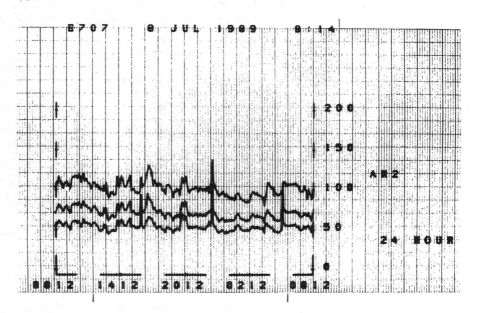

(b)

FIGURE 12.10 Two time-trend plots of systolic, mean, and diastolic pressure. The panel in (a) is for 8 hours; that in (b) is for 24 hours. Indicated across the bottom are the time of day at each of the tick marks. These plots show relatively stable blood-pressure trends over the time period.

- Systems can be upgraded easily. Only the software programs in read-only memory (ROM) need to be changed; in older analog systems, replacement of hardware was required.

12.3.2 Arrhythmia Monitoring—
Signal Acquisition and Processing

Although general-purpose computer-based physiological monitoring systems have not yet been adopted widely, computer-based ECG arrhythmia-monitoring systems have been accepted quickly. ECG arrhythmia analysis is one of the most sophisticated and difficult of the bedside monitoring tasks. Conventional arrhythmia monitoring, which depends on people observing displayed signals, is expensive, unreliable, tedious, and stressful to the observers. One early approach to overcoming these limitations was to purchase an arrhythmia-monitoring system operating on a time-shared central computer. Such minicomputer-based systems usually monitor 8 to 16 patients and cost at least $50,000. The newest bedside monitors, in contrast, have built-in arrhythmia-monitoring systems. These computers generally use a 16-bit architecture, waveform templates, and real-time cross-correlation techniques to classify rhythm abnormalities. Figure 12.11 shows the output from a modern bedside monitor. There are four ECG

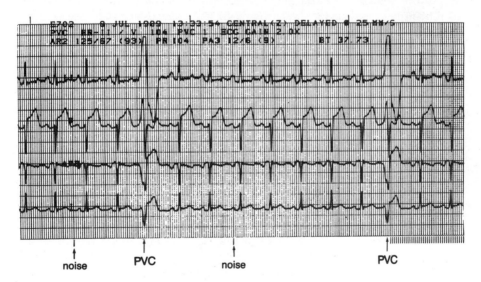

FIGURE 12.11 Four simultaneous lead tracings of ECG for a patient. The patient is having premature ventricular contractions (PVCs) at a rate of 1 per minute. (Two PVCs occur— one at the middle left and one at the right of the tracing.) The PVC is most apparent in lead II (top trace); it is much less apparent in lead V (second trace). Multiple-lead recording and computer access permit detection of a much wider variety of arrhythmias and also minimize the effect of artifacts (noise), which may occur in only one lead (as shown here in the bottom lead).

leads attached to the patient, and the computer has correctly classified a rhythm abnormality—in this case, a premature ventricular contraction (PVC). The bedside monitor also retains an ECG tracing record in its memory, so that at a later time a health professional can review the information.

Modern computer algorithms for processing ECG rhythms take sampled data, such as those shown in Figure 12.7, and extract features, such as the amplitude and duration of the QRS complex [Larsen and Jenkins, 1987]. The system performs feature extraction by searching the sampled data from beginning to end to locate the P wave, QRS complex, and T wave. A slope-detection strategy is often used to detect the quick upswing of the QRS complex—the rate of change in voltage (slope) is expressed as the difference between the values of two consecutive ECG data points. The algorithm compares the computed slope with a threshold value, and, if the threshold is exceeded, a trigger response signals the presence of a waveform edge. In some computer-based arrhythmia-monitoring systems, the user can adjust the threshold value, or QRS sensitivity.

Whereas the location of the QRS complex is relatively easy to detect using this slope-detection method, the P and T waves, because of their gentle slopes, are more difficult to recognize. Lack of reliable P-wave detection is one of the most serious limitations of computer-based arrhythmia monitors; the problem has not yet yielded to practical solution. Another major problem with automated waveform detection is attributable to noise in the signal. Movement of the patient frequently causes signal artifacts, which are seen on the ECG as steep slopes or transient spikes, both of which cause false trigger responses.

The Marquette 7700 series bedside monitor—from which waveforms shown in Figures 12.6, 12.9, 12.10, and 12.11 were derived—samples four leads simultaneously. Before performing the QRS detection step, the computer-based monitor searches for high-frequency noise or artifact. If the system finds artifact, the monitor displays the message "noise" on the screen and halts QRS detection for 2.5 seconds. Such processing helps to prevent the generation of many false alarms due to noise. When ECG monitoring begins, the computer-based bedside monitor initiates a *learning process* to determine which QRS waveform shape is seen most frequently. The learning process requires 16 beats from which to determine R–R intervals (the times between successive R waves) and to calculate the average interval. Waveforms are classified by shape. Of those waveforms with the most frequently occurring shape, the one having the longest R–R interval is designated the dominant shape. If at any time the dominant beat fails to occur within an interval of four beats, then the system seeks a new dominant beat by restarting the learning process.

As the system detects each new QRS complex, it performs classification by comparing the waveform with stored beats called *templates*; the cross-correlation process seeks beats of a similar shape. The first template stored is the dominant beat found in the learning process. Up to 15 template beats are stored and are used for cross-correlation. Series of beats are analyzed to classify rhythms. Once an abnormal rhythm has been identified, the system generates one of four levels of alarm, depending on the severity of the detected arrhythmia.

12.3.3 Commercial Development of Computer-Based Monitoring

Development of computer-based patient monitoring took place primarily in universities and medical schools and their affiliated hospitals. Later, as excitement about computer-assisted care in the ICU increased, commercial vendors became interested in marketing the technology. Several large, capable, and reputable manufacturers have supplied over 300 computer-based patient monitoring systems worldwide. These companies include Hewlett-Packard (which in 1987 controlled almost two-thirds of the market with its Patient Data Management System (PDMS)), Mennen Medical, Roche, Kontron, Siemens, Litton Datamedix, General Electric, Spacelabs, and EMTEK [Brimm, 1987]. Most products have tended to emphasize the acquisition and processing of physiologic data, without meeting the need to integrate relevant data from other sources in the hospital—the clinical laboratories, the radiology department, and the pharmacy. Currently, only a handful of successful integrated patient-monitoring systems is available commercially.

12.4 Information Management in the ICU

The goal of patient monitoring is to detect life-threatening events promptly, so that they can be treated before they cause irreversible organ damage or death. Care of the critically ill patient requires considerable skill, and necessitates prompt, accurate treatment decisions. Health-care professionals collect numerous data through frequent observations and testing, and more data are recorded by continuous-monitoring equipment. Physicians generally prescribe complicated therapy for such patients. As a result, enormous numbers of clinical data accumulate. Professionals can miss important events and trends if the accumulated data are not presented in a compact, well-organized form. In addition, the problems of managing these patients have been made even more challenging by economic pressures to reduce the cost of diagnostic and therapeutic interventions.

Continuity of care is especially important for critically ill patients, who are generally served by a team of physicians, nurses, and therapists, and whose data often are transferred from one individual to another (for example, the laboratory technician calls a ward clerk who reports the information to a nurse who in turn passes it on to the physician who makes a decision). Each step in this transmission process is subject to delay and error. The medical record is the principal instrument for ensuring the continuity of care for patients.

12.4.1 Computer-Based Charting

As we discussed in Chapters 2 and 6, the traditional medical record has several limitations. The problems of poor or inflexible organization, illegibility, and lack of physical availability are especially pertinent to the medical records of critically ill patients, due to the large number of data collected and the short time allowed for many treatment decisions.

The importance of having a unified medical record was demonstrated by a study conducted at Latter Day Saints (LDS) Hospital [Bradshaw et al., 1984]. Researchers kept detailed records of the data used by physicians to make treatment decisions in a shock–trauma ICU (Figure 12.12). The investigators were surprised to find that laboratory and blood-gas data were used most frequently (42 percent total), given that physiological bedside monitors are always present in the modern ICU. Clinicians' observations (21 percent) and drug and fluid-balance data (22 percent) also were used frequently. The bedside physiological monitor accounted for only 13 percent of the data used in making therapeutic decisions. These findings clearly indicate that data from several sources—not just those from the traditional physiological monitoring devices—must be communicated to and integrated into a unified medical record to permit effective decision making and treatment in the ICU.

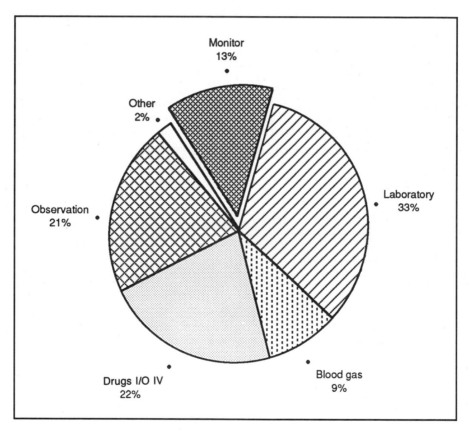

FIGURE 12.12 Pie chart indicating the variety of data physicians use when making treatment decisions in a shock–trauma intensive care unit. [I/O = input–output; IV = intravenous.] (*Source:* Reprinted with permission from Gardner, R. M., Sittig, D. F., and Budd, M. C. Computers in the intensive care unit: Match or mismatch? In Shoemaker, W. C., et al. (eds), *Textbook of Critical Care,* 2nd ed. Philadelphia: W. B. Saunders, 1989, p. 249.)

Effective computer-based charting in the ICU must support multiple types of data collection. As Figure 12.12 shows, a large percentage of the data is collected from typically manual tasks, such as administering a medication or auscultating breath or heart sounds. Furthermore, an instrument may present data in electronic form, yet require that a person note these data and write them in the chart. Thus, computer-based charting systems must be able to collect a wide variety of data from automated and remote sites, as well as from health-care providers at the bedside. Unfortunately, most computer-based charting systems have dealt with a limited subset (usually only the bedside monitoring) of the data that need to be charted.

Figure 12.13 illustrates the complexity of ICU charting. The chart must document the actions taken by the health-care staff, to meet both medical and legal requirements (items 1 and 2 in Figure 12.13). In addition, many of the data logged in the chart are used for management and billing purposes (items 3 and 4 in Figure 12.13). Many computer systems have ignored these requirements and thus have unwittingly forced the clinical staff to chart the same information in more than one place. Yet efficient

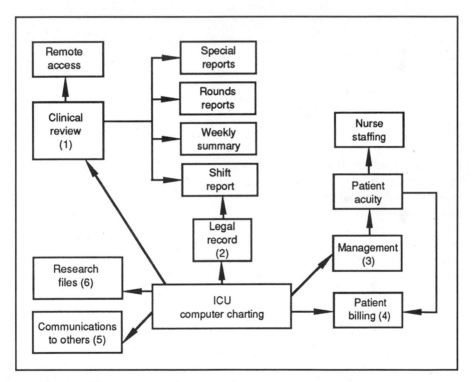

FIGURE 12.13 Block diagram showing the six major areas in which health-care professionals interact with computer-based ICU charting to make patient care more effective and efficient. See text for explanations of functions. (*Source:* Reprinted with permission from Gardner, R. M., Sittig, D. F., and Budd, M. C. Computers in the intensive care unit: Match or mismatch? In Shoemaker, W. C., et al. (eds), *Textbook of Critical Care,* 2nd ed. Philadelphia: W. B. Saunders, 1989, p. 249.)

management in hospitals is required, especially given the implementation of prospective-payment strategies (see Chapter 19). Hospitals now have strong incentives to evaluate and control the costs of procedures. As a result, it is necessary to know how ill the patient is, which in turn allows administrators to project nurse staffing needs and to account for the care of a patient by degree of illness. Communication (item 5 in Figure 12.13) with other departments within the hospital is mandatory. Access from office or home to clinical and administrative information is a great convenience to physicians. A computer-based record allows this type of communication. Because the computer-based ICU record is stored in the system, it is readily available for research purposes (item 6 in Figure 12.13). Anyone who has tried to retrieve data from manual patient charts for research purposes will recognize the value of this capability.

To meet the clinical management needs of critically ill patients, as well as to provide an adequate legal record, most patient data-management systems generate a variety of reports. At the LDS Hospital, in addition to the rounds report (shown in Figure 12.1), there is a variety of other reports. Figure 12.14 shows a nursing shift report for a patient. This 12-hour report documents the physiological data. The laboratory data are summarized in the upper section. A record of each drug given and each intravenous (IV) fluid administered is displayed in the lower section. The nurses who care for the patient are listed; the nurses place their initials next to their names to indicate that they have verified the data. Total fluid-intake data are derived from the IV data, and fluid-output data are summarized as well, allowing the system to calculate the net intake–output balance for the shift.

For the patient who is in the ICU for several days, a broader view of the course of the recovery process is essential. Thus, the system at LDS prepares weekly reports that summarize the data for each of the past seven 24-hour periods (Figure 12.15). The data already are stored in the computer, so no additional data entry is required to generate the report. A program abstracts and formats the data. Figure 12.16 shows a blood-gas report indicating the acid–base status of the patient's blood, as well as the blood's oxygen-carrying capacity. Note that, in addition to the numerical parameters for the blood, the patient's breathing status is indicated. Based on all these clinical data, the computer provides an interpretation. For life-threatening situations, the computer prompts the staff to take the necessary action. For example, if the level of a blood-gas measurement indicates that the patient is not getting enough oxygen, the system promptly notifies the laboratory staff, who are instructed to call the nurse or physician caring for the patient and to record whom they notified.

12.4.2 Calculation of Derived Variables

Increased sophistication of hemodynamic, renal, and pulmonary monitoring resulted in the need to calculate **derived parameters**; for the first time, ICU staff had to crunch numbers. At first, pocket calculators were used, with each step performed by a careful nurse. Then programmable calculators took over this task, making the computation simpler, faster, and more accurate. Soon these devices were replaced in turn by portable computers. Some of these systems provide graphical plots and interpretations.

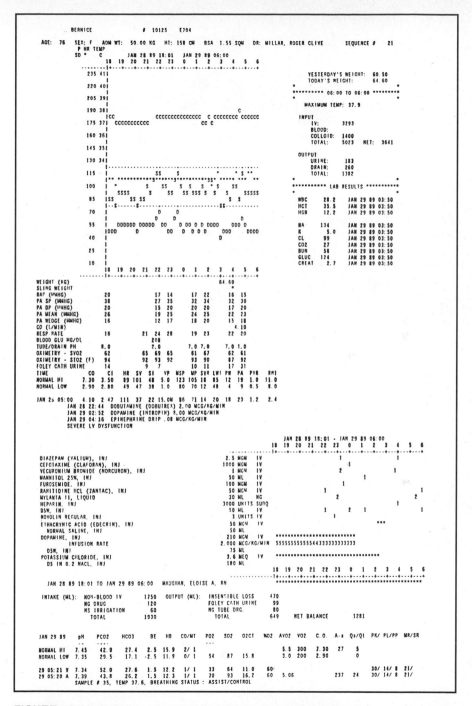

FIGURE 12.14 Shift report for a 12-hour ICU nursing shift produced by the HELP system at LDS Hospital. The report displays vital signs, laboratory-test results, and other patient data collected over a 12-hour period. (*Source:* Courtesy of LDS Hospital.)

12.4.3 Decision-Making Assistance

One mark of a good physician is the ability to make sound clinical judgments. Medical decision making traditionally has been considered an intuitive, as well as scientific, process. In recent years, however, formal methods for decision making have been applied to medical problem solving (see Chapter 3), and computer-assisted medical decision making has gained wider acceptance. Indeed, discussion of artificial intelligence (AI) is commonplace in medicine today (see the discussions of decision-support systems in Chapter 15). We now have the opportunity to use the computer to assist staff in the complex task of medical decision making in the ICU. For example, the HELP computer system at the LDS Hospital in Salt Lake City has been used effectively to assist in ICU decision making. The system collects and integrates data for the ICU patient from a wide variety of sources. The data are processed automatically by the HELP decision-making system to determine whether the new information, by itself or in combination with other data in the patient record (such as a laboratory result or a previously generated decision), should lead to a new medical decision. These computer-generated medical decisions are based on predefined criteria stored in the system's knowledge base.

The HELP decision-making system has been used in the following areas:

- *Interpretation of data;* for example, interpretation of breathing status based on blood-gas reports and hemodynamic parameters
- *Alerts;* for example, notification that a drug is contraindicated, at the time the drug is being ordered

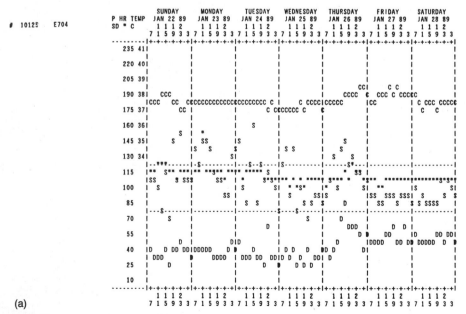

(a)

FIGURE 12.15 Two portions of a weekly (7-day) ICU report produced by the HELP system at LDS Hospital. The report provides a daily weight, fluid-balance, drug, and physiological-data summary for an individual patient. (*Source:* HELP System, LDS Hospital.)

			JAN 22	JAN 23	JAN 24	JAN 25	JAN 26	JAN 27	JAN 28
MORPHINE, INJ	MGM	IV	37.0	21.0	2.0			7.0	6.0
ACETAMINOPHEN, SUPP	MGM	RECT					1300	650	
DIAZEPAM (VALIUM), INJ	MGM	IV						10.0	5.0
CEFOTAXIME (CLAFORAN), INJ	MGM	IV							1000
GENTAMICIN, INJ	MGM	IV						60.0	60.0
CEFUROXIME (ZINACEF), INJ	MGM	IV	3000	3000	3000	3000	3000	3000	
DOBUTAMINE (DOBUTREX), INJ	MGM	IV	732	582	792	810	270	87	222
EPINEPHRINE DRIP, INJ	MGM	IV	22.20	11.46	3.96	0.00			1.53
VECURONIUM BROMIDE (NORCURON), INJ	MGM	IV	39	26	18	13	10	3	7
DOPAMINE, INJ	MGM	IV	648	492	420	396	522	864	738
METOLAZONE (ZAROXOLYN), TAB	MGM	NG					5.00		
NITROPRUSSIDE (NIPRIDE), INJ	MGM	IV	0						
AMRINONE (INOCOR), INJ	MGM	IV	0						
FUROSEMIDE, INJ	MGM	IV	80	80	80	80	120	80	280
MANNITOL 25%, INJ	ML	IV							50
ETHACRYNIC ACID (EDECRIN), INJ	MGM	IV							50
ACETAZOLAMIDE (DIAMOX), INJ	MGM	IV			250	250		250	
RANITIDINE HCL (ZANTAC), INJ	MGM	IV	150	100	150	150	150	150	150
MYLANTA II, LIQUID	ML	NG		60	30	120	90	60	180
MYLANTA, LIQUID	ML	NG			30	60			
HEPARIN, INJ	UNITS	SUBQ						3000	6000
HEPARIN FLUSH, INJ	UNITS	IV	400	300		300	500	200	100
ARTIFICAL TEARS (LACRIL), SOLUTION	GTTS	OPTH	6	4					
PLASMANATE 5%, INJ	ML	IV						250	1400
PACKED RBC	ML	IV					500		
ALBUMIN 25%, INJ	ML	IV	100	50	50	150			
PLATELETS (RANDOM DONOR)	ML	IV	400		150				
AMINOSYN 8.5%, INJ	ML	IV	311	621	472	529	608	1079	617
POTASSIUM	MEQ	IV	25.2	50.3	38.2	59.7	73.0	131.0	94.9
CALCIUM	MEQ	IV	3.1	6.2	4.7	5.3	5.7	9.9	5.8
MAGNESIUM	MEQ	IV	14.9	35.0	28.3	31.7	12.7	17.3	9.9
ZINC	MGM	IV	3.4	6.8	5.2	5.8	6.7	11.9	6.4
COPPER	MGM	IV	0.7	1.4	1.0	1.2	1.3	2.4	1.3
MANGANESE	MGM	IV	0.3	0.6	0.5	0.5	0.6	1.1	0.6
CHROMIUM	MCG	IV	6.8	13.7	10.4	11.6	13.4	23.7	12.7
CHLORIDE	MEQ	IV	20.8	41.6	31.6	35.4	35.0	50.6	47.5
ACETATE	MEQ	IV	24.9	49.7	37.8	42.3	41.5	69.7	52.2
PHOSPHATE	MEQ	IV	14.9	29.8	22.7	25.4	65.8	138.5	45.5
SULFATE	MEQ	IV	9.9	25.1	20.8	23.3	10.1	17.3	7.6
GLUCONATE	MEQ	IV	3.1	6.2	4.7	5.3	5.7	9.9	5.8
FAT EMULSION 10% (LIPOSYN), INJ	ML	IV							500
NORMAL SALINE, INJ	ML	IV	6	2		2	154	10	40
FAT EMULSION 20% (LIPOSYN), INJ	ML	IV	200	200	200	200	200	66	134
POTASSIUM CHLORIDE, INJ	MEQ	IV	67.9	78.0	183.7	51.9	51.6	104.3	17.6
D5W, INJ	ML	IV	410	215	25	150	5	10	
HETASTARCH (HESPAN), INJ	ML	IV					250	0	
MAGNESIUM SULFATE 50%, INJ	GM	IV	2.00						
NOVOLIN REGULAR, INJ	UNITS	IV	18	15					3

		JAN 22	JAN 23	JAN 24	JAN 25	JAN 26	JAN 27	JAN 28
INTAKE (ML):	BLOOD	400		150		500		
	COLLOID	100	50	50	150		250	1400
	NON-BLOOD IV	2783	3046	2707	2395	2254	3145	3293
	NG DRUG		60	60	180	90	60	180
	TOTAL	3313	3216	2967	2815	2874	3485	5023
OUTPUT (ML):	INSENSIBLE LOSS	937	946	943	873	1016	1077	939
	FOLEY CATH URINE	360	740	210	902	2950	895	183
	NG TUBE DRG.	50	200	80	125	40	75	260
	WATERSEAL DRG, 1	180	50					
	TOTAL	3918	3936	4023	2512	5226	2470	1382
NET BALANCE (ML):		-605	-720	-1056	303	-2352	1015	3641
WEIGHT (KG)		61.2	61.4	60.8	62.2	60.4	60.5	64.6
NUTRITIONAL:	NP ENERGY KCAL (IV)	1468	2143	1784	1803	1953	2813	2395
	TOTAL ENERGY KCAL (IV)	1573	2354	1944	1982	2160	3181	2605
	PROTEIN GM	26	53	40	45	52	92	52
	FAT GM	40	40	40	40	40	13	77
	CHO GM	315	513	407	413	456	789	464
	NP ENERGY/N2 KCAL/GM	367	238	254	257	244	200	266
	N2 IN GM	4	9	7	7	8	14	9

(b)

FIGURE 12.15 *Continued.*

L D S   H O S P I T A L   B L O O D   G A S   R E P O R T

STEVEN						NO. 10072	DR. STINSON, JAMES B.			RM E609
		SEX: M	AGE: 43							

JAN 05 89	pH	PCO2	HCO3	BE	HB	CO/MT	PO2	SO2	O2CT	%O2	AVO2	VO2	C.O.	A-a	Qs/Qt	PK/ PL/PP	MR/SR
NORMAL HI	7.45	40.6	25.9	2.5	17.7	2/ 1					5.5	300	7.30	22	5		
NORMAL LOW	7.35	27.2	15.7	-2.5	13.7	0/ 1	64	91	18.5		3.0	200	2.90		0		
05 04:36 V	7.43	34.5	22.7	-.4	11.5	2/ 1	42	76	12.3	40						30/ 28/ 5	20/
05 04:35 A	7.48	29.3	21.7		11.6	2/ 1	128	96	15.9	40	3.43			75	12	30/ 28/ 5	20/

SAMPLE # 37, TEMP 37.3, BREATHING STATUS : ASSIST/CONTROL
MILD ACID-BASE DISORDER
MODERATELY REDUCED O2 CONTENT
SUPRA-NORMAL PO2
PULSE OXIMETER SO2 96.0

| 04 04:20 V | 7.45 | 36.1 | 24.9 | 1.9 | 10.2 | 2/ 1 | 37 | 72 | 10.4 | 40 | | | | | | 26/ 20/ 5 | 21/ |
| 04 04:19 A | 7.49 | 31.6 | 24.0 | 2.0 | 10.2 | 2/ 1 | 90 | 95 | 13.7 | 40 | 3.36 | 353 | 10.50 | 111 | 18 | 26/ 20/ 5 | 21/ |

SAMPLE # 36, TEMP 37.5, BREATHING STATUS : ASSIST/CONTROL
MILD ACID-BASE DISORDER
SEVERELY REDUCED O2 CONTENT (13.7) DUE TO ANEMIA (LOW HB)
PULSE OXIMETER SO2 93.0

| 03 06:05 A | 7.44 | 35.8 | 24.1 | 1.0 | 11.7 | 2/ 1 | 91 | 95 | 15.7 | 40 | | | | 105 | | 26/ 22/ 5 | 23/ |

SAMPLE # 35, TEMP 37.0, BREATHING STATUS : ASSIST/CONTROL
NORMAL ARTERIAL ACID-BASE CHEMISTRY
MODERATELY REDUCED O2 CONTENT
PULSE OXIMETER SO2 93.0

| 02 04:16 V | 7.46 | 37.4 | 26.4 | 3.4 | 9.1 | 1/ 1 | 35 | 71 | 9.1 | 40 | | | | | | 32/ 25/10 | 20/ |
| 02 04:15 A | 7.51 | 32.4 | 25.8 | 3.9 | 9.5 | 2/ 1 | 91 | 95 | 12.8 | 40 | 3.29 | 237 | 7.20 | 109 | 17 | 32/ 25/10 | 20/ |

SAMPLE # 34, TEMP 37.1, BREATHING STATUS : ASSIST/CONTROL
MODERATE METABOLIC ALKALOSIS
SEVERELY REDUCED O2 CONTENT (12.8) DUE TO ANEMIA (LOW HB)
PULSE OXIMETER SO2 95.0

| 01 10:53 A | 7.47 | 37.0 | 26.8 | 4.0 | 11.1 | 1/ 1 | 77 | 94 | 14.7 | 60 | | | | 238 | | 36/ 27/10 | 20/ |

SAMPLE # 33, TEMP 37.7, BREATHING STATUS : ASSIST/CONTROL
MILD ACID-BASE DISORDER
MODERATELY REDUCED O2 CONTENT
PULSE OXIMETER SO2 93.0

| 01 03:59 V | 7.41 | 46.2 | 29.0 | 4.5 | 10.0 | 1/ 1 | 42 | 73 | 10.2 | 80 | | | | | | / /12 | 20/ |
| 01 03:58 A | 7.46 | 39.2 | 27.7 | 4.5 | 9.9 | 1/ 1 | 146 | 97 | 13.7 | 80 | 3.64 | 331 | 9.10 | 287 | 23 | / /12 | 20/ |

SAMPLE # 32, TEMP 38.4, BREATHING STATUS : ASSIST/CONTROL
MILD ACID-BASE DISORDER
SEVERELY REDUCED O2 CONTENT (13.7) DUE TO ANEMIA (LOW HB)
SUPRA-NORMAL PO2

| 01 00:39 A | 7.44 | 42.2 | 28.4 | 4.7 | 10.0 | 1/ 1 | 104 | 95 | 13.5 | 90 | | | | 386 | | / /10 | 20/ |

SAMPLE # 31, TEMP 38.9, BREATHING STATUS : ASSIST/CONTROL
MILD ACID-BASE DISORDER
SEVERELY REDUCED O2 CONTENT (13.5) DUE TO ANEMIA (LOW HB)
PULSE OXIMETER SO2 91.0

| 31 23:35 A | 7.42 | 42.4 | 27.2 | 3.2 | 10.1 | 1/ 1 | 63 | 87 | 12.3 | 65 | | | | 276 | | / / 5 | 20/ |

SAMPLE # 30, TEMP 39.0, BREATHING STATUS : ASSIST/CONTROL
MILD ACID-BASE DISORDER
MODERATE HYPOXEMIA
SEVERELY REDUCED O2 CONTENT (12.3) DUE TO ANEMIA (LOW HB)
PULSE OXIMETER SO2 83.0

| 31 16:00 A | 7.49 | 34.4 | 26.1 | 3.8 | 9.7 | 1/ 1 | 87 | 95 | 13.1 | 40 | | | | 111 | | / / 5 | 21/ |

SAMPLE # 29, TEMP 37.8, BREATHING STATUS : ASSIST/CONTROL
MILD ACID-BASE DISORDER
SEVERELY REDUCED O2 CONTENT (13.1) DUE TO ANEMIA (LOW HB)

PRELIMINARY INTERPRETATION -- BASED ONLY ON BLOOD GAS DATA.   ***(FINAL DIAGNOSIS REQUIRES CLINICAL CORRELATION)***
KEY: CO=CARBOXY HB, MT=MET HB, O2CT=O2 CONTENT, AVO2=ART VENOUS CONTENT DIFFERENCE (CALCULATED WITH AVERAGE OF A &V HB VALUES),
VO2=OXYGEN CONSUMPTION, C.O.=CARDIAC OUTPUT, A-a=ALVEOLAR arterial O2 DIFFERENCE, Qs/Qt=SHUNT, PK=PEAK, PL=PLATEAU, PP=PEEP
MR=MACHINE RATE, SR=SPONTANEOUS RATE.   *** SPECIMEN IDENTIFICATION: BLOOD (A=ARTERIAL, V=VENOUS, C=CAPILLARY, W=WEDGE);
FLUIDS (P=PLEURAL, J=JOINT, B=ABDOMINAL, S=ABSCESS); E=EXPIRED AIR;
ECCo2R (I=INFLOW, M=MIDFLOW, O=OUTFLOW)

KEEP FULL PAGE FOR RECORDS
(END)

FIGURE 12.16 A blood-gas report produced by the HELP system at LDS Hospital. The report shows the patient's predicted values, as well as the measured values. The computer provides a decision-making interpretation and alerting facility. Note that this report summarizes, in reverse chronological order, the patient's blood-gas status over the course of 1 week. (*Source:* Courtesy of LDS Hospital.)

- *Diagnoses;* for example, detection of hospital-acquired infections
- *Treatment suggestions;* for example, suggestions about the most effective antibiotics to order, when the microbiology laboratory reports a positive culture result

The ICU component of HELP is the most mature of the system's clinical applications. The basic requirements for data acquisition, decision support, and information reporting are similar for patients in the ICU and on the general wards of the LDS Hospital. The number of variables and the volume of observations that must be integrated, however, are much greater for patients in the ICU.

12.4.4 Response by Nurses and Physicians

Currently, bedside terminals are functioning in all ICUs at LDS Hospital, and nurses use a computer-based system to create nursing care plans and to chart ICU data. The goals of automation were (1) to facilitate the acquisition of clinical data, (2) to improve the content and legibility of medical documentation, and (3) to increase the efficiency of the charting process so that nurses could devote more time to direct patient care. Studies demonstrated that the number and quality of nursing care plans increased, and that the content and quality of nursing charts improved markedly [Bradshaw et al., 1988]. To date, however, the studies have not shown improvements in the efficiency of information management by ICU nurses (time savings) that could be credited to use of the system.

The failure to demonstrate time savings may be a result of several factors. First, the new system affected only selected aspects of the nursing process. For example, physiological and laboratory data were already acquired automatically, so the effects of these computer-based systems were not included in the analyses. Second, the computer-based charting system is not yet comprehensive; nurses still must perform some manual charting. Third, nurses do not always take advantage of the capabilities of the charting system. For example, they sometimes reenter vital signs that have already been stored in the computer. Fourth, the intervals of time saved may have been too small to be measured using the work-sampling methods employed in the studies. Fifth, these small savings in time are easily absorbed into other activities. Despite the lack of demonstrated improvement in efficiency, however, the nursing department at LDS is enthusiastic about using computers; surveys of the nursing staff have shown that nurses favor the prospect of using computers throughout the hospital.

Physician members of the LDS staff are also heavy users of the computer system. The information in the computer is more current and more readily available than information in the paper charts. Now, when physicians want to review laboratory and other data, they use a computer terminal, rather than searching for the paper record.

12.5 Current Issues in Patient Monitoring

The future of computer-based ICU monitoring systems is bright. Developments in bedside monitors have recently accelerated because of the availability of the microcomputer. Nonetheless, some important areas of research in patient monitoring have not yet been addressed effectively.

12.5.1 Data Validation

A major problem is how to ensure that the data entered into ICU data-management systems are valid representations of patient state, and are not the product of noise or errors in data collection or data processing. A system must provide feedback at various levels to verify correct operation, to carry out quality control, and to present intermediate and final results. As we discussed earlier, some **cross-validation** between signals is possible, but this process is performed by few of the bedside monitors used today. Some of the newer patient-monitoring devices, such as pulse oximeters that attach to the ear or finger and direct pressure-measuring systems, have built in noise-rejection algorithms to improve the quality of the data presented [Gardner et al., 1986]. Data validation, however, is one area of patient monitoring that still offers much opportunity for technological development and improvement.

12.5.2 Invasive Versus Noninvasive Monitoring

Physiological and biochemical parameters commonly used in monitoring can be measured by instruments and devices that are either invasive (require breaking the skin or entering the body) or noninvasive. After several decades of development of **invasive techniques,** the recent trend has been to design **noninvasive methods.** Much of the development of noninvasive technology can be attributed to the availability of microcomputers and solid-state sensors.

The development of inexpensive light-emitting diodes (LEDs), small solid-state light detectors, and new computer methods, for example, made possible the development of the pulse oximeter, an exciting example of noninvasive monitoring technology. By alternately shining red and infrared light from the LEDs through a finger or an ear, the device can detect the pulsations of blood and determine arterial oxygen saturation and heart rate [Severinghaus and Astrup, 1986]. Pulse oximetry is one of the most significant technological advances ever made in monitoring. The technology is reliable yet inexpensive; also, because it is noninvasive, it does not subject the patient to the discomfort, expense, and risks of invasive techniques (infection and blood loss, for example).

12.5.3 Continuous Versus Intermittent Monitoring

One of the persistent questions facing people who monitor patients is "Should I measure a parameter continuously, or is intermittent sampling enough?" A related question is, "How often do I make the measurement?" These questions have no simple answer. If we want to display an ECG signal continuously, we must sample the signal at a rate of at least twice the rate of the maximum frequency of interest in the signal (the Nyquist frequency; see Chapter 4). For an ECG, the sampling rate should be at least 200 measurements per second.

When **intermittent monitoring** (periodic measurement of blood pH value, for example) must be performed, the overriding concerns in determining sampling rate are how rapidly the parameter can change, and how long before a dangerous change will result in irreversible damage. Sudden heart stoppage or severe dysrhythmias are the most frequent causes of sudden death. Therefore, heart-rate and heart-rhythm monitors must function continuously and should sound alarms within 15 to 20 seconds after detecting a problem. Other physiological parameters are not as labile and can be monitored less frequently. For the most part, medical measurements are made intermittently, and even continuously measured parameters are displayed at intervals. For example, heart rate can change with each beat (by 0.35 to 1 second). To provide data that a human can interpret, however, a bedside monitor usually updates its display of the rate every 3 seconds.

12.5.4 Integration of Patient-Monitoring Devices

Most bedside patient-support devices, such as IV pumps, ventilators, and physiological monitors, are microcomputer-based. Each has its own display and, because each comes from a different manufacturer, each is designed as a standalone unit. As a result, it is common for a nurse or therapist to read a computer display from one of these devices and then to enter the data through a terminal into a different computer. The need to integrate the outputs of the myriad devices in the ICU is apparent. The absence of standards for medical-device communications has stymied the acceptance and success of automated clinical data-management systems. Because of the large number and variety of medical devices available, and the peculiar data formats, it is impractical to attach the growing number of bedside devices to computers by building special software and hardware interfaces. For these reasons, an IEEE committee (P1073) has been organized to write standards for the **Medical Information Bus (MIB)** [Gardner and Hawley, 1984; Franklin, 1988; Shabot, 1989].

Pilot work underway at LDS Hospital [Hawley et al., 1988] has shown that the use of a common bus system facilitates data acquisition from bedside devices such as pulse oximeters, ventilators, infusion pumps,[6] pH meters, and mixed venous oxygen-saturation monitoring systems. The MIB data-communications system tested at LDS Hospital permits connection of up to 255 devices on a network, and will be able to communicate with each of these devices every few seconds. The communications technology being developed will allow the connection of a variety of bedside devices to the computer, and the recording of these devices' data will be almost continuous (Figure 12.17). The potential for improvements in the accuracy and timeliness of data acquisition, as well as for labor savings, is enticing. We shall discuss the MIB in Chapter 20, when we consider major issues that affect the future of medical informatics.

12.5.5 Closed-Loop Control Systems

Closed-loop control devices use a computer to sense and control a physiological variable; they alter therapy directly without human intervention. A nonmedical example of a closed-loop control system is the thermostat on a heater. A sensor continuously measures the temperature of the air. When the temperature drops below the setpoint,

---

[6]An infusion pump is a device used to control the rate of delivery of intravenous drug so as to maintain a constant level of drug in the body.

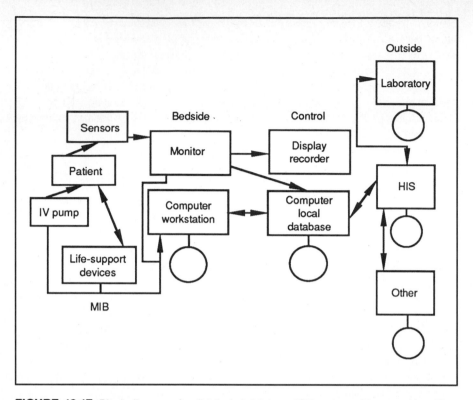

FIGURE 12.17 Block diagram of a distributed-database ICU system with networking. The database has been distributed to improve response time and reliability; the communications network has been implemented to enhance the integration function needed to care for the critically ill patient. [MIB = medical information bus, HIS = hospital information system, IV = intravenous.]

the heater turns on. When the temperature rises sufficiently, the heater shuts off. Sheppard and associates at the University of Alabama have shown the effectiveness of this type of device in controlling physiological parameters. They used a computer-controlled infusion pump to control the administration of sodium nitroprusside, a drug used to regulate blood pressure [Sheppard and Sayers, 1977; Sheppard, 1980]. These investigators have shown that the controller performed more effectively than did a nurse in regulating a constant blood pressure. The system works well under a wide range of clinical situations, and is designed with several fail-safe features. Closed-loop drug-delivery systems now are commercially available for controlling the infusion of oxytocin (a labor-inducing drug) and insulin and dextrose (used to control the level of glucose in the blood). In the future, closed-loop systems will control the delivery of other drugs and fluids, the administration of anesthesia, and the management of patients on ventilator therapy. Application of this type of technology is exciting because the computer may be able to provide more effective patient care while saving nursing time.

12.5.6 Open-Loop Treatment Protocols

The use of protocols—standardized plans for patient management—in the treatment of critically ill patients is not new. Protocols have been used for numerous applications, such as to guide therapeutic dosing so as to prevent adverse drug reactions, to suggest fluid management, to improve cardiac management of surgical patients, and to suggest therapy based on hemodynamic information. If these plans are encoded in the logic of a computer, the computer can analyze the patient data and recommend appropriate treatment. In a closed-loop system, as we discussed, the computer determines the appropriate action and acts directly to implement that action. However, given the complexity and inherent uncertainty of many medical decisions, the incompletely solved problem of data validation, and the dire consequences of error, it may be undesirable or impossible to relinquish complete control to the computer. Nonetheless, we should not ignore the superior computational ability and memory of the computer. Consequently, there is growing interest in the use of computers in **open-loop control systems,** in which the computer collects and analyzes data and generates recommendations or instructions, but human decision makers—such as physicians and nurses—evaluate the appropriateness of the advice before acting on it.

The Ventilator Manager (VM) program was an experimental system designed to interpret quantitative data collected in the ICU and to aid in managing the care of postoperative patients who were receiving mechanical ventilatory assistance [Fagan, 1985]. VM applied AI techniques to detect possible errors in data measurement and to suggest adjustments to therapy based on the patient's status over time and on long-term therapeutic goals. Developed as an experimental prototype, VM was not used to manage actual patients in the ICU. More recently, researchers at LDS Hospital implemented a program to manage the therapy of patients who have acute respiratory distress syndrome (ARDS) and who are enrolled in a controlled clinical trial [Sittig, 1987]. The system automatically generates therapeutic instructions to health-care providers from data input by the laboratory and by physicians, nurses, and respiratory therapists. The system has been used successfully to manage the care of several patients. The researchers' hypothesis is that the system can reduce the time required to initiate correct therapy, and can assist in managing the clinical trial.

12.5.7 Demonstration of the Efficacy of Care in the Intensive-Care Unit

ICU care is expensive. Given the current pressures to control health-care spending (see Chapter 19), there is growing concern about the cost-effectiveness of such care. In a 1984 study prepared for the Office of Technology Assessment, one researcher estimated that 15 to 20 percent of the nation's hospital budget, or almost 1 percent of the gross national product, was spent for ICU care [Berenson, 1984]. Unfortunately, the problems of assessing the benefit of each element in the ICU are many; to date, no definitive studies have been performed. It is difficult to identify and isolate all the factors in the ICU setting that affect patient recovery and outcome. Furthermore, as we mention in our discussion of technology assessment in Chapter 19, the ethical implications of withholding potentially beneficial care from patients in the control group of a randomized clinical trial make such studies difficult to perform. For the moment, we do not know what incremental benefit even the bedside monitor has for a patient. The value of a computer-based data-management system used in conjunction with monitoring devices is even more difficult to assess. One study from LDS Hospital reported that the implementation of a computer-based record-keeping system resulted in a 15-percent increase in the productivity of respiratory therapists [Andrews et al., 1985]; often, however, medical and nursing staff acceptance is the only clear indicator of value we have.

Another study that evaluated how nurses spend their time in caring for patients who have undergone open-heart surgery provided insight about how the computer may assist in improving nursing efficiency [Tolbert and Pertuz, 1977]. The authors concluded that automated patient monitoring should relieve nurses of some routine tasks, such as checking and charting vital signs. The extra time then could be used to provide more direct patient care, if necessary, or could be channeled into other productive tasks. A striking finding of both this study and an unpublished study conducted at LDS Hospital (Figure 12.18) was that nurses spend less than one-half of their time performing direct patient care.

In one attempt to assess the differences in patient outcome among major medical centers and with different treatment modalities, Knaus and associates developed an Acute Physiology and Chronic Health Evaluation (APACHE) scoring system [Knaus et al., 1986]. Scores assigned to patients are intended to stratify them prognostically by risk, so that different treatment programs can be compared more accurately. Fortunately, the data needed to derive the APACHE score are already available from computer-based monitoring systems [Shabot et al., 1987]. By using such systems to simplify data acquisition, we may be able to analyze variations in care and to determine optimal treatment strategies for critically ill patients.

12.5.8 Consensus Conference on Critical-Care Medicine

We can gain a perspective on what should be done to improve data management in critical-care medicine from a 1983 consensus conference organized by the National Institutes of Health (NIH) [Ayers et al., 1983]. Conclusions of the conference pointed out areas in treatment of critically ill patients that needed improvement. Many of these problems are amenable to computer assistance. Technical difficulties, errors in data interpretation, and increased interventions caused by continuous monitoring are potential nosocomial[7] hazards for ICU patients. Based on the findings of the conference, we identify eight areas in which computers can assist in the practice of critical-care medicine.

---

[7]Nosocomial hazards are dangers related to hospital care itself. A nosocomial infection, for example, is caused by exposure to infectious agents in the hospital environment.

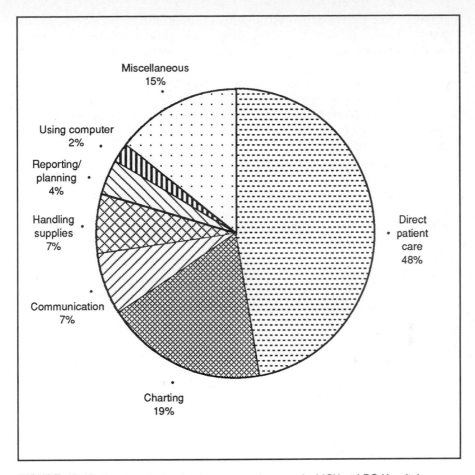

FIGURE 12.18 Pie chart indicating how nurses in a surgical ICU at LDS Hospital allocate their time among patient care, charting, communication, and other activities. Nurses spend only one-half of their time performing direct patient care. (*Source:* Reprinted with permission from Gardner, R. M., Sittig, D. F., and Budd, M. C. Computers in the intensive care unit: Match or mismatch? In Shoemaker, W. C., et al. (eds), *Textbook of Critical Care,* 2nd ed. Philadelphia: W. B. Saunders, 1989, p. 256.)

1. All ICUs should be capable of arrhythmia monitoring. Bedside physiological monitors using microcomputers now provide excellent arrhythmia monitoring.
2. Invasive monitoring should be performed safely. Computer-stored data on invasive events such as the insertion of an arterial catheter, analyzed in combination with data from the microbiology laboratory, can help to avoid infection (a major complication of invasive monitoring).
3. Generated data should be correct. The computer can check data as they are entered to verify that they are reasonable. Also, computer-based data communication and calculation are less subject to error than is work performed by human beings.

4. Derived data should be interpreted properly. The computer can assist in the integration of data from multiple sources. In addition, the computer can derive parameters and also can provide prompt, accurate, and consistent interpretations and alerts. For example, note in Figure 12.16 that oxygen consumption (VO_2) is calculated and displayed when data on arterial and venous blood gases and cardiac output are available (oxygen consumption was 353 ml/minute on 4JAN89 at 04:19).

5. Therapy should be employed safely. The computer can assist physicians by suggesting therapy, calculating appropriate drug doses, and flagging combinations of interacting drugs.

6. Access to laboratory data should be rapid and comprehensive. Computer networking provides fast access to all laboratory data, and can even interpret the results and provide alerts.

7. Enteral (tube-feeding) and parenteral (IV) nutritional support should be available. There are interactive computer programs that help physicians to prescribe care by assisting with the complex task of determining the appropriate volume and content of nutritional supplements.

8. Titrated[8] therapeutic interventions that use infusion pumps should be available. Closed-loop systems for controlling the administration of fluids and intravenous drugs can facilitate patient care and can provide an accurate record of the therapy.

The availability of microcomputers has greatly enhanced the ability to generate and process the physiological data used in patient monitoring. The use of computers in the ICU is still in its infancy, however. Many challenges remain in the exploration of ways with which the computer can be used effectively to integrate, evaluate, and simplify the complex data used in caring for critically ill patients.

Suggested Readings

Ginzton, L. E. and Laks, M. M. Computer aided ECG interpretation. *M.D. Computing*, 1:36, 1984.

> *This article summarizes the development of computer-based ECG interpretation systems, discusses their advantages and disadvantages, and describes the process by which a typical system obtains and processes ECG data.*

Shoemaker, W. C., et al. (eds). *Textbook of Critical Care*, 2nd ed. Philadelphia: W. B. Saunders, 1989.

> *This handbook will be of interest to the medical computer scientist who is exploring the use of computers in critical-care settings. It includes a chapter that summarizes the current status of medical practice in the ICU.*

Westenskow, D. R. Automating patient care with closed-loop control. *M.D. Computing*, 3:14, 1986.

> *This article provides an understandable discussion of closed-loop control theory and a brief summary of the medical applications of closed-loop systems.*

---

[8]Titration is a method for adjusting the concentration of a dissolved substance by observing a resulting effect. It is used as a method for adjusting the concentration of a drug to achieve the desired effect; for example, a nitroprusside infusion may be adjusted to control blood pressure within prespecified limits.

Wiederhold, G. and Clayton, P. D. Processing biological data in real time. *M.D. Computing*, 2:16, 1985.

This article summarizes the logical elements of real-time data acquisition and analysis. It contains a detailed discussion of signal acquisition, sampling frequency, and analog-to-digital conversion.

Questions for Discussion

1. Describe how the integration of information from multiple bedside monitors, the pharmacy, and the clinical laboratory can help to improve the sensitivity and specificity of the alarm systems used in the ICU.
2. Discuss three factors you must consider when deciding when and how often a physiological, biochemical, or observational variable should be measured and stored in a computer's database.
3. You have been asked to design part of an electronic exercise bicycle. Sensors in the handgrips of the bicycle will be used to pick up transmitted electrical signals reflecting the rider's heart activity. Your system then will display the rider's heart rate numerically on a liquid crystal display (LCD).
   a. Describe the steps your system must take in converting the heart's electrical signals (essentially a single ECG lead) to the heart rate displayed on the LCD.
   b. The resistance of the pedals can be controlled electronically by a microprocessor. Design a simple closed-loop system that dynamically adjusts (increases or decreases) the work for the cyclist based on heart rate. Draw a flowchart for how you might use the calculated heart rate to control the pedal resistance.
   c. How is the accuracy of your data affected by a rider's failure to maintain constant contact with the handgrips? What would happen if your algorithm were used with these inaccurate data? Suggest a second type of data you could collect to verify the accuracy of the handgrip heart-rate data.

13

Information Systems for Office Practice

Michael C. Higgins and Andrew B. Newman

After reading this chapter, you should know the answers to these questions:

- What unique characteristics of office-based medical practice must developers consider when designing computer systems for information management?

- What four classes of information are used by health professionals in office settings?

- Why have computer-based billing systems been widely accepted in physicians' offices, whereas systems for managing clinical information are still relatively uncommon?

- What types of computing services and software are currently available to help office-based physicians with information-management tasks?

- What economic, social, and technologic forces are driving the development of office computer systems?

13.1 The Office-Practice Setting

During the next decade, computers for use in doctors' offices will be one of the largest growth segments in the medical computer market. The quantity and complexity of the information processed during the care of patients are increasing as public and private insurance carriers require more documentation for reimbursement and as the profusion of new medical technology accelerates. With the development of inexpensive hardware and easy-to-use software, it is now possible to transfer some of this information-processing burden to machines.

Some form of automated data processing is used in a growing number of doctors' offices in this country. For the most part, these data-processing systems perform traditional billing functions; however, systems with broader functions are available. Physicians can purchase commercial software to search and access the medical literature, schedule appointments, manage inventories of drugs and supplies, and maintain medication lists and medical records. A few offices have automated most of their information-processing tasks, and thus approach the ideal of a completely paperless office.

This chapter explores the range of uses of computers in physicians' offices. Although virtually all the computer applications discussed in this book in principle could be applied in the office-practice setting, the organization of private practices, the types of services provided in office settings, the ways that ambulatory-care services are purchased, and the interactions between community practice and other segments of the health-care industry combine to make outpatient medicine a unique and rapidly changing environment.

13.1.1 An Overview of Physician Services

Of the 450,000 physicians who were actively caring for patients in the United States in 1985, three-quarters had office-based practices [U.S. Bureau of the Census, 1987]. These physicians provide a variety of services, ranging from routine care for self-limiting diseases to long-term treatment for chronic illnesses. More recently, outpatient facilities, such as emergency-care centers and same-day surgery clinics, have begun to provide services that previously were available only in hospitals.

Although much outpatient care is delivered by doctors who treat a broad spectrum of problems, the trend is toward greater specialization. In 1970, about 27 percent of office-based physicians were in general practice; by 1985, this percentage had dropped to 16 percent [U.S. Bureau of the Census, 1987]. Currently, family practitioners, pediatricians, obstetricians, gynecologists, dermatologists, and other office-based specialists constitute about one-half of the physicians who are actively practicing medicine in this country.

Partially as a result of such specialization, multiple health professionals often cooperate in caring for individual patients. For example, some office- or clinic-based physicians provide diagnostic services, such as radiologic examinations and simple endoscopic procedures. The physicians who perform these procedures play consulting roles, functioning as members of a patient-care team. In addition, many office-based physicians admit patients to local hospitals.

Data sharing and communication among the various health professionals involved in a patient's care are crucial. For example, surgeons and anesthesiologists, who constitute over 15 percent of the physicians in this country, typically maintain offices where they perform initial examinations and provide follow-up care. To care for their patients effectively, such physicians must be able to access the clinical information collected during hospitalization.

In 1985, patients made 636 million visits to office-based ambulatory-care physicians—an average of 2.7 visits by every person in the United States. This number probably will increase as the elderly population grows in proportion to the total population; men and women aged 65 years and older averaged over 4.8 visits per person [National Center for Health Statistics, 1988]. Many office visits are made by patients receiving treatment for chronic illnesses and other ongoing problems. The results of the 1985 National Ambulatory Medical Care Survey showed that only 17 percent of office visits were made by new patients. Established patients returning for treatment of old problems were responsible for about 60 percent of visits [National Center for Health Statistics, 1988].

In busy practices, physicians often see 25 or more patients per day. In comparison to episodes of hospitalization, these office encounters are brief—70 percent involve physician–patient contact of 15 minutes or less [National Center for Health Statistics, 1988]. Routine visits for follow-up care might last only 5 or 10 minutes; even detailed consultations typically last at most several hours. As a result, health-care professionals must collect, process, and record a large amount of information in a short period.

Given that outpatient visits are also relatively inexpensive, data entry and storage are high-overhead activities. Nonetheless, a complete record of past medical problems and treatments is necessary to ensure continuity of care for patients over time. The provision of high-quality health care often depends on the availability of information about patients' past problems and treatments. In fact, the retrieval of historical medical data is one of the critical information-management tasks in outpatient care.

13.1.2 Health-Care Financing

In dollar terms, hospital care accounts for the largest single portion of the annual health-care bill in the United States—about 40 percent of total health expenditures, or approximately $180 billion in 1986. Expenditures for physicians' services make up another 20 percent of the total. The remaining 40 percent pays for drugs, nursing-home care, medical appliances, and so on.

Of the $92 billion spent on physicians' services, private consumers paid for 70 percent of the charges, either directly (28 percent) or indirectly through private insurance (42 percent). Government programs (primarily Medicare and Medicaid) paid for the remaining 30 percent of the bill. By comparison, over 50 percent of hospital charges are paid through some form of public funding; only 9 percent of expenditures for hospital care were paid out of pocket by patients. As we shall see in Chapter 19, high and rapidly increasing health-care costs alarmed the government, third-party payers, and consumers alike. The resultant cost-containment measures, which were implemented in the 1980s, targeted hospitals in an attempt to slow the rate of growth, thus producing incentives to physicians to provide more services in outpatient rather than inpatient settings. Outpatient care will continue to gain prominence in response to the cost-containment measures that have been imposed on hospital care.

13.1.3 Health-Care Personnel

Physicians, nurses, and health-care workers perform a variety of information-management tasks related to patient care and business operation. Office personnel locate, retrieve, and update patients' medical records. Nurses collect and record baseline data, such as weight, temperature, and blood pressure, as well as much of the past medical history. Physicians gather additional data, form opinions about patients' problems, and devise treatment plans. This information becomes part of the visit note, which physicians either enter into the record directly or dictate for later transcription.

In addition to managing information related to patient care, health-care workers also must perform the day-to-day tasks related to running a small business and to ensuring that the practice remains profitable. Following each examination, clerical staff update the patient accounts and financial records and periodically generate bills for patients or for third-party payers. Given the growing demand for documentation and information by insurance companies and the increase in the number of patients covered by insurance, the management of financial information represents an increasing burden to physicians' practices.

Despite the fact that they are not information managers either by interest or training, health professionals in most physicians' offices are responsible for performing all information-management tasks. These duties compete with patient-care and other professional responsibilities. The business aspects of medical practices are particularly troublesome. By default, most private practices are run by physicians. This is true despite the paucity of business training in the typical medical-school curriculum and the differences in the motivations people have for entering the health-care professions and for entering business.

Typically, physicians hire support staff to assist them in many of the nonmedical aspects of office practice. Virtually every office has at least a receptionist who answers the telephone, registers patients, and handles some or all of the nonmedical paperwork. In addition, most offices employ, on a part-time basis, an accountant who oversees the accuracy of the financial records and prepares the tax reports. As a practice grows, additional office workers are added to the payroll. Larger practices may employ transcriptionists or data-entry personnel to record the physicians' progress notes, and may hire chart auditors who help to organize the content of the medical records. Group practices that employ several office workers usually hire an office manager who is responsible for making day-to-day business decisions and for supervising the nonmedical staff. It is not uncommon for office managers to have some formal business training. Typical office workers, however, have little training outside of what they learn from coworkers. Employee turnover often is so high that training new office personnel can account for a significant portion of the office expenses.

13.1.4 Implications for the Design of Computer-Based Office Systems

Several technologic, sociologic, and economic trends favor the development of computer systems for use by physicians in private practice. Rapid increase in the volume and complexity of medical knowledge, an aging population and the associated increase in chronic disease, and increasing documentary requirements by third-party payers create growing internal and external demands for gathering information. Furthermore, the trends away from general practitioners toward specialists, and away from solo practice toward partnerships and group practices, create a need for more effective storage and communication of information. The accessibility and legibility of the record also become crucial as more health professionals share medical data.

Vendors must design their systems to fit key characteristics of physicians' practices. Of necessity, most physicians are pragmatists who will adopt a new technology only if it improves the quality or reduces the cost of the services they provide. In addition, because of the time pressures they face, physicians may reject even a system with substantial benefits if using the system would increase the total amount of time spent on information-management tasks, or if setting up and learning the system would be excessively time consuming. The high turnover rate and limited training of most office workers further underscores the fact that computer systems must be simple to learn and use—only the largest of offices can afford to employ computer personnel whose sole responsibility is to operate the data-processing equipment used by the practice. These factors, combined with limited availability of capital for investment by small practices, place important constraints on the function, design, and price of office-based information systems. In physicians' offices, more than in any other medical setting, computer systems must be practical, inexpensive, and easy to use.

13.2 Information Management in Physicians' Offices

Health professionals in office-based practices manage four types of information:
1. The *medical information* describing history of illness, clinical findings, diagnoses, and treatments for individual patients
2. The *scientific information* applied by physicians while caring for patients
3. The *administrative and accounting information* involved in scheduling appointments, managing patient accounts, paying bills, collecting revenue, and performing the other tasks necessary to operate a small business
4. The *financial-management and practice-planning information* that physicians use to assess the status of their practices, including the magnitude of revenues and expenses, the numbers and types of procedures they perform, and the demographic composition of the patient populations they serve

13.2.1 Medical Information

The specific information used during an encounter between physician and patient differs depending on the purpose of the visit and on whether or not the patient has been seen before. The general classes of information, however, are common to almost all cases. For example, the patient's *past medical history* is pertinent to most evaluations. This historical information describes the patient's family and social history, as well as past medical events that are relevant to the physician's understanding and treatment of current problems. For the established patient, the physician or a nurse updates the historical information at the start of the encounter; Figure 13.1 shows a typical **medical-history form.**

If the purpose of the visit is assessment of a specific complaint, rather than a routine checkup, the physician will gather information about current symptoms and obtain a *history of the present illness.* The examination typically continues with a *review of systems,* during which the physician assesses various aspects of the patient's well-being by asking general questions about each of the body's major systems. The level of detail in this review depends on the physician's interviewing style, familiarity with the patient, and the nature of the examination. The **system-review form** in Figure 13.2 illustrates the type of information that is collected during this process.

The physician investigates significant abnormalities detected during the review of systems by performing a *physical examination.* For example, because the hypothetical patient summarized in Figure 13.2 displayed symptoms and signs of respiratory disease, the physician focused the subsequent physical examination on this patient's nose, throat, and lungs. The findings during the physical examination usually are documented on a form like that shown in Figure 13.3. Notice that the information collected during the physical examination is far more detailed than that collected during the history and review of systems. Much of the information can be recorded on checklists; however, some findings are more easily conveyed with illustrations (such as the location of the polyp in the patient's nasal passage noted in Figure 13.3) or with free text.

Occasionally, physicians perform diagnostic tests during office visits. They may, for example, examine blood samples under a microscope, take chest X-ray films, or administer special procedures, such as pulmonary-function tests. These tests sometimes generate diagrams or reports, such as the spirometer chart shown in Figure 13.4, which become part of the patient's medical record.

As we discussed in Chapter 2, physicians seem to apply an iterative strategy to medical diagnosis—findings on examination often prompt further questioning to rule-in or rule-out alternative hypotheses. Eventually, the physician reaches conclusions about the nature of the patient's problem, the need for further diagnostic testing, and the desirability of possible alternative treatments. These conclusions can be summarized on forms like those shown in Figures 13.5 and 13.6.

Not all information is available at the time of the patient visit. Many office practices routinely send specimens to independent laboratories for processing; the results of bacterial cultures and some laboratory tests may not be known until several days after the visit. Once the laboratory-test results are available, they must be added to the patient's medical record. Occasionally, a delayed finding will have therapeutic implications. In these cases, the physician may recall the patient for further evaluation or for alteration of treatment.

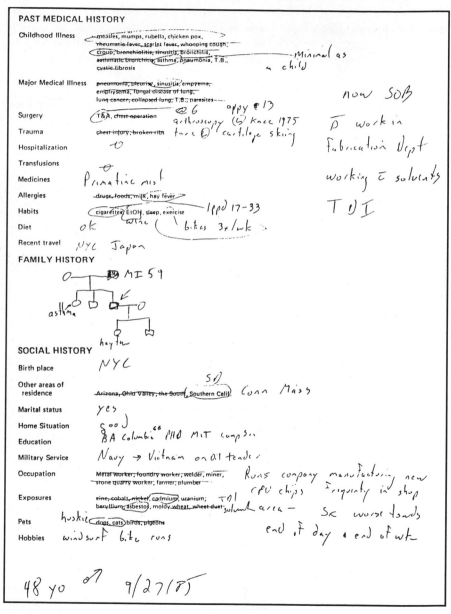

FIGURE 13.1 Physicians may use a checklist to guide their questioning when gathering information about relevant medical, family, and social history.

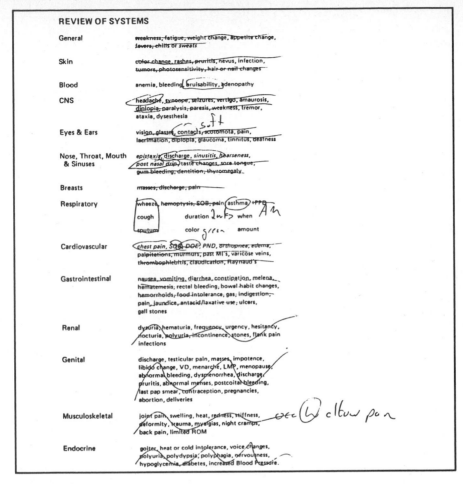

FIGURE 13.2 During the review of systems, physicians ask questions and collect data that pertain to each of the major systems of the body.

13.2.2 Scientific Information

Medical practice requires the management of general information as well as of patient-specific information—in principle, patient-care decisions reflect the application of medical science to individual cases. During a typical day, physicians raise a number of questions related to patient management: questions of medical fact ("What are the contraindications for drug X?"), questions of medical opinion ("What is the appropriate management for a patient with disease Y?"), and questions of nonmedical information ("What day-care services are available to the disabled elderly?"). Given the rapidly changing state of medical science, physicians cannot hope to know the answer to every question that arises during a patient visit, and they frequently seek information from a variety of outside sources [Covell et al., 1985].

Physical Examination

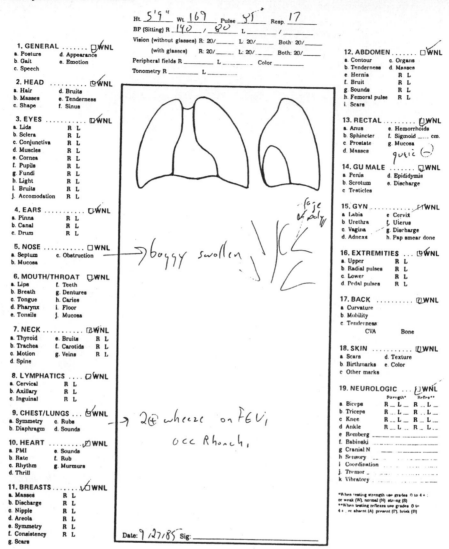

Ht. 5'9" Wt. 169 Pulse 8? Resp. 17
BP (Sitting) R 140 , 80 L ____ / ____
Vision (without glasses) R: 20/____ L: 20/____ Both: 20/____
(with glasses) R: 20/____ L: 20/____ Both: 20/____
Peripheral fields R _____ L _____ Color _____
Tonometry R _____ L _____

1. GENERAL .... ☐WNL
a. Posture   d. Appearance
b. Gait   e. Emotion
c. Speech

2. HEAD .... ☑WNL
a. Hair   d. Bruits
b. Masses   e. Tenderness
c. Shape   f. Sinus

3. EYES .... ☑WNL
a. Lids   R L
b. Sclera   R L
c. Conjunctiva R L
d. Muscles   R L
e. Cornea   R L
f. Pupils   R L
g. Fundi   R L
h. Light   R L
i. Bruits   R L
j. Accomodation R L

4. EARS .... ☐WNL
a. Pinna   R L
b. Canal   R L
c. Drum   R L

5. NOSE .... ☐WNL
a. Septum   c. Obstruction
b. Mucosa

→ boggy swollen

6. MOUTH/THROAT ☐WNL
a. Lips   f. Teeth
b. Breath   g. Dentures
c. Tongue   h. Caries
d. Pharynx   i. Floor
e. Tonsils   j. Mucosa

7. NECK .... ☑WNL
a. Thyroid   e. Bruits   R L
b. Trachea   f. Carotids R L
c. Motion   g. Veins   R L
d. Spine

8. LYMPHATICS .... ☐WNL
a. Cervical   R L
b. Axillary   R L
c. Inguinal   R L

9. CHEST/LUNGS ... ☑WNL
a. Symmetry   c. Rubs
b. Diaphragm   d. Sounds

→ 2⊕ wheeze on FEV₁
occ Rhonchi

10. HEART .... ☑WNL
a. PMI   e. Sounds
b. Rate   f. Rub
c. Rhythm   g. Murmurs
d. Thrill

11. BREASTS .... ☑WNL
a. Masses   R L
b. Discharge   R L
c. Nipple   R L
d. Areola   R L
e. Symmetry   R L
f. Consistency R L
g. Scars

12. ABDOMEN .... ☐WNL
a. Contour   c. Organs
b. Tenderness d. Masses
e. Hernia   R L
f. Bruit   R L
g. Sounds   R L
h. Femoral pulse R L
i. Scars

13. RECTAL .... ☐WNL
a. Anus   e. Hemorrhoids
b. Sphincter   f. Sigmoid ____ cm.
c. Prostate   g. Mucosa
d. Masses
quiec (−)

14. GU MALE .... ☐WNL
a. Penis   d. Epididymis
b. Scrotum   e. Discharge
c. Testicles

15. GYN .... ☑WNL
a. Labia   e. Cervix
b. Urethra   f. Uterus
c. Vagina   g. Discharge
d. Adnexa   h. Pap smear done

16. EXTREMITIES ... ☑WNL
a. Upper   R L
b. Radial pulses R L
c. Lower   R L
d. Pedal pulses R L

17. BACK .... ☑WNL
a. Curvature
b. Mobility
c. Tenderness
        CVA   Bone

18. SKIN .... ☑WNL
a. Scars   d. Texture
b. Birthmarks e. Color
c. Other marks

19. NEUROLOGIC ... ☐WNL
                Strength*   Reflex**
a. Biceps   R__L__ R__L__
b. Triceps   R__L__ R__L__
c. Knee   R__L__ R__L__
d. Ankle   R__L__ R__L__
e. Romberg   _____
f. Babinski   _____
g. Cranial N   _____
h. Sensory   _____
i. Coordination _____
j. Tremor   _____
k. Vibratory   _____

*When testing strength use grades 0 to 4 +:
or weak (W), normal (N) strong (S)
**When testing reflexes use grades 0 to
4 + : or absent (A), present (P), brisk (B)

Date: 7/27/85   Sig: _____

FIGURE 13.3 The physical examination form provides a checklist of common examinations and allows space for physicians to record their findings.

The dynamic nature of medical science is evident from the cornucopia of medical periodicals. Today, more than 20,000 journals are published each year in biomedicine alone. Conscientious physicians follow several of these journals to keep abreast of new developments pertaining to their practices. Doctors sometimes consult reference books when interpreting clinical findings or when planning therapy. One common reference is the *Physicians' Desk Reference* (PDR) [Medical Economics Company,

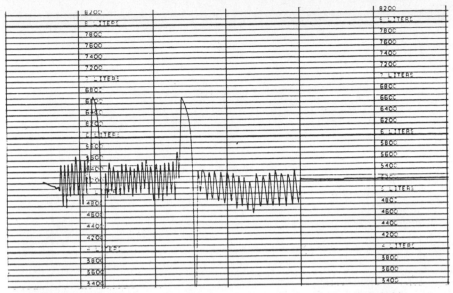

FIGURE 13.4 The results of spirometry and other diagnostic tests are included in patients' permanent records.

1988], a compendium of drug information as provided by the manufacturers that is published annually, with updates distributed on a more frequent basis. The standard medical textbooks, such as *Harrison's Principles of Internal Medicine* [Braunwald et al., 1987] and *Cecil Textbook of Medicine* [Wyngaarden and Smith, 1988] are published less frequently; however, a periodical textbook published by Scientific American is growing in popularity [Rubenstein and Federman, 1988]. Subscribers to *Scientific American Medicine* receive updates monthly. As we shall discuss in Chapter 14, physicians can search a variety of online bibliographic databases to find articles relevant to specific biomedical topics.

In addition to reading the published literature to stay current on developments in their field, and to obtain answers to specific questions, physicians converse and correspond with colleagues, attend conferences, and enroll in continuing medical-education courses. The development of commercial networks for the exchange of electronic mail and bulletin-board messages provides an additional mode for communicating important clinical information.

13.2.3 Accounting and Administrative Information

Keeping track of clinical and scientific information represents only part of the information-management burden. Although patient care is a major objective of medical practice, a doctor's office is also a business; physicians and their staff must attend to the financial and administrative aspects of running a small business. A large component of these tasks is related to the creation and maintenance of patient accounts for billing purposes.

Name _____ Age __48__ Birthdate __6/5/37__

Problem No.	Problems/Diagnoses		Code
(1)	Occupational Asthma		493
(2)	s/p torn (L) meniscus cartilage		
(3)	s/p Arthroscopic Repair (L) knee 1975		
(4)	Allergic Rhinitis		477
(5)	Sinusitus		

	Risk Factors		Surgery
(1)	Cigs 1ppd 17-33	(1)	T+A @ 6
(2)	Asbestos exp in Navy.	(2)	Appy @ 13
(3)	Asthma as a child	(3)	L meniscus cartilage 1975
(4)	TDI & Cadmium exposure		

FIGURE 13.5 Physicians may use a standard form to maintain lists of clinical problems and diagnoses.

Patient _____

		Date	5/10/85	5/24/85	8/27/85	9/27/85		
Bronchodilators								
	Oral	Theedur 300	B,D	B,D	B,D	B,D		
	Inhaled	AKoPKosol	B,D	B,D	B,D	B,D		
		Tornolate	B,D	B,D	B,D	B,D		
Steroids								
	Oral							
		Nasalide		2p H,D	2p H,D	2p B,D		
	Inhaled	Beclovent	4p g.d					
		Azmacort		4p T,D	4p T,D	4p T,Y		
Cromolyn			B,D					
Antibiotics								
Antihistamines								
Diuretics								
Miscellaneous		Moduretic	9/ A.m	9 A.m	9 A.m	7 A.m		
		K	B,D	B,D	B,D	B,D		
Nasal Passages				Boggy Swollen		oK		
BP				110/70				
Wheeze				=		=		
FEV₁								
Chest X-ray								
Eosinophils								
Aminophylline Level								

FIGURE 13.6 The medication-administration form provides a succinct record of a patient's medication history.

When patients arrive at the doctor's office, they are checked into the system. If the patient has not been seen before—which is the case in about one of five visits—the patient must register by providing basic demographic information (such as name, age, and gender), emergency contacts, address, telephone number, and insurance information. Figure 13.7 contains an example of a registration form used to collect this information. Office personnel then create a new chart and set up a patient account. Established patients often are asked to complete a shorter form to verify that the registration information has not changed since the last visit. At the end of the examination, the physician usually records the final diagnosis and indicates the services that were performed on an **encounter form** like those shown in Figures 13.8 and 13.9, and an office worker totals the charges.

The resolution of the resulting bill depends on the type and extent of the patient's insurance coverage. Patients pay for a substantial portion of outpatient medical costs directly. An increasing number of patients, however, are covered by public or private insurance. Regardless of whether the bill is sent to the patient or to an insurance company, the office must document the services provided (Figures 13.10 and 13.11). The preparation of this documentation is a labor-intensive process and usually is responsible for a major portion of the overhead in operating a doctor's office.

DATE_____

PATIENT REGISTRATION FOR MEDICAL RECORDS (PLEASE PRINT)

LAST NAME	FIRST	MIDDLE	SOCIAL SECURITY NO.	DATE OF BIRTH	AGE
Jober	Jonathan	Q	064-42-1691	6/3/37	48

HOME ADDRESS STREET	CITY	STATE	ZIP	HOME PHONE
1021 Cherry Ave.	Los Altos Hills	CA	94022	415 322-1236

SEX	MARITAL STATUS	SPOUSE NAME	REFERRED BY	OCCUPATION
M	⊗ S D W SEP	Susan	Dr. Rbt. Weed	Pres. Cheako Computers

EMPLOYED BY	EMPLOYER'S ADDRESS STREET	CITY	STATE	ZIP	PHONE NUMBER
Cheako Computers	100 Golden Way	Santa Clara	CA	95054	408 962-CHIP

POLICYHOLDER (IF DIFFERENT)	STREET ADDRESS	CITY	STATE	ZIP	RELATION TO PATIENT	PHONE NUMBER

IN CASE OF EMERGENCY CONTACT: NAME, HOME ADDRESS	HOME PHONE NUMBER	RELATION TO PATIENT
Sylvia Throckmorton 130 Hill Ct. La Honda	323-2126	sister

EMERGENCY CONTACT: BUSINESS ADDRESS	BUSINESS PHONE NUMBER

⚑ MEDICAL INSURANCE INFORMATION

COMPANY		POLICY NUMBER
Blue Cross of California Group 9164		102 345711
COMPANY		POLICY NUMBER
COMPANY		POLICY NUMBER

⚑ IF SOMEONE OTHER THAN PATIENT IS RESPONSIBLE FOR PAYMENT PLEASE COMPLETE THIS SECTION

NAME OF RESPONSIBLE PARTY	RELATION TO PATIENT
NA	

BILLING ADDRESS STREET	CITY	STATE	ZIP	PHONE NUMBER

BIBBERO SYSTEMS, INC.   •   PETALUMA, CA.   •   © 1983   FORM # 88-8420

FIGURE 13.7 New patients typically complete a registration form that provides basic demographic and billing information. Established patients may complete a shorter form to verify that the office's information is up to date. (*Source:* Form courtesy of BIBBERO SYSTEMS, Inc., Petaluma, California.)

The bill itself must describe the services for which payment is due. Typically, physician services are identified on an invoice by brief descriptions or by numeric codes. The widely used five-digit coding system developed for the California Relative Value Study [California Medical Association, 1969] is an example of the latter. In addition, third-party payment programs often require that the invoice include a medical justification for the performance of a service—a brief description or a code that identifies the diagnoses or problems that were treated. The **Ninth International Classification of Diseases–Clinical Modification (ICD-9-CM)** for encoding medical diagnoses is used frequently [Health Care Financing Administration, 1980]. Originally, the ICD-9-CM codes were developed to classify the diagnoses assigned to patients in hospital care; however, this system has been extended to incorporate the symptoms and nonspecific complaints with which patients in ambulatory care commonly present.

In addition to the description and justification of the services provided, third-party payers often require that invoices include information that is used to determine patient eligibility and level of reimbursement. For example, the date and site of the service and the identification of the provider usually are required on third-party invoices. Additional information is used to determine whether the patient is eligible for coverage under other programs. For example, the patient's age indicates whether Medicare can be billed. Similarly, many work-related injuries are covered under Workmen's Compensation programs or insurance policies carried by employers.

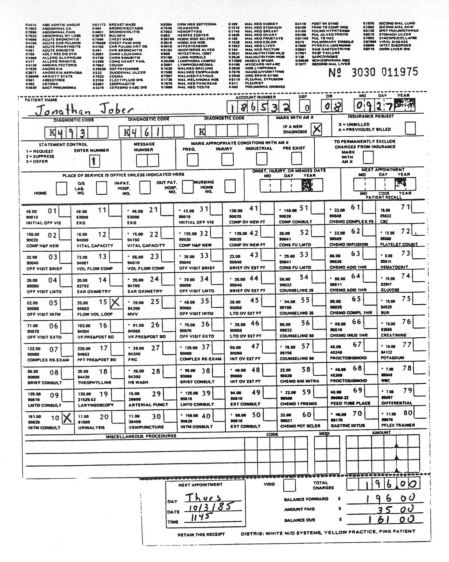

FIGURE 13.8 Physicians often use standard forms to indicate which services were provided during a patient visit.

The diversity of the third-party payment programs is reflected in the large number of invoice forms currently in use. Most private carriers accept the standard **Health Insurance Claim Form (HICF)** shown in Figure 13.12. The exceptions, however, include the Medicare and Medicaid programs, as well as several large private insurance companies. Therefore, an effective billing system, whether manual or automated, must be able to accommodate a variety of invoice formats. Moreover, the restructuring of both the private and public sectors of our health-care system

Patient: JOBER JONATHAN Q   DOB: 06-03-37   Sex: M   Rel: Self

JOBER JONATHAN Q   1021 CHERRY AVE   LOS ALTOS HILLS CA   94022
MD#:02 Acct frm Current   0.00   0.00   0.00   0.00 Date 01-24-89 or _____

Acct #:626 03 /   C   < CR >   D   Ticket #: 2753

INITIAL OFF VIS 90010 50 101	COMP IN OV 90020 18B 102	OFF VISIT BRIEF 90040 34 103	OFF VISIT LMTD 90050 44 104	OFF VISIT INTM 90060 55 105	OFF VISIT EXTD 90070 78 105	COMPLEX RE-EXAM 90080 130 107	BRIEF CONSULT 90300 95 108	LMTD CONSULT 90610 140 109	INTM CONSULT 90620 190 110
EKG 93000YB 53 111	VITAL CAPACITY 94000YB 20 112	VOL FLOW COMP 94001YB 78 113	EAR OXIMETRY 82792YB 28 114	FLOW VOL LOOP 94002YB 40 115	VF-PRE/POST BD 94004YB 122 116	PFT PRE/POST BD 94603YB 245 117	THEOPHYLLINE 84420YB 35 118	LARYNGOSCOPY 31525YB 359 119	URINALYSIS 81000YB 11 120
*EKG 93000YB 46 121	*VITAL CAPACITY 94150YB 15 122	*VOL FLOW COMP 94010YB 65 123	*EAR OXIMETRY 82792YB 20 124	*MVV 94200YB 33 125	*VG-PRE/POST BD 94060YB 91 126	*FRC 94240YB 39 127	*HE WASH 94350YB 25 128	*ARTERIAL PNCT 36600YB 15 129	*VENIPUNCTURE 36415YB 15 130
*INITIAL OFF VI 90010 48 131	*COMP IN OV 90020 136 132	*OFF VISIT BRIE 90040 25 133	*OFF VISIT LMTD 90050 39 134	*OFF VISIT INTM 90060 48 135	*OFF VISIT EXTD 90070 49 136	*COMPLEX RE EXA 90080 91 137	*BRIEF CONSULT 90300 95 138	*LMTD CONSULT 90610 125 139	*INTM CONSULT 90620 152 140
CONS FU LMTD 90641 50 152	*LIM CON FU 90541 40 153	FLEX SIG 45330YB 128 167	*FLEX SIG 45330YB 145 168	PFLEX TRAINR 90070 11 180	PEAK FLOW MTER 90070 25 221	*HOLTER MONITOR 93274 220 222	HOLTER MONITOR 93274 240 223	FLU INJECTION 90720 18 224	*PNEUMOVAX INJE 90749YB 18 225
*THERAPEUTIC IN 90782YB 18 181	INSTRUMENT TRAY 90970YB 30 227	PAP SMEAR 88150YB 14 228	PHLEBOTOMY 90085YB 40 229	PPD SKIN TEST 86580YB 14 230	STRESS TEST 94620 375 231	STOOL G/A/UC 89205YB 4 232	*THORACENTESIS 32000YB 101 233	THORACENTESIS 32000YB 125 234	TCENTESIS TRAY 99070YB 45 235
ABDOMINAL PAIN 7890 502	ABPA 1173 637	ALLERG RHINITIS 477 510	ANGINA PECTORIS 4139 511	ADLT RES DIS SY 769 504	ASBESTOSIS 501 515	ASTHMA 493 516	ARRYTHMIA 4279 620	BREAST MASS 61172 518	BRONCHIECTASIS 494 519
ACUTE BRONCHITI 4660 504	BRONCOILITIS 4661 520	CERVICALGIA 7866 621	CHEST MASS 7866 522	CHEST PAIN NOS 78650 523	CONG HEAR FAIL 4280 530	COPD 4960 622	COR PULMONALE 4169 623	COSTOCHONDRITIS 7336 624	COUGH 7862 531
DIVING ACCIDENT E9101 625	DRUG RASH 6930 626	DYSPNEA 7860 627	EDEMA 7823 534	ESOPHAGITIS 5301 536	FX RIB 807 628	HEADACHE 7840 538	HEMOPTYSIS 7863 539	HEMORRHOIDS 4558 629	HYPERTENSION 4019 543
IDIOFIBROS ALVE 5163 544	IRRIT COLON 5641 615	PURE HYPERCHOLS 2720 593	LUNG NODULE 5188 547	MAL NEO BREAST 1748 559	MAL NEO BR/LUNG 1628 550	MALAISE/FATIGUE 7807 552	MELANA 5781 631	MYOCARD INFARC 4108 567	MITRAL VALVE PR 3949 632
MUSCLE SPASM 72885 566	NAEVS VOM 7870 612	NASOPHARYNGITIS 460 633	PLEURAL EFFUSIO 5119 571	PLEURISY 511 572	PNEUMONIA ORGNE 483 573	SPNT PHELMOTHRA 5120 588	PUL ALVEO FROTH 5160 577	PULMONARY EMBOL 673 573	PULMO HYPERTENS 4160 576
PUL TB NEC 01192 578	PRIM TB COMP NO 0100 575	RESP FAILURE 7981 582	SARCOIDOSIS 1. 983	SCIATICA 7243 634	ACUTE SINUSITIS 461 507	CHRN SINUSITIS 4738 529	SLEEP APNEA 78035 635	SYNCOPE/COLLAPS 7802 580	URINARY TRACT I 5990 636

Serv/Diag not listed _____
Serv/Diag not listed _____
Serv/Diag not listed _____

    < CR >   Y   S   /

FIGURE 13.9 A bar-coded superbill provides a quick way to enter patient data at the end of a visit. Using a wand to highlight the patient's name, diagnosis, and charges, office personnel can enter all the information needed to produce billing statements and to update patient accounts.

suggests that significant changes in invoice formats are likely to occur in the future as reimbursement requirements continue to change. The billing system must be able to respond to these inevitable changes in billing procedures.

The work is not complete once the bill has been sent to the patient or to the third-party payer. Office workers must monitor the accounts receivable to identify patients who are delinquent in paying their bills. Private insurance companies and public

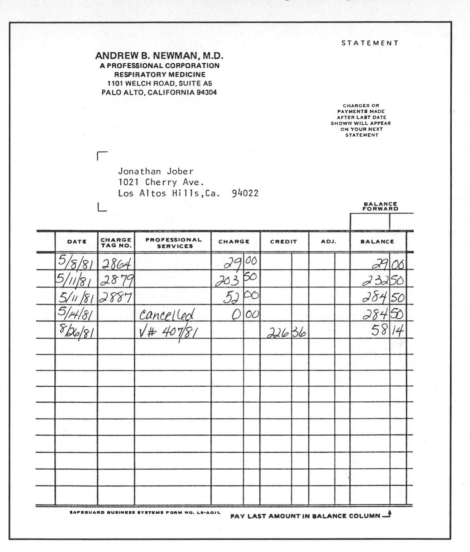

STATEMENT

ANDREW B. NEWMAN, M.D.
A PROFESSIONAL CORPORATION
RESPIRATORY MEDICINE
1101 WELCH ROAD, SUITE A5
PALO ALTO, CALIFORNIA 94304

CHARGES OR
PAYMENTS MADE
AFTER LAST DATE
SHOWN WILL APPEAR
ON YOUR NEXT
STATEMENT

Jonathan Jober
1021 Cherry Ave.
Los Altos Hills,Ca.   94022

BALANCE
FORWARD

DATE	CHARGE TAG NO.	PROFESSIONAL SERVICES	CHARGE		CREDIT		ADJ.		BALANCE	
5/8/81	2864		29	00					29	00
5/11/81	2879		203	50					232	50
5/11/81	2887		52	00					284	50
5/14/81		cancelled	0	00					284	50
8/26/81		√# 407/81			226	36			58	14

SAFEGUARD BUSINESS SYSTEMS FORM NO. LS-ADJL   PAY LAST AMOUNT IN BALANCE COLUMN ⬏

FIGURE 13.10 Bills typically are produced on a monthly cycle. They summarize the financial transactions that were recorded since the previous bill, including new charges, payments, adjustments for errors, and penalty charges.

agencies are supposed to process claims promptly. In fact, most government-sponsored programs are required by law to meet certain performance standards, which include the processing of invoices within a set period. Actual practice often falls short of this ideal. Government agencies and private insurance companies are large bureaucracies, and they often use outmoded data-processing procedures. One consequence is that valid invoices are misplaced or rejected erroneously. The claimant's only recourse is to track the status of each invoice so that rejected or misplaced claims can be resubmitted promptly.

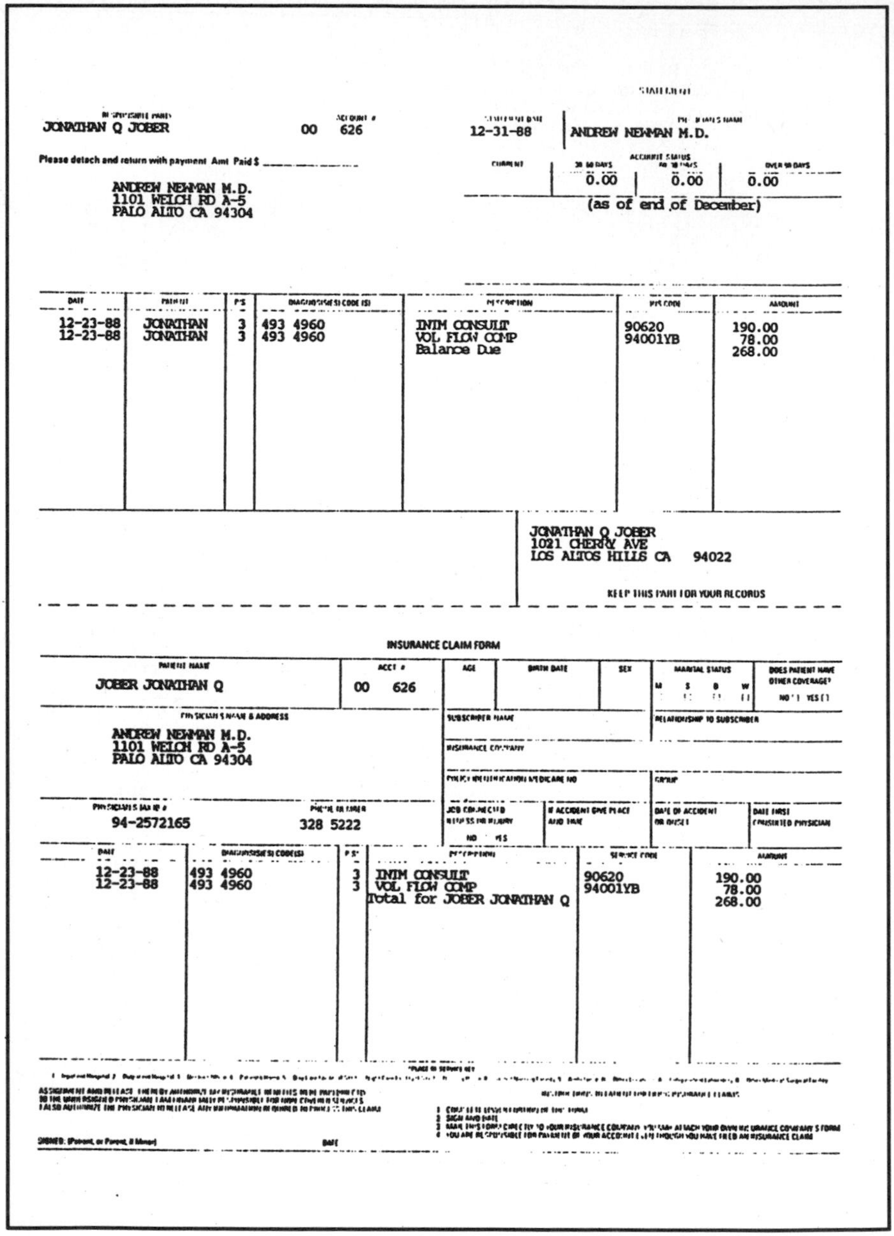

STATEMENT

JONATHAN Q JOBER   00   626   12-31-88   ANDREW NEWMAN M.D.

Please detach and return with payment Amt Paid $ _____

CURRENT   30-60 DAYS   ACCOUNT STATUS   OVER 90 DAYS
             60-90 DAYS
ANDREW NEWMAN M.D.   0.00   0.00   0.00
1101 WELCH RD A-5
PALO ALTO CA 94304   (as of end of December)

DATE	PATIENT	P'S	DIAGNOSIS CODE(S)	DESCRIPTION	PRT CODE	AMOUNT
12-23-88	JONATHAN	3	493 4960	INTM CONSULT	90620	190.00
12-23-88	JONATHAN	3	493 4960	VOL FLOW COMP	94001YB	78.00
				Balance Due		268.00

JONATHAN Q JOBER
1021 CHERRY AVE
LOS ALTOS HILLS CA   94022

KEEP THIS PART FOR YOUR RECORDS

INSURANCE CLAIM FORM

PATIENT NAME	ACCT #	AGE	BIRTH DATE	SEX	MARITAL STATUS	DOES PATIENT HAVE OTHER COVERAGE?
JOBER JONATHAN Q	00 626				M S D W	NO [ ] YES [ ]

PHYSICIAN'S NAME & ADDRESS   SUBSCRIBER NAME   RELATIONSHIP TO SUBSCRIBER
ANDREW NEWMAN M.D.
1101 WELCH RD A-5   INSURANCE COMPANY
PALO ALTO CA 94304

POLICY IDENTIFICATION/MEDICARE NO   GROUP

PHYSICIAN'S TAX #	PHONE NUMBER	JOB CONNECTED ILLNESS OR INJURY	IF ACCIDENT GIVE PLACE AND TIME	DATE OF ACCIDENT OR ONSET	DATE FIRST CONSULTED PHYSICIAN
94-2572165	328 5222	NO YES			

DATE	DIAGNOSIS CODE(S)	P'S	DESCRIPTION	SERVICE CODE	AMOUNT
12-23-88	493 4960	3	INTM CONSULT	90620	190.00
12-23-88	493 4960	3	VOL FLOW COMP	94001YB	78.00
			Total for JOBER JONATHAN Q		268.00

SIGNED: (Patient, or Parent, if Minor)   DATE

FIGURE 13.11 Computer-generated bills must include descriptions of the services provided, diagnostic and therapeutic codes, and an itemized listing of charges. Typically, these statements contain a section that is mailed back with the payment; they may also contain a form that the patient can submit directly to an insurance company for reimbursement.

PLEASE DO NOT
STAPLE IN
THIS AREA
➡

FORM APPROVED
OMB NO 0938-0008

HEALTH INSURANCE CLAIM FORM

(CHECK APPLICABLE PROGRAM BLOCK BELOW)

MEDICARE

| ☐ MEDICARE (MEDICARE NO) | ☐ MEDICAID (MEDICAID NO) | ☐ CHAMPUS (SPONSOR S SSN) | ☐ CHAMPVA (VA FILE NO) | ☐ FECA BLACK LUNG (SSN) | ☐ OTHER (CERTIFICATE SSN) |

PATIENT AND INSURED (SUBSCRIBER) INFORMATION

1. PATIENT'S NAME (LAST NAME, FIRST NAME, MIDDLE INITIAL)
JOBER JONATHAN Q

2. PATIENT'S DATE OF BIRTH
06 | 03 | 37

3. INSURED'S NAME (LAST NAME, FIRST NAME, MIDDLE INITIAL)
JOBER JONATHAN Q

4. PATIENT'S ADDRESS (STREET, CITY, STATE, ZIP CODE)
1021 CHERRY AVE
LOS ALTOS HILLS CA 94022

PATIENT'S SEX
MALE [X]   FEMALE ☐

INSURED'S ID NO (FOR PROGRAM CHECKED ABOVE, INCLUDE ALL LETTERS)
552 23 5845A

TELEPHONE NO 322 1236

7. PATIENT'S RELATIONSHIP TO INSURED
SELF [X] SPOUSE ☐ CHILD ☐ OTHER ☐

INSURED'S GROUP NO (OR GROUP NAME OR FECA CLAIM NO)

☐ INSURED IS EMPLOYED AND COVERED BY EMPLOYER HEALTH PLAN

9. OTHER HEALTH INSURANCE COVERAGE (ENTER NAME OF POLICYHOLDER AND PLAN NAME AND ADDRESS AND POLICY OR MEDICAL ASSISTANCE NUMBER)

10. WAS CONDITION RELATED TO
A. PATIENT'S EMPLOYMENT YES ☐ NO ☐
B. ACCIDENT AUTO ☐ OTHER ☐

11. INSURED'S ADDRESS (STREET, CITY, STATE, ZIP CODE)
SAME
SAME
TELEPHONE NO

11a. CHAMPUS SPONSOR'S
STATUS ☐ ACTIVE DUTY ☐ DECEASED ☐ RETIRED
BRANCH OF SERVICE

12. PATIENT'S OR AUTHORIZED PERSON'S SIGNATURE (READ BACK BEFORE SIGNING) I AUTHORIZE THE RELEASE OF ANY MEDICAL INFORMATION NECESSARY TO PROCESS THIS CLAIM I ALSO REQUEST PAYMENT OF GOVERNMENT BENEFITS EITHER TO MYSELF OR TO THE PARTY WHO ACCEPTS ASSIGNMENT BELOW

SIGNED _____ DATE _____

13. I AUTHORIZE PAYMENT OF MEDICAL BENEFITS TO UNDERSIGNED PHYSICIAN OR SUPPLIER FOR SERVICE DESCRIBED BELOW

SIGNED (INSURED OR AUTHORIZED PERSON)

PHYSICIAN OR SUPPLIER INFORMATION

14. DATE OF
15. ILLNESS (FIRST SYMPTOM) OR INJURY (ACCIDENT) OR PREGNANCY (LMP)
16. DATE FIRST CONSULTED YOU FOR THIS CONDITION
16a. IF PATIENT HAS HAD SAME OR SIMILAR ILLNESS OR INJURY, GIVE DATES
16b. IF EMERGENCY CHECK HERE ☐

17. DATE PATIENT ABLE TO RETURN TO WORK
18. DATES OF TOTAL DISABILITY   FROM _____ THROUGH _____
DATES OF PARTIAL DISABILITY   FROM _____ THROUGH _____

19. NAME OF REFERRING PHYSICIAN OR OTHER SOURCE (e.g. PUBLIC HEALTH AGENCY)
20. FOR SERVICES RELATED TO HOSPITALIZATION GIVE HOSPITALIZATION DATES   ADMITTED _____ DISCHARGED _____

21. NAME AND ADDRESS OF FACILITY WHERE SERVICES RENDERED (IF OTHER THAN HOME OR OFFICE)
22. WAS LABORATORY WORK PERFORMED OUTSIDE YOUR OFFICE? YES ☐ NO ☐ CHARGES

23. A. DIAGNOSIS OR NATURE OF ILLNESS OR INJURY. RELATE DIAGNOSIS TO PROCEDURE IN COLUMN D BY REFERENCE NUMBERS 1, 2, 3.
1. ICD-9 CM CODE 493 ASTHMA
2.
3.

EPSDT YES ☐ NO ☐
FAMILY PLANNING YES ☐ NO ☐

PRIOR AUTHORIZATION NO

24. A. DATE OF SERVICE FROM — TO	B. PLACE OF SERVICE	C. PROCEDURE CODE IDENTIFY	FULLY DESCRIBE PROCEDURES, MEDICAL SERVICES OR SUPPLIES FURNISHED FOR EACH DATE GIVEN (EXPLAIN UNUSUAL SERVICES OR CIRCUMSTANCES)	D. DIAGNOSIS CODE	E. CHARGES	F. DAYS OR UNITS	G. TOS	H. LEAVE BLANK
05-26-89	3	90620	*INTM CONSULT	1	151 50			
05-26-89	3	94010YB	*VOL FLOW COMP	1	65 65			

25. SIGNATURE OF PHYSICIAN OR SUPPLIER (INCLUDING DEGREES OR CREDENTIALS) (I CERTIFY THAT THE STATEMENTS ON THE REVERSE APPLY TO THIS BILL AND ARE MADE A PART THEREOF)

DATE 05-29-89

26. ACCEPT ASSIGNMENT (GOVT CLAIMS ONLY) (SEE BACK) YES ☐ NO [X]

28. YOUR SOCIAL SECURITY NO

29. YOUR PATIENT'S ACCOUNT NO 01 / 626
30. YOUR EMPLOYER ID NO

27. TOTAL CHARGE
217 15

28. AMOUNT PAID

29. BALANCE DUE

31. PHYSICIAN'S, SUPPLIER'S AND/OR GROUP NAME, ADDRESS, ZIP CODE AND TELEPHONE NO
ANDREW NEWMAN M.D.
1101 WELCH RD A-5
PALO ALTO CA 94304

PLACE OF SERVICE AND TYPE OF SERVICE (TOS) CODES ON THE BACK

APPROVED BY AMA COUNCIL ON MEDICAL SERVICE 8/83

Form HCFA-1500 (C-2) (1-84) Form OWCP-1500
Form CHAMPUS-501 Form RRB-1500

FIGURE 13.12 The majority of private third-party payers accept the standardized Health Insurance Claim Form (HICF), as well as their own special forms.

The business office performs a number of tasks in addition to the generation of bills and invoices. Payments must be made and recorded for the medical and office supplies, rent, utilities, license fees, and miscellaneous purchases. The delivery of medical care is labor-intensive, so payroll usually is the biggest single expense in the operating budget of a doctor's office. The numerous deductions required by federal and state laws greatly complicate payroll transactions. As we all know, there is a sizeable difference between a person's salary or wages and the amount that actually appears on the paycheck. This difference reflects the amounts withheld for federal and state income taxes and for the Federal Insurance Contributions Act (Social Security). Funds also may be withheld for state unemployment and disability programs, employer-sponsored insurance programs, union dues, various savings programs, and the repayment of salary advances.

Appointment scheduling is critical to the smooth operation of an office practice. For professional and financial reasons, physicians usually try to see as many patients as possible. An overly ambitious schedule, however, can seriously detract from the quality of patient care by restricting the time a physician spends on each case. Scheduling the appropriate number of patients is not a simple task. The time needed for a visit varies considerably among patients. Workups of new patients and comprehensive screening examinations require much more time than do follow-up visits for chronic problems by established patients.

Offices typically categorize visits according to complexity. When scheduling an appointment, the staff allocates a slot on the appointment log to allow for the average time required by a visit within a category. Of course, urgent visits by unscheduled patients, the unexpected complications that can arise during a patient visit, and the outside distractions that are part of the daily life of most physicians can disrupt the ideal prescribed by any schedule. Therefore, a schedule must be flexible enough to accommodate unexpected events without drastically increasing the time patients spend in the waiting room. Because it is not uncommon for patients to fail to keep appointments, some offices telephone each patient 1 or 2 days prior to a scheduled visit to remind the patient of the appointment and to verify that the patient intends to keep it.

13.2.4 Financial-Management and Practice-Planning Information

In addition to managing the information necessary for guiding day-to-day operations, the business office also must collect the data needed to analyze the financial health of the practice, to evaluate the efficiency of the practice's operation, and to predict future demands for resources. Most offices produce a financial report that describes the flow of cash into and out of the various bank accounts used by the business. Physicians use this cashflow report when making short-term expenditure decisions, as well as when planning major capital investments. In addition, the business office usually prepares periodic expenditure reports and income analyses, which show how money is spent and how revenue is generated. Together, these two reports provide a basis for judging the net productivity of a practice's various activities.

A variety of data can be collected to assess different aspects of operational efficiency. For example, office workers can monitor patient waiting times to evaluate the appropriateness of the appointment-scheduling procedure, or they can track the number of no shows (patients who fail to keep their appointments) to determine whether a policy of routinely reminding patients of their appointments is warranted. Similarly, periodic analysis of inventory levels provides useful information for deciding whether the inventory level on hand is appropriate.

Understanding who the patients are and what their needs are allows physicians to anticipate growth or shrinkage in number of visits and shifts in patient population that require changes in practice procedures, expansion or contraction of the practice, purchase of new equipment, and so on. Some useful measures are the number of active patients; the number of new patients; the distribution of patients by age, by gender, and by occupation; the frequency of each procedure performed; the revenue and expenses of services by volume; and the source and volume of referrals. Comparison of current and past measures may expose important trends that can affect the practice.

13.2.5 The Information-Management Process

We have examined four types of information managed in physicians' offices; now, we shall look at the information-management process. Figure 13.13 illustrates a patient's movement through a physician's office during a visit, and identifies the points at which different types of information are collected. The process begins when a patient calls and schedules an appointment. When the patient arrives at the office, the staff completes a registration form (Figure 13.7) and, if the patient is new to the practice, creates a medical chart. The patient is then sent to the examination or consultation room where the physician and other health-care personnel collect the bulk of the medical information (Figures 13.1, 13.2, 13.3, and 13.4). At the end of the visit, the physician documents in the medical record the important findings, diagnoses, and treatments prescribed (Figures 13.5 and 13.6). The patient returns to the front desk with a charge slip (Figures 13.8 or 13.9), which the staff uses to update his account. At this point, he may schedule a follow-up appointment, and may be given a bill for services (Figure 13.10). Once the patient leaves the office, he may contact the medical personnel to receive laboratory-test results or to ask questions about his progress. The business office sends monthly billing statements to patients that have outstanding balances (Figure 13.11), and some practices bill insurance companies directly. The cycle repeats each time the patient returns for treatment of new or ongoing problems.

13.3 Historical Perspective: Traditional Office Systems

Traditionally, office practices have used paper-based information systems—office workers manually complete forms like those shown in Figures 13.1 through 13.12. Despite growing pressures for automation, paper-based systems are still widely used.

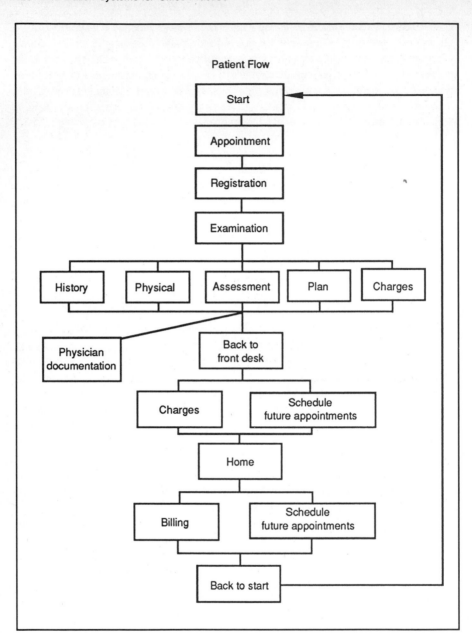

FIGURE 13.13 The information-management process begins when a patient calls a physician's office for an appointment. During the course of a visit, the patient registers at the front desk, is examined by a physician, then returns to the front desk to arrange payment for services and to schedule a follow-up visit, if necessary. Throughout the visit, health professionals collect and process a variety of information, which they use to provide medical care and to operate the business.

The first medical computer systems appeared in the 1960s. These systems automated patient billing and were operated by businesses that sold data-processing services to doctors' offices. The introduction of small affordable microcomputers, starting in the mid-1970s, made it possible for medical offices to own and operate computer systems. This section describes the capabilities of the traditional paper-based systems and these early computer-based medical-information systems.

13.3.1 Paper-Based Systems

Although limited in functionality, traditional paper-based systems are still widely used because they are moderately inexpensive and easy to use. The operation of these systems requires little training beyond learning how to decipher the handwriting of the other members of the staff. Moreover, within limits, a properly designed traditional paper system can be as flexible as are many of the computer-based information systems in use today.

At the core of a paper-based system are data-capture forms, such as the medical-history form (Figure 13.1) and the system-review form (Figure 13.2) discussed in the previous section. By standardizing the collection of information, the various encounter forms facilitate data storage and communication. Once the forms have been completed, they become part of the patients' permanent medical records. During subsequent visits, the physician can refer to them to obtain information about past medical problems and care. Provided that the person responsible for recording the data has legible handwriting, the information on these forms can be used by other members of the patient-care team as well.

On the other hand, as we discussed in Chapter 6, one serious disadvantage of the traditional patient chart is that it can be lost or misplaced. The chart that is incorrectly filed or hidden under a stack of old journals becomes a proverbial needle in a haystack. Because that missing chart contains all the medical information that has been collected for the patient, the consequences can be more than a minor inconvenience. The static organization and inflexible display of information are other shortcomings of the traditional paper chart.

Many medical offices use a paper-based **write-it-once system** for generating the bills that are sent directly to patients. After each visit, a clerical worker copies charges for services rendered to the patient from the encounter form (see Figure 13.8) onto a *ledger card*. When payments are received, these transactions are recorded as well. Each month, photocopies of the ledger cards showing unpaid balances are mailed to patients. More sophisticated write-it-once systems using carbon paper to generate **superbills** also are available (Figure 13.14).

From a cost perspective, a major shortcoming of paper-based systems is the labor required to produce third-party invoices. Office workers must copy the necessary information from the encounter forms and registration forms onto the appropriate invoice. In the case of copayments and deductibles, they also must enter the appropriate amounts and compute the unpaid balances. Besides being labor-intensive, reliance on transcription and manual calculation increases the likelihood of bookkeeping errors.

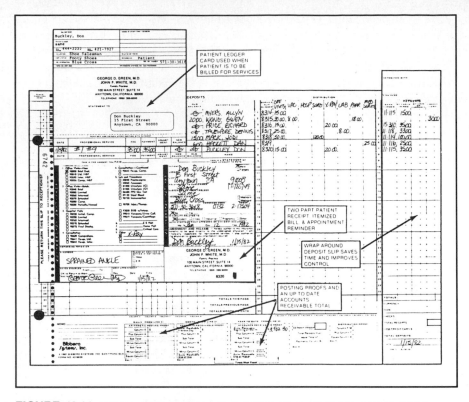

FIGURE 13.14 Using a carbon-paper write-it-once system, clerical personnel record transactions on a patient's bill; a duplicate entry is recorded on the patient's account ledger card. (*Source:* Provided courtesy of BIBBERO SYSTEMS, Inc., Petaluma, California.)

Accordingly, patient billing and production of third-party invoices were the first information-processing activities to be automated in physicians' offices.

13.3.2 Service Bureau Systems

In the late 1960s and early 1970s, before small affordable computer systems were available, data-processing businesses, called **service bureaus,** began to offer billing services to doctors' offices. Health-care workers in medical practices completed the appropriate registration and encounter forms; outside vendors processed these forms to produce the bills. Service bureaus could afford to use larger and more powerful computer systems because their fixed operating costs were spread over multiple doctors' offices. Furthermore, large service bureaus could employ professional programming staff and thus were more able to adapt to changes in third-party billing procedures. In addition to producing bills and invoices, early service bureaus also generated standard financial reports for their customers using data from the encounter forms.

Service bureaus are still common today despite the availability of low-cost computer hardware. Individual physicians' offices that use these services do not have to operate and maintain computer equipment—the clerical staff need only to learn to handle the paper forms. The major disadvantage of using a service bureau is that the medical practice loses some control over information—information that is vital to the practice's financial well-being. The practice can lose substantial revenue if the service bureau loses or fails to process encounter forms. Delay is another problem inherent in the use of an outside vendor in the processing of information. In the case of billing and invoice production, rapid turnaround time may not be crucial. On the other hand, health-care personnel must have timely access to medical information. For this reason, the use of outside vendors to enter and store clinical data usually is impractical.

13.3.3 Early Standalone Systems

In the mid-1970s, several companies introduced computer systems that were affordable even to practices comprising only two or three physicians. Although limited in capacity and functionality, these low-cost systems made it possible for doctors' offices to undertake most of the billing tasks performed by service bureaus. Initially, the available software was limited to adaptations of financial packages intended for use in small retail businesses, and thus was poorly suited for the medical setting. Eventually, however, system developers began to write software specifically designed to meet the needs of doctors' offices. Some of these systems are still in use today.

The Billing, Information, and Accounting System (BIAS) developed at the Eastern Kentucky Health Services Center is representative of these early standalone systems [Higgins, 1976]. BIAS was implemented on an IBM System 32 microcomputer. It allowed a single operator to enter and process all the financial information used by a clinic treating approximately 100 patients per day. Over a 10-year period, the annual cost of purchasing and maintaining the hardware and developing the software was approximately $10,000.

The early standalone systems were limited to traditional financial functions, such as production of bills and invoices, processing of payroll checks, and management of accounts-payable transactions. The presence of these systems in the doctor's office, however, demonstrated the potential utility of computers to the general medical community. The resulting awareness helped to stimulate interest in the development of simple applications in clinical information management. For example, computer generation of third-party invoices requires the entry of data describing the types of services provided to individual patients and the reasons why these services were performed. BIAS used this information to produce a brief summary of each patient's visit (diagnosis and services provided), which could be included in the medical record. The system also generated reports that summarized the services provided to patients who had certain key diagnoses.

13.4 Current Capabilities of Office-Information Systems

The introduction in the 1980s of powerful and affordable microcomputers made it financially feasible for even solo practices to own computer systems; the availability of a wide selection of medical software applications made owning a computer potentially useful. Capturing the status of office systems is difficult on a static medium such as the printed page. The field is changing rapidly, and the capabilities of the computer systems that are current as we write this chapter will be surpassed by the time you read it. This section describes the range of applications available to doctors' offices in the late 1980s. You can find software reviews and more detailed discussions in periodicals that specialize in this field. These periodicals publish surveys that will be of particular interest to students seeking up-to-date information about the capabilities of the systems currently available. See, for example, the *M.D. Computing* annual survey of medical software, which is cited in the Suggested Readings.

13.4.1 Systems Based on General-Purpose Software

A wide variety of general-purpose PC software is commercially available today. These programs can assist with many of the information-management tasks in a doctor's office. For example, clerical workers can use text-editing programs in the preparation of letters and reports. Physicians and other health professionals can access online databases of biomedical literature (see Chapter 14) using communication programs and commercial networks. Office workers can schedule patient visits using personal time-management software, and can keep track of inventories using spreadsheet programs. Accounting programs designed for small businesses can be used to manage the payroll and accounts-receivable transactions in a doctor's office. General-purpose database programs have been used to generate bills and insurance invoices in small practices [Quigley, 1984].

General-purpose software offers an inexpensive solution to many of the information-management problems encountered in a doctor's office. A PC with a hard disk and printer can cost as little as $2500, and the price of each software package usually is a few hundred dollars. The modularity of this approach makes it relatively easy to upgrade separate functions as new software becomes available. For example, an office can change an independent scheduling program without affecting the use of other applications programs.

A drawback of general-purpose software is that it must be custom-tailored to meet users' requirements. With the exception of word processors, none of these systems is ready to use. Physicians must assess their needs carefully and adapt the general-purpose software programs to meet their information-management requirements. Furthermore, general-purpose programs may not be powerful enough to fulfill specialized requirements. For example, although the reports generated by a database program probably are adequate to produce bills for patients, the formatting capabilities of the report generator may be unable to meet the more stringent requirements of third-party payment programs. Moreover, an accounting system may not be directly compatible with a billing system built from a database program. Therefore, when multiple programs are used, lack of integration can be an additional problem.

The adaptation and integration of the different systems is a nontrivial task. The success of these systems requires the dedication of at least one member of the practice who is willing to devote time and energy to overcoming the difficulties that result from the use of otherwise unrelated programs. Integrated software packages that combine database, spreadsheet, communication, word processing, and other capabilities are commercially available. These systems can provide greater versatility and convenience, once the system has been custom-tailored. They are, however, more difficult to learn and more expensive.

13.4.2 Systems Designed for Specific Medical Applications

The development of microcomputer technology expanded the functionality of the stand-alone systems that first appeared in the previous decade. Physicians now can purchase systems that fully integrate the basic financial functions, as well as perform most of the other peripheral data-management tasks, such as patient scheduling and inventory control. Specialized medical software is available to perform appointment scheduling, to maintain medication lists, to produce problem lists, to store medical records, to automate patient recall, to assist in practice analysis, and to generate referral letters. Such special-purpose systems tend to be relatively inexpensive and easy to use because each is designed to meet only a subset of the information-processing needs of small office practices. Accordingly, these systems may be limited in the range of functions they can perform or in the mode of use.

The *M.D. Computing* survey in the Suggested Readings lists more than 1000 medical software products marketed by 46 different vendors. Collectively, these commercial products can assist private practitioners and their staff with the following types of information-processing tasks:

- *Appointment scheduling.* A variety of electronic appointment books is available to assist office personnel in scheduling appointments. Typically, these programs allow workers to search for the next available slot by time required, physician, clinic area, and room. Larger practices can purchase more sophisticated systems to help coordinate the scheduling of constrained resources, such as physicians, nurses, examination rooms, and equipment. Scheduling systems also may generate lists of patients to be reminded of appointments, and may monitor the number of no shows.

- *Patient surveillance and recall.* Surveillance programs maintain a subset of clinical data—for example, demographic information, active problem list, current medication list, and preventive health information (immunization records, date of last Pap smear, date of last sigmoidoscopic examination, and so on). Office personnel can run the surveillance program periodically to identify patients for recall. The programs also print notification letters.

- *History taking.* Several history-taking systems are available to help physicians to obtain information about patients' medical histories and to identify medical problems (see also Chapter 18). The programs may ask general questions or may be tailored to specific subspecialty areas. Typically, they pose multiple-choice questions and use branching logic to pursue potential problems in greater detail. Physicians who have a significant number of patients who do not speak English may choose systems with foreign-language questionnaires and automatic translation of questions and answers to facilitate communication and to avoid misinterpretation.

- *Risk assessment.* Risk-assessment programs can help physicians to evaluate a patient's degree of health risk based on individual characteristics (such as age, gender, and weight) and the results of diagnostic tests. For example, cardiologists can use one system to estimate the risk of coronary-artery disease based on the results of treadmill stress tests. Other programs allow physicians to identify patients who are at high risk of developing coronary-artery disease based on risk factors, such as blood pressure, smoking behavior, and cholesterol levels.

- *Decision support.* The least sophisticated decision-support systems simply provide a fast and convenient means for physicians to reference diagnostic and treatment information for hundreds of medical conditions. More sophisticated systems can actively assist physicians in medical decision making. In Chapter 15, we shall discuss the conceptual issues underlying the development of computer-based systems for diagnosis and treatment planning, and we shall describe some well-known systems. Currently, most of these programs are still experimental. Several systems are available commercially, however, including DXplain, which produces ranked differential diagnoses based on patient characteristics and clinical findings (see Chapter 15), and Intellipath, which assists pathologists in the diagnosis of tissue specimens (Chapter 9).

- *Medication lists and prescription writing.* A variety of programs is available to assist physicians in the tasks of prescribing and writing prescriptions. They can provide references for drug interactions, maintain patients' medication lists, track patients' medication allergies, and assist in adjusting dosing recommendations for specific patients. These systems may automatically print out the prescriptions themselves and assist in monitoring and authorizing refill requests.

- *Patient education.* Verbal communication of physicians' instructions to patients is not always the most effective means of transferring information. Busy physicians may not have the time to explain their orders thoroughly; patients may fail to understand physicians' explanations or may forget what they are supposed to do and why they should do it. A number of programs are available that produce printed instructions for patients, some in multiple languages—for example, care instructions for common clinical conditions. Other programs summarize drug-use instructions and describe drug effects and side effects in easily understandable language. A different class of patient-education systems is designed to be used directly by patients. Patients can run these programs interactively to learn self-care for certain conditions. For example, Medical Logic International sells an interactive training program that teaches patients with diabetes mellitus to manage their disease safely and effectively.

- *Bibliographic retrieval.* As we shall discuss in Chapter 14, a wide selection of bibliographic databases and bibliographic-retrieval programs is available to assist health professionals in searching the medical literature. Systems such as BRS and

DIALOG provide capabilities for automatic dialup and logon. Some systems provide a common interface for searching—the program translates standard search terms into the proper syntax and search terms for the particular system being used. In this way, users avoid the need to learn multiple systems.

- *Communications.* Commercial networks not only allow access to bibliographic databases, but also facilitate communication among health professionals by providing access to electronic bulletin boards for the exchange of information and ideas related to general medical knowledge, to specific issues, and to special interest groups. In addition, electronic-mail facilities allow colleagues to exchange correspondence and to share data.

- *Computer-aided instruction.* Educational programs are available in a range of levels of sophistication, from simple drill-and-practice systems to case-management simulations. As we shall discuss in Chapter 17, these systems allow physicians to gain experience with a variety of different patient problems. Examples of the many systems available are programs that teach physicians to evaluate acid–base values, to manage arrhythmias, to treat alcoholics, to perform advanced cardiac life support, to evaluate chest pain, and to manage patients with hypertension. In some cases, physicians can receive credits for continuing medical education by completing computer-based courses.

- *Business systems.* Software is available to perform most of the business-related tasks of physicians' offices that we discussed in Section 13.2.3. Special-purpose programs can format and generate bills for patients and insurance companies, monitor accounts receivable and aging accounts, maintain accounts payable, administer the payroll, and assist in the creation of profit and loss statements and yearly budget projections.

One of the important features of office-practice programs is the use of modern graphical interface technology to simplify interactions between the operator and the machine. User interfaces built with graphics technology provide easy access to data and generally cause only modest reductions in speed of data retrieval. The *Clinical Experience* program, a prototype system developed by Innovative Medical Software for use on Apple Macintosh computers, is representative of the microcomputer-based systems available today; it provides a good illustration of the behavior of a user-friendly graphical-interface design.

A window like that shown in Figure 13.15 opens when the user selects the appropriate icon from an initial menu. A portion of the alphabetically ordered registration file is displayed on the left side of the window, and the user can scroll up or down to find the names of other patients in the file. After choosing the name of a specific patient in the list, the user can select icons to navigate to various parts of the medical record. Choosing the "Select Patient" icon brings the user to the problem list (Figure 13.16). This allows the physician to view the basic medical data and demographic information needed for immediate patient care. Selecting the "First Note" from the initial information display brings up the Initial History and Physical screen, which the physician can use to enter documentation collected during the first encounter (Figure 13.17a). By selecting from a menu of options, such as present illness, childhood illness, hospitalization, and physical examination, the

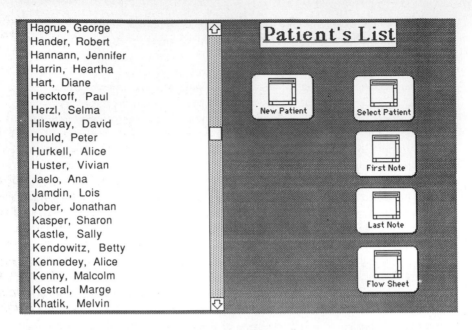

FIGURE 13.15 The initial screen of the *Clinical Experience* program allows users to access problem lists and visit notes for individual patients. (*Source:* Courtesy of Innovative Medical Software, Palo Alto, California.)

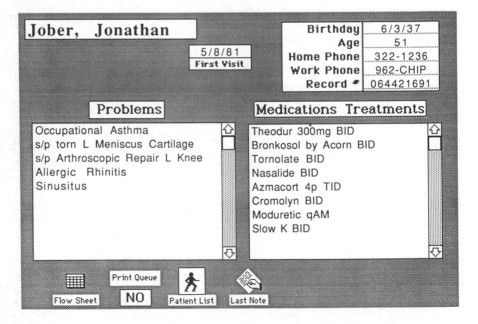

FIGURE 13.16 The problem list of *Clinical Experience* displays key medical and demographic information for an individual patient. (*Source:* Courtesy of Innovative Medical Software, Palo Alto, California.)

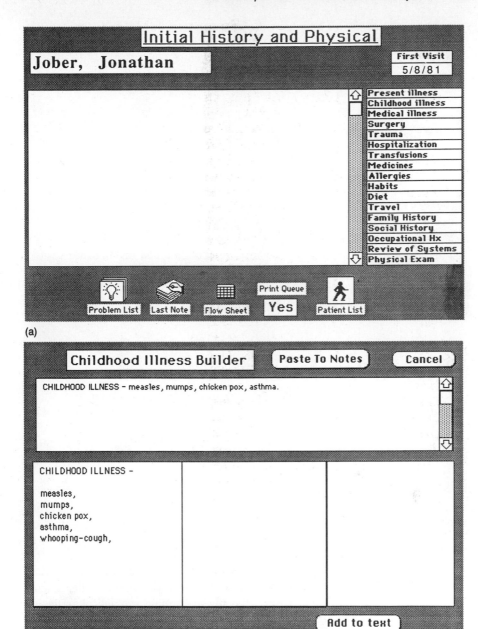

FIGURE 13.17 The *Clinical Experience* program allows users to enter an initial visit note with minimal use of the keyboard. (a) By selecting "Childhood Illness" from the menu at the right of the Initial History and Physical screen, the user brings up a form used to enter information about childhood illnesses. (b) When an item is selected from the menu of childhood illnesses (lower window), the information appears in the patient's list of illnesses (upper window). Once the entry is complete, the user can paste it into the Initial History and Physical note. (*Source:* Courtesy of Innovative Medical Software, Palo Alto, California.)

user can bring up screens that allow him to construct a progress note by using the mouse to select and enter appropriate terms (Figure 13.17b). Users can navigate the system and view the entire medical record by selecting icons. Because the user can enter most data by choosing items from predefined lists, keyboard data entry is minimized.

13.4.3 Comprehensive Systems

During the past decade, medical-record systems for ambulatory-care settings were developed in several academic institutions. We described the capabilities of some of these systems in Chapter 6. Commercial systems derived from these research endeavors are available; in the mid-1980s, the costs of such systems ranged from approximately $20,000 for practices of up to five physicians, to $200,000 for clinics with up to 40 physicians [Barnett, 1984]. The complexity of the software and the necessary hardware considerably increase the operating and maintenance costs of these systems. Nevertheless, commercially available systems such as TMR and COSTAR (see Chapter 6) do provide medical-record systems for use in outpatient clinics.

13.5 A Look to the Future

We have every reason to expect that the computer systems used in doctors' offices will continue to improve as new technology is developed and existing technology is applied more effectively. Moreover, the health-care industry itself is undergoing significant alterations in response to a variety of social, economic, and technical changes. This final section predicts the probable effect of these trends on the availability of information-processing systems for use in physicians' offices.

The inefficiency of available mechanisms for data entry currently limits the role of computers in doctors' offices. The entry of financial data is the major operating cost for the systems described in Section 13.4; most practices cannot afford the cost of using traditional keyboard-oriented procedures to enter medical information. Moreover, accessing medical information often is more difficult when data are stored electronically than it is when traditional paper-based record systems are used.

Unfortunately, direct approaches to data entry, such as machine understanding of handwritten forms or natural speech, probably will remain impractical for the immediate future. Several groups, however, are exploring alternative modes of data entry. One promising approach uses machine-readable bar codes to encode demographic information, as well as common diagnoses and procedures (Figure 13.9). Patient-specific encounter forms can be printed at the time of a visit. These encounter forms contain a bar code that identifies the patient, the physician, the date of the visit, and a menu of possible services. Nurses and physicians check off the services that are provided during the visit. Office personnel then can use a bar-code reader to enter the information from the encounter form in a fraction of the time required by conventional keyboard entry. This same approach can be extended to include a subset of the medical information collected during a visit. The development and widespread acceptance of coding schemes for recording medical information will allow for more efficient entry, storage, and retrieval of clinical information (see Chapter 2).

Changes in the health-care industry are likely to affect the use of computers in doctors' offices. The current trend is away from solo practice and toward partnerships and larger group practices. These larger business units can support more sophisticated information-management systems. Moreover, communication among the members of the same practice grows increasingly difficult as the size of the group increases. The standardization of record keeping enforced by a computer-based system will help to minimize the difficulties in data access and communication that arise as more and more physicians join group practices.

The use of computer-based information systems by hospitals, medical suppliers, drug companies, laboratories, and third-party payment programs is increasing at least as rapidly as is that by doctors' offices, thus raising the possibility of installing direct electronic links between doctors' offices and the organizations with which those offices must deal. For example, physicians soon may routinely access hospital data for the patients under their care from their offices via local-area networks, or exchange mail messages with their colleagues electronically. Already, physicians who subscribe to commercial networks can send messages to other subscribers throughout the national medical community. Soon, the computer may become as important a tool as is the telephone for dealing with colleagues and outside organizations.

As we mentioned in the introduction to this chapter, most of the applications discussed elsewhere in this book can be applied in the office setting. Researchers and software vendors are devoting significant time and resources to the development of systems for electronic publishing, computer-aided instruction for patients, clinical consultation, and other potential applications for outpatient care. Such systems will undoubtedly influence the future uses of computers in doctors' offices.

Suggested Readings

The sixth annual medical hardware and software buyers' guide. *M.D. Computing*, 6(6):334, 1989.

> *This extensive catalog provides an alphabetized listing of current medical software and product descriptions. The programs are cross-referenced by primary and secondary subject categories.*

Felts, W. Choosing office practice systems for billing, accounting, and medical record functions. *M.D. Computing*, 1(3):10, 1984.

> *The author reviews the ways in which computers can help physicians in private practice with business and clinical applications. He stresses the importance of analyzing the need for a computer system and of planning for implementation to maximize the benefits of automation.*

Gabrieli, E. R. Automated medical office records. *Journal of Medical Systems*, 11(1):59, 1987.

> *This paper describes a computer-based information system that accesses electronically stored patient records in client physicians' offices, automatically encodes their contents, and stores them in an online database. System support staff can then analyze the database to extract information that physicians can use in patient care and practice management.*

Oberst, B. B. and Long, J. M. *Computers in Private Practice Management.* New York: Springer-Verlag, 1987.

> This practical guide to office computer systems first discusses the use of computers in private practice and provides an introduction to computing hardware and software. The body of the text describes computer applications in eight major areas: administration, accounting, appointment scheduling and time management, patient care, marketing, practice management, hospital management, and medical-information management.

Schlager, D. D. A comprehensive patient care system for the family practice. *Journal of Medical Systems,* 7(2):137, 1983.

> This paper describes the design and function of a computer-based information system that serves a three-physician, two-office family practice medical group. The system stores all financial, pharmaceutical, scheduling, and medical data for the practice and for the affiliated clinical pharmacy.

Schneeweiss, R. Clinical applications of computers in office practice. *The Journal of Family Practice,* 19(1):54, 1984.

> This paper describes the design and operation of two custom-developed systems that perform clinical and business functions for two family practices.

Sellars, D. *Computerizing Your Medical Office.* Oradell, NJ: Medical Economics Company, 1983.

> This ''how to'' guide is one of many books and articles available to physicians who wish to acquire computer systems for their practices. It discusses common office computing applications and contains sections on assessing the need for a computer system and selecting the right system.

Stead, E. A. and Stead, W. W. Computers and medical practice: Old dreams and current realities. *M.D. Computing,* 2(6):26, 1985.

> This article briefly reviews the development of computer systems in medical care, then explains several of the uses of computers in medical practice.

Questions for Discussion

1. You are a partner in a three-physician private practice that is considering acquiring a computer system to perform certain information-management tasks. Discuss the important factors that you must consider when deciding whether your practice can benefit from the purchase of an office computer system.

2. Suppose that you run a family-practice clinic that has three examining rooms, one doctor's consultation office, and two work areas for nurses and clerical staff. Which type of system is more appropriate, a network of single-user personal computers or a larger machine with multiple terminals? How do the intended uses of the computer influence the selection and location of the machine(s)?

3. Suppose that a father takes his son to the doctor for a well-child examination and that the cost of the visit will be covered by the father's health-insurance plan. Describe the steps that the office staff must perform to process this financial transaction. Start with the patient's arrival at the office and end with the submission of the claim form.

4. List three reasons, other than cost, for the continued popularity of paper-based information-management systems in physicians' offices.

5. Discuss the advantages and disadvantages of using a service bureau for data processing versus acquiring and operating an inhouse system. How do these advantages and disadvantages affect the potential role of service bureaus for managing each of the four types of information discussed in Section 13.2?

6. Describe an appointment-scheduling procedure that could be implemented in a computer program. Take into account the reason for the visit, whether the patient is a new or returning patient, and other factors that influence the length of each visit. Discuss desirable features of an appointment system, identify the inputs and outputs to the system, and describe how the system will be used.

7. During a typical day, physicians often need answers to questions related to the care of individual patients. Discuss four ways by which computer technology can help physicians find the information they need.

8. Private insurance and government programs pay for the major portion of health care provided in physicians' offices. Discuss three ways in which the participation of these third-party payers affects information management in outpatient medicine.

9. Discuss two ways in which the development of graphics technology has affected the design of computer-based information systems. For each of the four types of information managed in physicians' offices (see Section 13.2), briefly describe one way that graphics technology can help health professionals to access or interpret the information.

14

Bibliographic-Retrieval Systems

*Elliot R. Siegel, Martin M. Cummings,
and Rose M. Woodsmall*

After reading this chapter, you should know the answers to these questions:

- How and why are bibliographic-retrieval systems used by health professionals?
- What are the problems associated with end-user searches, and how can they be solved?
- What are the features of a user-friendly search system?
- How may artificial-intelligence techniques be used someday to improve the performance and reduce the cost of bibliographic-retrieval systems?

14.1 The Information-Transfer Problem

As we stressed in Chapter 1, the name *medical informatics* refers broadly to issues in the storage, management, retrieval, and use of medical information. With the increasing recognition that it is folly to try to read, memorize, and recall all the information necessary for high-quality medical research and practice, health professionals have consistently sought new methods for dealing with the medical literature. For many years, they relied on personal (as well as institutional) libraries of books, journals, and articles to which they could turn when they needed information. It soon became clear, however, that the sheer volume of written material made the biomedical literature unusable without special auxiliary methods—indexes and, in recent years, computer systems with an ability to *search* the literature for pertinent references (which could subsequently be retrieved from personal journals or libraries).

This chapter deals with such computer systems. It describes how they have evolved from the written indexes that were, in the past, the only practical means for locating needed information. It also points the way to new developments that may revolutionize the ways in which we think about computer-based literature management.

14.1.1 Information Seeking and the Biomedical Literature

Scientists, educators, and physicians seek information in many ways. Direct personal communication with peers and experts frequently is the easiest way to gain assistance in problem solving. Within large organizations, technical communications often take place through a **gatekeeper.** The gatekeeper is a person who maintains a high level of external communication and, through contacts, keeps colleagues informed of new developments. Attendance at meetings and conferences also serves to keep individuals informed of recent developments in specialized fields of interest. The broadest and most comprehensive access to innovations and new knowledge, however, comes from an examination of the published literature. Traditional guides to the literature are printed indexes, catalogs, and abstracts that identify the subjects and authors of articles and books relevant to the reader's interest.

One problem is that the amount of literature continues to increase as biomedical research expands. De Solla Price has described the development of the biomedical literature in relationship to science and technology [De Solla Price, 1981]. He points out that, for more than 300 years, the learned literature has grown exponentially, doubling every 10 to 15 years. Today, in biomedicine alone, more than 20,000 journals are published annually, as are approximately 17,000 new books. The magnitude of this literature presents special problems of access because few institutions can hope to acquire more than a representative sample for their user communities. Therefore, it is important that the bibliographic apparatus not only list what is available, but also indicate where items are located.

14.1.2 Access to the Biomedical Literature: A Computer-Based Model

Increasingly, computer technology is being used to facilitate rapid and convenient access to biomedical literature. Vendors of secondary literature products and services (the indexing and abstract guides to the published primary literature) have been especially quick to realize the potential of computer technology as a means of dealing with the huge and rapidly growing files of data and information in biomedicine. The user community has been quick to respond as well.

MEDLINE, the National Library of Medicine's (NLM's) major bibliographic database, is a case in point. This computer-based system contains more than 900,000 references to the recent journal literature; backfiles to 1966 also are available for searching. From a handful of users in 1971, the MEDLINE network has expanded to include institutions in every state—about 9000 in all. The number of annual computer searches exceeds 4 million. This volume of activity confirms what health professionals have long known: The medical literature continues to be a vital link connecting research, education, and practice.

The NLM has built its information-retrieval system using references and abstracts taken from approximately 340,000 articles appearing in 3400 medical journals each year. Many of these references also appear in *Index Medicus,* produced monthly in printed form by the NLM. In general, however, **online bibliographic searching** has several advantages over conventional manual searching. It is much faster, it is more cost-efficient, and it allows for selective retrieval of items most relevant to user requirements. Perhaps most important, online searching permits comprehensive, complex searches that would be impossible to do using printed indexes (for example, searches to find articles dealing with two or more topics).

The benefits derived from MEDLINE vary with the nature of the request. Practitioners may search the literature for an article that will illuminate some puzzling phenomenon they have encountered in caring for a patient. A scientist or educator may require a comprehensive bibliography to survey a broad field of research. Whatever the purpose of the search, the requester receives a list of articles on the subject, including abstracts, if desired.

The same computer-based network used for online searching of the NLM's databases also can be used to request, by mail, copies of articles (or books, reports, audiovisual materials, and so on), the citations for which have been retrieved. Seven Regional Medical Libraries, covering all geographic areas of the United States, assist in providing documents or routing requests for them through the network (Figure 14.1). Requests are filled (photocopies for journal articles, original volumes for books) by an institution as close as possible to the requester; hard-to-find items are supplied by the Regional Medical Library or by the NLM itself.

14.2 Historical Development of Bibliographic-Retrieval Systems

The literature archived at the National Library of Medicine is an invaluable resource for medical practitioners and researchers. Without organization and a systematic means

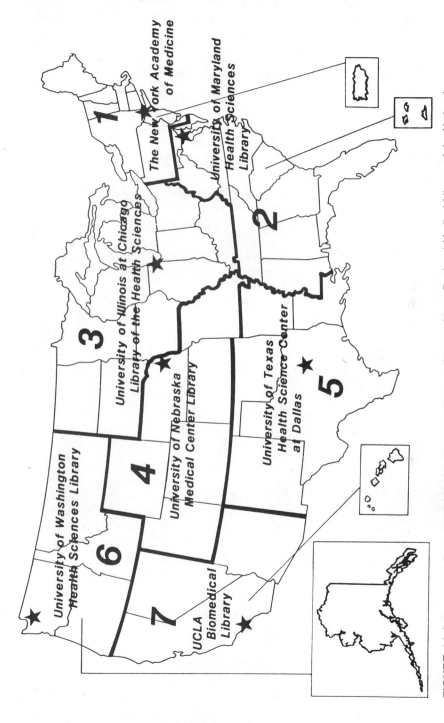

FIGURE 14.1 The United States is divided into seven regions, each served by a Regional Medical Library of the National Library of Medicine. (*Source:* Courtesy of the National Library of Medicine.)

for access, however, the information saved there would be unusable. For many years, printed indexes served adequately, guiding their users to relevant books and articles. As the volume of written material grew, these indexes evolved into today's **computer-based bibliographic-retrieval systems.**

14.2.1 From Printed Indexes to Online Access

The earliest bibliographies and guides to the scientific literature were started in the sixteenth century by people who had begun to collect printed books. No comprehensive index to the medical literature was available until the mid-nineteenth century, when Dr. John Shaw Billings (Figure 14.2) developed the *Index-Catalogue of the Library of the Surgeon General's Office. Index-Catalogue* included both books and periodicals. Books were listed under subject headings and the author's name, whereas the journal articles were presented under subject headings only. Subheadings were used to define the topics more clearly. More than 0.5 million books and 1.5 million journal articles were included in *Index-Catalogue* before it was terminated in 1961.

To maintain a current index to the rapidly developing medical literature, Billings also developed *Index Medicus*. This publication was first issued in 1879 and has been maintained with few interruptions for more than a century. *Index Medicus* provided

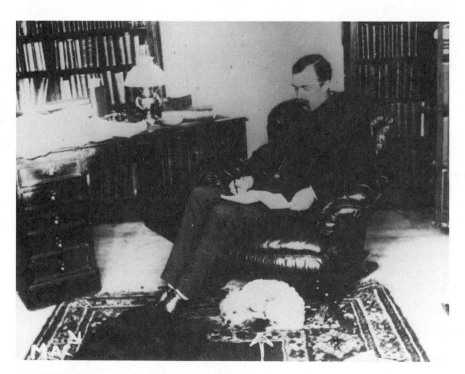

FIGURE 14.2 Dr. John Shaw Billings (1838–1913) began the work that has evolved into the present day *Index Medicus* and the National Library of Medicine. (*Source:* Photograph courtesy of the National Library of Medicine.)

both subject and author listings of journal articles, and soon became an indispensable guide to the world's medical literature (Figure 14.3). From 1927 to 1931, it appeared as the *Quarterly Cumulative Index Medicus,* sponsored jointly by the American Medical Association (AMA) and the Army Medical Library. Foreign-language titles of subject entries were translated into English. A rapid increase in scientific publications following World War II, however, caused delays in the indexing, making the *Index Medicus* less valuable for medical research. At that time, *Index Medicus* covered approximately 2000 journal titles comprising approximately 100,000 new articles each year.

Mechanization of the production of *Index Medicus* was undertaken in 1960. The manual card system was replaced by one using punched cards, enabling the use of sorters and collators for alphabetical filing. A special camera was used to photograph text at a rate of 200 cards per minute. True automation took place in 1964, when *Index Medicus* was produced for the first time by the NLM computer-based Medical Literature Analysis and Retrieval System (MEDLARS). The MEDLARS project pioneered the use of a computer-driven graphic-arts composing system (known as GRACE). These technical innovations made it possible to broaden the scope and coverage of the biomedical literature indexed by the library, and to shorten the time required to announce the literature's availability. All titles in foreign languages were translated into English, and indexers assigned as many subject headings as were required to characterize the content of the article.

A thesaurus entitled *Medical Subject Headings* (MeSH) was developed to provide the categorized lists of headings and subheadings (and cross-references) that made *Index Medicus* so useful (Figure 14.4). The MeSH vocabulary is routinely updated to reflect the constantly evolving vocabulary of biomedicine. NLM elicits assistance from professional societies to maintain an accurate set of terminology. Current NLM-sponsored research in developing a Unified Medical Language System (UMLS), based on MeSH, is directed toward making the myriad of other biomedical classification systems invisible while providing a single logical path to a broad range of biomedical information sources [Lindberg and Humphreys, 1989] (see Chapter 20).

Index Medicus has been produced successfully using computer technology for over 20 years; since 1971, the great volume of medical information contained in the MEDLARS system has been available through online access. At present, *Index Medicus* includes 2800 journal titles, together containing approximately 315,000 articles per year.

MEDLARS not only achieved the automated publication of *Index Medicus,* but also made possible the development of a computer-based search and retrieval service. Initially, this system allowed for batch-mode searching of MEDLARS references in response to an inquiry. Such individualized searches, however, were slow; they had to be formulated by a trained search analyst and then tediously keypunched before they could be submitted for processing. If the user wished to modify the original search formulation after seeing what was retrieved, an entire new round of processing was required. Even with a dozen search-formulation centers around the country, it was never possible to respond to more than about 20,000 search requests per year. In addition, the indexing was too limited to allow for complex, multisubject searching.

LEGIONELLA

Legionella species, serogroups and subgroups found in the environment in Singapore. Meers PD, et al.
Ann Acad Med Singapore 1989 Jul;18(4):375-8
Legionella: an infrequent cause of adult community acquired pneumonia in Dublin. Hone R, et al. **Ir J Med Sci** 1989 Sep;158(9):230-2

LEGIONELLOSIS

DIAGNOSIS

[Legionella dumoffii and Legionella pneumophila serogroup 5 isolated from 2 cases of fulminant pneumonia] Fujita I, et al. **Kansenshogaku Zasshi** 1989 Aug;63(8):801-10 (Eng. Abstr.) **(Jpn)**

ETIOLOGY

[Community-acquired pneumonia] Kemmerich B, et al. **Dtsch Med Wochenschr** 1989 Sep 29;114(39):1471-7 (Eng. Abstr.) **(Ger)**

LEGISLATION, VETERINARY

It's all in the states [news] Brody M.
J Am Vet Med Assoc 1989 Oct 1;195(7):880-1
[Veterinary Chief Inspection of Public Health. Harmonization of EEC legislation in the field of Veterinary Public Health] **Tijdschr Diergeneeskd** 1989 Oct 1; 114(19):1019-21 **(Dut)**
[Animal welfare legislation and animal experiments in Switzerland—effects and challenges] Steiger A.
Schweiz Arch Tierheilkd 1989;131(7):435-56 (35 ref.) (Eng. Abstr.) **(Ger)**

LEGUMES

Effect of bean intake on biliary lipid secretion and on hepatic cholesterol metabolism in the rat. Rigotti A, et al.
J Lipid Res 1989 Jul;30(7):1041-8

ANALYSIS

Reduction of aflatoxin content of infected cowpea seeds during processing into food. Ogunsanwo BM, et al.
Nahrung 1989;33(6):595-7

ENZYMOLOGY

Amine oxidase from Lathyrus cicera and Phaseolus vulgaris: purification and properties. Cogoni A, et al.
Prep Biochem 1989;19(2):95-112

MICROBIOLOGY

The cutworm Peridroma saucia (Lepidoptera: Noctuidae) supports growth and transport of pBR322-bearing bacteria. Armstrong JL, et al. **Appl Environ Microbiol** 1989 Sep; 55(9):2200-5
Requirement for chemotaxis in pathogenicity of Agrobacterium tumefaciens on roots of soil-grown pea plants. Hawes MC, et al. **J Bacteriol** 1989 Oct; 171(10):5668-71

ULTRASTRUCTURE

[Morphology of the seeds of Astragalus complanatus R.Br. and Astragalus on the scanning electron microscope] Ling Y. **Chung Kuo Chung Yao Tsa Chih** 1989 Feb;14(2):3-5, 61 (Eng. Abstr.) **(Chi)**

FIGURE 14.3 *Index Medicus* provides a structured method for finding recent articles dealing with a topic of interest. (*Source:* Courtesy of the National Library of Medicine.)

GENETIC ENGINEERING

E5.393.420+

only /hist /instrum /methods /psychol /trends /u
/vet; TEST-TUBE FERTILIZATION see FER7
is available

89; was GENETIC INTERVENTION 1973-88; v

use GENETIC ENGINEERING to search GEN
back thru 1973

see related
    ANIMALS, TRANSGENIC
    DNA, RECOMBINANT
    MICE, TRANSGENIC
X   GENETIC INTERVENTION
XU SEX PRESELECTION
XR BIOTECHNOLOGY
XR DNA, RECOMBINANT
XR INDUSTRIAL MICROBIOLOGY

GENETIC ENGINEERING OF PROTEINS see PR(
    E5.393.420.601

GENETIC INDUCTION see GENE EXPRESSION
    G5.331.380+

GENETIC INTERVENTION see GENETIC ENGI!
    E5.393.420+

GENETIC MARKERS

D24.185.101.387   G5.735.450

usually NIM; IM GEN only; coord with specific genetic feature (IM) if
pertinent; only /anal /blood-csf-urine

89; was GENETIC MARKER 1980-88

use GENETIC MARKERS to search GENETIC MARKER back thru 1980

see related
    CHROMOSOME MAPPING
X   CHROMOSOME MARKERS
X   DNA MARKERS
X   MARKERS, DNA
X   MARKERS, GENETIC

GENETIC SCREENING

E1.563.390   E5.318.370.580.120
G3.850.520.610.580.120   N1.224.458.527.125
N2.421.143.827.233.443.125

only /instrum /methods /trends /vet

78

see related
    HETEROZYGOTE DETECTION

GENETIC TECHNICS

E5.393+

do not use /man /methods /supply /util   CATALOG: do not use
/laboratory manuals

73

XR GENETIC COUNSELING

GENETIC TOXICITY TESTS see MUTAGENICITY TESTS
    E5.393.560+

+INDICATES THERE ARE INDENTED DESCRIPTORS IN MESH TREE STRUCTURES AT THIS NUMBER.

FIGURE 14.4 The *Medical Subject Headings* (MeSH) thesaurus provides a standardized set of hierarchically organized terms that are used for indexing articles. MeSH is now widely accepted internationally for this purpose. (*Source:* Courtesy of the National Library of Medicine.)

In the late 1960s, spurred by increasing demands for search services and a growing backlog of requests, the NLM undertook the development of a more rapid and widely accessible system. The result was the implementation of MEDLARS Online (MEDLINE) in October 1971. This system provided in-depth indexing with an enlarged vocabulary, as well as online retrieval in real time.

14.2.2 The NLM's MEDLINE System

Using MEDLINE, health professionals throughout the United States (and in several foreign countries) have immediate access to a database of about 6 million citations published since 1966. Access is through computer terminals (or microcomputers) that are linked to the NLM's computers by commercial telecommunications networks. More than 9000 hospitals, medical schools, medical-research institutions, government agencies, and commercial organizations in the United States have access to MEDLINE, and more than 4 million computer searches are done each year. In addition, several hundred foreign institutions are connected to the system.

MEDLINE is an *interactive system*; that is, the user identifies the journal-article references needed by carrying on a dialogue with the computer. The user types a query on the terminal keyboard, receives a response from the computer, and enters the next query based on the computer response. Any of the 15,000 **medical subject headings** in the MeSH thesaurus can be combined to search a specific subject. Users also can search by an author's name, words in the title or in the abstract of an article, publication date, language, specific journal title, or a combination of these elements.

After pertinent references are located, the author, title, and journal for each citation are printed at the user's location. English abstracts are available for over 60 percent of the citations from 1975 through the present. If a large number of references are retrieved, they can be printed overnight at NLM and mailed to the requester the next day. The entire online search usually takes less than 10 minutes.

In most institutions, the MEDLINE search is done by a trained *intermediary* who uses information provided by the search requester or ultimate end user. Ideally, end users should be able to negotiate their own searches at a terminal. Many people, however, are unwilling to learn the intricacies of access protocols, command languages, search-strategy formulation, and controlled vocabularies. These elements vary widely among the many existing databases, so it is not surprising that an infrequent user would be reluctant to expend the effort necessary to become proficient in searching. The recent availability of low-cost microcomputers and user-friendly front-end software, however, is beginning to change the status quo (see Section 14.4).

A variety of other MEDLARS databases is available for use by biomedical researchers, educators, and practitioners. These deal with toxicological and chemical information, health-planning and health-management literature, cancer-research information, and several other areas. About 20 separate NLM files useful for searching the published biomedical literature in the form of journal articles, books, and audiovisual materials are accessible online.

14.2.3 Other Biomedical Database Systems

You should be familiar with some of the other bibliographic databases that contain biomedical information, in addition to those produced by the NLM. These include the following:

- *BIOSIS Previews* is produced by Biosciences Information Service. Five million records with abstracts from 1969 to the present are available online, and approximately 40,000 are added monthly. The online counterpart to *Biological Abstracts,* BIOSIS screens some 9000 scientific journals covering worldwide literature on research in the life sciences, as well as books, monographs, and meeting and conference proceedings.

- *Excerpta Medica* is a broad-based information-retrieval service that indexes and abstracts biomedical and clinical literature. It produces 44 journals containing abstracts of articles published in the primary literature. Some 4500 journals are screened each year. Since 1974, 3.5 million records, with abstracts, have been entered into Excerpta Medica's online database, EMBASE.

- *PSYCHINFO,* produced by the American Psychological Association, covers the world's literature in psychology and related disciplines in the behavioral sciences. Over 950 journals and 1500 books, technical reports, and monographs are scanned each year. PSYCHINFO contains about 550,000 citations from 1967 to the present; its printed counterpart is *Psychological Abstracts.*

- *CA SEARCH,* produced by the Chemical Abstracts Service, provides international coverage of the chemical literature from more than 14,000 scientific and technical journals, as well as from conference proceedings, technical reports, books, and patents. Approximately one-third of the literature is biochemical. CA SEARCH's printed counterpart is *Chemical Abstracts.*

- *SCISEARCH/SOCIAL SCISEARCH* are the online counterparts of *Science Citation Index* and *Social Science Citation Index,* produced by the Institute for Scientific Information. The data they contain indicate the frequency with which published articles are cited, and they identify articles that are potentially related to one another because they cite the same reference. Furthermore, they provide a means for tracing subsequent work done on a subject.

14.2.4 Vending Online Database Services

Publicly available online databases in all fields grew in number from approximately 400 in 1979 to nearly 3700 in 1987 [Cuadra/Elsevier, 1988]. An estimated 10 percent are in disciplines pertinent to the information needs of the biomedical community. This rapid growth has been fostered by the existence of telecommunications networks that make it technologically and financially feasible to link users' terminals to remote computer centers or to host systems containing the databases.

Host systems may be owned and operated by the same organization that produces the database contents, as is the case for the NLM and the MEDLARS family of databases. More frequently, however, the host systems are commercial enterprises built specifically for the purpose of vending a database service to users. These vendors lease the databases from the producers and, in turn, charge their users according to the amount of information retrieved, user-system connect time, or some combination of these and related measures of use. **Vendor systems** typically contain a multitude of databases (some numbering in the hundreds) that are produced by a variety of organizations. In addition to providing users with a large number of choices, these electronic database "supermarkets" also allow significant economies of scale.

More than 550 public- and private-sector organizations vend database services. Among the largest serving the biomedical community are BRS Information Technologies, Dialog Information Services, NLM, Pergamon Orbit InfoLine, Paper-Chase, and Mead Data Central. CompuServe, a relative newcomer to the marketplace, is achieving a substantial base among individual users, rather than with institutions. The American Medical Association's AMA/NET also provides bibliographic-retrieval service to its users.

14.3 Contemporary Issues Affecting Bibliographic-Retrieval Systems

The potential benefits of using online databases are influenced markedly by the ease with which users can access the system and retrieve information. Organizations that build and maintain these databases must develop effective methods for accessing information.

14.3.1 Impediments to Information Access

Access to bibliographic-retrieval systems, especially in the educational setting, is impeded both by a lack of people's awareness of the systems and by the costs of using those systems.

To help overcome the first obstacle, we should ensure that students in the health sciences are informed of the availability and use of library resources in general, and contemporary computer-based bibliographic-retrieval systems in particular. Instruction can be provided by the institution's library staff or by knowledgeable faculty. Schoolman [Schoolman, 1982] and other analysts have predicted that the philosophical basis of medical education will shift from a memory-based system to an information-processing system in which students are expected to master the tools for locating and obtaining information for decision making, rather than simply to acquire facts. Such a trend would increase students' needs for training in the use of bibliographic-retrieval systems.

With greater awareness of the value of bibliographic-retrieval systems will come increased use of them. In the educational setting, this increased use could place even greater strain on library budgets that are already stretched thin, making it difficult for students to continue to receive free access to the literature required for their education and research. One solution to this problem may be for libraries to purchase subsets of bibliographic databases and to make them available locally on their own library computer systems. Such an approach generally could reduce the costs sufficiently, once the capital investment has been made, so that the library could offer individual searches without charge to students, faculty, and staff (see the discussion of Approach E in Section 14.4.1).

14.3.2 Emergence of End-User Searching

The traditional model of online searching centers on a highly trained information specialist or librarian who functions as a **search intermediary,** interpreting the information requirements of the search requester and translating these needs into the particular command language and vocabulary of the search system being used. System command languages vary and frequently are cryptic. It is therefore not surprising to find that until the past few years, 85 percent of the searches conducted on the NLM's MEDLARS network were performed by search intermediaries on behalf of requesting health professionals.

The ready availability and proliferation of relatively low-cost microcomputers and mass-storage devices—in combination with the introduction of user-friendly access—has had a revolutionary effect on bibliographic-retrieval systems and practices, as it has had on many other facets of the workplace and marketplace. For example, since user-friendly access to the NLM system was introduced in 1986, there has been a marked increase in the number of individual health professionals requesting personal codes to the NLM system so that they can carry out MEDLARS searches directly without the aid of a search intermediary, and the proportion of search sessions performed by end users has more than doubled. Significantly, nearly one-half of end users on the NLM system are physicians engaged in direct patient-care activities [Wallingford et al., 1989]. This statistic represents a more than seven-fold increase in code holders who are direct-care physicians since the introduction of user-friendly access. Student access has also contributed dramatically to the growth of end-user searches.

Some telecommunications networks, such as TYMNET and TELENET, have had their infrastructures in place since the early 1970s and thus far have been able to accommodate new users easily. New national networks, targeted specifically to the educational and research communities, provide additional capacities.

Database vendors have responded to the increased interest in end-user searching in two ways: by training users; and by designing systems that, while retaining as much as possible of the power of command-language systems, can be used by people who have no special training.

User Training

Most database vendors have developed short training courses geared specifically to the needs of **end-user searchers.** Some courses teach these new searchers a set of basic commands, using the conventional search system, that allow the user to retrieve "a few good citations" on relatively simple searches, and to interact more effectively with search intermediaries on more complex searches. Individualized instruction for the user-friendly services is mainly in the form of tutorials on a number of media, including paper, microcomputer diskette, and CD-ROM. Some vendors have produced videotapes explaining both search concepts and the retrieval system.

End-User Systems

An alternative approach to support end-user searching involves the development of user-friendly interfaces to the conventional bibliographic-retrieval system. A *user-friendly interface* is designed for use by individuals who are not computer specialists (or retrieval specialists in this case), who have had only limited training, and who might reject a system that is nonintuitive or complicated, or that uses unfamiliar jargon to communicate. In the case of bibliographic-retrieval systems, such interfaces may be simplified versions of their conventional counterparts, or may be brand new search systems. These interfaces generally use a few basic commands that are a subset of the more powerful and versatile conventional search systems used by the intermediaries, and they have human-engineering features that make them relatively nonthreatening to persons unfamiliar with computers. Brief menus or command nomenclatures that mimic standard English are the norm. Section 14.4 contains an overview of several currently available approaches to end-user searching.

Although the advent of end-user searching of bibliographic databases promises to facilitate and accelerate biomedical-information transfer, direct access is not without potential problems for end users, for the biomedical library community, and for database producers and vendors.

End-user searching is more convenient than is intermediary searching, and it allows end users to capitalize on their special knowledge of the subject matter. Furthermore, much of the required hardware, in the form of relatively low-cost microcomputers and peripherals, is already in place. However, a question remains: Will end-users, especially busy physicians, be willing to devote the time and effort required to learn to do their own searching, and will they continue to use this skill once the novelty has worn off? A user-friendly search system provides a simplified service, and does not incorporate all the refinements of the conventional search service. Thus, if the physician delegates searching to an office assistant who does not have the strong subject knowledge that might compensate for having fewer search features, the search results may be inferior to those obtained with the standard service mediated through the library staff. Increasing numbers of physicians are gaining and maintaining bibliographic-retrieval skills, however, and it now seems less likely that this problem will be a serious one.

Two primary concerns in the library community are the potential effect of end-user searching on the professional searcher's role, and the possibility of increasing demands on library resources. Will the librarians' perceived value be diminished by end users who perform their own searches, or will librarians' images be enhanced by a new appreciation for the professional services they provide? Will end-user searching stimulate greater use of intermediaries for the more complex searches? Will it stimulate greater use of a library's journal and book collections, thereby placing additional pressures on slender budgets for acquiring books and journals?

These issues remain largely unresolved and await the insight and data that time and experience will bring.

14.3.3 Improvement of Retrieval Relevance

Whether a literature search is conducted by an end user or by a search intermediary, the primary objective is to discriminate among documents and to retrieve only those relevant to the topic of interest. Improving retrieval relevance is a critical concern in the design of bibliographic-retrieval systems.

Index Terms and Text-Word Searches

A **bibliographic database** consists of a set of records, each of which uniquely characterizes a document in terms of author, publication source, and subject matter. The record serves as a surrogate for the actual journal article or book, and is intended to enable users to determine whether the document is relevant to their information needs, and, if it is, where the document can be obtained. Perhaps the most important element in this characterization involves the assignment of index terms, or descriptors, which help to define the content of a document. Precision is aided by controlled indexing vocabularies and thesauri that are internally consistent and hierarchically structured. The NLM's MeSH vocabulary has emerged as the de facto standard for biomedical indexing.

Online bibliographic-retrieval systems can rapidly perform complex sorting and matching of hundreds of thousands of file records using such search techniques as combinations of Boolean operators ("and," "or," and "not"). Retrieval relevance can be optimized by minimizing the occurrence of false positives (retrieval of irrelevant records) and false negatives (failure to retrieve relevant records). **Indexing** plays a crucial role in this process; effective assignment of index terms links documents that are related, discriminates broadly among subsets of documents within the entire file, and discriminates finely among individual documents.

The assignment of index terms by human indexers is highly labor-intensive and costly work. Accordingly, researchers are developing methods (drawing on techniques from the field of artificial intelligence) that can facilitate the mechanics of this process through automated indexing and classification. The goal is to develop computer programs that can "understand" the text of an article well enough to determine how the article should be indexed. Such systems promise not only to improve retrieval relevance, but also to decrease the cost of database production.

With the maturation of online bibliographic-retrieval systems, abstracts were added to the contents of many databases, and capabilities for text-word searching became increasingly prevalent. This system feature made it possible for the user to search and retrieve records on the basis of specific user-defined words appearing in the titles and abstracts (rather than indexing terms separately assigned by human readers). Familiarity with the precise terminology comprising a database's controlled indexing vocabulary was no longer a requisite for performing an adequate search. Some database vendors even made the terms of the controlled indexing vocabulary text-word searchable. Although **text-word searching** may increase the likelihood of retrieving false positives, the expanded size of the retrieval set also may increase the likelihood that a searcher—especially an end-user searcher—will locate a starting point appropriate for modifying the original search formulation, ultimately obtaining a highly relevant retrieval.

A specific type of text-word searching is found in **full-text databases.** These are databases that contain the text of a journal article, book, or newsletter, as opposed to bibliographic references. Captions to graphics and references generally are included, but the graphics themselves are not. Two medical full-text vendors are Mead Data Central (the MEDIS system) and BRS Information Technologies (the Colleague system). Both provide access to the full text of a number of medical journals, textbooks, and newsletters as well as to the familiar bibliographic databases, such as MEDLINE. In full-text searching, what becomes important is the spatial relationship of words or phrases to one another, rather than the coexistence of the words. Thus, a technique known as **proximity searching** is used. Although there are system variations, the user basically searches for words adjacent to each other, or within a specified number of words of each other. Full-text systems also allow the user to designate a particular portion of the text to be searched. When a reference is retrieved, the user first views only the portion of the text that contains the search terms, which are highlighted on the screen for ease of reading.

Satisfactory full-text searching requires that the user be aware of and use synonyms. The MEDIS system has an automatic stemming system that assists the user in retrieving root words with different endings. If a comprehensive search is required, a combination of full-text and controlled-vocabulary searching is desirable.

An explicit objective of text-word searching is to enable the user to interact with the system in customarily familiar ways. Other tools of the artificial intelligence (AI) community, such as natural-language interfaces and conceptual indexing techniques that semantically structure the contents of a database, have the potential to achieve this objective to an even greater extent. Potential applications of AI techniques to bibliographic-retrieval systems are discussed in more detail in Section 14.5.

Statistical Approaches to Information Retrieval

The use of statistical or probabilistic methods to rank and retrieve individual records in a database in terms of their likely relevance to the searcher has its origin in the pioneering work of Gerard Salton [Salton, 1971]. Recent research in the biomedical domain, carried out by Doszkocs using bibliographic databases [Doszkocs, 1983], and by Bernstein and Williamson using full-text databases [Bernstein and Williamson, 1984], has moved this work closer to everyday use.

Statistical approaches to information retrieval address the problem of retrieval relevance by performing a combinatorial or **closest-match search,** in which documents or full-text paragraphs that have all or some of the user-selected search terms are displayed in ranked sequence, with those most likely to be relevant to the searcher's question being shown first. Records judged relevant by the searcher may then be used to expand the search and to locate other items in the database that are similar. This process is aided by stemming algorithms (techniques for determining the *root* word in a search term) that take into account the special characteristics of medical terminology, thereby greatly enhancing the power of a system's thesaurus. At the heart of these systems, keyword stems and their text-word variants are automatically assigned unique weights based on inverse postings (values denoting their frequency in the database). Thus, the higher a search term's frequency in the database (for example, common words such as "the" and "a"), the lower its assigned weight. Conversely, more specific search terms are assigned higher weights by this algorithmic process.

Many of the same system features that are designed to yield relevant search results also serve to support user-friendly searching for end users. Typically, users are permitted to enter their search question as free-form English sentences or phrases. In fact, the phrase *natural-language query input* has been used by some system designers to label this capability. However, this process does not involve natural-language *understanding* in the sense that this term has come to be used in the computer-science community (where the term generally implies a rich model of the semantic content of a sentence). At times, the failure to make this distinction has been a source of confusion and disharmony.

In a similar sense, statistically based information-retrieval systems may appear "smart," but they are not "intelligent" in that they do not encode or understand the semantic meaning of the concepts in the articles. They do, however, offer the near-term promise of improving end users' access to bibliographic data, and of thereby increasing the likelihood that health practitioners can use the information contained in the referenced journal articles and books more readily to support their own intellectual decision-making processes.

Section 14.4 includes a detailed description of Doszkocs' CITE (Current Information Transfer in English) application system, and a depiction of an actual search session carried out on a prototype system (CITE/CATLINE) installed for operational use at the NLM from 1982 to 1987. It provides an example of the type of new search systems that are available [Benson et al., 1986; Zeichick, 1988].

14.4 Recent Advances in Bibliographic Retrieval

As we noted, the past several years have seen burgeoning growth in the development and availability of user-friendly search systems designed specifically for end-user searching of bibliographic databases. The appearance of these systems is in large measure a result of the invention of the microcomputer; these powerful tools are now available to many people, including to health professionals. Concomitantly, people expect that these devices will simplify and enhance their ability to deal with the day-to-day mundane tasks of home and office, as well as with more complex intellectual activities, including the timely and efficient retrieval of biomedical information. Hardware manufacturers, software developers, and both established and new entrants to the field of database vending have fostered these expectations. In many cases, these vendors have fulfilled their promises, creating a legion of end users performing their own searches on user-friendly systems.

14.4.1 End-User Search Systems

As a group, end-user search systems share a common set of objectives or characteristics in that they may be used with little or no formal training; they make use of a few basic commands or menus, enabling the novice user to get reasonably good results quickly; and they have human-engineering features that make them relatively nonthreatening to people who have only a rudimentary understanding of computer hardware, software, and programming languages. Despite this common set of objectives, significantly different approaches have been taken. Figure 14.5 illustrates these differences schematically.

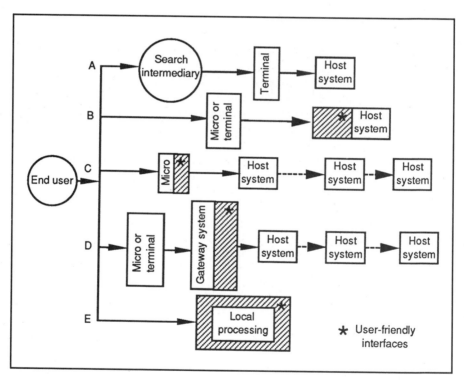

FIGURE 14.5 Alternative approaches to end-user searching. Approach A is the conventional search model; a search intermediary carries out the search on behalf of a requesting end user. Approach B incorporates a user-friendly interface that resides on the database vendor's computer system. In approach C, a user installs a user-friendly interface on his own microcomputer. In approach D, a user can access a number of computer systems with databases via a *gateway* computer system. Approach E supports end-user searching in local-processing mode; a user obtains the database contents as well as the search software for use on his own computer system.

Approach A is the conventional search model. A search intermediary carries out the search on behalf of a requesting end user. The vendor's host computer system provides a full range of searching features, including Boolean operators. Access to as many as 250 different databases in multiple disciplines, including biomedicine, may be available. Examples of these large-scale vendor systems include BRS Information Technologies, Dialog Information Services, NLM, and Pergamon Orbit InfoLine.

Approach B incorporates a user-friendly interface that resides on the database vendor's computer system. The end user logs on to the system via a telecommunications network, using either a microcomputer or a terminal. The searching features are typically a subset of the more elaborate options available in conventional search systems. Search choices are listed in a brief menu or are expressed in Englishlike commands. The user can do relatively straightforward author, title, and subject searches on the standard bibliographic records the databases comprise. Examples of these systems include BRS Colleague, Dialog's Knowledge Index, AMA/NET,[1] and Beth Israel Hospital's PaperChase.

Approach C also calls for end-user searching via online access to a remote computer system. In this approach, however, the user-friendly interface consists of a specially constructed software package that is purchased by the users and installed on their microcomputers. The software enables them to access one or more of the vendors' conventional search systems by using standardized procedures or menus. Differences among vendors' systems are thus made transparent to the user, allowing a novice or occasional searcher to move from system to system without concern for the host-system interface protocols. This approach to end-user searching is used by the Institute for Scientific Information's SCI-MATE (Universal Online Searcher) and NLM's GRATEFUL MED program, which is discussed in Section 14.4.3.

Approach D again calls for end-user searching via online access to a remote computer system. In this approach, however, the software that enables the end user to access one or more of the vendors' conventional search systems resides on a *gateway* computer system. The end user calls one telephone number and can access a number of computer systems with databases on myriad subjects. The search is charged to the user's credit card. No knowledge of the individual databases or search systems is needed; both database selection and searching are done with assistance of menus and prompts. This approach is especially practical for the user who conducts searches infrequently, because it is not necessary to obtain access codes, to maintain manuals, or to administer the use of the system. EasyNet, provided by Telebase Systems, is a gateway system that accesses a number of medical databases, including MEDLINE and Embase. It also is marketed under Western Union's label, InfoMaster, and as CompuServe's IQuest.

Approach E supports end-user searching in a standalone or local-processing mode: Users obtain the database contents as well as the search software for use on their

---

[1]Since 1987, AMA/NET has provided access to a variety of vendor services in the area of bibliographic retrieval. Access to basic AMA services is provided through Approach B. AMA/NET users can also search MEDLINE by accessing GRATEFUL MED (running on an NLM machine) via a gateway computer (Approach D).

own computer systems. The database contents may be obtained by downloading from a remote source, or by obtaining prepackaged subsets of database contents specifically intended for this purpose. Several biomedical-database producers, including BIOSIS, Excerpta Medica, and NLM, currently offer tape subsets. Examples of search software intended for standard microcomputer applications include SCI-MATE (Personal Data Manager) and BIOSIS's BioSuperfile. Software designed for use on larger computer systems includes BRS SEARCH, Cuadra Associates' STAR, Georgetown University's MINI-MEDLINE, and Beth Israel Hospital's PaperChase.

Other database-distribution techniques make use of the latest CD-ROM storage technology, in which large quantities of database contents are digitally encoded on 3.5-inch compact discs like those used in consumer market music systems now gaining widespread popularity. Recent years of MEDLINE are available in CD-ROM format from multiple vendors including: Aries Systems Corporation, BRS Information Technologies, Cambridge Scientific Abstracts, DIALOG Information Services, Digital Diagnostics, EBSCO Electronic Information, Online Research Systems, and SilverPlatter Information. Some vendors provide the entire database, 1 year per disc, for varying numbers of years; others have elected to provide a smaller subset of journals of clinical interest with a greater number of years on the disc [Rapp et al., 1989]. Several other biomedical databases, such as Embase (Excerpta Medica) and PsychLit (Psychological Abstracts), are available in CD-ROM format from these vendors.

14.4.2 The CITE/CATLINE System

The CITE/CATLINE system prototype is a user-friendly interface to the NLM's CATLINE database (online book catalog). The CITE/CATLINE prototype functioned as an online public-access catalog for visitors and staff at the NLM from 1982 to 1987[2] [Doszkocs, 1983]. As originally configured, the CITE/CATLINE prototype supports end-user searching in a local-processing mode, Approach E (see Figure 14.5), and—at least in theory—could support user-friendly remote database access, as in Approach B.

The CITE/CATLINE application has clearly demonstrated the feasibility of building a statistically based, user-friendly information-retrieval system; the relevance of its search retrievals is probabilistically determined by the system's internal algorithms. As such, CITE/CATLINE represents a new generation of bibliographic-retrieval systems that differs markedly from traditional search systems. We shall describe the key features of this system. Figures 14.6 through 14.11 illustrate a CITE/CATLINE search session.

Entering the Search Question

CITE/CATLINE has unique capabilities especially well suited to searching by end users. When a user types in a search in plain English (Figure 14.7), the system handles

---

[2]GRATEFUL MED, with its greater flexibility in searching multiple NLM databases, replaced CITE in the NLM reading room in 1987.

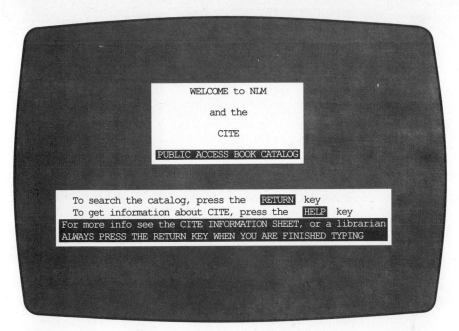

FIGURE 14.6 The CITE/CATLINE welcoming screen. The user-friendly information-retrieval system has an online help facility. (*Source:* Courtesy of the National Library of Medicine.)

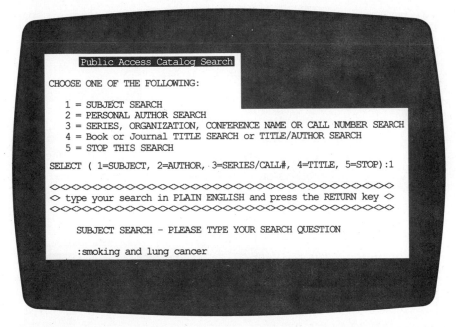

FIGURE 14.7 The CITE/CATLINE user selects "subject" search option; the user then enters a search question. (*Source:* Courtesy of the National Library of Medicine.)

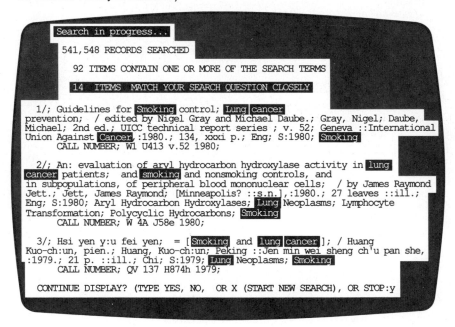

```
┌──────────────────────────────────────────────────────────────┐
│ Looking in the index for terms to use in searching...         │
│                                                                │
│ THE FOLLOWING 14 SEARCH TERMS ARE BEING PROCESSED FOR YOUR SEARCH: │
│                                                                │
│    RANK    TERM                                                │
│     1   SMOKING   (text word )                                 │
│     2       SMOKING   (medical subject heading )               │
│     3       CANNABIS   (medical subject heading )              │
│     4       TOBACCO   (medical subject heading )               │
│     5       HABITS   (medical subject heading )                │
│     6   LUNG   (text word )                                    │
│     7       LUNG   (medical subject heading )                  │
│     8       CARBON DIOXIDE   (medical subject heading )        │
│     9       CARDIOPULMONARY BYPASS   (medical subject heading )│
│    10   CANCER   (text word )                                  │
│    11       CANCER CARE FACILITIES   (medical subject heading )│
│    12       CERVIX NEOPLASMS   (medical subject heading )      │
│    13       CYCLOPHOSPHAMIDE   (medical subject heading )      │
│    14       CARCINOMA   (medical subject heading )             │
│                                                                │
│ TYPE THE RANK NUMBERS OF THE SEARCH TERMS YOU WANT TO USE      │
│ IN THEIR ORDER OF IMPORTANCE   OR TYPE ALL                     │
│ :                                                              │
│    2 6 10                                                      │
└──────────────────────────────────────────────────────────────┘
```

FIGURE 14.8 CITE/CATLINE displays candidate search terms selected from MeSH and text-word indexes; the user is given the option to rerank the terms. (*Source:* Courtesy of the National Library of Medicine.)

```
┌──────────────────────────────────────────────────────────────┐
│ Search in progress...                                         │
│                                                                │
│   541,548 RECORDS SEARCHED                                    │
│                                                                │
│     92 ITEMS CONTAIN ONE OR MORE OF THE SEARCH TERMS          │
│                                                                │
│     14  ITEMS  MATCH YOUR SEARCH QUESTION CLOSELY             │
│                                                                │
│  1/; Guidelines for Smoking control; Lung cancer              │
│ prevention;  / edited by Nigel Gray and Michael Daube.; Gray, Nigel; Daube, │
│ Michael; 2nd ed.; UICC technical report series ; v. 52; Geneva ::International │
│ Union Against Cancer, :1980.; 134, xxxi p.; Eng; S:1980; Smoking │
│    CALL NUMBER; W1 U413 v.52 1980;                            │
│                                                                │
│  2/; An: evaluation of aryl hydrocarbon hydroxylase activity in lung │
│ cancer patients;  and smoking and nonsmoking controls, and   │
│ in subpopulations, of peripheral blood mononuclear cells;  / by James Raymond │
│ Jett.; Jett, James Raymond; [Minneapolis? ::s.n.],:1980.; 27 leaves ::ill.; │
│ Eng; S:1980; Aryl Hydrocarbon Hydroxylases; Lung Neoplasms; Lymphocyte │
│ Transformation; Polycyclic Hydrocarbons; Smoking            │
│    CALL NUMBER; W 4A J58e 1980;                               │
│                                                                │
│  3/; Hsi yen y:u fei yen;  = [ Smoking  and  lung cancer ]; / Huang │
│ Kuo-ch:un, pien.; Huang, Kuo-ch:un; Peking ::Jen min wei sheng ch'u pan she, │
│ :1979.; 21 p. ::ill.; Chi; S:1979; Lung Neoplasms; Smoking  │
│    CALL NUMBER; QV 137 H874h 1979;                           │
│                                                                │
│ CONTINUE DISPLAY? (TYPE YES, NO,  OR X (START NEW SEARCH), OR STOP:y │
└──────────────────────────────────────────────────────────────┘
```

FIGURE 14.9 CITE/CATLINE displays the initial retrieval set. (*Source:* Courtesy of the National Library of Medicine.)

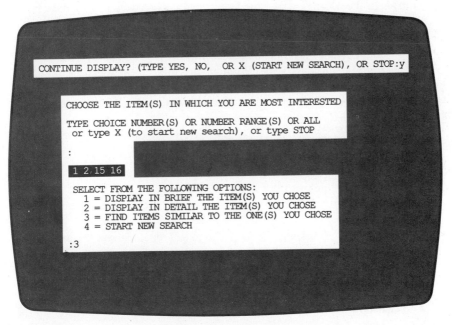

```
WOULD YOU LIKE TO SEE ONLY ENGLISH LANGUAGE ITEMS? Y/N:y

WOULD YOU LIKE TO SEE ONLY "CURRENT" BOOKS? Y/N:y

PLEASE ENTER EARLIEST PUBLICATION DATE (YEAR) OF INTEREST: 1975


  15/; National program coordination; /Office of Program Planning and
Evaluation, National Heart, Lung , and Blood Institute.; NIH publication
; no. 81-2181 - 81-2184; Bethesda, Md. ::U.S. Dept. of Health and Human
Services, Public Health Service, National Institutes of Health,:[1980]; 4 v. :
:ill.; Eng; S:1980; Cardiology; Hematology; Lung Diseases; Research
Support; Smoking ; United States; Vascular Diseases
     CALL NUMBER; WG 22 AA1 N3 1980;


  16/; Fighting the first cause of lung disease;  / American Lung
Association.; American Lung Association.    Annual; New York ::The
Association,: [1975?]; 17 p. ::ill., ports.; Eng; S:1975; Lung Diseases;
Smoking
     CALL NUMBER; W1 AM5629 1974/75;
```

FIGURE 14.10 The user responds to language and year prompts; CITE/CATLINE displays "current" records in English. (*Source:* Courtesy of the National Library of Medicine.)

```
CONTINUE DISPLAY? (TYPE YES, NO,  OR X (START NEW SEARCH), OR STOP:y


  CHOOSE THE ITEM(S) IN WHICH YOU ARE MOST INTERESTED

  TYPE CHOICE NUMBER(S) OR NUMBER RANGE(S) OR ALL
   or type X (to start new search), or type STOP

  :

  1 2 15 16

  SELECT FROM THE FOLLOWING OPTIONS:
    1 = DISPLAY IN BRIEF THE ITEM(S) YOU CHOSE
    2 = DISPLAY IN DETAIL THE ITEM(S) YOU CHOSE
    3 = FIND ITEMS SIMILAR TO THE ONE(S) YOU CHOSE
    4 = START NEW SEARCH

  :3
```

FIGURE 14.11 The CITE/CATLINE user selects the most relevant items to expand the search. (*Source:* Courtesy of the National Library of Medicine.)

text words and MeSH descriptors identically. Thus, for example, the user does not need to know that lung "neoplasm" is the accepted MeSH term for lung "cancer." The user also can search on multiple terms simultaneously. Unlike some conventional bibliographic-retrieval systems, CITE/CATLINE does not require that the user enter a single term at a time, and successively narrow or enlarge the retrieval set with Boolean operators; CITE/CATLINE's computational approach (described in the next section) allows the user to enter a search question consisting of a string of as many words as are necessary to define the subject matter sought.

Automated Selection and Ranking of Search Terms

Using the words entered by the user as the search question, CITE/CATLINE automatically builds and displays a ranked list of candidate search terms, which it selects from MeSH and from inverted files of text words in the book titles (Figure 14.8). The term ranks are based on the weighted frequency of the term in the database; the rarer the term, the higher the rank. Before the search is executed, the user can rerank the displayed terms and delete any that are inappropriate.

The Retrieval Set

CITE/CATLINE displays a closest-match set of retrieval records (Figure 14.9). The system never tells the user that the retrieval set is null (except for a *known-item search* in which, for example, a book by a particular author may not be present in the file). In contrast to many conventional bibliographic-retrieval systems, which simply display retrieved items in the order in which the latter were collected by the database producer, CITE/CATLINE has internal algorithms that determine the display sequence.

Items that have all or most of the search terms embedded within their title and descriptor list appear uppermost in the retrieval set. Within the set, items containing higher-ranked terms are displayed first. Within identically weighted groups of items, those with the most recent publication dates are shown first. Terms that caused a specific item to be retrieved are highlighted on the screen, so that the user can rapidly confirm the item's relevance (Figure 14.9).

Automatic User Prompts

During the course of the search, CITE/CATLINE automatically prompts the user with several options to improve the search result (Figure 14.10). Thus, if the user wishes to see more than the first three items retrieved, she can limit the resultant output by language or by year of publication. The user also is given the option of searching for additional items similar to those she judges most relevant (Figure 14.11). Other items containing the same MeSH terms or related call numbers are retrieved in this manner.

14.4.3 The GRATEFUL MED System

The GRATEFUL MED microcomputer software package is a user-friendly front-end to many of the NLM's databases, including all years of MEDLINE, CATLINE (catalog records for books and journals), AVLINE (audiovisual materials for health

education), AIDSLINE, CANCERLIT, HEALTH Planning & Administration, TOX-
LINE and TOXLIT (toxicology databases), CHEMLINE (a chemical dictionary file),
and DIRLINE (a directory of organizations that provide information for the general
public). An expert mode allows access to all (more than 20) NLM files. Direct access is also available to PDQ, a menu-driven database designed to assist physicians
in the treatment and referral of cancer patients, and to TOXNET, a group of factual
databanks (Hazardous Substances Databank, Registry of Toxic Effects of Chemical
Substances, and Chemical Carcinogenesis Research Information System).

An interactive search on the MEDLINE database generally requires about 10
minutes. A major goal of the GRATEFUL MED software is to reduce the time spent
connected to the mainframe computer, and hence the cost to the user. The software
is designed to allow the intellectual portions of the search process—that is, choice
of terminology, structuring of the search, and examination and assessment of the
retrieval—to take place on the user's microcomputer rather than on the mainframe
computer at the NLM. The only time spent on the mainframe is that needed to upload
(to send the search request from the microcomputer to the mainframe over telecommunications lines) and download (to receive the retrieval result at the microcomputer from the mainframe in the same way). Searches requiring a fairly small
retrieval—10 to 15 citations—can be done within a 2- or 3-minute connection to the
mainframe computer. Downloading of searches requiring large or comprehensive
retrieval requires time proportional to the result size.

Entering the Search

GRATEFUL MED uses a *form screen* to aid the user in structuring the search (Figure
14.12). The screen guides the user in entering author names, words from a journal
article (or book) title, and subjects. Searches generally are performed on a subject,
except when users are looking for a specific article or book already known to them.
GRATEFUL MED enters the logical connectors for the user. Words on a subject
line of the form screen are combined with the "or" connector; synonyms or like
concepts can be included in the search in this way. All lines on the form screen that
are used in the search are combined by the "and" connector.

The user has a choice of phrasing queries in his own language or using and selecting from MeSH headings, a complete list of which is contained in the software. Cross-
references—terms that lead to other terms for searching—are included in the list,
with the "real" term following in parentheses. The notation *N.B.* (nota bene) introduces
brief guidance for the selection of terms. Many MeSH terms have narrower *children*
terms that can be searched simultaneously with the broader *parent* term; these are
followed by a plus sign (+) (Figure 14.13). If the user chooses not to check his terms
against the available MeSH list, and uses a word that is not a MeSH heading, that
word is searched as a text word contained in the title or abstract of a journal article
(other fields are searched for books). Both text words and MeSH headings can be
combined in a search (Figure 14.14).

There are lines on the form screen to limit the search to English language only,
to review articles only, or to a particular journal title or set of titles in a personal
journal collection.

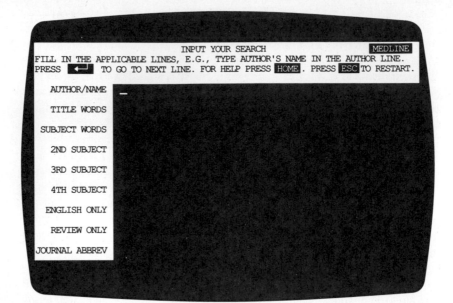

FIGURE 14.12 GRATEFUL MED input-form screen. (*Source:* Courtesy of the National Library of Medicine.)

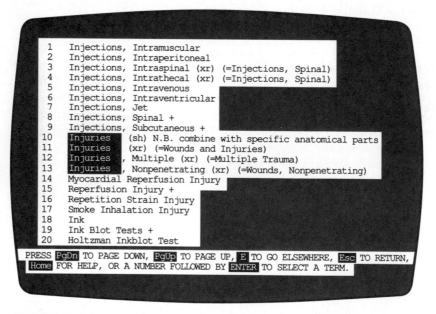

FIGURE 14.13 GRATEFUL MED screen of MeSH terms resulting from entering INJURIES on a subject line. The user can select terms by number and transfer them to the input form without rekeying. Selection guidance is provided by indication of cross-reference terms (xr), terms with narrower *children* terms available (+), and usage notes (N.B.). (*Source:* Courtesy of the National Library of Medicine.)

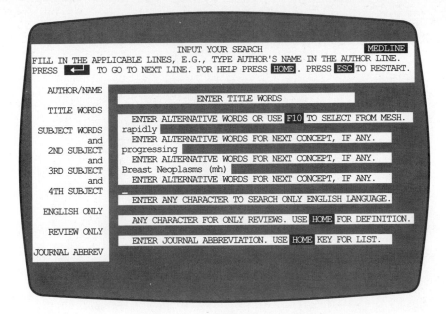

FIGURE 14.14 A search entered on the input-form screen. Term followed by (mh) was selected from lists of MeSH terms displayed in GRATEFUL MED. (*Source:* Courtesy of the National Library of Medicine.)

Uploading the Search and Downloading the Retrieval

In journal searching, the user has the option of retrieving abstracts or MeSH headings with the basic bibliographic information of author(s), title, and journal information. (There are no abstracts for books.) Once the user has made these decisions and is satisfied with the terminology and logic of the search, the telecommunications module contained in GRATEFUL MED is signaled to upload the search to the NLM computer. GRATEFUL MED automatically makes the appropriate telephone calls and network connections to the NLM machine. It then translates the information contained in the form screen to the command language of the mainframe system, so it is not necessary for the user to learn even the most basic commands. The results are downloaded to the user's microcomputer; if more information is retrieved than is needed, the user can terminate the search at any time.

Assessing the Retrieval

GRATEFUL MED reformats the retrieval citations into an easy-to-read display and presents them one at a time. The user is queried as to the relevance of each, and GRATEFUL MED records the response in order to determine which MeSH headings might be useful for finding additional citations of interest. These MeSH headings are then displayed for the user (Figure 14.15). In addition, because MEDLINE contains only 2 to 3 years of current data, the option to search the older material is then presented.

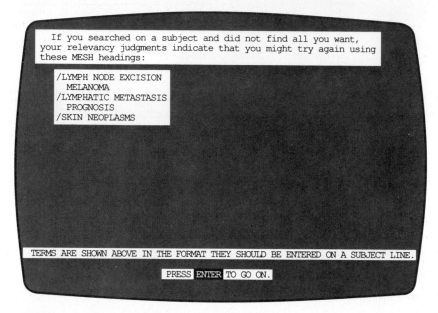

FIGURE 14.15 Suggested MeSH terms resulting from a search on the user's words *lymph, node, dissection,* and *melanoma* entered on the four subject lines of the GRATEFUL MED input form. (*Source:* Courtesy of the National Library of Medicine.)

An option to edit the search is also provided. If the user elects this option, the form screen is returned to view with the original input of the user and feedback for each individual line of the form screen, as well as the combination of terms. The user can add, delete, or correct a term (or terms), then resend the search to the NLM computer.

14.5 The Future of Bibliographic Retrieval

More than 20 years ago, the President's Science Advisory Committee's report on information transfer identified the fundamental task of the information-transfer chain as "the switching of information, not documents . . . the ultimate aim being to connect the user, quickly and efficiently, to the proper information and to only the proper information" [President's Science Advisory Committee, 1963]. Nowhere is this need more acute than in biomedicine, particularly in the practice setting, where the scope of the information that health practitioners require is determined not by circumscribed research interests but by the varied illnesses of the patients. In the practical sense, a busy practitioner cannot read and process the contents of all the documents relevant to a patient's problems that could be retrieved by searching a bibliographic database.

This need has spawned research to develop **information-synthesis databases,** as exemplified in biomedicine by early experiments on the Hepatitis Knowledge Base prototype [Bernstein et al., 1980]. This system provided specialized programs for locating information in a hierarchically organized network of text paragraphs describing the state of the art in hepatitis knowledge. The information was derived from the literature, but the individual paragraphs were written by knowledgeable scholars who had studied the most recent articles. Thus, the Hepatitis Knowledge Base could be viewed as a large, computer-oriented, online review article.

Clinical decision-support tools are similarly designed to provide practitioners with access to recent knowledge and expertise. Like the Hepatitis Knowledge Base, such systems store synthesized knowledge in the computer. However, these systems must store the knowledge in a form that permits the computer to *use* that knowledge to give advice. Only one system to date has explicitly based its knowledge representation on individual articles from the clinical literature [Rennels, 1987]. We shall describe this system, known as Roundsman, in Section 14.5.1. As such programs are refined and made generally available, they are likely to have a profound effect on how health professionals access information to make complex decisions (see Chapter 15).

Until systems such as these become widely available, we shall continue to need bibliographic-retrieval methods. Moreover, those methods will continue to play an important role in the knowledge acquisition that is a cornerstone of the development of knowledge bases such as those we have mentioned.

14.5.1 AI Techniques for Managing the Literature

Because AI research is inherently involved with issues in knowledge-base development and knowledge management (see Chapter 15), there are potentially strong links between AI and the computer-based management of biomedical literature. After all, the literature is a primary repository of biomedical knowledge. Thus, the transfer of the contents of that literature to online knowledge bases is likely to benefit from AI techniques for encoding knowledge in computers.

Recall from our discussion in Chapter 2 that a knowledge base includes information encoded so that the computer can *use* it to reach decisions and to offer custom-tailored analyses of specific problems. Yet, except for the Roundsman system, not one of the bibliographic-retrieval systems we have described in this chapter can do more than display textual information, which the user must interpret and apply appropriately. We can anticipate the day, however, when bibliographic-retrieval systems not only will help a person to locate a pertinent article, but also will help her to determine the applicability of its contents to a specific problem.

We envision at least three ways in which AI methods will find useful application in the field of literature management:

- *"Intelligent" retrieval assistance.* As we have described, a major challenge in system development is determining how best to describe the information for which a user is looking. Available interfaces have no understanding of medicine and therefore will blindly accept (and search with) any specification provided by a user, *even if a knowledgeable intermediary could have immediately seen a preferable search strategy.* As investigators better characterize the complex nature of expertise in searching the literature (an expertise that involves knowledge both of biomedicine and of the literature-search process), AI methods will provide a set of tools for implementing those insights in improved systems for online search assistance.

- *Expert advice systems based on literature references.* The notion of medical expert advice systems is gaining in popularity; these systems are described in Chapter 15. Such systems generally have used medical knowledge that is abstracted from the literature or derived by interviewing experts in the field of application. In contrast, the Roundsman research system [Rennels, 1987] explicitly codes the contents of individual articles, so the program can give advice about specific patients by quoting data from the literature. Figure 14.16 shows an example of the advice generated by this system. Note that the program is designed to critique a physician's proposed management plan for a patient with breast cancer by analyzing that plan in terms of empirical studies reported in the literature. Articles about breast cancer are separately represented in the knowledge base, and Roundsman has techniques for selecting relevant articles and identifying subsets of patients that were similar to the patient being managed by the physician-user.

- *Programs that "read" the literature.* Because medical knowledge is rapidly changing, it is a major challenge for both physicians and computer knowledge bases to be kept up to date. Problems in knowledge-base maintenance and currency frequently are cited as major limitations in the development of reliable computer-based advice systems. If the literature could be surveyed, analyzed, and *understood* by computer programs, however, then the process of knowledge-base maintenance

---

Roundsman's critique:

Peters67 employed non-randomized controls in a study conducted at Princess Margaret Hospital, Toronto. A set of patients who were treated by wedge resection and adjuvant radiotherapy (N=94) is contrasted to a second therapy group: radical mastectomy and adjuvant radiotherapy (N=247). In the group which received the first protocol the overall survival at five years was 0.76. For patients who underwent the second protocol the overall survival at five years turned out to be 0.72.

How well does the study generalize to your particular patient? We are not particularly concerned that one modality you propose may not be quite like what was done in the study ('wedge resection' here indicates excisional biopy, quadrant resection, or any technique to excise the primary.) More troublesome is that the study population was probably in a better prognostic stratum than your patient (the study used a pooled clinical stage I and II - so that's a slightly better prognostic group than your patient).

FIGURE 14.16 The Roundsman system uses a knowledge base of articles about breast cancer to generate a prose critique of a physician's treatment plan. (*Source:* Reprinted with permission from Rennels, G. D., et al. A computational model of reasoning from the clinical literature. *Computer Methods and Programs in Biomedicine,* 24:139, 1987.)

would be greatly facilitated. To understand written text, a computer system must have a capability for *natural-language understanding,* a major research topic in AI. As investigators make progress in this area, methods for merging new knowledge from the literature with existing biomedical knowledge bases may evolve. Natural-language understanding of a more limited form also will be needed for automated indexing of literature articles (see Section 14.5.4).

14.5.2 Human–Database Interfaces

As we discussed, the development of user-friendly interfaces is intended to make computers generally more accessible to people who have no special training. In the AI community, this work has tended to focus on how a computer can be programmed to "understand" natural-language commands and queries in much the same way as a well-informed human would. When available, these natural-language processing systems could be designed to function as interfaces to conventional bibliographic-retrieval systems, thereby greatly enhancing the utility of the bibliographic database for novice or occasional searchers.

14.5.3 Conceptual Indexing

Conceptual indexing organizes an information base by the *meaning* of the entries. In this context, the system actually understands the information it contains. Users must specify queries using the same representation of meaning as is used for storage of the contents of the information base; such queries are used to locate matching pieces of information. To the extent that the matching process is successful, retrieval relevance is greatly enhanced and false-positive retrievals are decreased [DeJong, 1983]. Traditional measures of system performance such as **precision** (ratio of relevant to irrelevant records retrieved) and **recall** (the ratio of relevant records retrieved to all relevant records in a database) should show corresponding improvement.

14.5.4 Automatic Indexing and Classification

In a conceptually organized information base, each new entry must be mapped to a representation of its meaning before it can be added to the information base. Although a meaning representation can be coded manually by humans who are subject-matter specialists (analogous to current database-indexing practices), the use of an intelligent system that is capable of reading and understanding the items to be added can potentially achieve greater indexing consistency and fewer errors. Such a tool also could yield substantial cost savings in a number of areas associated with the mechanics of database production.

The successful application of AI techniques to bibliographic retrieval awaits the solution of many of the same types of problems that confront the AI community in general. However, the special nature of bibliographic databases, consisting as they do of regularly structured items that are heavily indexed with regard to subject matter, could serve to render some of these problems more susceptible to resolution. For example, the preexistence of a well-developed and hierarchically structured indexing vocabulary, such as MeSH, should help to create a meaningful representation that characterizes and semantically structures the contents of a biomedical database. Thus, the bibliographic-retrieval environment can be an especially fertile ground for AI research, which in turn can yield substantial benefits for system users and producers.

Suggested Readings

Albright, R. G. *A Basic Guide to Online Information Systems for Health Care Professionals.* Arlington, VA: Information Resource Press, 1988.

> *This text, written for the practicing physician, provides information on available online avenues to the medical literature. It contains practical examples and directions for obtaining access to each system described, as well as easy-to-understand information on telecommunications technology.*

Haynes, R. B., et al. How to keep up with the medical literature: Parts 1–6. *Annals of Internal Medicine,* 105(1):149, 105(2):309, 105(3):474, 105(4):636, 105(5):810, 105(6):978, 1986.

> *This six-part series includes the following articles: I. Why try to keep up and how to get started, II. Deciding which journals to read regularly, III. Expanding the number of journals you read regularly, IV. Using the literature to solve clinical problems, V. Access by personal computer to the medical literature, and VI. How to store and retrieve articles worth keeping. The last two parts relate most closely to the issues in this chapter. The entire series provides an excellent overview of varied aspects of dealing with the medical literature.*

Meadow, C. T. and Cochrane, P. A. *Basics of Online Searching.* New York: Wiley, 1981.

> *This textbook covers the principles of online bibliographic searching; it does not discuss specific systems or databases. The section explaining set combinations is especially useful for those people who want to review Boolean logic.*

Smith, L. D. Artificial intelligence applications in information systems. In M. E. Williams (ed), *Annual Review of Information Science and Technology,* Vol. 22. Amsterdam: Elsevier, 1987.

> *This chapter, in an annual monograph on information science, provides both a historical perspective on the applications of AI in information science and a review of the recent literature.*

Williams, M. E. Electronic databases. *Science,* 228:445, 1985.

> *This article provides an overview of online databases, including bibliographic, full-text, and numeric databases. It describes database vendors and user-friendly front-ends, and discusses the role of artificial intelligence as related to online databases.*

Questions for Discussion

1. Explain the notion of an *information gatekeeper.* Name an organization with which you are familiar and in which such a gatekeeper exists. List three reasons why

it would be difficult to serve as gatekeeper for a large organization. Distinguish a gatekeeper from a bibliographic-retrieval intermediary.

2. As a learning exercise, obtain access to a bibliographic-retrieval system specifically designed for end-user searches. Plan and carry out a search on a topic of interest to you. Are the search results satisfactory? Did you find the material for which you were looking? Arrange to have the same search query replicated by an intermediary on a conventional bibliographic-retrieval system. Are the search results the same? Discuss what you have learned from this exercise.

3. Talk with an expert in online retrieval about a search you would like to do on a complex problem. Record the conversation you have with the expert while he or she helps you to devise a search strategy. Analyze the recording to identify the kinds of knowledge the expert used in giving you advice. How much was specific to the search system you were using? How much was based on the expert's understanding of the biomedical question you were asking? When you have formulated a model of the kind of knowledge needed to be an expert search intermediary, consider the nature of a computer-based consultation system that would help you with search formulation. Such tools often are cited as goals for the medical artificial-intelligence research community. Do you think it is reasonable to expect that such intelligent consultant programs can be built for the bibliographic-retrieval setting?

4. Look again at the Roundsman example in Figure 14.16. Remember that the paragraphs are not simply stored in the computer as shown. Rather, they are generated from sentence fragments based on the program's analysis of a specific patient and of the relevant literature. What kinds of "knowledge" does Roundsman apparently have? Based on this example, list some of the facts and skills to which the program evidently has access. Explain how the program might produce patient-specific analyses based on these facts. (If you have trouble answering this question, see [Rennels, 1987].)

5. The terms *false positive* and *false negative* were used in this chapter to describe the success of retrieval requests. Explain how the terms *sensitivity, specificity,* and *predictive value* also might be applied appropriately to the retrieval process (refer to Chapters 2 and 3). If a given search has too many false-positive retrievals, how might you as the searcher deal with the problem? What problems beyond your control might account for the difficulty?

6. What effect will the availability of search systems accessible to end users have on your information-seeking behavior? How might it change the way health professionals are educated? How might it change clinical practice?

7. How might AI tools and techniques be used to improve the performance of conventional bibliographic-retrieval systems? (Develop ideas not discussed in this chapter.) How might bibliographic retrieval be used as part of a decision-support system?

15

Clinical Decision-Support Systems

Edward H. Shortliffe

After reading this chapter,[1] you should know the answers to these questions:

- What are the three requirements for excellent decision making?
- What are the types of decision-support roles for computers in clinical medicine?
- How has the use of computers for clinical decision support evolved since the late 1950s?
- What concerns attracted researchers in this area to the field of artificial intelligence?
- What is a medical expert system?
- What influences account for the gradual improvement in professional attitudes toward use of computers for clinical decision support?
- What are the five dimensions that characterize clinical decision-support tools?
- What has been the role of human-factors research in the development of decision-support tools?
- What are the principal scientific challenges in building useful and acceptable clinical decision-support tools?
- What legal and regulatory barriers could affect distribution of clinical decision-support technologies?

---

[1]Portions of this chapter are based on Shortliffe, E. H. Computer programs to support clinical decision making. *Journal of the American Medical Association*, 258:61–66, July 3, 1987. Copyright 1987, American Medical Association.

15.1 The Nature of Clinical Decision Making

If you ask people what the phrase *computers in medicine* means, they often describe a computer program that helps physicians to make diagnoses. Although computers play numerous important medical roles, from the earliest days of computing people have recognized that computers might support physicians by helping users to sift through the vast collection of possible diseases and symptoms. This notion has been echoed in futuristic works of science fiction. In *"Star Trek"* episodes, for example, we see Dr. McCoy pointing a "tricorder" probe at an injured crew member to determine in a moment what is the problem and how serious is the damage. The prevalence of such expectations, coupled with a general societal concern about the influence of computers on interpersonal relationships and on job security, has naturally raised questions among health workers. Just what can computers do today to support clinical decision making? How soon will diagnostic tools be generally available? How good will they be? What will their effects be on the practice of medicine, on medical education, and on relationships among colleagues or between physicians and patients?

We can view the contents of this entire book as addressing medical data and decision making. In Chapter 2, we discussed the central role of accurate, complete, and relevant data in supporting the decisions that confront clinicians and other health-care workers. In Chapter 3, we described the nature of good decisions and the need for clinicians to understand the proper use of information if they are to be effective and efficient decision makers. Subsequent chapters have mentioned many real or potential uses of computers to assist with such decision making. Medical practice *is* medical decision making, so most applications of computers in medical care are intended to have a direct or tangential effect on the quality of health-care decisions. In this chapter, we bring together these themes by concentrating on systems that have been developed specifically to assist health workers in making decisions.

15.1.1 Types of Decisions

By now, you are familiar with the range of clinical decisions. The classical problem of diagnosis (analyzing available data to determine the pathophysiologic explanation for a patient's symptoms) is only one such decision task. Equally challenging, as we emphasized in Chapter 3, is the diagnostic *process*—deciding which questions to ask, tests to order, or procedures to perform, and determining the value of the results relative to associated risks or financial costs. Thus, diagnosis involves not only deciding what is true about a patient, but also what data are needed to determine what is true. Even when the diagnosis is known, there may be challenging management decisions that test the physician's knowledge and experience: Should I treat the patient or allow the process to resolve on its own? If treatment is indicated, what should it be? How should I use the response to therapy to guide me in determining whether an alternate approach should be tried or, in some cases, to question whether my initial diagnosis was incorrect after all?

Biomedicine is also replete with decision tasks that do not involve specific patients or their diseases. Consider, for example, the biomedical scientist who is using laboratory data to help with the design of her next experiment, or the hospital administrator who uses management data to guide decisions about resource allocation in his hospital. Although we focus on systems to assist with clinical decisions in this chapter, we emphasize that the concepts discussed generalize to many other problem areas as well. In Chapter 19, for example, we examine the need for formal decision techniques and tools in creating health policies.

The requirements for excellent decision making fall into three principal categories: accurate data, pertinent knowledge, and appropriate problem-solving skills. The data about a case must be adequate for making an informed decision, but they must not be excessive. Indeed, as we learned in Chapter 12, a major challenge occurs when decision makers are bombarded with so much information that they cannot process and synthesize the information intelligently and rapidly. Thus, it is important to know when additional data will confuse rather than clarify, and when it is imperative to use tools (computational or otherwise) that permit data to be summarized for easier cognitive management. The operating room and intensive-care units are classical settings for this problem; patients are monitored extensively, numerous data are collected, and decisions often have to be made emergently. Equally important is the *quality* of the available data. In Chapter 2, we discussed imprecision in terminology, illegibility and inaccessibility of records, and other opportunities for misinterpretation of data. Similarly, measurement instruments or recorded data may be simply erroneous; use of faulty data can have serious adverse effects on patient-care decisions.

Even good data are useless if we do not have the basic knowledge necessary to apply them properly. Decision makers must have broad knowledge of medicine, in-depth familiarity with their area of expertise, and access to information resources that provide pertinent additional information. Their knowledge must be accurate, with areas of controversy well understood, and questions of personal choice well distinguished from topics where a dogmatic approach is appropriate. Their knowledge must also be current; in the rapidly changing world of medicine, facts decay just as certainly as dead tissue does.

Good data and an extensive factual knowledge base still do not guarantee a good decision. Good problem-solving skills are equally important. Decision makers must know how to set appropriate goals for a task, how to use the heuristics of the hypothetico-deductive approach (see Chapter 2) to guide them in data collection, and how to make explicit the tradeoffs between costs and benefits of diagnostic procedures or of therapeutic maneuvers. The skilled clinician draws extensively on personal experience, and novice physicians soon realize that good clinical judgment is based as much on an ability to reason effectively and appropriately about what to do as it is on knowledge of the field or access to high-quality patient data. Thus, clinicians must develop a strategic approach to test selection and interpretation, understand notions of sensitivity and specificity, and be able to assess the urgency of a situation. Awareness of potential biases (see Chapter 3), and of the way they can creep into problem solving, also is crucial.

This brief review of issues central to clinical decision making serves as a fitting introduction to the topic of computer-assisted decision making—precisely the same topics are pertinent when we develop a computational tool for clinical problem solving. The programs must have access to good data, they must have extensive background knowledge encoded for the clinical domain in question, and they must embody an intelligent approach to problem solving that is sensitive to requirements for proper analysis, appropriate cost–benefit tradeoffs, and efficiency.

15.1.2 The Role of Computers in Decision Support

A **clinical decision-support system** is any computer program designed to help health professionals make clinical decisions. In a sense, *any* computer system that deals with clinical data or medical knowledge is intended to provide decision support. It is accordingly useful to consider three types of decision-support functions, ranging from generalized to patient-specific:

1. *Tools for information management.* Examples are hospital information systems (Chapter 7) and bibliographic-retrieval systems (Chapter 14). Specialized knowledge-management workstations are under development in research settings [Greenes, 1986]; these provide sophisticated environments for storing and retrieving clinical knowledge, for browsing through that knowledge much as we might page through a textbook, and for augmenting it with personal notes and information that we may later need for clinical problem solving. Information-management tools provide the data and knowledge needed by the clinician, but they generally do not help physicians to *apply* that information to a particular decision task. Interpretation is left to the doctor, as is the decision about what information is needed to resolve the clinical problem.

2. *Tools for focusing attention.* Examples are clinical-laboratory systems that flag abnormal values or that provide lists of possible explanations for those abnormalities, and pharmacy systems that alert providers to possible drug interactions [Tatro et al., 1975; Evans et al., 1986]. Such programs are designed to remind the user of diagnoses or problems that might otherwise have been overlooked. They typically use simple logic, displaying fixed lists or paragraphs as a standard response to a definite or potential abnormality.

3. *Tools for patient-specific consultation.* Such programs provide custom-tailored assessments or advice based on sets of patient-specific data. They may follow simple logic (such as algorithms), may be based on statistical theory and cost–benefit analysis, or may use numerical approaches only as an adjunct to symbolic problem solving. Some diagnostic assistants (such as Reconsider [Blois et al., 1981] and DXplain [Barnett et al., 1987]) suggest differential diagnoses or indicate additional information that would help to narrow the range of etiologic possibilities. Other systems (such as Internist-1 [Miller et al., 1982] and its successor QMR [Miller et al., 1986]) suggest a single best explanation for a patient's symptomatology. Still other systems provide therapy advice, rather than diagnostic assistance.

The boundaries among these three categories are not crisp, but the distinctions are useful in defining the range of capabilities that computers can provide to assist clinicians with making decisions. We have discussed systems of the first two types elsewhere in this book. For example, Chapters 6 through 13 all describe systems that contain and manipulate patient data that are of importance in reaching good clinical decisions. Chapters 14 and 16 discuss methods for accessing information, knowledge, and the accumulated experience of other clinicians and researchers. In the remainder of this chapter, we shall focus on the third category, patient-specific systems.

15.2   Historical Perspective

Since the earliest days of computers, health professionals have anticipated the time when machines would assist in the diagnostic process. The first articles dealing with this possibility appeared in the late 1950s [Ledley and Lusted, 1959], and experimental prototypes were shown to be accurate within a few years [Warner et al., 1964]. Several problems prevented the clinical introduction of such systems, however, ranging from the limitations of the scientific underpinnings to the logistical difficulties developers encountered when encouraging clinicians to use and accept the systems.

Two advisory systems from the 1970s provide a useful overview of the field's evolution prior to the last decade. These are de Dombal's system for diagnosis of abdominal pain [de Dombal et al., 1972] and Shortliffe's system for selection of antibiotic therapy [Shortliffe, 1976]. Since the late 1960s, de Dombal and his associates at the University of Leeds have been studying the diagnostic process and developing computer-based decision aids using Bayesian probability theory (see Chapter 3). Using surgical or pathologic diagnoses as the gold standard, they have emphasized the importance of deriving the conditional probabilities used in Bayesian reasoning from high-quality data that they have gathered by collecting information on thousands of patients [Adams et al., 1986]. Their system used sensitivity, specificity, and disease-prevalence data for various signs, symptoms, and test results to calculate, using Bayes' theorem, the probability of seven possible explanations for acute abdominal pain (appendicitis, diverticulitis, perforated ulcer, cholecystitis, small bowel obstruction, pancreatitis, and nonspecific abdominal pain). To keep the Bayesian computations manageable, the program made the assumptions of (1) conditional independence of the findings for the various diagnoses, and (2) mutual exclusivity of the seven diagnoses (see Chapter 3).

In one system evaluation [de Dombal et al., 1972], physicians filled out data sheets summarizing clinical and laboratory findings for 304 patients who came to the emergency room with abdominal pain of sudden onset (Figure 15.1). The data from these sheets became the attributes that were analyzed using Bayes' rule. Thus, the Bayesian formulation assumed that each patient had one of the seven conditions and selected the most likely one on the basis of the recorded observations. Had the program been used directly by emergency-room physicians, results could have been available, on average, within 5 minutes after the data form was completed. During the study, however, the cases were run in batch mode; the computer-generated diagnoses were saved for later comparison to (1) the diagnoses reached by the attending clinicians, and (2) the ultimate diagnosis verified during surgery or through appropriate tests. In contrast to the clinicians' diagnoses, which were correct in only 65 to 80 percent of the 304 cases (with accuracy depending on the individual clinician's training and experience), the program's diagnoses were correct in 91.8 percent of the cases. Furthermore, in six of the seven disease categories, the computer was

Abdominal Pain Chart

NAME		REG NUMBER	
MALE/FEMALE AGE		FORM FILLED BY	
PRESENTATION (999, GP, etc)	DATE		TIME

PAIN

SITE

ONSET

PRESENT

RADIATION

AGGRAVATING FACTORS
movement
coughing
respiration
food
other
none

RELIEVING FACTORS
lying still
vomiting
antacids
food
other
none

PROGRESS
better
same
worse
DURATION

TYPE
intermittent
steady
colicky

SEVERITY
moderate
severe

HISTORY

NAUSEA
yes   no

VOMITING
yes   no

ANOREXIA
yes   no

PREV INDIGESTION
yes   no

JAUNDICE
yes   no

BOWELS
normal
constipation
diarrhoea
blood
mucus

MICTURITION
normal
frequency
dysuria
dark
haematuria

PREV SIMILAR PAIN
yes   no

PREV ABDO SURGERY
yes   no

DRUGS FOR ABDO PAIN
yes   no

♀ LMP

pregnant

Vag. discharge

dizzy/faint

EXAMINATION

MOOD
normal
distressed
anxious

SHOCKED
yes   no

COLOUR
normal
pale
flushed
jaundiced
cyanosed

TEMP   PULSE

BP

ABDO MOVEMENT
normal
poor/nil
peristalsis

SCAR
yes   no

DISTENSION
yes   no

TENDERNESS

REBOUND
yes   no

GUARDING
yes   no

RIGIDITY
yes   no

MASS
yes   no

MURPHY'S
+ve   −ve

BOWEL SOUNDS
normal   absent   +++

RECTAL — VAGINAL TENDERNESS
left
right
general
mass
none

INITIAL DIAGNOSIS & PLAN

RESULTS
amylase
blood count (WBC)
computer
urine
X-ray
other

DIAG & PLAN AFTER INVEST

(time   )

DISCHARGE DIAGNOSIS

History and examination of other systems on separate case notes

UPS/4462/7/82

FIGURE 15.1 de Dombal and coworkers developed this specialized datasheet to standardize the collection of clinical data for the diagnosis of abdominal pain. Physicians filled out the sheet as they examined a patient, and the data were converted to a format suitable for entering the findings into the diagnostic advice program. (*Source:* Courtesy of F. T. de Dombal, M.D.)

more likely to assign the patients to the correct disease category than was the senior clinician in charge of the case. Of particular interest was the program's accuracy regarding appendicitis—a diagnosis that is often made incorrectly. In no cases of appendicitis did the computer fail to make the correct diagnosis, and in only six cases were patients with nonspecific abdominal pain incorrectly classified as having appendicitis. Based on the actual clinical decisions, however, more than 20 patients with nonspecific abdominal pain underwent unnecessary surgery for an incorrect diagnosis of appendicitis, and six patients with appendicitis were observed for more than 8 hours before they were finally taken to the operating room.

With the introduction of microcomputers and the acquisition of geographically diverse probability data for abdominal pain, de Dombal's system began to achieve widespread use over the last decade. Because it deals with an important but narrowly defined area of medicine for which probability data are available and definitive diagnostic criteria exist, it remains one of the best examples of how the Bayesian approach can be applied effectively for useful decision support in routine clinical settings.

A different approach to computer-assisted decision support was embodied in the MYCIN program, a consultation system that deemphasized diagnosis to concentrate on appropriate management of patients who have infections [Shortliffe, 1976]. MYCIN's developers found that straightforward algorithms or statistical approaches were inadequate for this clinical problem, in which the nature of expertise was poorly understood and even the experts often disagreed about how best to manage specific patients, especially before definitive culture results became available. As a result, the researchers were drawn to the field of **artificial intelligence (AI)**, the subfield of computer science that has focused on symbolic manipulations rather than numerical calculations. A variety of design considerations led them to select AI methodologies. They wanted the system to be useful to physicians so they chose a problem domain in which physicians err frequently. In addition, MYCIN had to be acceptable to physicians. Therefore, the system was designed (1) to explain the advice it offered, (2) to justify its performance using simple English sentences, (3) to learn new information through interactions with experts, (4) to encode knowledge in a modular format (thus facilitating modification of the knowledge base), and (5) to have prompts, answers, and volunteered information that matched its users' needs. Previous computer decision aids that did not meet these criteria generally had been poorly accepted by physicians—even those that performed well in problem solving. MYCIN's developers thought that the system had to be perceived as a clinical *tool,* rather than as a replacement for the primary physician's own reasoning.

Knowledge of infectious diseases in MYCIN was represented as production rules, each containing a "packet" of knowledge obtained from collaborating experts (Figure 15.2). A **production rule** is simply a conditional statement that relates observations to associated inferences that can be drawn. MYCIN's power was derived from such rules in a variety of ways:

- The program determined which rules to use and how to chain them together to make decisions about a specific case.

Rule507

IF: 1) The infection which requires therapy is meningitis,
      2) Organisms were not seen on the stain of the culture,
      3) The type of the infection is bacterial,
      4) The patient does not have a head injury defect, and
      5) The age of the patient is between 15 years and 55 years

THEN: The organisms that might be causing the infection are
      diplococcus-pneumoniae and neisseria-meningitidis

FIGURE 15.2 A typical rule from the MYCIN system. Rules are conditional statements that indicate what conclusions can be reached or actions taken *if* all elements of a specific set of conditions are found to be true. In this rule, MYCIN is able to conclude probable bacterial causes of infection if the five conditions in the premise are all found to be true for a specific patient. Not shown are the measures of uncertainty that are also associated with inference in the MYCIN system. (*Source:* Courtesy of Section on Medical Informatics, Stanford University.)

- The rules often formed a coherent explanation of MYCIN's reasoning—those that applied to the current decision were displayed in response to users' questions (Figure 15.3). Although rules were stored in a machine-readable format, English translations could be displayed.
- By removing, altering, or adding rules, system developers could modify the program's knowledge structures rapidly, without explicitly reprogramming or restructuring other parts of the knowledge base.

The developers evaluated MYCIN's performance on therapy selection for patients with blood-borne bacterial infections [Yu et al., 1979a], and for those with meningitis [Yu et al., 1979b]. In the latter study, MYCIN gave advice that compared favorably to that offered by experts in infectious diseases. MYCIN, however, is best viewed as an early exploration of methods for capturing and applying ill-structured expert knowledge to solve important medical problems. The program was never used clinically, in large part because the technology in the 1970s was unable to support a program of MYCIN's size on a cost-effective machine with acceptable response times; nonetheless, it paved the way for a great deal of research and development in the 1980s. In fact, the development of **expert systems,** and the commercialization of the rule-based approach in a variety of nonmedical fields during the early 1980s, evolved from MYCIN and from related systems developed during the 1970s [Hayes-Roth et al., 1983].[2]

[2]The research results and influence of medical AI experiments during the 1970s and 1980s were due in large part to support for the field through the SUMEX-AIM computing resource. Located at Stanford University, SUMEX-AIM has been shared by investigators in biomedical AI throughout the country who have accessed it over computer networks. It was supported by the Division of Research Resources, National Institutes of Health and, more recently, by the National Library of Medicine.

In this series, how many of the cultures were positive for the e.coli   {*typical system prompt*}
(ORGANISM-1)?

** WHY   {*request from user to determine motivation for question*}

[i.e. WHY is it important to determine the number of cultures which were   {*system's rephrasing of the WHY*
positive for the organism?]   *question, and answer*}

[1.0] This will help to determine whether there is significant disease
associated with this occurrence of the organism.
    It has already been established that
        [1.1] the culture was taken from a sterile source
        [1.2] the number of cultures in the series is greater than 2
    Therefore, if
        [1.3] the number of cultures which were positive for ORGANISM-1
            is greater than 2
    Then there is suggestive evidence (.5) that there is significant disease
            associated with this occurrence of the e.coli (ORGANISM-1).
        [RULE049]
        ** WHY   {*repeated WHY to determine relevance of previous explanation*}

[i.e. WHY is it important to determine if there is significant disease
associated with this occurrence of the organism?]

[2.0] This will help to determine a diagnosis for which the infection should
be treated.
    It has already been established that
        [2.1] the infection is not one of: primary-bacteremia, meningitis
        [2.2] for some current culture of the patient it is true that the site
                of the culture is blood
    Therefore, if
        [2.3] there is significant disease associated with this occurrence of
                the organism
    Then
        it is definite (1.0) that the diagnosis for which the infection should
        be treated is secondary-bacteremia
        [RULE103]

FIGURE 15.3 Two examples of MYCIN's explanation capabilities. User input is shown in boldface capital letters and follows the double asterisks. The system expands each "WHY" question (enclosed in square brackets) to ensure that the user is aware of its interpretation of the query. (*Source:* Courtesy of Section on Medical Informatics, Stanford University.)

Despite these early research successes, software tools in the 1970s were rarely used by health personnel and were viewed with some skepticism. The subsequent evolution in attitudes has been due in large part to three influences: (1) the emergence of microcomputers and easy-to-use software, with the concomitant demystification of computers and a general sense in society that such machines are manageable and useful; (2) the growing distress among health professionals regarding the amount of information they need in order to practice medicine well; and (3) the increasing fiscal pressure to practice cost-effective medicine, which leads practitioners to consider carefully the clinical utility and reliability of tests, procedures, and therapies—especially when the latter are expensive or risky.

Current enhanced opportunities for progress in the field of clinical decision support derive from several sources, including the rapid growth of awareness of and interest in computers and information-management systems, the growing usefulness of medical information systems for helping professionals to solve other biomedical-research and health-care problems, and the continuing rapid development of the technological base (the computers themselves, and the methods for interacting with them). The growing recognition of medical informatics as a distinct biomedical discipline is further evidence of the evolving attitudes toward computing by health-care professionals [Association of American Medical Colleges, 1986].

Gradual changes in attitudes, and increasing acceptance of the *notion* of computer-based decision tools for health-care professionals, are not, of course, in themselves adequate to ensure developmental progress and the adoption of new information-management facilities. Current enthusiasm will sour rapidly if the products of research are not responsive to real-world needs and sensitive to the logistical requirements of the practice settings in which clinicians work.

15.3 A Structure for Characterizing Clinical Decision-Support Systems

If we are to assess adequately any new clinical decision-support tool, or to under-stand the range of issues that can affect the chances for successful implementation, we must have an organizational structure for considering such programs. One approach is to characterize decision-support systems along five dimensions: (1) the system's intended function, (2) the mode by which advice is offered, (3) the consultation style, (4) the underlying decision-science methodology, and (5) the factors related to human–computer interaction. As this spectrum of considerations suggests, excellent decision-making capabilities do not guarantee system utility or acceptance.

15.3.1 System Function

Decision-support programs generally fall into two categories: those that assist physicians with determining *what is true* about a patient (usually the correct diagnosis, as in de Dombal's system), and those that assist with decisions about *what to do* for the patient (what test to order, whether to treat, or what therapy plan to institute—as in MYCIN). Many systems assist clinicians with both activities (for example, diagnostic programs often help physicians to decide what additional information would be most useful in narrowing the differential diagnosis for a given case), but the distinction is important because advice about what to do for a patient cannot be formulated without balancing of the costs and benefits of actions. Determination of what is true about a patient, based on a fixed set of data that is already available, can theoretically be made without consideration of cost and risk. Thus, a "pure" diagnostic program leaves to the user the task of deciding what data to gather, or requires a fixed set of data for all patients. As all practitioners know, however, it is unrealistic to view diagnosis as separable from the process of choosing from the available options for data collection and therapy. Moreover, many physicians believe that the majority of questions about which they seek consultation deal with what they should *do* rather than with what is true about a patient given a fixed data set.

15.3.2 The Mode for Giving Advice

Like the abdominal-pain program and MYCIN, most decision-support programs have assumed a passive role in giving advice to clinicians [Reggia and Tuhrim, 1985]. Under this model, the physician must recognize when advice would be useful, and then must make an explicit effort to access the computer program; the decision-support system waits for the user to come to it. The physician then describes a case by entering data, and requests a diagnostic or therapeutic assessment.

There are also systems that play a more active role, providing decision support as a byproduct of monitoring or of data-management activities; such systems do not wait for physicians or other health workers specifically to ask for assistance. Examples of such programs include the hospital information system HELP [Warner, 1979; Pryor et al., 1983b] and the medical record system RMRS [McDonald et al., 1984]. As we shall describe in Section 15.5.3, HELP can generate advisory reports based on combinations of patient-specific data contained in its database. Thus, as data regarding a patient's laboratory-test results, drug therapy, and radiologic studies are gathered and are stored in the computer, HELP uses prespecified combinations of conditions to generate patient-specific advice or warnings. RMRS monitors outpatient medical records stored online, and sends clinically indicated reminders to physicians—for example, when a patient is due for an immunization or needs to have a previously abnormal laboratory-test value rechecked. A great appeal of such systems is their ability to give assistance to clinicians without requiring laborious data entry by the physicians themselves. Such capabilities are possible only because the system's decision logic is integrated with a comprehensive database of patient information that is already being gathered from diverse sources within the health-care institution. Because physicians generally do not request assistance from such systems, but instead receive it whenever monitored patient data warrant it, one challenge is to avoid generating excessive numbers of warnings for minor problems already likely to be understood. Otherwise, such "false-positive" advisory reports can generate antagonistic responses from users and can blunt the usefulness of those warnings that have greater clinical significance.

15.3.3 Consultation Style

Passive decision-support systems have tended to operate under one of two styles of interaction: the *consulting model* or the *critiquing model*. In the **consulting model,** the program serves as an advisor, accepting patient-specific data, asking questions, and generating advice for the user about diagnosis or management. For example, MYCIN and the general medical diagnostic programs DXplain [Barnett et al., 1987] and Internist-1/QMR [Miller et al., 1986] use the consulting approach.

In the **critiquing model,** on the other hand, the physician comes to the computer with a preconceived notion of what is happening with a patient or what management plan would be appropriate. The computer program then acts as a sounding board for the user's own ideas, expressing agreement or suggesting reasoned alternatives. Because the critiquing model requires a much more complex dialog, such systems are difficult to build. One example is ATTENDING, a program that critiques a patient-specific plan for anesthetic selection, induction, and administration after that plan has been proposed by the anesthesiologist who will be managing the case [Miller, 1986]. Such critiquing systems meet many physicians' desires to formulate plans on their own but to have those plans double-checked occasionally before acting on them.

The critiquing model also can be applied in an active monitoring setting. For example, the HELP system monitors physicians' drug-therapy decisions, and can suggest alternate approaches that may be preferable [Evans et al., 1986]. Another example is an experimental adaptation of ONCOCIN, a system for clinical oncology data management in which physicians record their observations and therapeutic plans using a graphical flowsheet displayed on a computer's screen [Hickam et al., 1985a; Shortliffe, 1986]. As we describe in Section 15.5.2, ONCOCIN was developed to follow the consulting model, and to advise physicians regarding the proper chemotherapy plan for patients being treated on a research protocol. The system was later adapted in one experiment such that, if it noted potential problems with a user's own therapy plan, it would initiate a critiquing dialog regarding alternatives [Langlotz and Shortliffe, 1983]. When the physician's plan was in agreement with the computer's assessment of the situation, however, this version of the program would simply continue its monitoring function and would not interrupt the user, who was filling out the interactive graphical flowsheet.

15.3.4 Underlying Decision-Science Methodology

A wide variety of techniques has been used in the design and implementation of decision-support systems. The simplest logics have been problem-specific algorithms designed by clinicians and then encoded for use by a computer. Although such algorithms have been useful for triage purposes and as a didactic technique used in journals and books where an overview of a problem's management has been appropriate, they have been largely rejected by physicians as too simplistic for routine use [Grimm et al., 1975]. In addition, the advantage of their implementation on computers has not been clear; the use of simple printed copies of the algorithms generally has proved adequate [Komaroff et al., 1974]. A noteworthy exception is a large computer program first described in the early 1970s and in continued use at the Beth Israel Hospital in Boston [Bleich, 1972]; it uses a detailed algorithmic logic to provide advice regarding the diagnosis and management of acid–base and electrolyte disorders.

Although additional techniques such as mathematical modeling, pattern recognition, and the analysis of large databases have been used in experimental decision-support systems [Shortliffe et al., 1979], the predominant methods have been drawn from Bayesian statistics, decision analysis, and AI. Because computers were traditionally viewed as numerical calculating machines, people had recognized by the 1960s that they could be used to compute the pertinent probabilities based on observations of patient-specific parameters (as long as each had a known statistical relationship to the possible disease etiologies). Large numbers of **Bayesian diagnosis programs** have been developed in the intervening years, many of which have been shown to be accurate in selecting among competing explanations of a patient's disease state [Reggia and Tuhrim, 1985]. As we mentioned earlier, among the largest experiments have been those of de Dombal and associates in England [de Dombal et al., 1972]; their Bayesian system for the diagnosis of acute abdominal pain runs on microcomputers and has been used extensively in British emergency departments.

Because most decisions in medicine require weighing the costs and benefits of actions that could be taken in diagnosing or managing a patient's illness, researchers also have developed tools that draw on the methods of decision analysis [Weinstein and Fineberg, 1980]. **Decision analysis** adds to Bayesian statistics the notion of decision trees and of *utilities* associated with the outcomes that could occur in response to interventions (see Chapter 3). One class of programs is designed for use by the analysts themselves; such programs assume a detailed knowledge of decision analysis and would be of little use to the average physician [Pauker and Kassirer, 1981]. A second class of programs uses decision-analysis concepts within systems designed to advise physicians who are not trained in these techniques. In such programs, the underlying decision models generally have been prespecified. Thus, the program's usefulness is limited to those cases that correspond closely to the decision tree provided [Gorry et al., 1973].

Since the early 1970s, a growing body of researchers has been applying AI techniques to the development of diagnostic and therapy-management consultation programs [Szolovits, 1982; Clancey and Shortliffe, 1984; Miller, 1988]. We have already discussed the MYCIN system, an important early example of work in this area. AI is closely tied to psychology and to the modeling of logical processes by computer. Psychological studies of how medical experts perform problem solving [Elstein et al., 1978; Kuipers and Kassirer, 1984] therefore have been influential in medical AI research. Of particular pertinence is the subfield of AI research that is concerned with expert systems [Duda and Shortliffe, 1983]. An expert system is a program that symbolically encodes concepts derived from experts in a field and uses that knowledge to provide the kind of problem analysis and advice that the expert might provide. Because clinical decision making inherently requires reasoning under uncertainty, medical expert systems have necessarily incorporated formal or ad hoc numerical schemes for dealing with partial evidence and with uncertainty regarding the effects of proposed interventions. These complement the **heuristic** techniques characteristic of AI systems.

15.3.5 Human–Computer Interface

There is perhaps no omission that accounts more fully for the impracticality of early clinical decision tools than the failure to deal adequately with the logistical, mechanical, and psychological aspects of system use. Often, developers have concentrated primarily on creating systems that can reach good decisions. Yet researchers have shown repeatedly that an ability to make correct diagnoses, or to suggest therapy similar to that recommended by human consultants, is only one part of the formula for system success [Shortliffe, 1982].

Logistical Considerations

Many potential users of clinical decision-support tools have found their early enthusiasm dampened by programs that are cumbersome to access, slow to perform, and difficult to learn to use. Systems can fail, for example, if they require that a physician interrupt the normal pattern of patient care to walk down the hall to a terminal and to follow complex or time-consuming startup procedures. Lengthy interactions, or ones that fail to convey the logic of what is happening on the screen, also discourage use of the program. With patient information increasingly available on clinical data-management systems, health professionals are likely to be particularly frustrated if the decision tool requires the manual reentry of information available on other nearby computers.

Solutions to such problems require sensitivity during the design process and, frequently, resolution of inadequacies at the institutional level. For example, linking computers to one another so that they can share data requires implementation of an overall networking strategy for the hospital or clinic (see, for example, the scenario with which we began Chapter 1). In many hospitals, however, departmental systems have grown up independently, and connecting them to coordinate functions can be complex and expensive. Many observers believe that decision-support programs are most likely to be accepted when such tools are integrated with routine data-management functions within an office or institution. If the physician is using the computer routinely to store and review data, and if that same machine can provide advice that is transparently integrated with its data-management function, a major barrier to the use of decision tools will have been overcome [Shortliffe, 1986].

Mechanical Considerations

The mode of interaction with the computer is an important determinant of any program's success. Computer programs have traditionally presumed keyboard typing for entering data or asking questions—a requirement that has accounted for much of the resistance to computer use among physicians. Many experimental decision-support tools require keyboard-based interactions to this day. Yet increasing numbers of programs are using successful alternate interactive techniques that allow the user to avoid typing and are intuitive to learn. Examples include light pens, mouse pointing devices, and touch-screens. We are also beginning to see early tools for speech understanding; these suggest that physicians may soon be able to talk to computers through a microphone when performing well-specified tasks, thereby avoiding manual interaction altogether.

Psychological Considerations

The mechanics of interaction described in the previous section are only a small part of the total relationship that develops between a computer and its user [Shneiderman, 1986]. The content and appearance of what is shown on the screen are also crucial determinants of a system's success. Many of the issues are psychological and require ongoing research. For example, the development of inexpensive graphical display screens, which permit interactions based on pictures as well as on text, has already revolutionized the way in which developers think about gathering and display-ing information [Shortliffe, 1986]. A related issue of particular importance to decision-support systems is the need for such programs to explain the basis for their advice. Regardless of whether the system uses text justifications or adds clarifying drawings on the screen, an explanation capability is mandatory to encourage physician accep-tance [Teach and Shortliffe, 1981]. The requirement that explanations be provided reflects a simple need to display tact when offering advice, and also acknowledges that the users are ultimately making the decision and are using the computer pro-gram as an adjunct, as they would use a textbook, journal, or other informational aid. Decision-support tools should provide enough information to allow physicians to determine whether their assessments are likely to be valid for specific patients.

15.4 Scientific Issues in the Construction of Decision-Support Tools[3]

Despite significant research progress since the idea of computer-based medical decision-support systems first emerged, several barriers remain that continue to limit the effective implementation of such tools in clinical settings. As we implied earlier, these obstacles include unresolved questions of both science and logistics. Rapid technological progress in recent years, especially in the development of powerful but inexpensive single-user computers that provide intuitively pleasing interactive en-vironments, suggests that effective and accepted decision-support tools will soon be widely available for application to well-defined clinical problems.

15.4.1 How to Acquire and Validate Patient Data

As we emphasized in Chapter 2, few problems are more challenging than is the development of effective techniques for capturing patient data accurately, completely, and efficiently. You have read in this book about a wide variety of techniques for data entry, ranging from keyboard typing, point-and-select techniques (light pens, mice, and fingertips), and speech input, to methods that separate the clinician from the computer (such as mark-sense forms, real-time data monitoring, and intermediaries who transcribe written data for use by computers). All these methods have limita-tions, and health-care workers frequently state that their use of computers will be limited unless they are freed of the task of data entry and can concentrate instead on data review and information retrieval [Shortliffe, 1989]. Even if computers could accept unrestricted speech input, there would be serious challenges associated with properly structuring and encoding what was said, so that ambiguity could be avoided. Otherwise, spoken input becomes a large free-text database that defies semantic

---

[3]Portions of this section are based on Shortliffe, E. H. Computers in support of clinical decision making. In Kelley, W. N. (ed), *Textbook of Internal Medicine*. Philadelphia: J. B. Lippincott, 1988, p. 37.

interpretation. Many workers believe that some combination of speech and graphics, coupled with integrated data-management environments that will prevent the need for redundant entry of information into multiple computer systems within a hospital or clinic, are the key advances that will attract busy clinicians and other health workers to use computer-based tools.

15.4.2 How to Represent Medical Knowledge

Among the ongoing research challenges is the need to refine further the computational techniques for encoding the wide range of knowledge used in problem solving by medical experts. Although techniques such as *frames* or *rules* now exist for storing factual or inferential knowledge, several complex challenges remain. For example, physicians use mental models of the three-dimensional relationships among body parts and organs when they are interpreting data or planning therapy. Representing such anatomical knowledge and performing spatial reasoning by computer have proved to be particularly challenging. Similarly, human beings have a remarkable ability to interpret changes in data over time, assessing temporal trends and developing models of disease progression or the response of disease to past therapies. Researchers continue to develop computer-based methods for modeling such tasks.

Another kind of expertise, often poorly recognized, but clearly important to optimal knowledge management by computer-based tools, is the human skill inherent in knowing how to use what is known. In medicine, we often call this skill "good clinical judgment," and we properly distinguish it from the memorization of factual knowledge or data from the literature. It is similarly clear that simply giving computers extensive factual knowledge will not make them skilled in a field unless they also are expert in the proper application of that knowledge. It is in this area particularly that improved understanding of the psychology of human problem solving is helping researchers to develop decision-support tools that more closely simulate the process by which expert clinicians move from observations to diagnoses or management plans.

15.4.3 How to Acquire Medical Knowledge

People who have attempted to encode the knowledge for a medical decision-support system by simply reading a textbook or journal articles can attest to the complexity of translating from the usual text approach for communicating knowledge to a structure appropriate for the logical application of that knowledge by a computer. The problem is not unlike that of identifying what you as a reader need to do to interpret, internalize, and apply properly the wealth of information in a book such as this. Researchers are devising methods that will facilitate the development and maintenance of medical knowledge bases, especially in light of the rapid pace at which medical knowledge has evolved in recent decades. Many workers have formalized the techniques by which experts should be interviewed, hoping to determine, in a structured fashion, the way in which skilled practitioners are solving problems and precisely what knowledge they are bringing to bear. More recently, investigators have developed computer programs that acquire the knowledge base for a decision-support program by interacting directly with the expert, thereby avoiding the need for a computer programmer as intermediary [Musen et al., 1987].

15.4.4 How to Provide Transparency of Function

A frequent concern expressed by health-care workers is the fear that decision-support tools will become the standard of care, usurping the very independence and flexibility that attracted these professionals to medical careers in the first place. As early as 1973, researchers began to emphasize the importance of explanation capabilities as a means of clarifying the computer's role as an advisor, rather than as a replacement for clinicians' own decision-making skills [Gorry, 1973]. Subsequently, formal studies showed that physicians did indeed place a high value on decision-support tools that could explain the basis for their advice, thereby allowing the user to assess the appropriateness of the recommendations [Teach and Shortliffe, 1981]. This need to provide explanations has accounted in large part for the appeal of AI methods, since they explicitly suggest ways of representing and communicating the symbolic and conceptual aspects of a complex domain such as medicine. In recent years, workers have examined methods that allow a merging of statistical and symbolic methods so that the rigor of Bayesian uncertainty management can be combined with the transparency of AI representation techniques. Much research remains to be done in this promising area.

15.4.5 How to Validate Both Knowledge and System Performance

Many observers are horrified when they imagine what they might have to do to validate and maintain the currency of large clinical knowledge bases. After all, medical knowledge is advancing at a rapid pace, and an advisory system that uses yesterday's knowledge may fail to provide the best advice available for a patient's problem. Although researchers with limited goals have been willing to take on responsibility for short-term knowledge-base maintenance in support of their scholarly activities, it is likely that professional organizations or other national bodies will in time need to assume responsibility for the currency and integrity of large clinical knowledge bases.

When a knowledge base is well validated, developers still face challenges in determining how best to evaluate the performance of the decision-support tools that use the knowledge. When a gold standard of performance exists, formal studies can compare the program's advice with that accepted standard of "correctness." This technique is especially pertinent for diagnostic tools, where biopsy, surgery, or autopsy data can be used as an appropriate gold standard. In the case of therapy-advice systems, however, the gold standard is more difficult to define. Even experts may disagree about the proper way to treat a specific patient, and there can seldom be a realistic controlled trial that attempts to show which approach is right in any absolute sense. For this reason, workers have experimented with techniques that compare the recommendations of a therapy-management program with those of experts [Yu et al., 1979b; Hickam et al., 1985a]. With proper controls, such studies can be useful, although they have shown that even experts in a field generally do not receive perfect marks when assessed by their peers. The problem of evaluation remains a ripe area for further research.

15.4.6 How to Integrate Decision-Support Tools

As we have emphasized in discussing many of the computer applications described in this book, the successful introduction of decision-support tools is likely to be tied to these tools' effective integration with routine data-management tasks. We need more innovative research on how best to tie knowledge-based computer tools to programs designed to store, manipulate, and retrieve patient-specific information. We explained how the HELP system includes decision-support functions that are triggered to generate warnings or reports whenever an internally specified set of conditions holds for a given patient. As hospitals and clinics increasingly use multiple small machines optimized for different tasks (see the example scenario in Chapter 1), however, the challenges of integration are inherently tied to issues of networking. It is in the electronic linking of multiple machines with overlapping functions and data needs that the potential of distributed but integrated patient data processing will be realized.

15.4.7 How to Encourage Use of Decision-Support Tools

Finally, there remain serious challenges related to implementing even the best of systems in clinical environments such that they will be welcomed and used routinely by clinicians. For example, one analysis suggested eight reasons why physicians resist the idea of decision-support systems: (1) fear of loss of rapport, (2) fear of loss of control, (3) inertia, (4) nonacceptance of machine capabilities, (5) suspicion of AI, (6) fear of legal liability, (7) distaste for data entry, and (8) belief that they are too old to learn computer technology [Shortliffe, 1989]. On the other hand, clinicians generally welcome simple information-retrieval programs that satisfy their thirst for information, and they recognize the need for effective chart control. These important factors warrant attention in system design. They also suggest the importance of improved education of health professionals regarding the computer's potential role.

15.5 Illustrative Examples of Clinical Decision-Support Systems

To illustrate the status of current systems and the ways in which new hardware technologies have affected the evolution of decision-support tools, we shall discuss selected features of three well-known decision-support systems. Internist-1/QMR supports diagnostic problem solving in general internal medicine, ONCOCIN provides therapeutic recommendations for cancer treatment, and HELP integrates decision-support functions with a generalized environment for information and data management.

15.5.1 Diagnosis: The Internist-1/QMR Project

Internist-1 is a large diagnostic program that has been under development at the University of Pittsburgh School of Medicine since the early 1970s [Miller et al., 1982]. It contains knowledge of almost 600 diseases and of nearly 4500 interrelated *findings* and *disease manifestations* (signs, symptoms, and other patient characteristics). On average, each disease is associated with between 75 and 100 findings. The task of diagnosis would be straightforward if each disease were associated with a unique set of findings. Most findings, however, are associated with multiple disease processes, often with varying levels of likelihood. Clinicians have long recognized the infeasibility of performing simple pattern matching to make difficult diagnoses. On the other hand, it would be equally difficult to collect conditional probabilities (such as those used by de Dombal's diagnosis program) for all the diseases and findings in Internist-1's knowledge base—particularly because many of the 600 disease syndromes are rare. For these reasons, the developers of Internist-1 created an ad hoc scoring scheme to encode the relationships between specific findings and diseases.

To construct the knowledge base, the senior physician on the project (a clinician with over 50 years of practice experience), other physicians, and medical students have worked together, considering each of the encoded diseases. Through careful literature review and case discussions, they determine the list of pertinent findings associated with each disease. For each of these findings, they assign a *frequency weight* (FW) and an *evoking strength* (ES), two numbers that reflect the strength of the relationship between the disease and the findings (see Figure 15.4). The FW is a number between 1 and 5, where 1 means that the finding is seldom seen in the disease, and 5 means that it is essentially always seen (see Table 15.1). The ES reflects the likelihood that a patient with the finding has the disease in question, and that the disease is the cause of the finding (see Table 15.2). An ES of 0 means that the disease would never be considered as a diagnosis on the basis of this finding alone, whereas an ES of 5 means that the finding is pathognomonic for the disease (that is, *all* patients with the finding have the disease).[4]

In addition, each finding in the knowledge base is associated with a third number, an *import* number that has a value between 1 and 5 (see Table 15.3). The import number captures the notion that some abnormalities have serious implications and must be explained, whereas others may be safely ignored. Internist-1 uses the import number to handle *red herrings* (minor problems that are not explained by the current disease process). This familiar clinical-diagnosis problem is not handled well by formal statistical approaches.

Based on these simple measurements, Internist-1 then uses a scoring scheme that is similar to the hypothetico-deductive approach we described in Chapter 2. The physician enters an initial set of findings; then the program determines an initial differential

---

[4]The knowledge base also encodes relationships between pairs of diseases, and these relationships are similarly described using FWs and ESs. Thus, if disease A always leads to disease B, then the FW of A given B is set to 5. The ES depends on whether disease B could develop other than through disease A. If everyone with disease B must have had disease A first, then the ES of the relationship also is 5.

TABLE 15.1 Interpretation of Frequency Weights

Frequency Weight	Interpretation
1	Listed manifestation occurs rarely in the disease
2	Listed manifestation occurs in a substantial minority of cases of the disease
3	Listed manifestation occurs in roughly one-half of the cases
4	Listed manifestation occurs in the substantial majority of cases
5	Listed manifestation occurs in essentially all cases—that is, it is a prerequisite for the diagnosis

Source: Reprinted with permission from Miller, R. A., Pople, Jr., H. E., and Myers, J. D. INTERNIST-1: An experimental computer-based diagnostic consultant for general internal medicine. *New England Journal of Medicine,* 307:468, 1982.

Disease profile for

ECHINOCOCCAL CYST <S> OF LIVER

ES	FW	
1	2	CHEST PERCUSSION DIAPHRAGM ELEVATED UNILATERAL
1	2	COUGH
1	1	FECES LIGHT COLORED
0	2	FEVER
1	3	HEPATOMEGALY PRESENT
1	2	JAUNDICE
1	2	LIVER CONTAINING LARGE PALPABLE MASS <ES>
1	1	LIVER CONTAINING LARGE PALPABLE MASS <ES> FLUCTUANT
1	1	LIVER DISTORTED OR ASYMMETRICAL
1	1	LIVER ENLARGED MASSIVE
1	2	LIVER ENLARGED MODERATE
1	2	LIVER ENLARGED SLIGHT
1	2	LIVER TENDER ON PALPATION
1	1	PRESSURE ARTERIAL DIASTOLIC LESS THAN 60
1	1	PRESSURE ARTERIAL SYSTOLIC LESS THAN 90
1	1	RHONCHI DIFFUSE

FIGURE 15.4 A sample disease profile from Internist-1/QMR. The numbers next to the findings represent the evoking strength (ranging from 0 [nonspecific] to 5 pathognomonic) and the frequency weight (ranging from 1 [rare] to 5 [always seen]). Only an excerpt from the disease profile for echinococcal cysts is shown here. (*Source:* Reprinted with permission from Miller, R. A., Masarie, F. E., and Myers, J. D. Quick Medical Reference (QMR) for diagnostic assistance. *M.D. Computing,* 3(5):34, 1986.)

TABLE 15.2 Interpretation of Evoking Strengths

Evoking Strength	Interpretation
0	Nonspecific—manifestation occurs too commonly to be used to construct a differential diagnosis
1	Diagnosis is a rare or unusual cause of listed manifestation
2	Diagnosis causes a substantial minority of instances of listed manifestation
3	Diagnosis is the most common, but not the overwhelming, cause of listed manifestation
4	Diagnosis is the overwhelming cause of listed manifestation
5	Listed manifestation is pathognomonic for the diagnosis

Source: Reprinted with permission from Miller, R. A., Pople, Jr., H. E., and Myers, J. D. INTERNIST-1: An experimental computer-based diagnostic consultant for general internal medicine. *New England Journal of Medicine,* 307:468, 1982.

TABLE 15.3 Interpretation of Import Values

Import	Interpretation
1	Manifestation is usually unimportant, occurs commonly in normal persons, and is easily disregarded
2	Manifestation may be of importance, but can often be ignored; context is important
3	Manifestation is of moderate importance, but may be an unreliable indicator of any specific disease
4	Manifestation is of high importance and can only rarely be disregarded (as, for example, a false-positive result)
5	Manifestation absolutely must be explained by one of the final diagnoses

Source: Reprinted with permission from Miller, R. A., Pople, Jr., H. E., and Myers, J. D. INTERNIST-1: An experimental computer-based diagnostic consultant for general internal medicine. *New England Journal of Medicine,* 307:468, 1982.

diagnosis. Based on the current set of hypotheses, the program selects appropriate questions to ask, choosing from several strategies, depending on how many diseases are under consideration and how closely matched they are to the available patient data. The program considers the cost and risks of tests, as well as the benefits, and asks for simple historical and physical-examination data before recommending laboratory tests or invasive diagnostic procedures. An important feature, not previously implemented in diagnostic programs, is Internist-1's ability to set aside some of the findings not well explained by the current differential diagnosis and to return to them later after making an initial diagnosis. Thus, Internist-1 can diagnose multiple co-existent diseases, and does not make the assumptions of mutual exclusivity and completeness that have characterized most Bayesian diagnostic programs.

Using these simple knowledge structures and weighting schemes, Internist-1 has demonstrated impressive diagnostic performance. In one study, the developers tested the program on 19 difficult diagnostic cases taken from a major clinical journal [Miller et al., 1982]. The 19 patients had a total of 43 diagnoses, of which Internist-1 correctly identified 25. By comparison, the physicians who had cared for the patients in a major teaching hospital made 28 correct diagnoses, and the expert discussants who presented the cases before a large audience prior to the publication of each case in the journal correctly identified 35 diagnoses. Although Internist-1 missed several of the difficult cases (as did the physicians and discussants), the test patients had problems that were drawn broadly from across all problems in general internal medicine—no other diagnostic program would have been able to deal effectively with more than a small subset of these cases.

Internist-1 runs on only large, mainframe computers and therefore is not suited for widespread use by practitioners. In the 1980s, the program was adapted to run on microcomputers as QMR (Quick Medical Reference) [Miller et al., 1986]. Unlike Internist-1, which was developed to provide only patient-specific diagnostic advice, QMR can serve health professionals in three modes. In its basic mode, QMR is an expert consultation system that provides advice much as Internist-1 did (using essentially the same knowledge base and scoring scheme). QMR can also be used as an electronic textbook, listing the patient characteristics reported to occur in a given disease or, conversely, reporting which of its 600 diseases can be associated with a given characteristic. Third, as a medical spreadsheet, it can combine a few characteristics or diseases and determine the implications. For example, the user can specify two apparently unrelated medical problems and obtain suggestions about how coexisting diseases could, under the right circumstances, give rise to both problems (Figure 15.5).

15.5.2 Patient Management: The ONCOCIN System[5]

ONCOCIN is an experimental system developed in the early 1980s at Stanford University using the SUMEX-AIM resource. The system was designed to assist oncologists (cancer specialists) with the management of chemotherapy (drug therapy) for patients who have cancer and are participating in formal protocol-based clinical trials. It was developed to meet the need for a comprehensive computer system that could provide protocol guidance while enhancing the management of clinical trial data in both university and community settings.

ONCOCIN runs on powerful, relatively small, dedicated computers. Its developers believed that advisory tools would appeal to physicians only if the programs were in routine use at the times when decisions had to be made. Therefore, the program was designed to replace the traditional paper flowsheet filled out by oncologists as they track a patient's progress over a course of chemotherapy. After a physician has seen a patient, he uses an ONCOCIN workstation that presents the familiar flowsheet

[5]Portions of this section are based on Shortliffe, E. H. and Hubbard, S. M. Information systems for oncology. In DeVita, V. T., Hellman, S., and Rosenberg, S. A. (eds), *Cancer: Principles and Practice of Oncology*. Philadelphia: J. B. Lippincott, 1989, pages 2403–2412.

Associations List

Pulmonary Disease and DIARRHEA Chronic

Pairs of diseases consistent with Entered Finding and Topic

Atelectasis
caused-by Carcinoid Syndrome Secondary to Bronchial Neoplasm

Eosinophilic Pneumonia Acute <LOEFFLER>
caused-by Hookworm Disease

Pulmonary Legionellosis
predisposed-to-by Immune Deficiency Syndrome Acquired <AIDS>

Pleural Effusion Exudative
caused-by Pancreatic Pseudocyst

Pneumococcal Pneumonia
predisposed-to-by Immune Deficiency Syndrome Acquired <AIDS>

Pulmonary Hypertension Secondary
caused-by Progressive Systemic Sclerosis
or co-occurring-with Schistosomiasis Chronic Hepatic

Pulmonary Infarction
predisposed-to-by Carcinoma of Body or Tail of Pancreas
or predisposed-to-by Carcinoma of Head of Pancreas
or caused-by Hepatic Vein Obstruction

Pulmonary Lymphoma
coinciding-with Lymphoma of Colon
or coinciding-with Small Intestinal Lymphoma

FIGURE 15.5 A sample associations list from QMR. QMR permits the physician to request exploratory searches of the knowledge base for associations that might be clinically relevant. For example, as shown here, the physician has asked for pulmonary diseases that may also be associated with chronic diarrhea. The resulting lists, which QMR generates dynamically, can be useful "memory joggers" for physicians who might otherwise overlook the suggested relationships. (*Source:* Reprinted with permission from Rennels, G. D. and Shortliffe, E. H. Advanced computing for medicine. *Scientific American,* October 1987, p. 159.)

on a graphics display monitor (Figure 15.6). The patient's flowsheet is displayed so that the physician can review old data and enter new ones. He can enter all the data using a mouse pointing device, so he does not need to type. To enter a data element, he selects the appropriate box on the flowsheet. A register (a mouse-selectable numeric keypad) appears on the screen; then the physician uses the mouse to indicate the proper value. When he selects the word "done," the register disappears and the entered

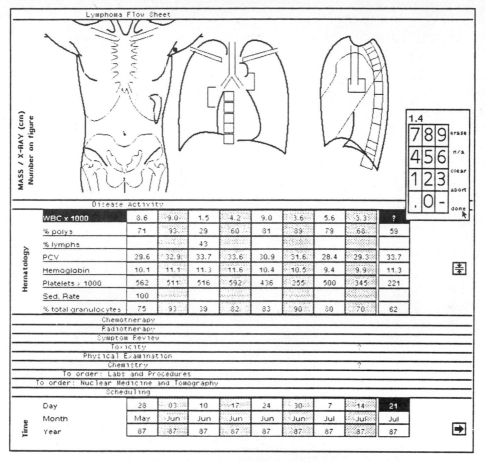

FIGURE 15.6 The ONCOCIN flowsheet uses menus and registers to facilitate data entry. The physician enters data (in this case, a white-blood-cell count) by using a mouse to select a box on the flowsheet. A register appears on the screen; the physician then uses the mouse to indicate the proper value (in this case, 1.4 thousand per cubic milliliter). When he selects the word "done," the register disappears and the entered value appears in the appropriate box on the flowsheet. The physician can use the graphical portion of the flowsheet to indicate, by drawing, the areas of disease involvement (in this case, a left axillary lymph node and the spleen). (*Source:* Courtesy of Section on Medical Informatics, Stanford University.)

value appears in the appropriate box on the flowsheet. The physician can use a graphical portion of the flowsheet to indicate, by drawing, the areas of disease involvement. In Figure 15.6, the sections labeled MASS/X-RAY and HEMATOLOGY have been opened. The TIME section opens automatically to show the dates that correspond to the columns of data that are displayed in the opened sections.

Although these features of ONCOCIN could be used for the routine management of oncology outpatient data, regardless of whether patients were participating in clinical trials, a principal goal of the system is to assist physicians with determining complex

Lymphoma Flow Sheet									
Mass / X-ray									
Disease Activity									

Hematology

WBC x 1000	8.6	9.0	1.5	4.2	9.0	3.6	5.6	3.3	1.4
% polys	71	93	29	60	81	69	79	68	59
% lymphs			43						
PCV	29.6	32.9	33.7	33.6	30.9	31.6	28.4	29.3	33.7
Hemoglobin	10.1	11.1	11.3	11.6	10.4	10.5	9.4	9.9	11.3
Platelets x 1000	562	511	516	592	436	255	500	345	221
Sed. Rate	100								
% total granulocytes	75	93	39	82	83	90	80	70	62
BSA (m2)	1.71	1.68							
Arm assignment									
Combination Name	MACOP-B	MACOP-B	MACOP-B	MACOP-B	MACOP-B	MACOP-B	MACOP-B	MACOP-B	MACOP-B
Cycle #	1	1	1	1	1	1	1	1	1
Subcycle	week 1	week 2	week 3	week 4	week 5	week 6	week 7	week 8	week 9
Visit type	TREAT	TREAT	TREAT	TREAT	TREAT	TREAT	TREAT	TREAT	TREAT

CHEMOTHERAPY (includes non-cytoxic drugs)

Methotrexate 400 MG/M2				700				700	
Doxorubicin 50 MG/M2	85		55		85		85		55
Cytoxan 350 MG/M2	600		390		600		600		390
Vincristine 1.4 MG/M2		2.0		2.0		2.0		2.0	
Prednisone 75 MG	75	50	50	75	75	75	75	75	75
Bleomycin 10 U/M2		17				17			
Folinic Acid 15 MG				15				15	
Septra DS 2 TABLETS	2	2	2	2	2	2	2	2	2
Ketoconazole 200 MG	200	200	200	200	200	200	200	200	200
Hydrocortisone 100 MG						100			
Sodium Bicarbonate 3000 MG				3000				3000	
Cum. Bleomycin (mg/m2)						20			
Cum. Doxorubicin (mg/m2)	50		82		132		181		213

Radiotherapy									
Symptom Review									
Toxicity									
Physical Examination									
Chemistry									
To order: Labs and Procedures									
To order: Nuclear Medicine and Tomography									
Scheduling									

Time

Day	28	03	10	17	24	30	7	14	21
Month	May	Jun	Jun	Jun	Jun	Jun	Jul	Jul	Jul
Year	87	87	87	87	87	87	87	87	87

FIGURE 15.7 ONCOCIN displays its chemotherapy dosing recommendations in the right-most column of the CHEMOTHERAPY section of the flowsheet. The CHEMOTHERAPY section, unlike the sections used by the physician when he is entering data, is filled out by ONCOCIN based on patient-specific data, as well as on a knowledge base of information regarding the treatment protocol in which the patient is enrolled. (*Source:* Courtesy of Section on Medical Informatics, Stanford University.)

chemotherapy plans. As clinical data are entered on the graphical flowsheet, they are passed to a program that uses them, plus knowledge about the protocol or treatment program, to consider whether chemotherapy should be administered on this visit, and, if it should be, whether dosage adjustments are indicated. This decision-support program, known as the Reasoner, then displays its recommendations in the appropriate column on the flowsheet when the physician opens the section labeled CHEMOTHERAPY (Figure 15.7). Thus, ONCOCIN provides recommendations by assisting the physician with filling out the therapy-plan portion of the flowsheet. Because ONCOCIN uses current and past data to guide its assessment of the appropriate protocol-directed treatment for the current visit, it knows what information it needs to make an informed recommendation. Therefore, although the physician may enter data on the flowsheet in whatever order appears most natural, and does not need to fill in all items on the standard form, ONCOCIN indicates unobtrusively what information it requires by displaying question marks in areas of particular interest. In Figure 15.6, for example, question marks indicate that ONCOCIN needs to know the white-blood-cell (WBC) count and would like the physician to open and fill out the TOXICITY and CHEMISTRY sections.

In addition to knowing the rules for chemotherapy administration in specific clinical trials, ONCOCIN keeps track of the data required by the protocol and provides reminders to the physician when laboratory studies or radiologic examinations are indicated. Two sections of the graphical flowsheet deal with test ordering (see the two unopened sections labeled TO ORDER in Figure 15.7). Selected items are used to generate order forms, which are printed and used by the scheduling desk when the patient is arranging for subsequent appointments. When the clinic visit ends, ONCOCIN also produces a hardcopy flowsheet, similar to the traditional paper document, which is placed in the patient's chart for backup and review. The entire interaction between ONCOCIN and the physician generally requires less than 5 minutes.

It would be impractical if ONCOCIN had to be reprogrammed every time a new protocol were developed. The program's developers therefore devised a second system that can be used by clinical researchers to enter the details of new protocols and to refine existing protocols. This *knowledge-entry system,* known as OPAL, also takes advantage of the graphical capabilities of the computer workstation. After a cancer specialist has described a protocol using OPAL, special programs create a corresponding knowledge base that ONCOCIN can use when it helps physicians to manage specific patients enrolled in that protocol [Walton et al., 1987]. The expert using OPAL does not need to understand either computer programming or the internal organization of ONCOCIN's knowledge base. Instead, she describes the overall organization and temporal sequence of the steps in the protocol, using a flow diagram that is intuitive to understand and create (it is based on the diagrams that appear in many hardcopy protocol documents; Figure 15.8). OPAL interprets the pictures that she creates and translates that knowledge to a form that ONCOCIN can use. Protocol details that are not captured in these diagrams (information about drug doses, dose attenuation, timing of drug administration, and criteria for aborting cycles or deleting specific agents) are entered using a second part of OPAL, a logical sequence of fill-in-the-blank forms (Figure 15.9).

15.5.3 System Integration: The HELP System

You have already learned a great deal about the HELP System, the integrated hospital information system developed at LDS Hospital in Salt Lake City over the past 2 decades. In Chapter 6, you learned about its data query language and its ability to generate alerts when abnormalities in the patient record are noted. In Chapter 7, we again described HELP, comparing it to other hospital information systems and

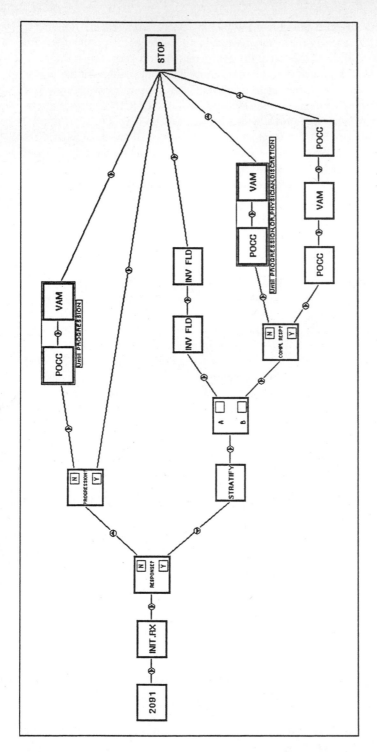

(a)

492

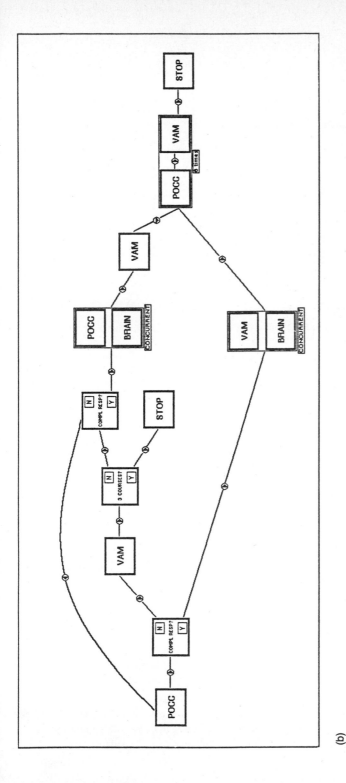

(b)

FIGURE 15.8 A clinical researcher can use OPAL to describe the overall schema of an ONCOCIN protocol using the graphical environment shown here. She creates the individual boxes using mouse selections, and then positions and joins them as desired. (a) The top-level schema for protocol 2091 (used in the treatment of small-cell lung carcinoma) indicates that all patients are first managed using a standard initial treatment (INIT.RX). Patients who respond to the initial treatment participate in an experiment to determine whether involved-field irradiation is an adequate alternative to further (perhaps indefinite) treatment with POCC and VAM chemotherapies in patients who have had a complete or partial response to the drugs (note the randomization between arms A and B). (b) The subschema corresponding to the box labeled INIT.RX in part (a). Patients first receive a cycle of POCC chemotherapy. Those having a complete response then receive VAM chemotherapy with concurrent brain irradiation, whereas those without a complete response to POCC receive up to three cycles of alternating POCC and VAM, stopping earlier if they demonstrate a complete response. [POCC = procarbazine, vincristine, cyclophosphamide, and CCNU; VAM = VP-16, adriamycin, and methotrexate.] (*Source:* Courtesy of Section on Medical Informatics, Stanford University.)

493

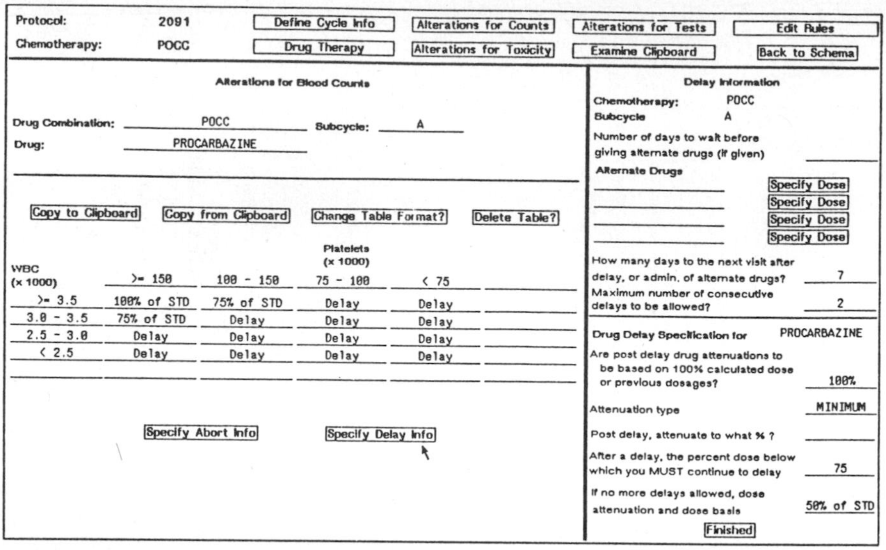

FIGURE 15.9 The expert has used the mouse and a series of OPAL's menus to indicate the appropriate response to combined reductions in white-blood-cell (WBC) and platelet counts when treating with procarbazine in POCC chemotherapy. For example, a platelet count less than 75,000 per cubic milliliter requires a delay in therapy even if the WBC count is normal. The subform at the right defines the proper management of such delays. The top of the form provides access to other forms used for protocol definition. (*Source:* Courtesy of Section on Medical Informatics, Stanford University.)

outlining its internal organization. Indeed, HELP could have been mentioned in almost any chapter in this book, because it has incorporated applications and methodologies that span nearly the full range of activities in medical informatics [Kuperman and Gardner, 1988].

Refer to Figure 7.5, and recall that HELP adds to a conventional medical-record system a monitoring program and a mechanism for storing decision logic in "HELP sectors" or logic frames. Thus, patient data are available to users who wish to request specific information, and the usual reports and schedules are automatically printed or otherwise communicated by the system. In addition, there is a mechanism for *event-driven* generation of specialized warnings, alerts, and reports. HELP's developers have created a specialized language named PAL for writing medical knowledge in HELP sectors. Figure 6.17 shows one such sector and its representation in the PAL language.

Whenever new data become available about a patient, regardless of the source, the system checks to see whether they match the criteria for invoking the logic of a HELP sector. If so, the system evaluates the entire sector to see whether it is relevant for the specific patient. The logic in these sectors has been developed by clinical experts working with medical information scientists. Decisions generated by successful sectors may be, for example, alerts regarding untoward drug actions, interpretations of laboratory tests, or calculations of the likelihood of diseases. The decisions are communicated to the appropriate people through the terminals of the hospital information system or on written reports, depending on the urgency of the decision and the location and functions of the person for whom the report is intended.

The creation and maintenance of HELP sectors is a major challenge, as is the construction of any large knowledge base. Thus, HELP developers have sought ways to represent and display sector knowledge more intuitively using a *HELP frame language*. The resulting knowledge frames encode information that may be useful not only to HELP, but also to other knowledge systems (Figure 15.10). For example,

```
Title: Pneumonia diagnosis (7.141.1)
Type: Diagnosis
Author: Peter Haug.
Date: 12/12/86
Message: "<disease_prob (val: #.##)>Pneumonia (history)".
Variables: chest_pain as (DO YOU HAVE CHEST_PAIN?),
        cough as (HAVE YOU HAD A COUGH WITH THIS ILLNESS?),
        fever_or_chills as MAX(fever, chills)
        where fever is (HAVE YOU RECENTLY HAD A FEVER?)
        and chills is (HAVE YOU HAD CHILLS RECENTLY?)
        if Exist (fever) or Exist (chills),
                                •
                                •
                                •
Statistics:    for fever_or_chills with TPR(YES, 0.85;  NO, 0.15),
               and FPR(YES, 0.3;  NO, 0.7),
               for cough with TPR(YES, 0.9;  NO, 0.1),
               and FPR(YES, 0.2;  NO, 0.8),
                                •
                                •
                                •
Evoking Criteria: If chest_pain EQ YES or fever EQ YES or chills EQ YES or cough EQ YES.
Logic:       disease_prob = 0.014.
        If Exist(fever_or_chills) then disease_prob=Bayes(disease_prob, fever_or_chills).
        If Exist(cough) then disease_prob = Bayes(disease_prob, cough).
                                •
                                •
                                •
        If disease_prob LT 0.014 then finish.
Ask:  Patients(fever, chills, cough) Hierarchical.
Urgency: 5/9
Gold Standard: If ICD_pneumonia and pneumonic_infiltrate
References: Harrison's Principals of Internal Medicine. Braunwald E., et al (editors)
Validation: Tested experimentally (DD method)
```

FIGURE 15.10 This diagnostic frame (sector) for pneumonia in the HELP system was written with the general-purpose HELP decision editor. The frame is processed if the criterion in the *Evoking Criteria* field is met. The *Ask* field indicates which information the frame may collect interactively. The *Urgency* field indicates the relative urgency of recognizing this disease. The *Gold Standard* field specifies criteria available by the time of discharge that would prove the existence of the disease being modeled. *References* refers to literature support for the frame, and *Validation* indicates the degree of evaluation to which the frame has been subjected. (*Source:* Reprinted with permission from Kuperman, G. J. and Gardner, R. M. *The HELP System: A Snapshot in Time.* Salt Lake City, UT: Department of Biophysics, LDS Hospital, 1988.)

HELP knowledge frames developed for event-driven logic on the main HIS computers have also been adapted at the University of Utah for use in a medical educational tool known as Iliad [Warner et al., 1988]. The Iliad frame representation has introduced the concept of *clusters* for dealing with conditionally dependent findings, which often describe important pathophysiologic concepts. Analysis of the Internist-1/ QMR knowledge base has shown that QMR's knowledge structures capture similar notions in their assigned values for evoking strengths [Lincoln et al., 1988].

HELP serves as a superb example of how the integration of decision support with other system functions can heighten a program's acceptance and encourage its use. Several studies (see, for example, [Evans et al., 1986]) have demonstrated the beneficial effect of HELP's decision logic on clinical measurements at LDS Hospital. Alerts and warnings are produced through the normal collection of patient data; transcription of data for reuse in secondary settings is avoided through the full integration of the computing environment. As we discussed in Chapter 7, HELP and other systems are evolving toward more distributed architectures, with microcomputers serving as workstations and data being shared over local-area networks. This large project at the University of Utah has served as an important model of how decision support through integrated data monitoring can bypass many of the traditional barriers to the use of computers for clinical decision support.

15.6 Decision Support in the Decade to Come

After 25 years of research on medical decision-support systems, investigators have learned a great deal about the difficulties inherent in the task, and about the complex barriers to successful implementation of programs. Systems in the first two categories mentioned at the beginning of this chapter (tools for information management and for attention focusing) are now widely available commercially. Systems in the third category (patient-specific consultation tools for use by physicians) are also beginning to appear, although they tend to deal with narrow medical problems and to integrate poorly with patient databases or other computer systems. Exceptions are active monitoring programs such as HELP [Warner, 1979; Pryor et al., 1983b] and RMRS [McDonald et al., 1984], which integrate decision support with medical-record systems. Both these systems have been in routine use in their home institutions for over 10 years, and HELP is now available to other hospitals as well. HELP's decision-support functions have been shown to influence beneficially the clinical practices of physicians at the hospital where this system was developed [Evans et al., 1986]. The few commercially available systems that follow the passive consultation model of decision support have tended not to emphasize the importance of the human–computer interface. As we have described, this lack can greatly limit the appeal of these systems to physicians.

In the research setting, several intriguing prototype systems for patient-specific decision support have appeared, some of which have been used clinically in controlled environments [Reggia and Tuhrin, 1985; Clancey and Shortliffe, 1984; Miller, 1988]. House staff and faculty at the University of Pittsburgh and other sites are beginning to test the diagnostic capabilities of QMR [Miller et al., 1986]. ONCOCIN is in limited use to assist with the management of patients being treated on research protocols in the oncology clinic at Stanford [Shortliffe, 1986], and is being adapted for eventual dissemination to private oncology offices. ATTENDING has been tested by anesthesia residents at Yale [Miller, 1986]. DXplain has been made available nationally via the computer network of the American Medical Association [Barnett et al., 1987]. Computer-based consultations regarding acid–base and electrolyte disorders are routinely available at Beth Israel Hospital, using a program developed in the early 1970s [Bleich, 1972]. Taken together, these and other programs have great promise, but there are still major challenges to be overcome before integrated tools with broad clinical capabilities will be widely available [Schwartz et al., 1987]. The field of AI, which has attracted commercial attention recently as expert systems have been successfully implemented in industry, has produced only a handful of narrowly focused commercial biomedical products [Aikins et al., 1983; Weiss et al., 1981]. Much of the medical AI work has concentrated on limited research questions, and only recently have large systems for direct use by physicians entered field testing.

At the same time, the educational potential of decision-support systems has been recognized [Association of American Medical Colleges, 1986]. First, and most simply, physicians learn by using decision aids such as those described in this chapter (particularly if the programs provide useful explanations of the basis for their assessments). Second, the systems are also being explicitly adapted and enhanced for teaching purposes (see Chapter 17). A new set of problems arises when system developers attempt to simulate the skills of a good clinical teacher [Clancey and Shortliffe, 1984]. New technologies, such as computer-controlled videodisc players that provide still-frame or motion-picture images (of radiologic studies, histologic sections, and the like), can clearly enhance the learning experience for system users. Direct links from teaching tools to large information resources such as MEDLINE also hold great educational promise. Such links may be accomplished by computer networks or by widespread distribution of the information on low-cost storage media such as CD-ROM.

15.6.1 Legal and Regulatory Questions

It may already have occurred to you that there are legal implications inherent in the development and use of such innovations. As we mentioned in Chapter 5, formal legal precedents for dealing with clinical decision-support systems are lacking at present. Several observers have noted that a pivotal concern is whether the courts will view the systems under negligence law or product liability law [Miller et al., 1985]. Under negligence law (which governs medical malpractice), a product or activity must meet reasonable expectations for safety. The principle of strict liability, on the other hand, states that a product must not be harmful. Because it is unrealistic to require that decision-support programs make correct assessments under all circumstances—we do not apply such standards to physicians themselves—the determination of which legal principle to apply will have important implications for the dissemination and acceptance of such tools. A related question is the potential liability borne by physicians who could have accessed such a program, who chose not to do so, and who made an incorrect decision when the system would have suggested the correct one. As with other medical technologies, precedents suggest that physicians will be liable in such circumstances if the use of consultant programs has become the *standard of care* in the community.

Questions have also arisen regarding the validation of decision-support tools prior to their release. The evaluation of complex decision-support tools is challenging; it is difficult to determine acceptable levels of performance when there may be disagreement even among experts with similar training and experience. There is often no such thing as *the* correct answer to a clinical question. Evaluations of medical decision-support tools [Miller et al., 1982; Reggia et al., 1984; Hickam et al., 1985a; Yu et al., 1979b] have suggested appropriate methods for assessing the adequacy of medical consultation systems before these tools are introduced for routine use.

What then should be the role of government in prerelease regulation of medical software? Current policy of the Food and Drug Administration (FDA) indicates that such tools will not be subject to federal regulation if a trained practitioner is assessing the program's advice and making the final determination of care [Young, 1987]. On the other hand, programs that make decisions directly controlling the patient's treatment (for example, closed-loop systems that administer insulin or that adjust intravenous infusion rates or respirator settings; see Chapter 12) are viewed as medical devices subject to FDA regulation.

15.6.2 Future Directions for Clinical Decision-Support Systems

Trends for decision-support research and development in the decade ahead are becoming evident. We shall examine several research subjects that will affect the evolution of decision-support tools.

First, there is growing interest in merging AI methods with classical statistical and decision-analytic techniques. Early rivalries among workers in these fields led to recognition of potential synergies among methodologies. For example, researchers are developing detailed causal models that can encode both mechanisms of pathophysiology (when known) and empirical statistical data regarding the frequency with which intermediate states lead to particular outcomes.

Second, workers are investigating the problem-solving techniques used by experts, which will influence greatly the features that will be incorporated into decision-support tools. We now know, for example, that experts often reason from first principles to solve unfamiliar problems. The role of basic models in our decision-support tools thus is taking on new importance. Such studies also identify when basic knowledge is needed, both for explanation and for problem solving. Psychologic research suggests that experts often make decisions using high-level, associational knowledge but, when asked to defend their decisions, resort to basic mechanistic knowledge that they had, but did not use, when solving the problem. Such studies also suggest ways to teach the domain knowledge while providing consultation, and how to avoid the cognitive biases that afflict human problem solvers.

Third, there is increasing recognition of the need to develop methods for providing anatomic and structural knowledge in a form that is useful to a decision-support system. Experts clearly use such information routinely when they solve both diagnostic and therapeutic problems, but our methods for encoding it are weak at best. Similarly, we need proven methods for reasoning about temporal issues when assessing a disease or judging a patient's response to therapy. Current systems tend to view the patient at a specific point in time, and have limited sensitivity to the time course of disease. Developers of systems that must function in settings where management of temporal issues is mandatory (such as ONCOCIN, which follows patients with cancer throughout their courses of therapy) have tended to create custom-tailored temporal-reasoning methods that may not generalize well to other problem areas.

Finally, changes in hardware technology will continue to have a major influence on the field's development. The falling cost of computers with large memories, rapid processing speeds, and large peripheral storage will make powerful decision-support tools more accessible and more affordable. Similarly, high-density bit-map display graphics, plus novel interactive devices, will have a profound effect on the systems' modes of interaction with users. In a similar vein, networking technologies will support sharing of patient data among distributed computer systems. As the medical infrastructure for computing and communications evolves, integration of decision-support tools into routine clinical care will improve. Many observers believe that such integration will be required before decision-support programs will be used in any but the most limited clinical settings.

15.6.3 Conclusions

The future of clinical decision-support systems inherently depends on progress in developing useful programs and in reducing logistical barriers to implementation. Although ubiquitous computer-based aids that routinely assist physicians in most aspects of clinical practice are still the stuff of science fiction, progress has been real and the potential remains inspiring. Early predictions about the effects such innovations will have on medical education and practice have not yet come to pass [Schwartz, 1970], but growing successes support an optimistic view of what technology will eventually do to assist practitioners with processing of complex data and knowledge. The research challenges have been identified much more clearly [Schwartz et al., 1987; National Library of Medicine, 1986b; Shortliffe, 1984b], and the implications for health-science education are much better understood. We have learned, for example, that the computer literacy of students can be increasingly assumed, but that health-science educators must teach the conceptual foundations of medical informatics if their graduates are to be prepared for the technologically sophisticated world that lies ahead.

Equally important, we have learned much about what is *not* likely to happen. The more investigators understand the complex and changing nature of medical knowledge, the more clear it becomes that trained practitioners will always be required as elements in a cooperative relationship between physician and computer-based decision tool. There is no evidence that machine capabilities will ever be equal to the human mind's ability to deal with unexpected situations, to integrate visual and auditory data that reveal subtleties of a patient's problem, or to deal with social and ethical issues that are often key determinants of proper medical decisions. Considerations such as these will always be important to the humane practice of medicine, and practitioners will always have access to information that is meaningless to the machine. Such observations argue cogently for the discretion of physicians in the proper use of decision-support tools.

Suggested Readings

Buchanan, B. G. and Shortliffe, E. H. (eds). *Rule-Based Expert Systems: The MYCIN Experiments of the Stanford Heuristic Programming Project*. Reading, MA: Addison-Wesley, 1984.

> *The MYCIN system, developed to provide assistance in selection of antibiotic therapies, provided a set of generalized methods that were broadly applied in other domains. Later, these methods were enhanced by the Stanford researchers to investigate research topics in computer-aided instruction, computer-supported knowledge acquisition, and other areas. This edited collection summarizes the MYCIN-related experiments performed at Stanford between 1972 and 1982.*

Clancey, W. J. and Shortliffe, E. H. (eds). *Readings in Medical Artificial Intelligence: The First Decade*. Reading, MA: Addison-Wesley, 1984.

> *This collection of 20 key articles deals with the first 10 years of research on the application of AI techniques in biomedicine. Comprehensive overviews of all the major systems from the 1970s are provided.*

Duda, R. O. and Shortliffe, E. H. Expert systems research. *Science*, 220:261, 1983.

> *By the early 1980s, there was a rapidly growing interest in AI and in the potential use of expert systems. This article is a concise overview of the expert systems field at that time.*

Ledley, R. S. and Lusted, L. B. Reasoning foundations of medical diagnosis. *Science*, 130:9, 1959.

> *This classic article provided the first influential description of how computers might be used to assist with the diagnostic process. The flurry of activity applying Bayesian methods to computer-assisted diagnosis during the 1960s was largely inspired by this provocative paper.*

Medical Decision Making, Philadelphia: Hanley and Belfus (published bimonthly).

> *This excellent journal frequently includes important papers dealing with the use of computers for decision support.*

Miller, P. L. *Selected Topics in Medical Artificial Intelligence*. New York: Springer-Verlag, 1988.

> *This edited collection updated the Clancey and Shortliffe volume (cited previously). It includes several key papers on medical AI that were written during the 1980s.*

Reggia, J. A. and Tuhrim, S. (eds). *Computer-Assisted Medical Decision Making* (Volumes 1 and 2). New York: Springer-Verlag, 1985.

> *This excellent collection includes several of the seminal papers on computer-assisted medical decision making. The articles represent all the major research paradigms in the field.*

Schwartz, W. B. Medicine and the computer: The promise and problems of change. *New England Journal of Medicine*, 283(23):1257, 1970.

> *A senior clinician from Boston wrote this frequently cited article, which assessed the growing role of computers in health care. Twenty years later, many of the developments*

anticipated by Schwartz had come to pass, although the rate of change was slower than he had predicted.

Shortliffe, E. H Testing reality: The introduction of decision-support technologies for physicians. *Methods of Information in Medicine,* 28:1, 1989.

> *This editorial summarizes the reasons for physicians' resistance to the introduction of computing technologies in general and of decision-support tools in particular. The discussion is based on a market-research study in which physicians' opinions were solicited.*

Warner, H. W. *Computer-Assisted Medical Decision-Making.* New York: Academic Press, 1979.

> *After over 15 years of the HELP system's development had been completed, Warner wrote this subject overview. Many of the examples are drawn from his group's experience at the University of Utah.*

Questions for Discussion

1. Researchers in medical AI have argued that there is a need for more expert knowledge in medical decision-support systems, but developers of Bayesian systems have argued that expert estimates are inherently flawed and that advice programs must be based on solid data. How do you account for the apparent difference between these views? Which view is valid? Explain your answer.

2. Explain the meanings of Internist-1/QMR's frequency weights and evoking strengths. What does it mean if a finding has a frequency weight of 4 and an evoking strength of 2? How do these parameters relate to the concepts of sensitivity, specificity, and predictive value that were introduced in Chapters 2 and 3?

3. Let us consider how de Dombal and other developers of Bayesian systems have used patient-care experience to guide the collection of statistics that they need. For example, consider the database in the following table, which shows the relationship between two findings (f_1 and f_2) and a disease (D) for 10 patients.

Patient	f_1	f_2	D	$-D$
1	0	1	0	1
2	0	1	1	0
3	0	1	0	1
4	1	1	1	0
5	1	1	1	0
6	1	1	0	1
7	1	0	1	0
8	1	1	1	0
9	1	0	0	1
10	1	1	1	0

In the table, $-D$ signifies the absence of disease D. A 0 indicates the absence of a finding or disease, and a 1 indicates the presence of a finding or disease. For example, based on the database presented, the probability of finding f_1 in this population is $\frac{7}{10} = 70$ percent. Refer back to Chapters 2 and 3 as necessary in answering the following questions:

   a. What are the sensitivity and specificity of each of f_1 and f_2 for the disease D? What is the prevalence of D in this 10-person population?

b. Use the database to calculate the following probabilities:
- $p[f_1|D]$
- $p[f_1|-D]$
- $p[f_2|D]$
- $p[f_2|-D]$
- $p[D]$
- $p[-D]$

c. Use the database to calculate $p[D|f_1 \text{ and } f_2]$.

d. Use the probabilities determined in part (b) to calculate $p[D|f_1 \text{ and } f_2]$ using a heuristic method that assumes that findings f_1 and f_2 are conditionally independent given a disease and the absence of a disease. Why is this result different from the one in part (c)? Do you see why it has generally been necessary to make this heuristic approximation in Bayesian programs?

4. You have read about both the MYCIN consultation system from the 1970s and the ONCOCIN system from the 1980s. Discuss how the design of each was affected by the available hardware and software technology. In particular, how might MYCIN have differed if today's hardware had been available a decade earlier? Suggest interface designs for MYCIN that would heighten usability and acceptance, using today's graphical workstations.

5. In an evaluation study, ONCOCIN provided advice that was approved by experts in only 79 percent of cases [Hickam et al., 1985a]. Do you believe this performance is adequate for a computational tool that is designed to help physicians make decisions regarding patient care? What safeguards, if any, would you suggest to ensure the proper use of such a system? Would you be willing to visit a particular physician if you knew in advance that she made decisions regarding treatment that were approved by expert colleagues less than 80 percent of the time? If not, what level of performance would you consider adequate?

6. We have stressed the importance of explanation capabilities in decision-support systems. Suppose you were building such a system for a modern computer with graphical capabilities similar to those of the machine used for ONCOCIN. Suggest ways in which you might use the modern graphical features to present the explanations.

16

Clinical Research Systems

Gio Wiederhold and Leslie E. Perreault

After reading this chapter, you should know the answers to these questions:

- What are the six steps of the clinical research cycle?
- What characteristics distinguish prospective and retrospective studies? What are the advantages and disadvantages of each type of study?
- How do randomization, blinding, and long-term followup reduce the chance of obtaining biased study results?
- What techniques can researchers use to handle the inevitable problem of missing data?
- What problems do researchers encounter when analyzing datasets that have been pooled from multiple sources?
- Which aspects of data management and analysis are supported by current computer-based research systems?

16.1 The Clinical Research Process

Rapid advances in the state of medical science in recent years have greatly improved the ability of physicians to care for their patients. Armed with knowledge of diseases and disease manifestations, diagnostic radiology and laboratory techniques, and an arsenal of drugs, procedures, and medical devices, health professionals have increasing power to prolong life, to alleviate symptoms, and to cure underlying disease. Nevertheless, much variability exists in patients' likelihoods of contracting disease and in their responses to treatment—the relation between intervention and outcome is uncertain. When choosing and tailoring therapies for individual patients, clinicians must rely on the *intuitive* aspects of medical practice, as well as on their knowledge of physiologic principles and medical science.

The goal of **clinical research** is to advance the state of medical science—to add to the base of knowledge that guides health professionals in caring for individual patients—and thus, ultimately, to improve the practice of medicine. Clinical researchers collect and analyze medical data to gain a better understanding of diseases and of disease manifestations, to uncover relationships between medical interventions and short- and long-term outcomes, to identify subsets of patients that have different medical prognoses, and to assess the effectiveness of new technologies relative to standard therapies.

In many scientific disciplines, researchers can investigate problems by conducting carefully controlled laboratory experiments. Ethical and practical concerns, however, limit experimentation in medical care. In certain situations, researchers can conduct experiments to compare the effects of alternative interventions in different groups of patients. For example, there are currently no generally accepted treatments for many types of cancer; physicians may treat patients with these diseases in conjunction with experimental protocols that are designed to determine the effectiveness of various therapies. Occasionally, clinicians must interrupt such a research protocol because preliminary results indicate that one treatment produces significantly better outcomes.

In general, clinical researchers must be content with observing interventions and the resulting outcomes as physicians try alternative therapies to help patients regain health. Physicians record clinical data in medical charts and in large clinical databases, which researchers can then analyze. Researchers rely on the collection of large numbers of data and the use of statistical techniques to untangle the effects in these uncontrolled experiments.

Two of the central tasks of clinical research are data management and data analysis. In this chapter, we shall discuss computer-based systems that support these activities. Computers also can help researchers to conduct the experiments; for example, they may automatically screen patient information to determine eligibility in ongoing experiments, or they may evaluate patient data and suggest appropriate treatment at each step of complicated treatment protocols. Someday, clinical research systems may scrutinize large databases of patient data to discover possible relationships, to form hypotheses, and to generate models for analysis. Today, however, automated discovery systems are still at the frontier of work on clinical research systems.

16.1.1 The Experimental Cycle

Clinical research, like all experimental sciences, typically comprises the following steps:

1. *Problem formulation.* Clinical researchers use knowledge gained through education and experience to identify gaps and inconsistencies in the existing scientific knowledge base, and thereby to pose interesting and tractable research questions.
2. *Hypothesis generation.* Once they have identified a problem, researchers develop a hypothesis to explain their observations.
3. *Experimentation.* Investigators and clinicians systematically gather data through experimentation, observation, and measurement of physical phenomena.
4. *Model development.* Research epidemiologists develop a testable model that relates the observed outcomes to their causes.
5. *Hypothesis testing.* When analyzing data, statistical researchers test the model using the data that they have collected. Parameters obtained from the analysis provide measures of the strength of the hypothesis and the fit of the model.
6. *Evaluation and dissemination.* Finally, the researchers evaluate the study methodology, assess the quality of the underlying data, and disseminate the newly acquired knowledge.

Figure 16.1 illustrates the cyclic nature of the clinical research process: Researchers' knowledge and experience suggest potentially fruitful experiments, and facilitate formation of a hypothesis, generation of a model, and interpretation of observations. In turn, the knowledge gained through experimentation is incorporated into the knowledge base, thus forming the basis for future research. Typically, a variety of specialized researchers (clinicians, statisticians, epidemiologists, and so on) cooperate to complete the research process.

The idealized cycle shown in Figure 16.1 implies an orderly progression from step to step. Actually, research never follows these steps cleanly, and there are many interactions and refining iterations among the steps. For example, hypothesis formulation typically occurs interactively with observation; rarely can we pinpoint the exact moment when a new hypothesis is formed (although we always can identify the time at which a hypothesis is first stated formally). Likewise, model building often entails successive refinements to identify a causal mechanism that best explains the observations. Furthermore, our initial beliefs about the likelihood of alternative models determine which data we choose to collect.

16.1.2 Prospective Versus Retrospective Research

We classify clinical research in two major categories: prospective and retrospective studies. The crucial methodological difference is whether or not the investigators collect new data for analysis. In **prospective studies,** researchers define the experimental conditions before collecting any data. Based on the expected magnitude of the response and the **sample attrition rate,** they calculate the sample size necessary to produce statistically significant results. They specify the parameters of the study, define methods for enrolling subjects, design protocols for delivering alternative treatments,

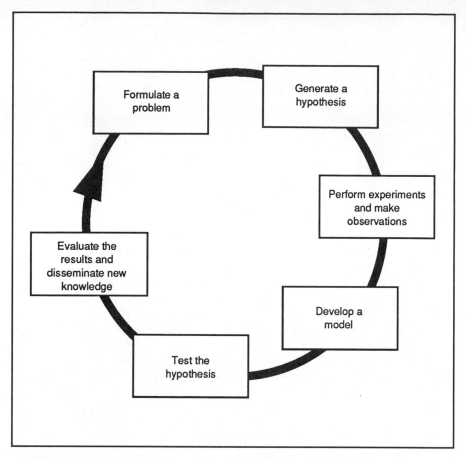

FIGURE 16.1 Clinical research is a cyclic process. Researchers' knowledge and experience suggest interesting experimental problems and facilitate hypothesis formation, model generation, and observation interpretation. New knowledge gained through experimentation is incorporated into the knowledge base, thus shaping the direction of future research.

and define the criteria for measuring outcomes. Only after they have completely planned the experiment do the researchers begin to enroll study subjects and start to collect data for later analysis.

In **retrospective studies,** clinical researchers analyze existing datasets, rather than collecting new observations. Sometimes, they can use datasets that were collected for other clinical studies. Often, they conduct **chart reviews** to glean research data from clinical records. Investigators performing retrospective studies also must specify the experimental parameters and define the criteria for including observations in the study. Because the data were not collected with the goals of this experiment in mind, however, the values for some variables of interest typically are unavailable, and the sample population may not represent the ideal study population.

The most desirable form of clinical research is the **randomized clinical trial (RCT),** a type of prospective experiment in which patients are randomly assigned to alternate groups, and are treated according to a **study protocol.** Investigators collect data and compare the results obtained from each group to determine whether patients who receive different interventions experience significantly different outcomes. The most common design for a clinical trial is the *parallel design*—an experimental group is treated with a new therapy and the results are compared with those from a control group that received the standard therapy or no treatment at all. A second design is the *crossover design,* in which each patient receives all treatments sequentially. The order of the treatments, however, is varied.

RCTs are attractive because they are designed to avoid **experimental bias**—differences in experimental outcome that are caused by factors other than the experimental therapy. One example of such a bias is a difference in the initial health statuses of the subpopulations under investigation. Once the likelihood of bias has been minimized, researchers can use statistical techniques to assess the amount of sampling variability and therefore the probability that the study result was obtained by chance. Well-designed RCTs use three techniques to minimize bias: randomization, blinding, and follow up.

Randomization minimizes the chance of obtaining biased results due to noncomparability of the treatment groups. When they are enrolled, subjects are randomly assigned to one of the groups; a table of random numbers often is used. This process eliminates the **selection bias** that can result if patients, physicians, or administrators can influence which type of treatment a particular patient receives. For example, selection bias occurs if investigators consciously or subconsciously assign patients with better prognoses to the group receiving the treatment that they believe—and wish to prove—is most effective. Randomization also minimizes the likelihood that the sample populations will vary significantly with respect to some as-yet-unknown characteristic that is correlated with outcome.

Blinding reduces the chance of bias from a second source—subtle and unrecognized differences in quality or style of treatment, patient response, or physician evaluation. In *single-blind studies,* patients do not know which treatment they are receiving. They may, for example, receive a placebo instead of an active drug. In *double-blind studies,* neither subject (patient) nor observer (researcher) knows to which group the subject belongs, thus avoiding systematic bias in the way treatments are given or in the way results are reported. In many cases, blinding is difficult; for instance, blinded studies of medical versus surgical treatment are impossible. *Unblinding* is likely to occur if one therapy has characteristic side effects. Complex treatments that require the physician to modify the therapy based on the patient's degree of response to previous therapy can be at best blind to only the patient. Blinding is most important when experimental outcomes require subjective judgments, such as determining the extent of disease or the degree of discomfort. Blinding is least important when endpoints are clearcut; such an endpoint is death within the study period.

Follow up is necessary to ensure thorough collection of results. Even when trials are appropriately randomized and blinded, bias may arise due to attrition. Investigators may be unable to collect follow-up data if patients discontinue treatment or move away. If dropouts are systematically related to the therapy or disease—for example, if patients stop taking treatments because they experience side effects or because they believe that the treatment is not working—then failure to include these data in the analysis will bias the results of the study because the occurrence of side effects or of lack of response will be underreported. The collection of follow-up data for long-term studies is a costly process.

Well-designed and properly conducted RCTs produce the least bias when testing a hypothesis—they are the gold standard for clinical research. Ideally, all clinical studies could be designed as RCTs; however, this ideal is impossible to achieve for several reasons. First, RCTs are time consuming and expensive to conduct. For extended studies, researchers must enroll several times as many patients as will be needed for the analysis because of attrition. Second, ethical considerations prohibit conducting clinical trials in which one treatment is clearly superior to another, or in which one alternative is already known to have clearly deleterious effects. For example, it would be unethical to assign subjects randomly to smoking and nonsmoking groups to test the extent of the effect of smoking on mortality. In addition, investigators must monitor prospective clinical trials to ensure that patients are not placed at a disadvantage by participation. If ongoing analysis demonstrates that one treatment is better than another, then part or all of the trial may be abandoned. For example, researchers decided not to complete a clinical trial to test the effects of an anti-AIDS drug when the results of preliminary analyses showed that patients who received the drug had significantly lower death rates than did patients who received an inactive placebo drug [Barnes, 1986].

Retrospective studies provide an alternative to RCTs. If a suitable database exists, researchers can avoid the long and expensive process of enrolling qualified patients and collecting data. The disadvantages of retrospective research stem from the fact that the experimental database was not created with the specific study goal in mind. In databases that have been collected for clinical rather than research purposes, many variables of interest to researchers (including potentially confounding variables) will not have been collected because they seemed not clinically relevant. Furthermore, investigators have no control over the manner in which interventions were applied and data were recorded. Hidden biases often exist because patients in the database were included for reasons unrelated to the study. For instance, patients with a poor prognosis may not have been given a costly treatment. Potential biasing of the samples makes it more difficult for researchers to interpret study results.

Despite their limitations, retrospective studies are often more appropriate than RCTs are. They are inexpensive relative to RCTs and pose no ethical problems because they do not affect which treatment a patient receives. Seldom can researchers enlist more than a few hundred patients for a prospective clinical trial. Thus, they are limited in their ability to investigate rare cases. On the other hand, clinical databases often include thousands of patients. Retrospective studies are appropriate as preliminary investigations designed to evaluate whether more rigorous studies are warranted.

16.1.3 Computers and Clinical Research

Various types of professionals participate in the clinical research process: the physicians, nurses, and other health-care providers who administer treatments and collect data; the medical-records personnel who enter, store, and retrieve data; the epidemiologists and statisticians who model the problem and analyze the data; and the patients themselves, as subjects in the experiments. A database provides a basis for the communication of shared information. The larger the study, the greater the need for computers to assist in the research process. If there are more subjects, there are more data to collect, manage, and analyze. Often, large clinical trials need to track patients over a course of many years so that delayed outcomes can be recorded. Clinical researchers may use database-management systems (DBMSs; see Chapter 4) to help in the tasks of data entry, multiuser access to data, and long-term maintenance of stored information.

Information systems with a research orientation also may include direct links to statistical-analysis programs. Clinical researchers use a variety of graphical and statistical techniques to analyze databases once the latter have been assembled. **Statistical packages** are collections of programs that can be invoked to perform calculations on input and to produce reports. Statistical packages for data analysis are well developed, and a number of commercial vendors compete in the delivery of accurate, comprehensive, and user-friendly packages. The biomedical data-analysis package, BMDP (originally BMD), was developed with support from the National Institutes of Health (NIH). The Statistical Package for the Social Sciences (SPSS) and Statistical Analysis System (SAS) are two other well-known packages.

Statistical packages typically provide a variety of capabilities:

- *Descriptive statistics* provide statistical summaries of the data. They are useful for exposing underlying patterns, and can help researchers to identify exceptional cases and errors in the data. The most common descriptive statistics are simple measures such as counts, averages, minima, maxima, ranges, standard deviations, and cross-tabulations. These statistics can be calculated for all subjects or for subgroups of interest (Figure 16.2). Common variables for grouping patients include demographic variables (for example, age and gender), disease categories (for example, stage of disease), and treatment parameters (for example, membership in treatment or control group).
- *Graphical presentations* portray relationships among variables for visual inspection. Scatterplots illustrate the degree of correlation between two variables and can suggest whether the underlying relationship is linear or has a more complicated form (Figure 16.3a). Bar graphs can display frequencies, and pie charts can show the percentage shares of a total by population subgroup or by attribute value (Figure 16.3b). For time-oriented data, time-series plots—which show events as they occur in sequence over time—can expose cyclic relationships and trends over time (Figure 16.3c).
- *Analytic statistical techniques* are used to explore and quantify postulated relationships among observations and variables. For example, researchers can apply

VARIABLE	N	MEAN	STANDARD DEVIATION	MINIMUM VALUE	MAXIMUM VALUE	STD ERROR OF MEAN	SUM	VARIANCE	C.V.
AGE	20	26.60000000	1.50087694	25.00000000	29.00000000	0.33560629	532.0000000	2.25263158	5.642
HGT	20	67.15000000	3.80131556	62.00000000	76.00000000	0.85000000	1343.0000000	14.45000000	5.661
WGT	20	144.05000000	23.86690067	110.00000000	183.00000000	5.33680123	2881.0000000	569.62894737	16.568

VARIABLE	N	MEAN	STANDARD DEVIATION	MINIMUM VALUE	MAXIMUM VALUE	STD ERROR OF MEAN	SUM	VARIANCE	C.V.
				—— SEX=F ——					
AGE	10	26.50000000	1.64991582	25.00000000	29.00000000	0.52174919	265.0000000	2.72222222	6.226
HGT	10	64.20000000	1.54919334	62.00000000	67.00000000	0.48989795	642.0000000	2.40000000	2.413
WGT	10	124.20000000	9.02835041	110.00000000	137.00000000	2.85501508	1242.0000000	81.51111111	7.269
				—— SEX=M ——					
AGE	10	26.70000000	1.41813649	25.00000000	29.00000000	0.44845413	267.0000000	2.01111111	5.311
HGT	10	70.10000000	2.96085573	65.00000000	76.00000000	0.93630479	701.0000000	8.76666667	4.224
WGT	10	163.90000000	15.66631205	132.00000000	183.00000000	4.95412286	1639.0000000	245.43333333	9.558

FIGURE 16.2 SAS's MEANS procedure computes and prints out elementary descriptive statistics, including number of observations, mean, standard deviation, minimum value, maximum value, and range.

clustering algorithms to identify subgroups of observations with similar characteristics. Or they can use multiple-regression techniques to estimate the effect of therapy and combinations of treatments on the outcome, independent of variables such as age, gender, and baseline health status.

Researchers use descriptive statistics to search for unexpected events and to support the generation of hypotheses. Graphical presentations extend the capability of descriptive statistics, and they can elucidate hypotheses about trends and correlations among variables. Analytic methods are used primarily to verify hypotheses.

16.2 Fundamental Issues of Data Collection and Analysis

Computer-based clinical research systems provide investigators with tools for acquiring, maintaining, and analyzing clinical information. The use of a computer, however, does not guarantee high-quality research. In this section, we shall review fundamental issues of data selection and representation—issues that are critical, albeit not unique, to the use of computer-based research systems. In addition, we shall discuss important aspects of data quality, and shall describe the special problems that can arise when we use sets of data that have been pooled from multiple sources. We shall close the section with a brief discussion of linear models for statistical analysis.

16.2.1 Description of Clinical Events

Three types of elements are necessary to describe a clinical event adequately for research purposes: (1) variables that identify which events are being studied, (2) variables that describe the study intervention and the experimental outcome, and (3) potentially confounding variables that could affect the experimental outcome.

Identification Variables

Identification information allows researchers to associate each observation with a unique clinical event. An individual datum (for example, "128") is meaningless unless it can be associated with a particular patient (Janice Chase, medical record number 123-456-789), a particular study parameter (systolic blood pressure), and a particular time (01JAN90, 02:14).

The choice of identifying information must be specific enough to identify each observation uniquely within a set of data. For example, if we are studying the effect of an antihypertensive drug on blood pressure and plan to measure systolic blood pressure several times during the course of the study, we must save enough identification information to distinguish among multiple measurements. We might label the three observations BP1, BP2, and BP3. Alternatively, we might record the time at which each measurement was taken.

A patient-oriented hierarchy of identification information is typically used for storing clinical information in computer-based medical records.

- *Patient.* Each patient in a database must have a unique identifier. Common choices are medical record number, Social Security number, or patient's name and birthdate.
- *Visit.* Clinical databases that accumulate patient data over a period of years typically contain information collected during multiple clinical encounters. Thus, each observation is associated with a particular visit (or examination or test) on a specific date.
- *Parameter.* Each observation is associated with an identifier that specifies which parameter was measured (for example, systolic blood pressure, serum potassium level, white-blood-cell count, or stage of disease).

Time is a critical element for the identification of clinical data. Many clinical studies are longitudinal—that is, they observe patients over extended periods. Therefore, the timing of the event must be recorded with the data that describe that event. Investigators may record times with more or less precision, depending on the purpose of the study. In many cases, the calendar date of the observation is sufficient. For other studies, however, researchers might need to pinpoint the time of an event to the minute or to the second. For example, in a study of the effects of anesthetic drugs, it might be crucial to record the exact time at which a drug enters the patient's blood stream. In most patient-care settings, that time is difficult to obtain accurately. Therefore, we might settle for an approximate time, such as the scheduled drug-administration time. Likewise, laboratory-test values are most appropriately associated with the time

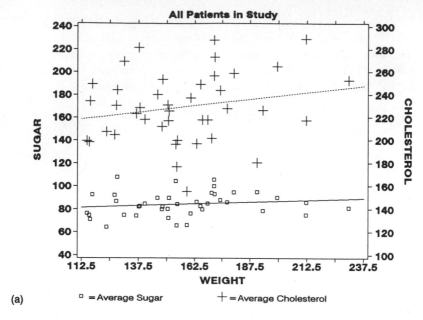

(a)   □ = Average Sugar   + = Average Cholesterol

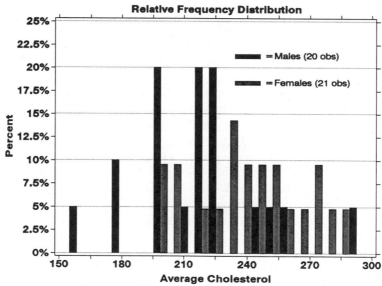

(b)

FIGURE 16.3 Graphical techniques visually portray relationships among data. Researchers using the MEDLOG system can create (a) a scatterplot to show correlations between blood-sugar level and weight and between cholesterol level and weight for patients in a study population; (b) a bar graph to show frequency distributions of average cholesterol level for men and women in a study group; and (c) time-oriented plots of a patient's cholesterol level, blood-sugar level, and weight on successive visits (see next page). (*Source:* Figures courtesy of Information Analysis Corporation.)

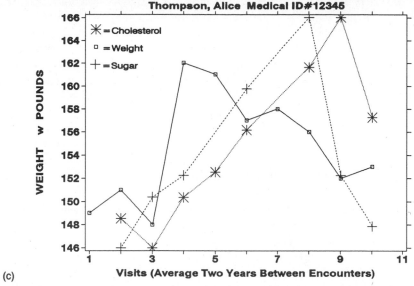

(c)

FIGURE 16.3 *Continued from previous page.*

the specimen was taken. This information is not always recorded accurately, and we might substitute the time the test was ordered or the time the specimen was received in the laboratory.

Primary and Confounding Variables

The *primary variables* of interest in a clinical experiment are those that describe the intervention under investigation and those that describe the outcome. For example, we might form the hypothesis that patients who receive an antihypertensive drug will have significantly lower blood pressure than will those who do not take the drug. The primary variables will include pre- and postintervention blood pressures and an indicator to distinguish patients in the study group from those in the control group. In addition, a host of other factors can affect the experimental outcome—for example, the patient's age, gender, weight, and baseline health status all might affect his blood pressure. To separate the effects of these *confounding variables* from the effect of the drug itself, we must collect data on these factors and include them in the analysis. The distinction between primary variables and confounding variables is related to the analytic model under consideration, and thus depends on the goals of the research.

16.2.2 Data Representation

Data are represented in a variety of forms in a clinical database. Some measurements are best stored as numeric data values. Other information may be encoded according to a classification scheme (for example, the ICD-9-CM coding scheme for clinical diagnoses [National Center for Health Statistics, 1978]) or may be stored as free text. The choice of representation determines the types of operations that the computer can perform on the data. Most statistical procedures operate on numeric data. As we discussed in Section 2.4.1, the interpretation of unstructured data is complicated, and automatic summarization may be impossible. In general, computer programs can read in and write out uncoded information, but cannot analyze that information. Thus, uncoded data are unsuitable for clinical research. Some of the most common data types used in clinical research are the following:

- *Real numbers* are used to record the values of variables that may take on continuous values—for example, values of laboratory-test results or measurements of physical size.

- *Integers* often are used to record numeric data that assume discrete values—for example, age in years, or number of previous pregnancies.

- *Character strings* allow the storage of textual data such as name and address, or free-text comments concerning a patient visit. These values typically are not used in computation. Rather, they are stored and displayed without interpretation.

- *Coded variables* are used for data values that can be classified into well-defined categories. For example, gender might be coded as "M" or "F," or as "0" or "1." Likewise, researchers might encode patients' discharge diagnoses according to the ICD-9-CM coding scheme or by diagnosis-related group (DRG).

- *Dates* often are given a special representation that facilitates the computation of time intervals. SAS, for example, translates and stores each date as the number of days before or after the base date of January 1, 1960. If the system stores all dates—including the current date—using this same representation, then data-manipulation programs can calculate time differences. For example, if patients' birthdates are stored in the database, a computer program can compute patients' ages using the relationship $age = (TODAY - birthdate) \div 365.25$.

Choice of representation depends on a data element's intended use. For example, we can think of blood pressure as a single value (for example 125/83). Often, however, researchers may record systolic pressure and diastolic pressure as two separate variables because they want to analyze these values independently. A patient's address is another complex variable. Data managers may choose to record the entire address as a single character-string variable. If they plan to perform analysis by patient location, however, they should store information on city, state, or zip code separately.

Each data value can be associated with the specific time at which the value was measured. Often, however, the information of interest is related to the *interval* between the current measurement and a previous observation. We might wish to compute the absolute difference, the rate of change (such as "average weight increase of 150 grams per day"), or a qualitative measure of change in state (for example, "improving" or "stable"). Sometimes, the mean value is the best summarization of an interval. At other times, the maximum or minimum values, or both, are most relevant to the analysis. In any case, we often can perform an operation on two or more instantaneous point events to create new types of data that can be associated with time intervals.

16.2.3 Aspects of Data Quality

Once data are stored in a database, we can assess the quality of the database on at least three dimensions: correctness, completeness, and consistency. *Correctness* refers to the accuracy with which events are recorded and entered into the computer. *Completeness* refers to the prevalence of omitted events and missing observations. *Consistency* refers to uniformity in the meaning of data encodings within the database.

Correctness

Data quality is compromised if values are measured incorrectly or if data-entry errors result in storage of incorrect data values. To verify that the data recorded in the database represent the true state of the world, data-system designers often create feedback loops. By comparing the stored data with an independent source of the information, they can detect and correct discrepancies. For simple demographic information, the best validation technique is to print out the data and to ask the patient to verify that they are correct. Patients are rarely included in the loop for the collection of medical information. More often, the health-care workers who collect the information are asked to verify its correctness. For example, they may be asked to countersign printouts of orders and observations that have been entered into the computer. In a busy environment, giving such signatures quickly becomes a formality, especially when the reports contain observations that do not immediately affect patient treatment. For instance, in clinical laboratories, all results may be reported under the signature of the pathologist in charge, although it is obvious that the pathologist has not personally verified each value.

A common method for assessing the correctness of clinical research databases is to compare their contents with the information recorded in the traditional medical record. This procedure is labor intensive and costly; therefore, only a sample of records is reviewed to obtain an estimate of error rates, or to detect patterns of errors.

The incidence of data-entry errors can be reduced by encouraging data-entry personnel to recheck the values they have entered before proceeding to a new screen, by presenting information in alternate form (for example, by displaying the text definition of a coded field), and by performing automatic checks for data type, acceptable range, logical consistency, and so on (see the discussion of error prevention in Chapter 6).

Completeness

The problem of missing data is even more serious than is that of data-entry errors. We usually can assume that data-entry errors occur randomly. Thus, they will not bias the results of the study, although they will reduce the statistical significance of the measured effects. On the other hand, there are often systematic reasons why certain data have not been recorded. We might infer that patients did not return for scheduled follow-up treatments because earlier treatments were effective. If this assumption is correct, then ignoring the missing observations will weaken the observed effect of treatment on outcome. On the other hand, patients may not have returned for follow up because the treatments were ineffective. In this case, failure to correct for missing observations would result in overestimation of the effectiveness of the treatment.

Clinical researchers can use one of three fundamentally different approaches to handle the problem of missing data:

1. *Eliminate patient records that have missing elements.* Indiscriminate application of this approach may leave insufficient data for the planned analysis. As we discussed previously, the elimination of records is likely to bias the results of the study, because the revised data set describes the more regular events or cases, and omits patients who experience problems that may be related to the treatment.

2. *Calculate missing data from neighboring observations in a series.* Researchers can estimate a missing datapoint in a time sequence by calculating the sequence's average or by performing linear interpolation from two adjacent datapoints. When the difference is great, however, the average is apt to be misleading. The application of more complicated functions can help in some cases, but generally is more likely to introduce further problems. For example, if a patient was too ill to be tested, then the missing value is likely to be an extreme, rather than an average, value. Whenever missing values are estimated, subsequent computations must adjust the number of **degrees of freedom** used in the analysis because the computed data value provides no new information. Current statistical packages do not allow users to alter the degrees of freedom, and hence overestimate the significance of the experimental results.

3. *Infer missing data from related findings.* A human decision maker can infer missing data values from related information if she has knowledge about the underlying disease processes and about the natural courses of the diseases. She might examine several datapoints and infer what other information must be true at that point in time. For example, she might infer that a patient whose X-ray film shows dense areas in the lungs, whose sputum culture is positive for pneumococcus, and who has a high fever also had an elevated white-blood-cell count, because these symptoms typically coexist in patients with pneumonia. Likewise, she can infer missing information by examining patterns of data over time. For example, if pneumonia was confirmed by X-ray examination at one point in time, she can infer that the patient also had pneumonia during the intervening intervals in which the patient's temperature and white-blood-cell counts were abnormal. If the patient receives a treatment to relieve symptoms without effecting a cure, the physician might infer the continued existence of the disease. Researchers have experimented with methods for automatically abstracting higher-level concepts from low-level data [de Zegher-Geets et al., 1988]. This approach, however, has been applied to only limited problem areas.

Masked data also complicate the interpretation of the contents of databases. Some treatments simply alleviate symptoms without curing the underlying disease. If we assume that symptoms indicate disease, and if only the values of these variables are recorded in the database, then important information about the patient's true state is missing.

Consistency

Consistency is a third major parameter of data quality. In a consistent database, comparable data values have the same interpretation across patients and over time. Usually, there is little problem in obtaining consistent measurements of objective variables, such as temperature, height, and weight. However, the measurement of many medical data—for example, degree of functional activity, severity of illness, or extent of disease—depends on the subjective judgment of the observers (Figure 16.4). A clinical database may reflect significant inter- and intraobserver variation. As discussed in Chapter 6, the development of standard medical terminology and the explicit definition of subjective values is critical if computers are to store and manipulate meaningful data.

16.2.4 Problems with Collaborative Studies and Pooled Databases

Collecting sufficient data of high quality is problematic. Some studies—those in which, for example, the relationships among study variables are weak—require extremely large samples of patients. Long-term studies are subject to a high rate of attrition. For investigations of many diseases, a single researcher, or a single institution, sees too few patients with the disease to verify an experimental hypothesis. For these reasons, multiple institutions may join to create databases to be pooled and to participate in **cooperative clinical trials**. Although multiinstitutional studies solve the difficulty of gathering sufficient data, they aggravate problems of data inconsistency. Research centers must define a common vocabulary—a uniform descriptive set of variables that encompasses disease stratification, disease activity, interventions, and outcomes—to characterize patients for collaborative cross-center studies. In addition, they must establish and enforce common protocols for data collection and verification.

To formalize the study of many diseases, some professional societies have established coding committees. For example, the American Rheumatism Association defines over 400 data elements that describe attributes of the various rheumatic disease processes. These descriptors range from demographic information to symptoms, signs, laboratory-test values, diagnoses, and therapies. To evaluate adherence to the standards, the coding committees conduct periodic checks. Coders from one institution visit other sites to establish consistency and to recode selected data. Typical rates of disagreement reported from such validation programs range from 5 to 30 percent per record.

One way to build a large database is to pool smaller databases from several independent studies. Although pooling increases the overall sample size, data quality tends to suffer. The individual studies may have used different criteria for inclusion of patients in the experiment. For example, patients who were extremely ill might have been excluded from some studies, or the various clinics might be serving different age groups. Data collected by independent research groups also might differ semantically. For example, clinicians might use broader or narrower subjective assessments when determining diagnosis or assessing stage of disease. Finally, because the specific data sets were collected to satisfy different objectives, some studies may be missing values for one or more variables of interest. Even if the participating institutions agree to collect a minimum set of data elements, researchers may devote less effort to collecting information that is peripheral to their own study; thus, these

NCOG TOXICITY CRITERIA

		0	1	2	3	4
Pulm.	Radiation pneumonitis	None	X-ray changes. Minimal or no symptoms.	Moderate symptoms. No specific rx. required	Severe sx. Corticosteroid rx. initiated	Irreversible, severe disability
	PFT	None	25-50% decr. in Dco or VC	>50% decrease in Dco or VC		
	Clinical	None	Mild Sx	Moderate Sx	Severe Sx - Intermit. O_2	Assisted vent or continuous O_2
Cardiac		None	ST-T changes	Atrial arrhythmias	Mild CHF	Severe or refract CHF
		None	Sinus tachy >110 at rest	Unifocal PVC's	Multifocal PVC's	ventric tachy
				PEP/LVET >.42	Pericarditis	Tamponade
Neuro	PN	None	Decr DTR's or Absent Ankle Jerk	Absent DTR's excluding ankle jerk	Disabling sensory loss PN weakness (foot drop)	Resp dysfunction 2° to weakness
			Mild paresthesias	Mod. paresthesias	Severe paresthesias	Ileus
			Mild Constipation	Severe constipation	Severe PN pain	Paralysis - confining
				Mild weakness	Obstipation	pt to bed/wheelchair
					Severe weakness (<60% of normal	
					Bladder dysfunction	
	CNS	None	Mild anxiety	Severe anxiety	Confused or manic	Seizures
			Mild depression	Mod depression	Severe depression	Suicidal
			Mild headache	Mod headache	Severe headache	Coma
			Lethargy	Somnalence	Cord dysfunction	Brain necrosis
				Tremor	Confined to bed due to CNS dysfunction	Cord transection
				Mild hyperactivity	Leukoencephalopathy	
				Lhermitte's sign		
Skin		None	Slight erythema; Dry desquamation	Brisk erythema	Moist desquamation	Necrosis
Hair		None	Limited hair loss	Mod hair loss	Severe hair loss	Total alopecia

FIGURE 16.4 Oncologists can refer to Northern California Oncology Group (NCOG) definitional guidelines when assessing toxicity due to chemotherapeutic agents for patients on NCOG protocols. The development of such guidelines promotes consistency in the encoding of data values. [PFT = pulmonary function test, PN = peripheral nervous system, CNS = central nervous system.] (*Source:* Courtesy of the Northern California Oncology Group.)

variables may have a higher incidence of missing values and the values may be recorded less accurately.

16.2.5 The Linear Statistical Model

Once the data have been collected, researchers must develop a testable model that relates the observed outcomes to underlying causes. Such a model represents a possible relationship among the measured variables. For example, researchers may propose a causal relationship between an experimental intervention (medical, surgical, or behavioral) and a health outcome (probability of death, likelihood of experiencing a treatment-related complication, long-term functional status, and so on). They may postulate that certain patient characteristics are related to the chance of acquiring a disease; for example, they might propose that the risk of heart disease is a function of gender, age, smoking behavior, exercise history, family history, blood pressure, and cholesterol level.

The outcome variable is called the **dependent variable,** because its value *depends on* the experimental intervention and on the characteristics of the patient. In a study of an antihypertensive drug's effect on blood pressure, for example, the dependent variable could be systolic blood pressure after 6 months (or another appropriate measure, such as diastolic blood pressure). The variables that are believed to affect the outcome are called **independent variables.** The independent variables in this study are factors that can affect blood pressure, including

- *DRUG*, a variable that is set to 1 if the patient receives the drug, and to 0 if not
- *CHL*, the patient's total cholesterol level (in milligrams per deciliter)
- *WGT*, the patient's weight (in kilograms)
- *SEX*, a variable that is set to 1 for men, and to 0 for women
- *AGE*, the patient's age (in years)

A linear model relating the effects of the independent variables on the change in blood pressure (*ChBP*) has the following form:

$$ChBP = b_1 DRUG + b_2 CHL + b_3 WGT + b_4 SEX + b_5 AGE + \text{error}$$

where b_1, b_2, b_3, b_4, and b_5 represent the effects on blood pressure of the antihypertensive drug, cholesterol level, weight, gender, and age, respectively.

The general form of a linear statistical model is

$$y = b_1 x_1 + b_2 x_2 + \ldots + \epsilon$$

where y is the dependent variable, the x_is are the independent variables, $[b_1 \ldots b_n]$ are the values of the coefficients, and ϵ is the **error**—the variance in y that cannot be explained by the variance in the x_is. The objective of the analysis is to determine the values of the coefficients $[b_1 \ldots b_n]$—that is, the magnitude of the effects of each of $[x_1 \ldots x_n]$ on y. Clinical researchers typically apply statistical techniques to determine the values and to assess the statistical significance of these coefficients.

Researchers encounter a variety of problems when building and testing models. Among the most common problems are the following:

- *Omitted variables.* Important variables that affect outcome may not have been recorded (for example, nutrition history) or may be unobservable (for example, genetic makeup). Failure to include variables with significant effects increases the uncertainty of the results of the study.

- *Incorrect model specification.* Researchers may make incorrect assumptions of linearity when, in fact, more complex relationships are appropriate. For example, increasing the dose of a drug initially might produce a steady increase in the effectiveness of the drug therapy. At some threshold level, however, the body will be unable to metabolize additional drug—thus, administering more drug will provide no increase in therapeutic benefit.

- *Large unexplained variance.* Often, medical relationships are characterized by **weak models** in which many variables have small effects on the outcome; no single variable can explain a large portion of the result, and much of the difference in outcome remains unexplained even after all likely predictors have been identified. For example, risk factors for breast cancer include a family history of breast cancer, no births, exposure to ionizing radiation, early menarche, late menopause, obesity, and chronic cystic disease of the breast. Even after we have accounted for these and other known risk factors, however, whether a particular woman will eventually develop breast cancer will still be uncertain.

- *Correlation among independent variables.* Some predictor variables may be closely related (for example, low socioeconomic status often is correlated with poor nutrition). If several highly correlated variables are included in the model, then disentangling their separate effects on outcome is difficult. As a consequence, the estimates of their coefficients may fail to reach statistical significance.

In all these cases, researchers may respond by building more complex models.

16.3 History of Clinical Research Systems

The development of computer-based systems to support clinical research is inexorably intertwined with the development of the medical record. By the late 1950s, researchers were already transcribing clinical data from paper medical records and were using computers' superior data-processing power to perform statistical analyses. Storage and processing were costly; therefore, data elements were selected carefully. Furthermore, poor reliability and limited storage capacity forced investigators to store their data offline on punch cards or magnetic tape; the data were loaded only for the analysis itself. As a result, most clinical research was limited to the analysis of a few variables collected from small sample populations.

In the early 1960s, two related developments changed the scope of clinical research activities. The development of time-sharing operating systems (see Chapter 4) allowed multiple users to share data and programs and to communicate with the computer interactively. The availability of magnetic-disk storage devices enabled rapid and shared access to relatively large data files. The ability to manage large numbers of data encouraged the development of packages of statistical analysis programs, such as BMD, PSTAT, SPSS, and SAS. Researchers used these packages to perform complex statistical analyses, to generate reports, and to display data graphically—they had only to specify the names of the procedures and the variables of interest. In addition to statistical routines, these packages also provided utilities for reformatting data files, sorting observations, creating subsets, and updating data files. Recently, many of these packages have been rewritten for use on PCs, putting sophisticated data-analysis capabilities in the hands of individual researchers.

As clinical research gained prominence, computer systems were developed that aided not only in data management and analysis, but also in other aspects of the clinical research process. One example was ACME, which supported the development of the Time Oriented Database (see Section 16.4.1). These systems permitted, for the first time, direct interaction between clinicians and computer, and produced many insights that contributed to the field of medical informatics [Crouse and Wiederhold, 1969]. To satisfy the data-collection and audit requirements for evaluation of new drugs, pharmaceutical companies adapted commercial database systems or developed in-house systems to monitor the data-collection process carefully. These systems created detailed audit trails by recording with every piece of data the identity of the data collector, the information source, and the date and time of acquisition.

Increases in the number and complexity of RCTs have produced a growing need for computer systems to support the management of the experiments themselves. For example, a Protocol Selection Module (PSM) helps clinicians to identify appropriate clinical trials for their cancer patients from among the hundreds of ongoing studies being conducted by the Eastern Cooperative Oncology Group, a cooperative research group composed of over 400 institutions ranging from community-based practices to specialized cancer centers [James et al., 1986]. PSM matches patient characteristics with study-eligibility requirements and performs formal eligibility verification before registering a patient in an RCT. Another research system, the Boston University Tracking System, was designed to track and schedule subjects for follow-up interviews during a long-term clinical trial, thus facilitating more complete collection of follow-up data [Coffman et al., 1987].

Other systems have been developed to assist clinicians in providing treatment in adherence to complicated protocols. For example, Wirtschafter and associates implemented a consultant-extender system that enables community physicians participating in the Alabama Breast Cancer Project to deliver chemotherapy to patients who have breast cancer [Wirtschafter et al., 1985]. The computer generates patient-specific protocol forms that indicate the data to be collected, the recommended doses of drugs, and the appropriate rules for drug administration. The system monitors patients' responses to therapy and modifies its recommendations on a visit-by-visit basis using an encoded clinical algorithm. Similarly, oncologists at the Stanford University Medical Center use the ONCOCIN system (see Chapter 15) to treat their patients in accordance with cancer-chemotherapy protocols [Shortliffe, 1986]. Expert critical-care physicians at the LDS Hospital in Salt Lake City developed detailed protocols for the management of patients in the ICU who were receiving experimental therapy for Acute Respiratory Distress Syndrome (ARDS). The protocols, which were implemented on an existing hospital information system (the HELP system; see Chapters 7 and 15), were used to generate treatment instructions and to remind physicians and nurses of the need to perform diagnostic tests [Sittig, 1987].

As computer-based medical records become more common, the body of clinical data readily available for research grows. Many data in the medical record are of potential interest to clinical researchers because they represent information about patient characteristics, medical interventions, and medical outcomes. Currently, some institutions are adapting their medical-record systems to support research as well as patient care. For example, the Beth Israel Hospital in Boston has implemented a system called ClinQuery to allow researchers to retrieve the records of patients who meet specified criteria (age, gender, diagnosis, surgical procedure, length of hospital stay, and so on) [Safran et al., 1989].

Computer-based systems capable of managing and analyzing clinical information are just beginning to be marketed commercially. It is not clear, however, to what extent clinical researchers will rely on these commercial DBMSs. Lack of modularity in the design of current generation DBMSs makes major adaptation impossible. Furthermore, the development and manipulation of databases on mainframe computers are complex and costly undertakings. The availability of database software that runs on microcomputers and that can be integrated with PC-based statistical packages for data analysis is making it easier and more economical for researchers to perform clinical investigations.

16.4 Current Clinical Research Systems

Computer systems that support clinical research offer three basic options: (1) databases developed inhouse, (2) databases available commercially, and (3) specialized systems for clinical research.

Do-it-yourself systems offer researchers the most flexibility; the systems can be custom-tailored to meet the goals of the research project. This option, however, rarely produces comprehensive clinical research systems. Typically, utilities for data sharing, quality control, and backup are primitive or nonexistent, because the development of these programs would divert resources away from the primary research. Many of the currently available systems were developed inhouse to support specific clinical research projects. Today, however, inhouse development must promise a significant improvement over commercial databases and special-purpose clinical research systems if it is to warrant the risk and the investment in money and time.

General commercial DBMSs require little programming and adequately support data entry, retrieval, and long-term storage. A plethora of products is available for use on various computers ranging from microcomputers to mainframes. Statistical analysis tends to be poorly supported by commercial systems; most such systems support little more than the computation of averages. Researchers typically must extract subsets of data from the DBMS, then use these subsets as input to general statistical packages.

Specialized database and analysis systems have been developed to support clinical research. We shall briefly describe six systems in this third category: the MEDLOG system; the American Rheumatism Association Medical Information System (ARAMIS); the Duke University Cardiovascular Disease Database; the Eastern Cooperative Oncology Group (ECOG) and the Cancer and Leukemia Group B (CALGB) system; PROPHET; and CLINFO+. These systems incorporate many services that are necessary for clinical research. They are, however, more costly initially than are general statistical packages.

16.4.1 MEDLOG

MEDLOG is an interactive, time-oriented database system used to store and analyze longitudinal clinical data [McShane and Fries, 1988]. Adapted in 1982 by the Information Analysis Corporation, MEDLOG is the microcomputer-based version of Time Oriented Database (TOD), a database-management system developed at Stanford University School of Medicine under ACME during the 1970s to support clinical research on mainframe computers [Weyl, 1975]. In addition to software for entering, updating, storing, and retrieving clinical information, MEDLOG provides built-in statistical programs for data analysis, and supports the creation of data files for analysis using standard statistical packages. The system's representation and syntax explicitly recognize the importance of the time dimension in clinical observations, a feature lacking in traditional statistical-support systems.

TOD was originally developed to facilitate clinical research on chronic disease. Thus, the TOD (and MEDLOG) databases are structured to store patient information that has been collected over the course of multiple clinic visits. Conceptually, these data are organized in a two-level hierarchy—the first level corresponds to patients, whereas the second level corresponds to these patients' clinic visits. Each datapoint is defined by three coordinates: patient, variable, and time point (visit). Figure 16.5 graphically represents the three-dimensional structure of MEDLOG's time-oriented databases.

MEDLOG stores data values in a set of linked data files. For data entry and retrieval of individual patient information, data items are stored in a file that is organized by patient. This organization is similar to the traditional paper-chart approach to recording clinical data. For analysis purposes, data elements are grouped by variable to provide rapid access to all values of a particular variable (Figure 16.6). Because two file systems are used, access time is minimized for both individual and aggregate data operations. Data are transferred from the entry files to the analysis files using a batch utility program, which is typically run daily.

A common feature of MEDLOG and TOD is the importance placed on the time dimension. For example, researchers can use basic commands to instruct the system to retrieve records in which a particular parameter changes by a specified percentage within a specified time window, or in which the parameter increases or decreases by a specified amount following a specified event. Both MEDLOG and TOD were designed to be used by medical researchers who do not have knowledge of computer programming; users can perform retrieval operations by responding to prompts and selecting options from menus.

Both MEDLOG and TOD are schema-driven systems. As we discussed in Chapter 4, a schema is a machine- and human-readable description of the contents of the databases. The schema contains information on each variable's data type, units of

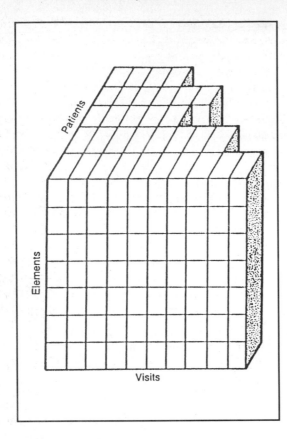

FIGURE 16.5 Conceptually, MEDLOG's time-oriented databases represent three-dimensional cubes of information. Researchers can access each datapoint by specifying three coordinates: patient, variable, and time point (visit). (*Source:* Reprinted by permission of the *Western Journal of Medicine.* Fries, J. F. and McShane, D. J. ARAMIS (The American Rheumatism Association Medical Information System)—A prototypical national chronic-disease data bank, 1986, December, 145, 801.)

measurement, range limits, and coding requirements. Researchers use the schema (indirectly through the applications programs) to access data by name rather than by location, and thus are insulated from changes in the underlying structure of the database. In addition, the applications programs can refer to the schema when doing error checking, performing calculations, and formatting information for output.

MEDLOG supports a variety of applications for creating databases, for selecting subgroups of observations and variables for analysis, and for performing statistical analyses. For example, the database administrator uses an interactive procedure to give MEDLOG the information it needs to construct the database schema. Programs allow the administrator to organize groups of variables for data entry in simple tabular form or on custom-formatted entry screens. Data-entry personnel can enter new data and can produce listings of patient data. Researchers can make subgroups for comparison or create files that contain subsets of observations and variables for analysis. In addition, a variety of statistical procedures (such as calculation of frequencies and means, and survival analysis) and display programs can be applied to produce statistics and graphical presentations of features of the underlying data. Recent additions to MEDLOG include double-entry verification, audit-trail logs, a report-writing facility, and presentation-quality graphics.

Patient-ID	pH	pCO$_2$	pO$_2$	NA	K	CL
123-132	7.44	39	111	131	3.7	95
142-633	7.41	36	137	134	5.6	105
208-926	7.39	41	126	141	4.1	101
214-411	7.45	42	131	137	4.4	97
286-004	7.40	37	120	133	3.9	93

Patient-ID	123-132	142-633	208-926	214-411	286-004
pH	7.44	7.41	7.39	7.45	7.40
pCO$_2$	39	36	41	42	37
pO$_2$	111	137	126	131	120
NA	131	134	141	137	133
K	3.7	5.6	4.1	4.4	3.9
CL	95	105	101	97	93

FIGURE 16.6 The data-transposition process reorganizes patient data so that each record in the data file contains the values associated with a single variable, rather than those associated with a single patient.

16.4.2 ARAMIS

The American Rheumatism Association Medical Information System (ARAMIS) is a nationwide database system developed by researchers at the Stanford University Medical Center in the early 1970s [Fries and McShane, 1986]. The system was founded on the premise that solutions to the problems of chronic diseases require large databanks of high-quality longitudinal data to support long-term studies of health outcomes. Thus, ARAMIS databases contain information about the long-term clinical courses of patients who have arthritis and rheumatic diseases and who have been observed in the clinical setting. Over the years, ARAMIS researchers have gathered detailed information on over 22,000 patients who have made more than 183,000 clinic visits to 17 institutions [McShane and Fries, 1988]. These data are stored in longitudinal clinical databases.

ARAMIS originally used TOD for data management and analysis. Beginning in 1985, however, the research group began to convert the TOD databases on the main-frame computer to MEDLOG databases on microcomputers. Today, ARAMIS researchers use TOD, MEDLOG, and a PC version of SAS to conduct studies on rheumatic disease. ARAMIS includes not only the clinical data and the programs to manipulate these data, but also a set of evolving investigational methods for studying chronic-disease databanks. The staff researchers carry out and publish about 40 studies each year.

16.4.3 Duke University Cardiovascular Disease Database

Since the early 1970s, Rosati and colleagues at Duke University Medical Center have been developing a clinical research database of information on patients who have documented or suspected ischemic heart disease [Rosati et al., 1975]. Similar to ARAMIS, the Duke project supports the long-term collection of data on patients who have chronic diseases. Its goal is to produce a rich database that is a tool for long-term research and for clinical management of individual patients.

The cardiovascular database contains several thousand variables, including demographic, history, and physical-examination data, as well as data on symptoms, signs, cardiac rhythms, hematology and chemistry studies, ECG recordings, X-ray examinations, exercise testing, echocardiography, and cardiac catheterization. Computer-generated forms prescribe the data to collect and are used by the health-care staff as the latter work up patients who are treated in the coronary-care unit or who are admitted for diagnostic catheterization. Clerical personnel enter the results and findings into the system, which generates summary notes automatically. After discharge, the researchers interview patients (or their families) annually to collect follow-up information on functional status, complications, medications, and survival, or on cause of death.

The cardiovascular database can be used to explore general research questions; many studies have used it to examine the relationship between various risk factors and patient outcomes. One research strategy is to segment patients into homogeneous subgroups that have common clinical courses or similar probabilities of disease or death. In one such study, researchers examined 23 clinical characteristics in 3627 consecutive, symptomatic patients referred for cardiac catheterization between 1969 and 1979. They identified nine factors that were important in estimating the likelihood that a patient had significant coronary-artery disease [Pryor et al., 1983a]. Clinicians can use estimates such as these when interpreting tests and selecting among alternative therapies (see the discussion of clinical prediction rules in Chapter 3). In a more recent study, researchers used the database to study changes over time in the relative efficacy of surgical versus medical treatment of coronary-artery disease [Pryor et al., 1987].

The database is also used to improve the care of individual patients. Based on history and physical examination data and the results of diagnostic tests, such as cardiac catheterization, the system generates *prognostigrams* that describe the expected outcome for a new patient based on the experience of similar patients in the database (Figures 16.7 and 16.8). These prognostigrams are generated automatically for tread-

```
                                                      Patient, Sample
                                                            Z99999

              HISTORY AND PHYSICAL EXAMINATION FINDINGS

Age ................................................................. 60
Sex ............................................................... Male
Type of chest pain ............................................ Typical
Course of chest pain ........................................... Stable
Average number of episodes of pain per week ......................... 2
Experiences nocturnal chest pain .................................. No
Duration of CAD (in months) ......................................... 2
Previous history of MI ........................................... Yes
History of smoking (smokes now OR > 1/2 pack/day in past 5 yrs) . Yes
History of Hyperlipidemia .......................................... No
History of Diabetes mellitus ...................................... No
History of Hypertension .......................................... Yes
History of Cerebral vascular disease .............................. No
History of Peripheral vascular disease ............................ No
History of Congestive heart failure ............................... No
NYHA Severity code for CHF (1-4) .................................N/A
Systolic BP (in mm Hg) ............................................ 150
Presence of Carotid bruit ......................................... No
Presence of S3 gallop ............................................. No
Cholesterol level (Enter '0' if you don't know) .................... 0
Cardiomegaly -- generalized or left vent. enlargement ............ No
STTW changes on ECG ............................................... No
Diagnostic Q-Waves on ECG ........................................ Yes
Presence of Intraventricular conduction disturbance............. None
Presence of PVC'S on 12-lead resting ECG ......................... No

                     CATHETERIZATION FINDINGS

Ejection Fraction (%) .............................................. 41
Mitral Insufficiency Grade (0=NO OR 1-4) ........................... 0
Left Main Stenosis (%) ............................................. 0
Stenosis of Proximal LAD (%) ...................................... 75
Number of diseased vessels (1-3) ................................... 3
```

FIGURE 16.7 Researchers at Duke University Medical Center have developed a model to classify patients in clinical subgroups with similar prognosis, based on data stored in the computer-based medical record. This report displays a subset of one patient's data, including medical history information, physical findings, and the results of cardiac catheterization. (*Source*: Courtesy of David Pryor, M.D., Duke University Medical Center.)

mill tests; physicians may request reports for cardiac catheterization. The estimated probabilities of survival for medical and surgical treatments are calculated using a statistical model that has been developed and validated by Duke researchers.

16.4.4 The ECOG/CALGB System

The Division of Biostatistics and Epidemiology at the Dana Farber Cancer Institute of the Harvard School of Public Health provides data-processing and data-analysis services to research groups that conduct RCTs, primarily the Eastern Cooperative Oncology Group (ECOG) and the Cancer and Leukemia Group B (CALGB) [McFadden, 1988]. The system supports every aspect of the clinical research process, from data collection, updating, and error checking, to data retrieval and analysis. Although most of the software is general purpose, the overall system was specifically designed to support the activities of cooperative research groups. The system's flexible modular architecture allows researchers to incorporate new group studies and to add new data formats quickly.

```
                                      NAME:   Patient, Sample
                                      HX NO: Z99999
                                      DUKE MD:   Duke
                                      CATH DATE:  12/20/88



                    PROGNOSTIC EVALUATION

                 DUKE CARDIOVASCULAR DATABANK

         The  predicted  survival  after  surgical  and  nonsurgical
      therapy for this patient is given below:



                  Estimated Probabilities of Survival
                  --------- -------------- -- --------

                          Medical              Surgical
                          -------              --------

            6-Month        0.96                  0.95
            1-Year         0.94                  0.95
            2-Year         0.89                  0.94
            3-Year         0.84                  0.93
            4-Year         0.79                  0.92
            5-Year         0.75                  0.91




      Note:  Estimates  for  surgical treatment are based  on  patients
             undergoing non-emergent aortocoronary bypass surgery.
             Estimates are based on cardiovascular death only.




                         Reviewed by:


                         _____
```

FIGURE 16.8 This prognostigram provides estimates of a patient's medical and surgical prognosis based on the experience of similar patients whose data are stored in the Duke University Cardiovascular Disease Database. (*Source*: Courtesy of David Pryor, M.D., Duke University Medical Center.)

Health professionals at member institutions complete computer-generated data forms each time they see a study patient. They send the forms to the group's statistical center, where the forms are logged and checked for completeness. In addition, data managers perform extensive manual checking to ensure that the data have been recorded accurately and consistently. They verify, among other things, that the patient was eligible for the study, that the treatment was given according to protocol, that all required data items were completed, that drug toxicities were reported correctly, and that there was adequate documentation to evaluate tumor response to therapy. Queries about the data and requests for more information are sent back to the contributing institution.

The statistical center updates the patient files nightly by running the updating program in batch mode. Interactive updating is also possible for corrections that must be made immediately. During an update run, the computer may calculate new data items—for instance, survival time. Both the calculated items and the primary items are checked with automated error-checking procedures, including type, range, and logical-consistency checking. The system also checks that values have been provided for all required fields, and generates exception reports that describe the data errors that have been detected. Once the data managers have corrected errors and resolved discrepancies, the new input data are merged into the master study data files. These study files are stored in a relational-database structure, using the INGRES DBMS. Multiple backup copies of the data files are created and are stored in remote locations to allow recovery of data in the event of hardware or software failure.

Two features of the system allow users to retrieve and manipulate data easily: the Data Dictionary and the BCROSS data-retrieval system. The *schema files* of the Data Dictionary specify the data formats, field widths, and allowable values that are used by the editing, updating, and retrieval programs. Applications programs refer to information in the Data Dictionary; thus, the structure of the database can grow dynamically without user applications being affected. Users can easily access the data and are insulated from changes in data formats and record structures. A database administrator is responsible for managing the Data Dictionary and maintaining the data files. The system builds data-entry screens automatically by accessing the Data Dictionary.

The BCROSS retrieval system is a collection of programs that allows users to retrieve data in the study data files, without having detailed knowledge about data formats and without writing INGRES data-retrieval routines. To specify the desired output, the user indicates the study or studies of interest, and enters a list of the data items to be retrieved. The BCROSS software refers to the Data Dictionary to locate the data, then creates an output data file. In addition to the output data file, the system generates a description file that contains information about the formats and labels associated with the retrieved data. Report-generation and data-analysis programs refer to the description file. Researchers can analyze the databases using programs such as SPSS, the IMSL subroutine library, and many specialized programs developed inhouse for analysis of clinical-trial data.

16.4.5 PROPHET

The PROPHET system was developed and maintained by Bolt Beranek Newman, Inc., and is supported by funding from the Division of Research Resources of the NIH [Raub, 1984]. PROPHET was designed to support research on interactions between chemical substances and biological processes. It provides pharmacologists, immunologists, endocrinologists, and other researchers in the life sciences with computational tools for managing and analyzing chemical and biological data. Researchers can use the DBMS to store and manipulate scientific spreadsheets and graphic data (including three-dimensional configurations). They can perform statistical and mathematical data analyses, and they can create and manipulate biological and molecular models. The system also provides access to the GenBank Genetic Sequence Data Bank and other databases. In addition, PROPHET's tabular data structures can be used to store clinical information. Investigators have used the system to conduct a variety of clinical studies, including studies of maternal mortality and of Legionnaires' disease. PROPHET currently runs on the Sun-3 family of workstations; a microcomputer version of the system is sold commercially as RS/1.

16.4.6 CLINFO+

The CLINFO+ system for clinical research was developed by the Rand Corporation under NIH sponsorship and is now supported and maintained by Bolt Beranek Newman, Inc. [King, 1986]. Originally designed as a tool for research on clinical protocols, the system has evolved to meet the demands of more general biomedical research. CLINFO+ supports the storage and retrieval of time-oriented data and provides software for performing worksheet calculations and manipulations, as well as basic statistical computations. It also provides links to pass data to statistical packages for more sophisticated analysis and a procedural language for programming specialized data-manipulation procedures.

16.5 The Future of Clinical Research Systems

The ongoing development of new drugs, surgical procedures, and medical devices is rapidly expanding the range of therapies that physicians can use to treat their patients. At the same time, the availability of the new technologies raises questions concerning their relative efficacy, safety, and cost-effectiveness. In addition, the increasing importance of chronic diseases (such as cancer, atherosclerosis, arthritis, emphysema, and cirrhosis) in terms of population morbidity and mortality creates a need to determine the risk factors for, evolution over time of, and effective treatments of these diseases. Thus, there is a growing demand for the collection and analysis of large bodies of clinical data. The existence of online databases will facilitate research on new approaches to analyzing clinical data. To address this increasing demand, researchers are developing methods for automating both the summarization of medical records and the discovery and validation of new medical relationships.

16.5.1 Automated Abstraction from Clinical Data

As we discussed in Section 16.2.3, missing data pose a significant problem for clinical researchers; the indiscriminate application of traditional statistical methods to incomplete sets of data carries a danger of producing biased results. Clinicians are able to piece together a view of a patient's health status over time by reasoning about the underlying disease processes and the manifestations of the disease. Because a single disease can be associated with multiple abnormal findings, many clinical data are correlated. Thus, much redundant information exists, even in incomplete medical records. The automated abstraction of higher-level conceptual entities—diseases and syndromes—from low-level data (such as laboratory-test values and physical findings) could help to reduce the problem of missing data, which is so common in clinical research.

Investigators on the RADIX Project at Stanford University have used several artificial-intelligence (AI) techniques to identify higher-level disease processes from the primitive observations recorded in a patient database. One prototype system was designed to summarize a patient's health status over time in terms of high-level disease descriptions, such as renal failure, urinary-tract infection, and glomerulonephritis [Downs et al., 1986]. The program searched the data in the database, detected abnormal values, generated hypotheses to explain the findings, examined evidence for and against the high-level diseases, and estimated for each clinic visit the likelihood that disease was present at the time (see Figure 6.8).

Later, the researchers tried an alternative approach. The IDEFIX system uses a three-level hierarchy of abnormal primary attributes (APAs), abnormal states, and diseases to derive increasingly abstract medical concepts from the primitive observations [de Zegher-Geets et al., 1988]. IDEFIX first infers the existence of APAs from the values of stored data elements, based on the normal ranges and expected values of the laboratory tests and physical findings. In the next step, the system determines the existence of abnormal states from sets of APAs. Finally, it draws conclusions about the presence of diseases by examining combinations of abnormal states. IDEFIX also provides a mechanism that allows the existence of previous episodes of illness or past history of disease to affect the likelihood that disease is present at the current time.

The objectives of research in automated abstraction are three: (1) to deal with data overload by reducing many data items to a much smaller number of items of information, (2) to compute automatically the intensity and certainty associated with each finding, and (3) to mitigate problems caused by missing data. As clinical databases grow, automated intelligent processing will become essential.

16.5.2 Automated Discovery of Medical Relationships

The availability of large databases of online clinical information creates a temptation to researchers to sift the data in search of as-yet-unrecognized relationships. Investigators can use existing data-analysis programs to graph correlations, to plot the values of variables over time, to match and compare summary statistics for patient subpopulations, and so on. The results of some of these analyses may suggest interactions among variables, and may spur the researcher to generate new hypotheses. Because this practice carries some risk of discovering correlations that occur purely by chance, researchers should use only part of a database for hypothesis generation, and should use the remaining data for subsequent confirmation of the relationships.

The development of automated discovery programs would allow investigators to comb existing databases to generate hypotheses for later verification. One such program, RX, succeeded in replicating many known medical relationships, including some findings not previously known to the investigators [Walker and Blum, 1986].

The program used data from 1700 patients in the ARAMIS database. RX consisted of two parts: a discovery module and a study module. The discovery module identified possible causal relationships in patient records by looking exhaustively at time-lagged, nonparametric correlations among variables. The output of the module was a list of possible relationships ranked by the strength of their correlations. This ranked list was then passed to the study module, which tested the hypotheses by performing biostatistical studies. Later work on the RADIX project combined two approaches: the development and application of statistical tools for exploratory data analysis, and the development of AI techniques that apply medical knowledge and reasoning strategies, and thus emulate the reasoning of a physician while examining patient records.

In summary, technological advances in computer hardware and software have decreased the costs of data storage and processing, and thus have reduced the barriers to long-term storage of rich clinical data. The development of new techniques for analyzing longitudinal data also encourages the creation and maintenance of large clinical databases. In the future, such databases will become increasingly valuable resources as researchers rely on computers to capture, store, and analyze large numbers of clinical data.

Suggested Readings

Bailar, J. C. When research results are in conflict. *New England Journal of Medicine*, 313:1080, 1985.

> *This editorial describes the differences in sample populations and study methodologies that could explain why two large prospective clinical trials reached opposing conclusions about the effect of postmenopausal hormones on cardiovascular morbidity. (See the Wilson and Stampfer articles described later in this section.)*

Blum, R. L. and Wiederhold, G. Studying hypotheses on a time-oriented clinical database: An overview of the RX project. In Reggia, J. A. and Tuhrim, S. (eds), *Computer-Assisted Medical Decision Making*, vol 2. New York: Springer-Verlag, 1985.

> *This article describes RX, a computer program that uses statistical techniques to generate and test hypothetical relationships in the data. The program automates a skeletal subset of the knowledge-acquisition cycle depicted in Figure 16.1.*

Feinstein, A. R. An additional basic science for clinical medicine: I. The constraining fundamental paradigms; II. The limitations of randomized trials; III. The challenges of comparison and measurement; IV. The development of clinimetrics. *Annals of Internal Medicine*, 99(3):393, 99(4):544, 99(5):705, 99(6):843, 1983.

> *This series of four articles defines the conceptual basis for biomedical research, describes the limitations of the scientific method and randomized trials with respect to clinical research, and suggests methods for improving the quality of subjective clinical data.*

Fries, J. F. and McShane, D. J. ARAMIS (The American Rheumatism Association Medical Information System)—A prototypical national chronic-disease data bank. *Western Journal of Medicine*, 145:798, 1986.

> *This article discusses the reasons for maintaining chronic-disease databases, describes the development of the time-oriented database-management systems TOD and MEDLOG, and outlines the evolution of the ARAMIS system.*

Ingelfinger, J. A., et al. *Biostatistics in Clinical Medicine*, 2nd ed. New York: Macmillan, 1987.

> *The final two chapters of this book discuss criteria for evaluating the design, conduct, and analysis of clinical trials, and describe the application of published results to the care of individual patients. The bulk of the book prepares physicians to use and understand probability and statistics in diagnosis, treatment, and case followup. Each chapter presents at least one detailed clinical problem, then explains the quantitative methods that can be used to solve the problem.*

King, C. Data management systems in clinical research. In Javitt, J. (ed), *Computers in Medicine: Applications and Possibilities*. Philadelphia: W. B. Saunders, 1986.

> *This chapter describes general data-management systems, statistical packages, and specialized clinical-research systems, including dBase II, SAS, MEDLOG, and CLINFO. Other chapters in the book discuss the uses of computers in medical decision making, maintenance of medical records, automated history taking, bibliographic retrieval, and medical education.*

Pryor, D. B., et al. Clinical databases: Accomplishments and unrealized potential. *Medical Care*, 23:623, 1985.

> *The authors discuss the organization and characteristics of clinical databases, describe several successful systems, and review databases used for clinical research, patient care, and technology assessment. The article includes an extensive bibliography of references on clinical databases.*

Stampfer, M. J., et al. A prospective study of postmenopausal estrogen therapy and coronary heart disease. *New England Journal of Medicine*, 313:1044, 1985.

> *This article describes the methodology and results of a prospective study of the effects of estrogen therapy on the risk of coronary-artery disease in postmenopausal women. The study of over 121,000 female nurses, aged 30 to 50 years, found that the use of postmenopausal estrogens protected women against severe coronary-artery disease.*

Wiederhold, G. *Databases for Health Care*. New York: Springer-Verlag, 1981.

> *The author defines database terminology, explains the concepts of schemas and data models, and summarizes the basic database operations: entry, storage, retrieval, and presentation of data. He then describes current and future uses of health-care databases, including clinical-research applications. The appendix presents several examples of databases used in health-care settings.*

Wilson, P. W. F., Garrison, R. J., and Castelli, W. P. Postmenopausal estrogen use, cigarette smoking and cardiovascular morbidity in women over 50. *New England Journal of Medicine*, 313:1038, 1985.

> *This article describes the methodology and results of a prospective study of the influence of estrogen use on morbidity from cardiovascular disease. The study of over 1234 postmenopausal women, aged 50 to 83 years, found that the administration of female hormones (estrogens) substantially increased the rates of cardiovascular morbidity from stroke and myocardial infarction.*

Questions for Discussion

1. List examples of descriptive statistics, graphical presentations, and analytic statistical techniques. For what purposes are each of these techniques best suited?
2. Create a sample database that contains information on the heights, weights, and ages of 20 teenagers. Calculate simple descriptive statistics to summarize the data. Do you think your sample is typical of the overall population? Do the statistics

suggest questions for further investigation? Sketch a bar graph and a pie chart to illustrate one aspect of the data. Which presentation is more informative? Explain all your answers.

3. Briefly outline a study methodology for a prospective clinical trial to evaluate the effect of birth-control pills on a woman's risk of having a stroke or myocardial infarction. (You may wish to refer to the Stampfer and Wilson articles in the Suggested Readings.) Identify an appropriate sample population and specify the procedures for assigning subjects to subgroups and for collecting data. Indicate the dependent and independent variables in your experiment.

4. Discuss the ethical implications of using experimental therapies to treat terminally ill patients. Address the arguments for and against allowing dying patients voluntarily to take drugs with unknown benefits and side effects.

5. Discuss two advantages and two disadvantages of performing retrospective analyses on data pooled from multiple independent studies.

6. Why are missing data so common in clinical research? Why might statistical analyses of incomplete data sets produce biased results? How can researchers handle the problem of missing data?

17

Computers in Medical Education

Edward P. Hoffer and G. Octo Barnett

After reading this chapter, you should know the answers to these questions:

- What are the advantages of computer-aided instruction over traditional lecture-style instruction in medical education?
- How can computer-based simulations supplement students' exposure to clinical practice?
- How has computer-aided instruction evolved as a result of advances in computer hardware and software?
- What are the distinguishing features of drill-and-practice programs, computer-based simulations, and intelligent tutoring systems?
- What are the significant barriers to widespread integration of computer-aided instruction into the medical curriculum?

17.1 The Role of Computers in Medical Education

To practice medicine effectively, physicians must have rapid access to the contents of a large and complex medical knowledge base, and they must know how to apply these facts and heuristics to form diagnostic hypotheses and to plan and evaluate therapies. Thus, the goals of medical education are to convey a body of specific medical facts and to instruct students in general problem-solving strategies. Medical educators are increasingly aware of the need for all medical students to learn to use information technology for accessing and managing medical information—both patient-specific clinical data and more general scientific knowledge. Computers also can play a direct role in the education process; students may interact with educational computer programs to acquire factual information and to learn and practice medical problem-solving techniques. In addition, practicing physicians may use computers to expand and reinforce their professional skills throughout their careers. The application of computer technology to education is often referred to as **computer-aided instruction (CAI)**.

17.1.1 Changing Medical Practice and the Medical-School Curriculum

We can best appreciate the potential role of computers in medical education by considering the limitations of the typical medical-school curriculum with respect to ongoing changes in the state of medical knowledge and in the medical-practice environment. As we discussed in Chapter 14, the volume of medical knowledge is increasing rapidly. The medical literature documents our continuing progress in understanding the risk factors, causes, and manifestations of diseases, and the effects of various therapies on medical outcomes.

In recent years, clinical medicine has encompassed an enormous growth in the number of diagnostic procedures that physicians can perform, many costly and some dangerous for the patient. Likewise, the therapeutic armamentarium has become vastly larger, more complex, more expensive, and more hazardous to the patient. When choosing from a wide array of alternative drugs, physicians must understand the indications, contraindications, and possible side effects of the drugs, and they must avoid prescribing interacting combinations of drugs. At the same time, growing pressure to control health-care costs creates additional demands on physicians; today, health professionals must consider not only efficacy and risk to the patient, but also cost of the care, when choosing tests for a diagnostic workup and when planning treatments.

The traditional medical-school curriculum emphasizes the rote memorization of medical facts, and students typically are evaluated based on their ability to recall these facts. This practice is prevalent, even though factual recall is only one of the skills necessary for competent medical practice. Students tend to focus their learning on acquiring the information needed to pass the examinations. In the process, they may neglect the development of problem-solving skills that are crucial to medical practice, yet are rarely tested.

A second weakness of the traditional medical curriculum is its heavy reliance on the lecture method of teaching. Students assume the role of passive recipients of knowledge, even though educational theory suggests that people retain information better when they seek it actively, through questioning, reasoning, and experimentation. The increasing heterogeneity of entering medical-school classes has made the lock-step lecture-dominated strategy increasingly anachronistic. The primary reason for this emphasis on lecture-style teaching is logistic; faculty believe that it is simply too expensive to provide individual instruction to every student in a medical-school class.

Medical students learn clinical-practice skills by observing and eventually by participating with teams of physicians caring for patients on the wards of teaching hospitals. Growing concern about professional liability, however, has decreased the opportunity for students to assume meaningful responsibility for patients. Another factor that makes clinical education more difficult today than it was a generation ago is the disappearance from the teaching hospital of patients with less than critical disease, or with illnesses that illustrate many of the "typical" medical diseases. The teaching hospital has become predominantly a large intensive-care unit. A high proportion of its beds are filled by patients with acute cardiopulmonary disease. Many patients are chronically ill with multiple diseases, and many patients are terminally ill. In an era of cost containment, few patients are admitted to hospitals for a pure diagnostic workup; thus, many valuable teaching opportunities have been eliminated.

Medical school, internship, and residency are the first steps in a lifelong educational commitment. Physicians must prevent atrophy of existing skills and knowledge, and must continue to acquire new knowledge, to keep up with the rapidly changing field. To gain the mandatory continuing medical education (CME) credits, practitioners incur large expenses for course-enrollment fees, transportation, lodging, and time lost from medical practices. These problems were recognized by many medical educators; however, before the advent of powerful and inexpensive computers (and of communication networks), there was little opportunity to rectify the weaknesses of the typical course in continuing medical education.

How are students and experienced practitioners to acquire and maintain the knowledge necessary to function effectively in today's complex and rapidly changing medical environment? The response of the typical medical-school faculty has been to add more factual knowledge to the curriculum. Many thoughtful educators now realize that simply giving medical students more to learn is counterproductive; a better educational policy is to encourage students to become self-motivated and enlightened learners—to shift from a system dominated by a concern with remembering information to an environment in which students learn basic strategies for problem solving and techniques for accessing information as they need it. Some educators believe that the computer, with its superior memory and information-processing capabilities, will play a powerful role in this process.

This philosophy was embodied in the 1984 report by the Panel on the General Professional Education of the Physician (GPEP) of the Association of American Medical

Colleges. The GPEP report recommended that medical schools take the lead in applying information science and computer technology to medical learning, and promote the use of computers in medical schools [Association of American Medical Colleges, 1984]. No longer is it sufficient for medical schools to teach a static body of facts. Instead, students must learn to think, to solve problems, and to make decisions—they must learn to learn.

17.1.2 Advantages of Using Computers in Medical Education

The use of computers in education provides a means to avoid the limitations of fact-based, lecture-oriented teaching. The use of educational computer programs in the curriculum offers students the opportunity for active, independent learning, without substantially increasing the burden on faculty. Eventually, CAI will become an integral part of primary education in medical, nursing, and pharmacy schools. Furthermore, computer-based education systems can facilitate continuing education, can provide a means for assessing competency for licensing and recertification, and (in conjunction with monitoring and surveillance systems) even may provide a mechanism for integrating ongoing education with the patient-care process.

The following characteristics of CAI offer advantages over traditional methods of medical instruction and evaluation:

- *Interactive learning.* Well-written CAI materials force students to make choices and to answer questions. Students must think about and actively solve problems, rather than passively collect facts, as they often do when attending a lecture or when skimming a written page.

- *Immediate, student-specific feedback.* Because they are interactive, CAI programs can evaluate student responses and can provide immediate feedback on the correctness of the responses. Well-written programs provide justifications for correct answers; some programs may explain why a student's answer is incorrect. In addition, the privacy of the interaction frees students to learn without fear of being criticized or penalized for making mistakes.

- *Individually tailored instruction.* CAI is self-paced and is tailored to the abilities of individual students. Students can select materials to focus learning on areas of weakness. Most programs provide some form of help on request from the student— for example, students typically can interrupt a case simulation to request help in interpreting data and in deciding which action to pursue next. More sophisticated programs can detect student weaknesses by evaluating the student's responses, and can offer help when it appears to be needed, even if the student is unaware of that need. Self-administered exercises also remove limitations related to the availability of teachers. Thus, students can learn at their own convenience.

- *Objective testing.* CAI programs can test students' knowledge and problem-solving skills objectively and reproducibly. Students can use the results of testing for self-evaluation, or faculty can track and record student performance with minimal effort.

- *Entertaining.* Good CAI programs are fun to use! Students often learn more effectively when the interaction is entertaining as well as instructional, because they are motivated to continue the interaction. This aspect of education is often neglected—although not by the best teachers.

CAI also can relieve some of the problems inherent in teaching clinical medicine through experience on the wards of teaching hospitals. For example, CAI allows experimentation. The use of simulations allows students to develop and practice patient-care skills without danger or inconvenience to real patients. It provides greater scope for problem solving and decision making, and allows students to try "what-if" exercises. In computer-based simulations, the student can assume full clinical responsibility for patients (albeit simulated patients). Thus, students learn the effects of interventions through *doing,* rather than simply by reading or being told. Such experiences may create stronger and more lasting effects than do traditional learning techniques.

Computer-based simulations allow students to manage a greater number and variety of patient cases than are typically seen in teaching hospitals. In addition, CAI programs can simulate prototypical, as well as unusual or complex, cases. For the student on the wards for the first time, a patient with several major diseases who is receiving multiple medications can be overwhelming. Simulations can be designed to exemplify a single disease; students can tackle more complex cases as they gain experience.

Simulations also allow students to manage cases as diseases evolve over time. A student's ability to follow a patient does not need to be limited by the length of time a student is assigned to a particular rotation or by the patient's length of stay in the hospital. This ability to learn about disease evolution is particularly important for teaching the management of chronic disease, which is becoming a major part of medical practice due to the increase in the elderly population.

Finally, standard cases can be used to assess problem-solving competency according to objective criteria. A student can compare her own performance on these cases with that of her peers, as well as with that of experts. Furthermore, faculty can use performance on clinical simulations as a measure of the student's mastery of problem-solving skills. The National Board of Medical Examiners has been developing simulation programs with the plan that such simulations might be used in the board certification of physicians (see Section 17.4.1).

CAI, like every new methodology, is often challenged to prove its superiority over more established teaching methods. Lack of firm data to demonstrate such superiority has been one factor preventing the wider acceptance of CAI. Nonetheless, we know that one indication of success is acceptance by users. From its earliest days, CAI has been well accepted by most students and practitioners. In a recent study of 1200 sessions with CAI programs at the Massachusetts General Hospital, users judged 62 percent of the interactions as superior to lectures or textbooks, and rated only 8 percent as inferior. In 15 percent of the cases, the users thought the methods of teaching were too different to be compared [Hoffer et al., 1986].

Rarely is problem solving taught explicitly in the typical medical curriculum. Therefore, setting up experiments to compare the *effectiveness* of various methods of teaching problem solving is difficult. Several researchers, however, have performed studies to gain more objective proof of efficacy. For example, Hoffer and colleagues published a small study that demonstrated that nurses learned advanced cardiac life support more effectively from a computer program than they did from lectures [Hoffer et al., 1975]. The authors also demonstrated that CAI programs can favorably affect physician behavior. A study of the use of CAI in five community hospital emergency departments found that the appropriate use of medications emphasized in the programs rose substantially after the CAI material was made available [Hoffer, 1975]. Not all such studies have had such gratifying results. For example, researchers at the University of Wisconsin found that performance on patient simulations correlated only weakly with students' grades on final examinations and ward rotations, except on the most complex computer cases [Friedman et al., 1978]. Physicians' patterns of test ordering and therapy selection in a related study, however, were similar in computer simulations and in actual patient-care situations [Friedman, 1973].

17.2 A Historical Look at Computer-Aided Instruction

Pioneering research in CAI was conducted in the late 1960s at three primary locations: Ohio State University (OSU), Massachusetts General Hospital (MGH), and the University of Illinois. Earlier attempts to use computers in medical instruction were hindered by the difficulty of developing programs using low-level languages and the inconvenience and expense of running programs on batch-oriented mainframe computers. With the availability of time-sharing computers, these institutions were able to develop interactive programs that were accessible to users from terminals via telephone lines.

CAI research began at OSU in 1967 with the development of Tutorial Evaluation System (TES). TES programs typically posed constructed-choice, true–false, multiple-choice, matching, or ranking questions, then immediately evaluated the student's responses. The programs rewarded correct answers with positive feedback. Incorrect answers triggered corrective feedback, and, in some cases, the student was given another opportunity to respond to the question. If a student was not doing well, the computer would suggest additional study assignments or direct the student to review related materials.

In 1969, TES was incorporated into the evolving Independent Study Program (ISP), an experimental program that covered the entire preclinical curriculum and was designed to teach basic medical-science concepts to medical students [Weinberg, 1973]. Although the ISP did not use CAI in a primary instructional role, students in the program relied heavily on a variety of self-study aids and used the computer intensively for self-evaluation. The use of COURSEWRITER III, a high-level authoring language, facilitated rapid development of programs. By the mid-1970s, TES had a library of over 350 interactive hours' worth of instructional programs.

Beginning in 1970, Barnett and colleagues at the MGH Laboratory of Computer Science developed CAI programs to simulate clinical encounters [Hoffer et al., 1986]. The most common simulations were case-management programs that allowed students to formulate hypotheses, to decide which information to collect, to interpret data, and to practice problem-solving skills in diagnosis and therapy planning. By the mid-1970s, MGH had developed more than 30 case-management simulations, including programs for evaluation of comatose patients, for workup of patients with abdominal pain, and for evaluation and therapy management for problems such as anemia, bleeding disorders, meningitis, dyspnea, secondary hypertension, thyroid disease, joint pain, and pediatric cough and fever.

The MGH laboratory also developed several programs that used mathematical or qualitative models to simulate underlying physiologic processes, and thus to simulate changes in patient state over time and in response to students' therapeutic decisions. The first simulation modeled the effects of warfarin (an anticoagulant drug) and its effects on blood clotting. The system challenged the user to maintain a therapeutic degree of anticoagulation by prescribing daily doses of warfarin to a patient who has a series of complications and who was taking medications that interacted with warfarin. Subsequently, researchers developed a more complex simulation model to emulate a diabetic patient's reaction to therapeutic interventions.

About the same time, Harless and researchers at the University of Illinois were developing a system called Computer-Aided Simulation of the Clinical Encounter (CASE), which simulated clinical encounters between physician and patient [Harless et al., 1971]. The computer assumed the role of a patient; the student, acting in the role of practicing physician, managed the patient's disease from onset of symptoms through final treatment. Initially, the computer presented a brief description of the patient; then the student interacted with the program using natural-language queries and commands (Figure 17.1). The program was able to provide logical responses to most student requests. This feature added greatly to the realism of the interaction, and CASE programs were received enthusiastically by students. The TIME system, under development by Harless and researchers at the National Library of Medicine (NLM), extends CASE's approach to incorporate videodisc technology (see Section 17.4.2).

CAI programs proliferated on a variety of hardware, using a Babel of languages. A 1974 survey of the status of medical CAI identified 362 programs written in 23 different computer languages, ranging from BASIC, FORTRAN, and MUMPS, to COURSEWRITER III and PLATO. Little sharing of programs among institutions was possible because the task of transferring programs was typically as large as writing the material de novo. Thus, there was little opportunity to share the substantial costs of developing new CAI programs. The lack of portability of systems and the extreme expense of system development and testing served as barriers to the widespread use of CAI.

The establishment of a NLM-sponsored, nationwide network in 1972 was a significant event in the development of CAI in medicine because it allowed users throughout the country to access computer-based educational programs easily and relatively inexpensively. Previously, the programs created at OSU, MGH, and the University of Illinois were available to users in selected regions, over voice-grade telephone lines. Poor quality of transmission and high costs, however, combined to limit access to CAI programs by distant users. Acting on the recommendation of a committee of

COMPUTER: It's a Tuesday morning, the middle of a cold January. You have seen three patients in the clinic and now a fourth person is waiting for you in your office. The woman---middle-aged, white, brown hair---is sitting at the side of your desk as you open the door. Her features seem worn, and she is slightly underweight. She looks up and smiles at you with a minimum of enthusiasm and effort.

STUDENT: **What brings you to see me?**

COMPUTER: Well, I'm just tired all the time. I don't ever feel like I'm rested and all my energy is gone.

STUDENT: **How long has this been going on?**

COMPUTER: About six months ago I started feeling tired all the time. I finally felt like I had to do something about it.

STUDENT: **What did you do?**

COMPUTER: Are you still talking about my being tired?

STUDENT: **Yes.**

COMPUTER: Well, I've been taking vitamins, but they don't seem to help. Maybe you can give me something stronger.

STUDENT: **Is there anything else bothering you?**

COMPUTER: I guess my only real complaint is that I am tired all the time. I just don't have any energy at all anymore.

STUDENT: **Do you have any trouble sleeping?**

COMPUTER: I sleep like a log ... eight or nine hours every day.

<student presses a key on the terminal keyboard that indicates Physical Examination>

STUDENT: **Vital signs.**

COMPUTER: Temperature: 98.6. Pulse: 96. Respiration: 20.

STUDENT: **Tongue.**

COMPUTER: Tongue examination: Red, some atrophy of the papillae; full movement.

STUDENT: **Neck examination.**

COMPUTER: Neck: Trachea central; thyroid not palpable. No lymph node enlargement; no abnormal pulsation.

STUDENT: **Heart auscultation.**

FIGURE 17.1

COMPUTER: Heart auscultation: Auscultation performed in all appropriate positions. Normal sinus rhythm. Rate of 80/ min. S1 and S2 of good quality. No extra sounds, murmurs, rubs.

<*student presses the key that indicates History*>

STUDENT: Have you ever had any trouble with your heart?

COMPUTER: I've never had any heart trouble at all that I know of.

STUDENT: Has anyone in your family ever had heart trouble?

COMPUTER: No one in my family has ever been bothered by heart trouble.

<*student presses a key to return to the Physical Examination*>

STUDENT: Abdomen.

COMPUTER: Abdomen inspection: symmetrical, normal contour. No visible dilated veins, scars, or other abnormality.

<*student presses the key that indicates Laboratory*>

STUDENT: Complete blood count.

COMPUTER: Complete blood count: red blood cell count, 2.5 million; hemoglobin, 8.5 gm; hematocrit, 26; white blood cell count, 5100. Differential: neutrophils, 58; eosinophils, 2; basophils, 1; monocytes, 4; lymphocytes, 35.

STUDENT: Color of urine.

COMPUTER: Urine appearance: Yellow, clear.

STUDENT: PBI.

COMPUTER: Protein bound iodine: 6 mg.

STUDENT: Gastric analysis.

COMPUTER: Gastric analysis: fasting. 0 free acid; 10 mEq/l total; 45 minutes after histamine; stimulation: 0 free acid; 30 mEq/l total.

<*student presses the key that indicates Treatment*>

COMPUTER: Please type your diagnosis.

STUDENT: Pernicious anemia.

COMPUTER: Please prescribe your treatment.

STUDENT: Vitamin B12

COMPUTER: After three weeks symptoms begin to vanish.

FIGURE 17.1 A student using the CASE system, developed at the University of Illinois, assumes the role of a practicing physician in simulated encounters between physician and patient. The student poses natural-language queries to the system, which interprets the question and responds as best it can. This transcript is an example of such an interactive session. (*Source:* Reprinted with permission from Harless, W. G., et al. CASE: A computer-aided simulation of the clinical encounter. *Journal of Medical Education*, 46:443, 1971. The journal is now published under the name *Academic Medicine.*)

the Association of American Medical Colleges, the Lister Hill Center for Biomedical Communications of the NLM funded an experimental CAI network. Beginning in July 1972, the CAI programs developed at the MGH, OSU, and the University of Illinois Medical College were made available from these institutions' host computers over the NLM network using communication lines of the Tymshare network. During the first 2 years of operation, 80 institutions used the programs of one of the three hosts. The high demand for network use prompted the NLM to institute a stepped charge, first $2.50 and then $5 per hour of use, but use continued to rise. Having exhausted the funds set aside for this experiment, the NLM announced that the experimental phase would be terminated and that it would discontinue financial support for the network after May 1975.

As a vivid testimony to the value placed on the educational network by its users, MGH and OSU continued to operate the network as an entirely user-supported activity. The MGH programs are currently available nationwide and in foreign countries over the Telenet communications network. This service is available around the clock, 7 days per week; access to a terminal or personal computer that supports modem communications is the only hardware requirement. In addition, since November 1983, the MGH programs have been offered as the CME component of the American Medical Association's Medical Information Network (AMA/NET). AMA/NET provides to subscribing physicians a variety of services in addition to the CME programs, including access to information databases, to the clinical and biomedical literature, to the DXplain diagnostic decision-support tool (see Chapter 15), and to electronic-mail services. By 1986, approximately 100,000 physicians, medical students, nurses, and other people had used the MGH CAI programs over a network, with about 150,000 total contact hours.

During the early 1970s, medical schools around the country began to conduct research in CAI. One of the most interesting programs was the PLATO system (Programmed Logic for Automated Teaching Operations) developed at the University of Illinois. PLATO used a unique plasma-display terminal that allowed presentation of text, graphics, and photographs, singly or in combination. An electrically excitable gas was used to brighten individual points on the screen selectively. The system also included TUTOR, a sophisticated authoring language, to facilitate program development. By 1981, authors had created 12,000 hours of instruction in 150 subject areas. The programs received heavy use at the University of Illinois; some of them also were used at other institutions that had access to the system. The high cost of PLATO, and the need for specialized terminals and other computer hardware, however, limited the widespread dissemination of the system.

Research on medical applications of artificial intelligence (AI) stimulated the development of systems based on models of the clinical reasoning of experts. The explanations generated by computer-based consultation systems (for example, why a particular diagnosis or course of management is recommended) can be used in computer-based education to guide and evaluate students' performance in running patient simulations. The GUIDON system is one of the most provocative examples of such an intelligent tutoring system. GUIDON used a set of teaching-strategy rules, which interacted with an augmented set of diagnostic rules from the MYCIN expert system (see Chapter 15) to teach students about infectious diseases [Clancey, 1986]. Subsequently, researchers reorganized and extended MYCIN's knowledge base to form the NEO-MYCIN system by adding explicit knowledge about the process of diagnosis. The NEOMYCIN knowledge base was then used by GUIDON2 to teach students about diagnostic strategies (see Section 17.4.5).

Researchers at the University of Wisconsin applied a different approach to the simulation of clinical reasoning. Their system is used to assess the efficiency of a student's workup by estimating the cost of the diagnostic evaluation [Friedman et al., 1978]. In one of the few successful field studies that demonstrated the clinical significance of a simulated diagnosis problem, Friedman found significant levels of agreement between physicians' performance on simulated cases and actual practice patterns [Friedman, 1973]. Of considerable interest is the commitment of the National Board of Medical Examiners (NBME) to proceed with Friedman's original work by establishing a nationwide delivery system of computer-based evaluation and learning centers. Friedman's simulation model was the prototype for the CBX system, which is being developed by the NBME and will be used to test students' diagnostic skills in the National Board Part III examination (see Section 17.4.1).

The development of PCs, authoring systems, and network technology removed some of the barriers to program development and dissemination, and more CAI software became available. PCs provide an affordable and relatively standard environment for the development and use of CAI programs. The use of networks for program distribution has a number of major advantages. As a two-way medium, it permits users and courseware authors to exchange comments. This interchange is invaluable for finding program bugs and for improving the programs. It also facilitates frequent updating and enhancement of programs. Because users access the software stored on the host computer, the programs are easy to update and the newly modified version is immediately available to all users.

Network distribution is not without its limitations, however. A major disadvantage is the cost of network access. For example, the communications costs incurred by users of the MGH Education Network are nearly equal to the costs of hardware and course development incurred by the MGH host institution. Furthermore, the variety of terminals used over a network limits the program's ability to use graphics or any other techniques that depend on specific terminal characteristics. For these reasons, other modes of program distribution are attracting increasing interest.

A number of publishing firms are presently distributing medical programs (educational and other) via floppy disks. The MGH laboratory has arranged with the Williams & Wilkins Company to publish the programs currently distributed via the MGH Education Network for use on Apple and IBM personal computers as the RxDx series. *Scientific American Medicine* has published case-management problems on floppy disk (DISCOTEST). Likewise, a quarterly journal called *Cyberlog* began distributing programs on floppy disk for Apple and IBM-series computers in the summer of 1985. These programs contain tutorials, case studies, and a series of tools, or calculation aids, that can be used by physicians for independent study. The Universities of Washington and Georgia each distribute case-management problems on floppy disks. In addition, faculty at a number of different medical schools have developed and distributed single examples of medical computer-based educational material on floppy disks. Most of the general-circulation medical journals currently carry advertisements for CAI material on floppy disk, and some software reviews have appeared in the *New England Journal of Medicine,* in the *Annals of Internal Medicine,* and in other respected journals. The unaccredited material is of uneven quality, however, and a peer-review process is needed urgently.

17.3 Fundamental Issues in Computer-Aided Instruction

The goals of medical education are to teach students specific facts and information and to teach strategies for applying this knowledge appropriately to the situations that arise in medical practice. Thus, students must learn about physiological processes, and must understand the relationships between their observations and these underlying processes. They must learn to perform medical procedures, and they must understand the effects of different interventions on health outcomes. Medical-school faculty employ a variety of strategies for teaching, ranging from the lecture-based one-way transmission of information to the interactive Socratic method of instruction. In general, we can view the teaching process as the *presentation* of a situation or a body of facts that contains the essential knowledge that students should learn; the *explanations* of what are the important concepts and relationships, how can they be derived, and why are they important; and the *strategy* for guiding the interaction.

The goals of instruction and the choices among teaching strategies are reflected in the overall design of CAI programs (fact-oriented drill-and-practice approach versus process-oriented simulation approach) and in the structure and style of the interaction between student and program (relative control of student versus program in structuring the interaction, and degree of guidance provided by the system).

17.3.1 Types of Computer-Aided Instruction Systems

The earliest computer-based education programs were based on the **drill-and-practice** method of teaching. These programs were essentially electronic implementations of programmed-learning texts. Typically, they presented a medical case or other textual material, then posed a series of questions that tested students' understanding of the material. Some of these programs used **branching questioning** to tailor the interaction to the student: The authors of programs anticipated possible answers and designated the next question to ask, given a student's answer. For example, if the student answered incorrectly, the program could ask more questions on the same subject, or could present another similar case. Conversely, if the student demonstrated clear understanding of the material, then the program would automatically move on to new material. Thus, the system's behavior depended on the branching algorithm and on the history of the student's actions.

Simulations are the basis for most CAI programs used today. These programs are designed to help a student learn by *doing.* They emphasize learning procedures and problem-solving strategies. Simulation programs now are available to help students learn to take medical histories, to diagnose illnesses, to perform clinical procedures (such as advanced cardiac life support), and to manage patient care over time. As we discussed in Section 17.1.2, students can use computer-based simulations to experiment and to learn from errors in reasoning and judgment without jeopardizing the well-being of real patients. Furthermore, students can gain experience managing patients with rare conditions, thus gaining familiarity with medical problems to which they might not otherwise be exposed.

Simulation programs may be either *static* or *dynamic*. Under the static simulation model, each case presents a "patient" who has a *predefined* problem and set of characteristics. Figures 17.2 through 17.6 illustrate the interaction between a student and the RxDx sequential-diagnosis program on abdominal pain. The student interrogates the computer about history, physical findings, and laboratory-test results to reach a diagnosis. At any point in the interaction, the student can interrupt data collection to ask the computer "consultant" to display the differential diagnosis (given the information that has been collected so far), or to recommend a data-collection strategy. The underlying case, however, remains static. On the other hand, dynamic simulation programs simulate changes in patient state over time and in response to students' therapeutic decisions. Thus, unlike those in static simulations, the cases of a dynamic simulation *evolve* as the student works through them. These programs

---

THE PATIENT IS A 56 YEAR-OLD MALE.
HE CAME TO THE EMERGENCY DEPARTMENT BECAUSE OF MODERATE EPI-
GASTRIC PAIN THAT STARTED OVER A MONTH AGO.

You may now examine your patient.

Item Number: 100 CHARACTER OF PAIN—BURNING
Item Number: 102 HOW LONG DO THE PAINS LAST?—MOST OF THE TIME, OCCA-
SIONALLY EASES
Item Number: 103 HAVE YOU EVER BEFORE HAD THIS KIND OF PAIN?—SEVERAL
YEARS AGO
Item Number: 107 VOMITING—YES
Item Number: 108 FEVER—NONE
Item Number: 109 DIARRHEA—NO
Item Number: CONSULTANT

FIGURE 17.2 This transcript shows the first part of an interaction between a student and the sequential-diagnosis program on abdominal pain (which is operational at MGH and is available over the MGH Educational Network or as part of the RxDx series of floppy disks published by Williams & Wilkins). The student is presented with a brief description of a patient with abdominal pain; he then collects information by selecting items from a list of almost 100 different signs, symptoms, or laboratory tests. The computer program provides immediate responses to each request. The text entered by the student is underlined for purposes of illustration. (*Source:* Courtesy of the Laboratory of Computer Science, Massachusetts General Hospital.)

```
ITEM INFO
BEST TESTS
CONSIDER
DISCRIMINATE
LEADING DIAGNOSES
TEACHING
EVIDENCE
RETURN TO MAIN PROGRAM
```

FIGURE 17.3 This menu shows the choices available to students using the sequential-diagnosis program on abdominal pain. At any time, the student can interrupt the computer to request a consultation—see the last entry in Figure 17.2. The computer program can provide information about the characteristics and potential usefulness of each item of information, and can give general guidance about how to work up a patient who has that specific type of problem. In addition, using a statistical model of clinical reasoning, the computer can provide a differential diagnosis (given the information available at that time), and can recommend the "best tests"—those items that have the highest potential value for clarifying the differential diagnosis. (*Source:* Courtesy of the Laboratory of Computer Science, Massachusetts General Hospital.)

```
CONSULTANT option: LEADING DIAGNOSES

The current leading diagnoses and their probabilities are as follows:

1) 901  PEPTIC ULCER (GASTRIC DUODENAL)        86
2) 905  ACUTE GASTRITIS                         4
3) 908  CHRONIC PANCREATITIS                    2
4) 904  GASTRIC CANCER                          1
```

FIGURE 17.4 The sequential-diagnosis program displays its list of leading diagnoses. This is the computer model's interpretation of the most likely diagnoses given the information collected thus far. The probabilities are crude approximations, because the underlying model is simplistic and is based on conditional probabilities that have been derived from experts, rather than from clinical studies. The text entered by the student is underlined for purposes of illustration. (*Source:* Courtesy of the Laboratory of Computer Science, Massachusetts General Hospital.)

help students to understand the relationships between actions (or inactions) and patients' clinical outcomes. To simulate a patient's response to intervention, the programs explicitly model underlying physiologic processes, often using mathematical models.

17.3.2 Constrained Versus Unconstrained Responses

The mechanism for communication between student and CAI program can take one of several basic forms. At one extreme, students may select from a constrained list of responses that are valid in the current situation (such as the set of answers to a

```
Item Number: 304  TENDERNESS TO PALPATION—EPIGASTRIC
Item Number: 509  STOOL EXAMINATION—BROWN; HEMOCCULT NEGATIVE
Item Number: 306  REBOUND TENDERNESS AND INVOLUNTARY
                  GUARDING—NO
Item Number: 303  ENLARGED ORGAN(S) OR MASS IN ABDOMEN—
- - - - - - - - -     NO MASSES OR ENLARGED ORGANS
Your Attending would like to know what you think is the leading diagnosis.
Enter the number of your diagnosis: 902 PEPTIC ULCER (GASTRIC/DUODENAL)
She is pleased—you are on the right track.
The current evidence strongly supports your conclusion.
```

FIGURE 17.5 The sequential-diagnosis program requests the student's primary diagnostic hypothesis. The student then collects further information. The computer-based model is tracking the interaction, updating its internal differential diagnosis with each new item of information as the latter is collected by the student. When the probability of the most likely diagnosis crosses a threshold, the computer interrupts the student and asks that the student enter his primary diagnostic hypothesis. The text entered by the student is underlined for purposes of illustration. (*Source:* Courtesy of the Laboratory of Computer Science, Massachusetts General Hospital.)

```
THE PATIENT IS A 22 YEAR-OLD MALE.
HE CAME TO THE EMERGENCY DEPARTMENT BECAUSE OF MODERATE
LEFT UPPER QUADRANT PAIN THAT STARTED WITHIN THE LAST 24 HOURS.
- - - - - - - - - -
You may now examine your patient.
Item Number: 100  CHARACTER OF PAIN—BURNING
Item Number: 103  HAVE YOU EVER BEFORE HAD THIS KIND OF PAIN?
                  —NEVER BEFORE
Item Number: 107  VOMITING—NO
Item Number: 109  DIARRHEA—YES; CHRONIC
Item Number: CONSULTANT
- - - - - - - - - -
CONSULTANT option: LEADING DIAGNOSES

The current leading diagnoses and their probabilities are as follows:

1) 934  IRRITABLE BOWEL SYNDROME      23
2) 921  ACUTE APPENDICITIS            16
3) 901  RUPTURED SPLEEN               11
4) 915  REGIONAL ENTERITIS            10
- - - - - - - - - -
CONSULTANT option: BEST TESTS

1) 104  TRAUMA
2) 126  HAVE YOU NOTICED ANY STOOL ABNORMALITY
3) 306  REBOUND TENDERNESS AND INVOLUNTARY GUARDING
4) 111  WEIGHT
5) 304  TENDERNESS TO PALPATION
```

FIGURE 17.6 In this session, the student is using the sequential-diagnosis program as a consultant on abdominal pain. The student has collected several items of information, and has requested a consultation regarding the computer's suggested diagnostic hypothesis and set of "best tests." The text entered by the student is underlined for purposes of illustration. (*Source:* Courtesy of the Laboratory of Computer Science, Massachusetts General Hospital.)

multiple-choice question). At the opposite extreme, students are free to query the program and to specify actions using entirely unconstrained natural language. An intermediate approach is to provide a single, comprehensive menu of possible actions, thus constraining choices in a program-specific, but not in a situation-specific, manner.

The use of a predefined, explicit vocabulary has two disadvantages: (1) it *cues* the user (suggests ideas that otherwise might not have occurred to him) and (2) it detracts from the realism of the simulation. On the other hand, programs that provide students with a list of actions that are allowable and reasonable in a particular situation are easier to write, because the authors do not need to deal with unanticipated responses. Furthermore, the use of a constrained vocabulary will be less frustrating to students who may otherwise have difficulty formulating valid interactions.

The use of free-text input works best in well-defined domains or in circumscribed contexts in which a student's responses are easy to anticipate and interpret. Thus, if the program asks, "What antibiotic would you prescribe for this patient?" it needs to be prepared to handle only a relatively small number of possible responses. In general, both laboratory tests and drug therapies can be handled relatively easily using natural language. On the other hand, the range of possible medical-history questions is so large that anticipating even the most logical set of student inquiries is difficult—devising any scheme that deals reliably with all possible inputs is impossible. Questions and actions related to the physical examination fall closer to the feasible range, although a student will almost certainly overtax the capabilities of the system if she uses an obscure eponym (such as "Sicar's sign"), or states an inquiry in a novel way (for example, "Is there puffiness around the ankles?" rather than, "Is there pedal edema?"), or asks about an unusual finding (such as webbed fingers) in a patient case in which such a finding would usually not be considered. Students quickly become discouraged if the system fails to recognize what seem to be legitimate inquiries, and they have little tolerance for learning how to state an inquiry in a way that the computer can understand.

17.3.3 Structured Versus Unstructured Interactions

CAI programs also differ by the degree to which they impose structures on a teaching session. In general, drill-and-practice and branching systems are highly structured. The system's responses to students' choices are specified in advance; students cannot control the course of an interaction directly. On the other hand, some CAI programs create an exploratory environment in which students can experiment without guidance or interference. Each of these approaches has advantages and disadvantages. For example, drill-and-practice programs are highly focused to teach important concepts. At the same time, they do not allow students to deviate from the prescribed course or to explore areas of special interest. Conversely, programs that provide an exploratory environment and that allow students to choose any actions in any order encourage experimentation and self-discovery. Without structure or guidance, however, students may waste time following unproductive paths and may fail to learn important material. Thus, unguided exploration can be an inefficient approach to learning.

17.3.4 Feedback and Guidance

Closely related to the structure of an interaction is the degree to which a CAI program provides feedback and guidance to users. Virtually all systems provide some form of feedback—for example, they may supply short explanations of why answers are correct or incorrect, present summaries of important aspects of cases, or provide references to related materials. Many systems provide an interactive help facility that allows students to ask for hints and advice.

More sophisticated systems allow the student to take independent action, but may intervene if she strays down an unproductive path or acts in a way that suggests a misconception of fact or inference. Such **mixed-initiative systems** allow students freedom, but provide a framework that constrains the interaction and thus helps students to learn more efficiently. Some researchers make a distinction between coaching systems and tutoring systems. The less proactive *coaching* systems monitor the session and intervene only when the student requests help or makes serious mistakes. *Tutoring* systems, on the other hand, guide a session aggressively by asking questions that test a student's understanding of the material and that expose errors and gaps in the student's knowledge. Mixed-initiative systems are the most difficult type of program to create because they must have models both of the student and of the problem to be solved.

17.3.5 Use of Graphics and Video

One of the most exciting new developments in CAI is the use of interactive videodisc technology to integrate images with computer-based teaching programs. Interactive videodiscs provide a means to combine information from a variety of media—for example, video footage of patient appearance, X-ray and other radiographic images, histology slides, explanatory text, and so on. In some areas of medicine, such as cardiology, auditory material also is important; such auditory material also can be saved on videodisc.

Abdulla at the University of Georgia [Abdulla et al., 1984], Friedman at the University of Wisconsin (see Section 17.4.1), and Harless at the Lister Hill Center of the NLM (see Section 17.4.2) are several of the researchers developing imaginative teaching programs based on videodisc technology. One of the major factors limiting the development of interactive videodisc programs is the significant expense involved in producing high-quality images.

17.3.6 Authoring Systems

Courseware development is a labor-intensive and time-consuming process. The ability of subject-matter experts to develop courseware within a reasonable time frame depends on the availability of good authoring systems. An **authoring system** allows the expert to focus on the content of the teaching program and to be less concerned with the details of writing a computer program. Thus, an authoring system is a specialized, high-level programming language with its own set of commands, functions, and utilities. Most currently available authoring languages are designed for a fairly stereotyped, frame-oriented, question-and-answer interaction. Examples of commercial authoring languages are McGraw-Hill's Interactive Authoring System and Boeing's Scholar-Teach, both written for the IBM PC. These simple systems allow a potential author to begin course design quickly, without having to worry about the complex housekeeping tasks that must be performed to get the material online. Convenience and simplicity have their price, however: Simple authoring systems greatly constrain the style and complexity of the teaching programs that users can develop, and most of these systems cannot be extended to support novel capabilities. On the other hand, authoring systems that exploit more of the power of the computer tend to be sufficiently complex that a would-be program author must devote considerable time to learning how to use them; the more complex the interaction, and the more powerful the authoring language, the more difficult it is for a neophyte author to master the programming resources without the help of a specialist in the language. The ideal authoring system would be multilayered, allowing new authors to create simple frame-oriented programs, yet permitting programming experts to add graphics, to create real-time simulations, and to add complicated physiological and disease models.

17.4 Examples of Recently Developed Computer-Aided Instruction Systems

In the past decade, CAI programs have proliferated rapidly. Undoubtedly, this increase in activity reflects the availability of personal computers. Today, virtually all medical schools use computers in some capacity to facilitate medical education. Many of the current CAI programs are simulations that allow students to diagnose and manage patient cases. The newest programs combine a variety of media—text, graphics, video, and sound. In this section, we shall describe several examples of current CAI programs. For discussions of additional systems, you can consult the proceedings of the Symposium on Computer Applications in Medical Care (SCAMC), which is cited in the Suggested Readings.

17.4.1 CBX

Computer-Based Examination (CBX) is a microcomputer-based simulation program under development by the National Board of Medical Examiners [Clyman and Melnick, 1987]. The developers plan eventually to use CBX to assess physicians' clinical knowledge and behavior during Part III of the National Board Examination. These examinations are required for licensure for medical practice and are intended to ensure that physicians are competent to practice general medicine without supervision. The goal of CBX is to provide an objective means for assessing the quality of a physician's behavior in situations that closely mimic the clinical environment.

CBX places the physician in the position of primary caretaker for a patient in a medical environment. Once presented with a clinical scenario, the physician can assess and manage the patient's condition by collecting medical-history information, conducting a physical examination, performing procedures, ordering diagnostic tests, ordering therapies, and calling in outside consultants. Almost all such requests are made through free-text entry of orders on a hospital order sheet. In addition, thousands of medical images are available on videodisc for interpretation and review, including those from X-ray films, ECG recordings, and slides of tissue specimens. The patient's condition evolves dynamically during the simulation, reflecting both the passage of time and the physician's therapy-management strategy; likewise, the results of tests and other clinical information reflect the patient's changing condition. CBX records the timing and sequencing of the physician's actions for later evaluation according to criteria defined by a group of expert physicians.

17.4.2 TIME

Researchers on the Technological Innovations in Medical Education (TIME) project of the Lister Hill National Center for Biomedical Communications combine interactive videodisc and speech-recognition technologies to create complex, realistic simulations that can be used by an instructor working with a group of medical students [Harless et al., 1986]. Each case study visually portrays a patient's medical and social conditions. The instructor uses uncued verbal commands to take the patient's history, to order tests and procedures, to review patient data, and to admit and discharge the patient from the hospital. Thus, together, instructor and students manage the medical workup and treatment of the simulated patient.

A typical case shows an introductory scene, then freezes the action in a *wait state*. The wait state is the students' cue to take action of some kind. Using a specified set of vocal inquiries and commands, the instructor interviews the patient, directs the diagnostic workup, and manages treatment. The videodisc allows students to witness a variety of scenes that depict past events related to the present illness and to current experiences in the hospital. Other scenes include significant portions of the physical examination, X-ray films, and so on. The instructor can interview the patient directly or can use the command word "thoughts" to hear what the patient is thinking—a feature designed to increase students' awareness of patients' emotional and mental states.

Each TIME case contains multiple *decision points,* or situations during the simulation that have uncertain outcomes. Thus, cases are not completely predictable and can unfold in a variety of ways. The program randomly chooses among the possible outcomes using a table of probabilities associated with the decision point. The probabilities of the various outcomes change dynamically during the case, depending on the students' behavior in making relevant inquiries and in choosing appropriate interventions. The case study ends following an outcome scene that describes the eventual fate of the patient (for example, complete recovery or subsequent return to the hospital). At this point, the program provides feedback on various aspects of the group's performance. For example, it describes the correctness of the diagnosis, the proportion of critical information obtained during the session, and the cost of the patient's hospital stay.

Prior to running the program, a user must train the system to recognize a vocabulary of 135 control words. This training session takes about 30 minutes to complete. The computer saves the voice patterns of the user as he speaks each word. These patterns are then used by the computer to recognize and interpret spoken commands when the simulation is run.

17.4.3 HeartLab

Developed by researchers at the Harvard Medical School, HeartLab is a simulation program designed to teach medical students to interpret the results of auscultation of the heart, a skill that requires regular practice on a variety of patient cases [Bergeron, 1989]. Physicians can diagnose many cardiac disorders by listening to the sounds made by the movement of the heart valves and by the movement of blood in the heart chambers and vessels. HeartLab provides an interactive environment for listening to heart sounds as an alternative to the common practice of listening to audio tapes. It was written for the Apple Macintosh and uses that machine's sound synthesizer to simulate the heart sounds of interest. A student wearing headphones can compare and contrast similar-sounding abnormalities, and can hear the changes in sounds brought on by changes in patient position (sitting versus lying down) and by physician maneuvers (such as changing the location of the stethoscope).

The student can run the program in each of three modes: laboratory, patient-case analysis, and review. In laboratory mode, the student selects from menus to control a synthesizer that can produce heart sounds with a variety of rates and rhythms, augmenting these with gallops, clicks, and murmurs (Figure 17.7). Accompanying graphics represent the heart sounds visually and indicate the optimal location on the chest wall for placement of the stethoscope to hear particular sounds. In patient-case–analysis mode, the system generates patient cases of varying severity. The student uses a mouse pointing device to position a stethoscope on the chest wall, then attempts to diagnose the cardiac anomaly based on the results of auscultation. If the student fails to reach the correct diagnosis, the program suggests appropriate lessons for review. In review mode, the program presents a variety of topics pertinent to the cardiovascular physical examination using text and graphics. A similar program, EKGLab, allows students to practice the interpretation of ECGs.

17.4.4 ElectricCadaver

The Advanced Media Research Group at Stanford University is exploring the creation of integrated media documents that link text, computer graphics, video images, and sound. ElectricCadaver, one product of this research, allows medical students to learn about anatomical structure and physiological function by exploring a database of digitized anatomical images, including photographs of classic dissection slides, microscopic views of tissues, radiographic images, and labeled line drawings [Freedman, 1989]. Students navigate through the system by activating graphical controls to rotate images to alternative views, to zoom in and out for closer and wider views, to examine slides of histological structures, and to compare radiographic images with views of gross structures.

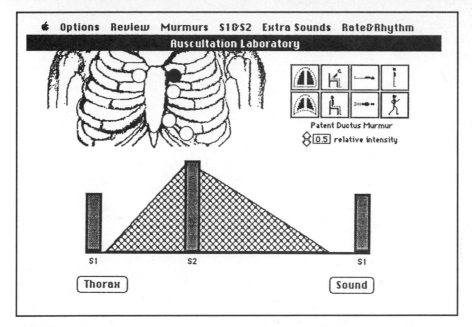

FIGURE 17.7 When running the HeartLab simulation program in laboratory mode, students can experiment with the heart sounds associated with a variety of cardiac anomalies. In this case, the user is experimenting with the murmur of a patent ductus arteriosis. The program portrays a graphical representation of the heart sound, as well as producing the sound itself on the computer's synthesizer. (*Source:* Courtesy of Dr. Bryan Bergeron.)

Images are displayed on two screens: Bit-mapped line drawings and text are displayed on a computer monitor, and photographic and radiographic images stored on videodisc are displayed on a television monitor. The image base is accessible by region of the body (head, thorax, abdomen, and so on) and by system (skeleton, cardiovascular system, nervous system, and so on). A collection of interactive illustrations also is available. Students can explore the effects of facial-nerve damage, for example, by selecting a nerve on the drawing, and viewing the corresponding image of a real patient with damage to that nerve (Figure 17.8). Likewise, students can use a mouse pointing device to probe an image of the hand of a patient with sensory nerve damage, testing various locations on the hand for pressure sensitivity. In addition to providing an environment for undirected exploration, ElectricCadaver includes a tutorial that teaches fundamental elements of anatomy and provides mechanisms for testing and for self-evaluation.

17.4.5 GUIDON

Researchers began developing the GUIDON system at Stanford University beginning in the mid-1970s; the first version of the system was operational by early 1979 [Clancey, 1984]. The goal of GUIDON was to convey to students the expertise embodied in a rule-based expert system. GUIDON used the knowledge base of the

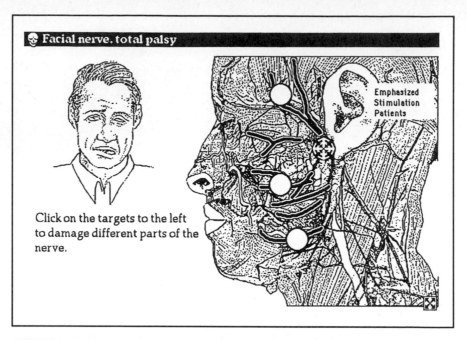

FIGURE 17.8 Students using the ElectricCadaver system can explore a database of digitized anatomical images to learn about human anatomical structure and physiological function. This figure shows a dynamic diagram that was designed to illustrate the effects of facial-nerve damage. The student uses a mouse pointing device to "damage" part of the nerve (near the earlobe). Immediately, the program displays on the computer monitor a drawing showing the effects of the damage, and presents on a television monitor a photographic image of a real patient with damage to that nerve. (*Source:* Courtesy of Vesalius, Inc.)

MYCIN system (see Chapter 15) to teach important parameters and rules for the diagnosis of meningitis and bacterial infections of the blood. In addition, GUIDON contained about 200 domain-independent *teaching rules*. These rules embodied strategies for teaching, and they determined what the system would do at each step. For example, when the program determined that MYCIN could draw a conclusion of interest based on the available information, the teaching rules determined whether GUIDON presented a conclusion, gave a summary, or asked the student to suggest a hypothesis.

The separation of domain knowledge and teaching knowledge allowed GUIDON to be used with any EMYCIN system.[1] This approach represented a significant advance over traditional CAI methodology because GUIDON's knowledge was reusable and could be adapted to new applications. Thus, the researchers were able to plug

---

[1]EMYCIN is the general expert-system shell that was extracted from the MYCIN system—that is, it is MYCIN without the knowledge base of domain-specific rules.

in the knowledge bases from the SACON and PUFF systems, and the same GUIDON program was able to tutor students about structural-analysis problems and the interpretation of pulmonary-function tests.

Although it was adequate for the purpose of diagnostic consultations, the MYCIN knowledge base was missing knowledge that was necessary to *teach* students about diagnosis of infectious diseases. For example, the knowledge base contained no information about diseases that cause symptoms similar to those of meningitis and bacteremia, and contained little support knowledge to justify the diagnostic rules. Furthermore, MYCIN's reasoning process differed from physicians' diagnostic inference process—MYCIN performed a top-down search through a prescribed set of diseases, while exhaustively collecting information. Physicians, on the other hand, form hypotheses based on partial evidence, then strategically collect information to refine the diagnosis.

In the early 1980s, researchers reorganized and greatly expanded MYCIN to create NEOMYCIN, another medical diagnosis program that addresses many of MYCIN's limitations with respect to teaching [Clancey, 1986]. The NEOMYCIN knowledge base contains knowledge of competing diseases and rules that embody explicit strategies for hypothesis formation, causal reasoning, and grouping and discriminating among competing hypotheses (Figure 17.9). Thus, the revised teaching system, GUIDON2, is able to access the strategic knowledge contained in NEOMYCIN's knowledge base to teach students about strategies for diagnostic reasoning [Rodolitz and Clancey, 1989].

17.5 The Future of Computers in Medical Education

Despite the strong arguments that have been made in support of computer-based medical education, progress in developing exciting programs and in the national dissemination of the existing programs has been agonizingly slow. This lagging development and diffusion are attributable to the difficulty and expense of writing CAI programs, to the lack of support for program development within institutions, and to the barriers to sharing programs among institutions.

Courseware development is labor intensive and time consuming. Initially, faculty members must devote considerable time to understanding and gaining expertise in the art of creating computer-based CAI programs; both the approach and the materials are significantly different from those used in preparing lectures. Even after this hurdle has been overcome, program development is a lengthy process. Often, there is a significant lead-time of many months before any results are seen. The time between the formulation of a concept and the delivery of a completed program can easily be 1 full year if the program is of any depth or complexity.

The development of improved tools for coursework authoring that can gain widespread acceptance is a high-priority need. Such tools could reduce the startup time for and speed the process of program development. The ideal authoring language

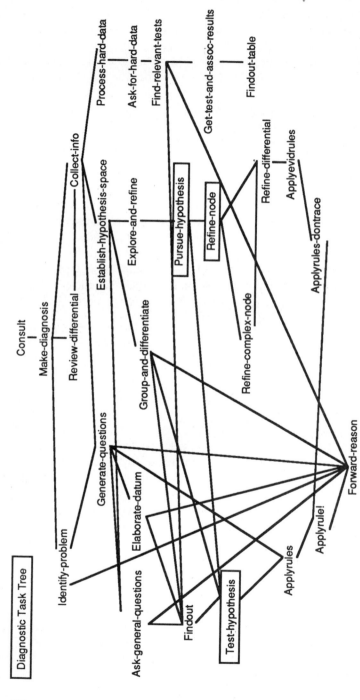

FIGURE 17.9 This tree diagram shows the structure of diagnostic tasks in NEOMYCIN. For example, problem identification, review of the differential diagnosis, and information collection are subtasks of making a clinical diagnosis. (*Source:* Courtesy of Dr. William J. Clancey.)

would combine simplicity for novice coursework writers and power for experts, and would be widely available to faculty at many institutions. In addition, the production of educational-support materials on videodisc, and the development of an extensive library of visual and graphical material to be shared among CAI authors, would help individual developers to avoid much redundant work.

At schools where CAI has played a major role, there usually has been a highly visible advocate for its use. Such an advocate, however, will not be successful unless other faculty take the time to learn about the computer programs, and to participate in the introduction of CAI in the curriculum. In most medical schools, such support is absent, usually because of lack of interest and commitment from the dean and senior faculty. To encourage medical-school faculty to become involved in courseware development, medical schools must develop an appropriate reward system. For example, instructors who author high-quality courseware should receive credit for their work when promotion and tenure decisions are made.

The high costs of software development would be more justifiable if the completed CAI programs were shared widely, thus reducing the cost per hour of instruction; however, relatively little sharing has taken place. One reason is simple lack of familiarity of many medical-school faculty with the medium. There has been little opportunity to have a medical CAI program published or, until recently, even reviewed in the standard literature. It is difficult to learn what computer-based medical educational programs are available, what hardware and software are required, what the cost is likely to be, what evaluation has been carried out, and who has used the programs and with what success. One of the more promising developments is the decision of a number of medical journals to publish software reviews.

Another barrier limiting the transfer of programs is the lack of a standard approach to program development. Medical schools cannot afford to acquire the software and hardware necessary to run every program of interest. PCs provide a relatively standard and inexpensive medium for the development and use of CAI systems, and several promising authoring systems are being developed. However, there is still a troublesome divergence of both hardware platforms and software tools that makes universal sharing difficult, if not impossible. To promote courseware sharing, leading medical schools could form a consortium to establish standards for program development. If such a consortium were to commit to the use of compatible hardware and one (or several) standard authoring systems, then programs written at one institution could be used elsewhere. The authoring systems should be designed to permit faculty at other institutions to modify the programs, a key factor in overcoming the "not-invented-here" syndrome that frequently limits courseware acceptance. The development of local-area networks within institutions and wide-area network communications linking geographically disparate institutions also encourages sharing of programs and facilitates access by physicians practicing in the community.

An important aspect of courseware development that is often overlooked is the integration of computer-based materials with the curriculum. Currently, most CAI materials are treated as supplementary material; they are placed in libraries, and are used by students or physicians on their own initiative. This is a valid use, and the programs serve as valuable resources for the students who use them; however, an educator can use CAI materials more effectively by integrating them into the standard curriculum. For example, programs might be assigned as laboratory exercises or used as the basis of a class discussion. One of the barriers to integration is the initial high cost of acquiring sufficient computing resources. The cost of the computer equipment has fallen substantially in recent years; nonetheless, the cost of enough PCs to accommodate the entire school would be a major item in the curriculum budget of a school. This consideration will grow less important as more students purchase their own PCs.

In summary, computer-based educational systems have the potential to help students to master subject matter and to develop problem-solving skills. Properly integrated into the medical-school curriculum and into the information systems that serve health-care institutions and the greater medical community, CAI can become part of a comprehensive system for lifelong education. The challenge to researchers in CAI is to develop this potential. The barriers to success are both technical and practical. To overcome them, we require both dedication of support and resources within institutions, and a commitment to cooperation among institutions.

Suggested Readings

Association of American Medical Colleges. Physicians for the twenty-first century (Report of the Panel on the General Professional Education of the Physician and College Preparation for Medicine). *Journal of Medical Education,* 59:1, 1984.
>   *This report by the Association of American Medical Colleges presents recommendations to medical schools about curriculum changes that are necessary to prepare physicians-in-training to meet the challenges of the current health-care environment.*

Kingsland III, L. C. (ed). *Proceedings of the Thirteenth Annual Symposium on Computer Applications in Medical Care.* Washington, D.C.: IEEE Computer Society Press, 1989.
>   *The proceedings of an annual conference on applications of computers in health care, this volume (as well as others in the series) contains articles on much of the current research in CAI.*

Piemme, T. E. Computer-assisted learning and evaluation in medicine. *Journal of the American Medical Association,* 260:367, 1988.
>   *This article traces the development of CAI in the United States, and discusses reasons for the slow growth and acceptance of this technology.*

Starkweather, J. A. The computer as a tool for learning. *Western Journal of Medicine,* 145:864, 1986.
>   *This overview article describes current major projects in CAI and discusses directions for the further development of the field.*

Questions for Discussion

1. You have decided to write a computer-based simulation about the management of patients who have abdominal pain.

a. Discuss the relative advantages and disadvantages of the following styles of presentation: (1) a frame-oriented question-and-answer format, (2) a controlled vocabulary program focusing on the differential diagnosis, (3) a simulation in which the patient's condition changes over time and in response to therapy, and (4) a program that allows the student to enter free-text requests for information and that provides responses.

b. Discuss two issues that you would expect to arise during the process of developing and testing the program.

c. For each approach outlined in part (a), discuss how you might develop a model that could be used to evaluate the student's performance in clinical problem solving.

d. What are the virtues and limitations of including visual material in a teaching program? How can you integrate the technology of the computer-based program and the presentation of the visual material?

2. Consider a simulation that is designed to teach a student how to develop the differential diagnosis of a patient who has abdominal pain. Develop a strategy and a vocabulary that will allow the computer to recognize the variety of inquiries that the student might make regarding what the character of the pain was, and what the results of a detailed physical examination were.

3. Create a simple transcript consisting of 10 exchanges of a hypothetical session between a student and each of the following programs:

a. A branching-questioning program

b. A coaching program

c. A tutoring program

4. What barriers inhibit the dissemination of computer-based medical education programs from one institution to another? Discuss three factors that could encourage sharing among institutions.

5. Discuss the relative merits of the computer being "in control" of the teaching environment, with the student essentially responding to computer inquiries, versus those of having the students being "in control," and thus having a much larger range of alternative courses of action.

6. Discuss the issues that the National Board of Medical Examiners will face when it attempts to use computer-based simulations to assess clinical competency for medical licensure.

18

Health-Assessment Systems

Morris F. Collen

After reading this chapter, you should know the answers to these questions:

- How can health-assessment systems improve the health of a population and reduce health-care costs?

- What criteria should program developers use to select screening tests for inclusion in multiphasic health-testing programs?

- What are the major functions performed by health-assessment information systems?

- How can self-administered questionnaires and interactive computer programs be used to collect medical-history information directly from patients?

- How have questions of financing and lack of third-party reimbursement for health examinations inhibited widespread acceptance of automated health-assessment systems in the United States?

18.1 Health-Assessment Systems: An Overview

Over the last 40 years, increasing interest in personal health promotion, disease prevention, and health maintenance has inspired health-care providers to develop systematic methods for providing health-assessment examinations. The application of computing technology and the use of automated instruments to perform laboratory tests and other diagnostic procedures provided a means for health-care institutions to perform large numbers of health examinations quickly and efficiently. After initial enthusiasm in the 1950s and 1960s, however, interest in automated multiphasic testing programs subsequently declined. The number of programs has been decreasing in the United States since the late 1970s, although the programs are still widely used in Japan and in France. Currently, most multiphasic testing programs in the United States are operated by health-maintenance organizations (HMOs) and industrial corporations.

In this chapter, we shall first discuss the reasons for the development of health-assessment systems and the primary functions of the computer-based information systems that support them. In the latter part of the chapter, we shall summarize the historical development of health-assessment systems, and shall discuss reasons for the decline in use of this technology in the United States. In particular, we shall examine the economic factors that discouraged widespread acceptance of health-assessment systems as a means for providing preventive health care.

18.1.1 The Systematic Approach

A **health assessment** is a survey examination of a presumably well person. It generally includes a medical history, a physical examination, and performance of tests and procedures to evaluate health status, to identify health risks, and to detect abnormalities that may indicate asymptomatic or undiagnosed diseases. Patients typically undergo such assessments at prescribed intervals as part of a health-maintenance program.

A **health-assessment system (HAS)** is a systematic approach to providing health assessments to an entire patient population. The testing process is tailored to address the health-care needs of target groups of patients. Often, HASs use computers to support data processing, data storage, and the communication of information. A **multiphasic health-testing program** expresses this general approach explicitly; patients visit a series of stations that have been set up to collect medical-history information, to perform selected tests and procedures, and to conduct physical examinations (Figure 18.1). Usually, nurse practitioners and paramedical personnel perform preliminary examinations and refer patients with unusual findings to physicians for more extensive workups (Figure 18.2).

A typical multiphasic testing facility includes stations for (1) registration of patients; (2) collection of medical-history information; (3) measurement of physiological parameters (such as height, weight, pulse rate, blood pressure, ocular tension, auditory and visual acuity, pulmonary function, and muscular fitness); (4) specimen analyses (hematology and clinical chemistry tests, urinalysis, stool analysis for occult blood); (5) electrocardiography (and sometimes physician-supervised cardiovascular testing

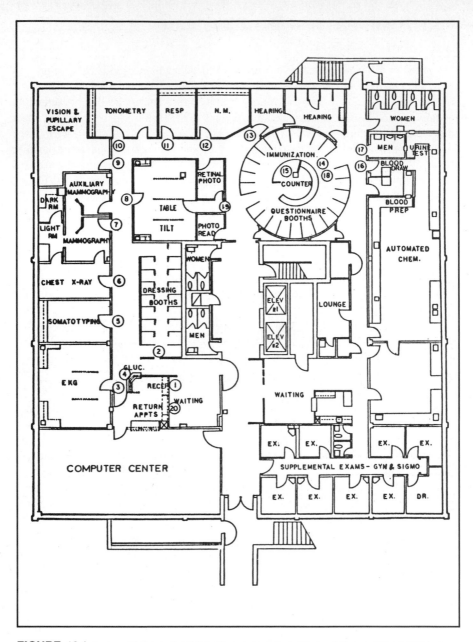

FIGURE 18.1 In a multiphasic health-testing program, patients visit a series of stations designed to collect information that is used in the health-assessment process. The floorplan of the original Oakland Kaiser-Permanente multiphasic health-testing system illustrates the clockwise flow of patients through the facility, from registration at the reception desk (station 1) to scheduling of follow-up appointments (station 20). (*Source:* Courtesy of Kaiser-Permanente Hospitals.)

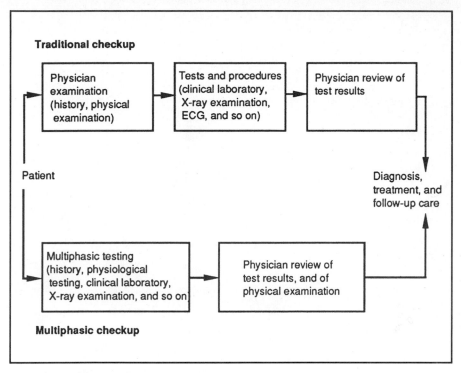

FIGURE 18.2 Flow of patient information differs in multiphasic and traditional health checkups. In traditional checkups, physicians collect medical history and examine patients, then order selected tests and procedures to gather additional medical data. In multiphasic checkups, physiological testing, laboratory testing, and other standard procedures are completed prior to examination by a physician.

by ergometry or treadmill); (6) chest X-ray examination and mammography (in women); (7) physical examination by a physician, physicians' assistant, or nurse practitioner (including rectal examination, and pelvic examinations and cervical Pap tests for women); and (8) review and explanation of results.

Automated multiphasic health-testing systems (AMHTs) use automated instruments to analyze laboratory specimens, and use computers to facilitate many aspects of the health-assessment process, including the collection and storage of medical data, and the generation of summary reports (Figure 18.3). In addition, some systems use computer-based decision rules to identify patients whose test results exceed prescribed limits, to produce lists of possible diagnoses, to suggest follow-up diagnostic tests, and to refer patients to physicians for more extensive workups.

The mere use of computers and automated equipment in a multiphasic testing program is not sufficient to qualify an HAS as an *automated* multiphasic health-testing program—the crucial component of an AMHT is the **health-assessment information system (HAIS),** which performs many of the functions of larger medical infor-

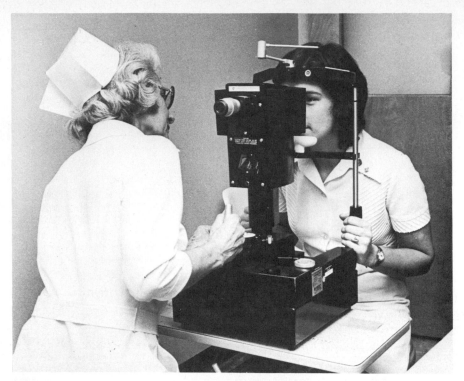

FIGURE 18.3 Measurement of ocular tension is one of the tests routinely performed in multiphasic health-testing programs. (*Source:* Photograph courtesy of Kaiser-Permanente Hospitals.)

mation systems, including maintenance of computer-based medical records, clinical decision support using advice rules, and appointment scheduling, patient recall, registration, and other operational tasks of HASs. The term **automated multiphasic health-testing services (AMHTS)** has been applied to an expanded AMHT, which provides adjunctive services within a health-care delivery system, such as patient triaging, health counseling, patient education, and preventive health maintenance.

18.1.2 Applications and Objectives

HASs have been used for a variety of purposes, the most common of which are the following:
- To provide periodic health checkups
- To obtain baseline health assessments for new enrollees to a health-care delivery system
- To perform prehospitalization workups
- To perform occupational health assessments and risk evaluations, often from mobile, self-contained testing units (such testing usually includes special-purpose tests for safety hazards, such as exposure to noise, radiation, dusts, or chemicals; also,

screening tests for non–work-related conditions, such as hypertension and diabetes, often are included)

- To perform testing to satisfy administrative requirements—for example, preemployment examinations, school entrance examinations, and periodic employee health examinations; HASs also are used to screen out persons unfit for military service and to identify high-risk applicants for life insurance

The primary motivations for using HASs are (1) to decrease morbidity, disability, and mortality in the patient population; and (2) to reduce total medical costs through more efficient use of health-care resources. The objectives of HASs are to improve health through early detection of abnormalities in asymptomatic populations, identification of subpopulations of patients who are at high risk for treatable diseases, and periodic monitoring of patients with known health problems. In turn, the objectives of early detection and treatment of disease are to reduce morbidity and the costs of medical care.

The operational costs of an HAS depend on the number of tests performed, number of personnel employed, facility design, amortization rate of capitalized equipment, cost of supplies, cost of facility maintenance, and so on. The most critical of factors for determining the unit cost per examination (which determines the charge to users) are the HAS workload (that is, the number of examinees per day), the degree of automation of equipment (which influences the number of personnel required to operate and manage the system), and the facility's design (which affects the efficiency of the program).

Because health-care delivery is a labor-intensive process, HASs can reduce total costs by substituting automated procedures for manual procedures and by using paramedical personnel, rather than physicians, whenever possible. Cost per examination is further reduced because the systematic approach and the use of automated equipment improve the efficiency of the operation of an HAS. An institution can perform more examinations per day with an HAS than with the traditional system of health-care delivery. Thus, the fixed costs of the HAS can be spread over a larger number of patients. In addition, automated data processing increases the efficiency of health-care personnel and the reliability of information processing by reducing the rate of data-acquisition errors and by hastening the turnaround time of summary reports to physicians.

In general, small HAS programs are unable to afford the large capital investment in automated equipment and therefore remain almost entirely manual operations. Larger HASs—those that examine more than 50 persons per day (or 1000 per month)—can spread the costs of acquiring computers and computer-based instruments over enough patients to attain an acceptable cost per examination. For such a large HAS, it usually is desirable to have a dedicated space and information system, which can be custom-tailored to meet the objectives of the HAS and, more specifically, the needs of the target population.

18.1.3 Criteria for Selection of HAS Tests

Appropriate selection of diagnostic tests and procedures is critical to the success of an HAS. The developers of an HAS must identify a battery of tests that has been custom-tailored to the needs of the target population. Different diseases occur with different frequencies in the young, in middle-aged adults, and in older adults; therefore, a different set of tests will be appropriate for each age group. Likewise, tests selected for personal health assessments will be different from those used for assessments that are sponsored by a corporation or by the military.

A system for personal health assessment should test for medical conditions that meet three criteria. First, the condition should be an important health problem for an individual or the community; that is, it should have a significant effect on the quality or length of life. Thus, an HAS should test both for conditions that are potentially disabling or life-threatening (for example, hypertension and breast cancer) and for conditions that impair the quality of life (for example, decreased hearing acuity and anxiety). Second, the condition should be prevalent in the target population, because testing for rare conditions will result in an exorbitant cost per positive test. Third, appropriate health-care services should be available for the condition, whether these be further diagnostic services, curative or rehabilitative services, or health and psychosocial counseling.

Once the HAS designers have determined the conditions for which they can and should test people, they must select the specific tests and procedures that can detect these conditions. To be a valuable tool, a test must be a highly sensitive indicator, and the cost per positive test result must be acceptable to users. Ideally, the test should detect disease in asymptomatic individuals. The cost per true-positive test result usually is the key criterion for test selection. As we discussed in Chapter 3, however, adjusting the defining limits for "normal" and "abnormal" results changes the percentage of test results that are classified as true positives versus false negatives, and as true negatives versus false positives. When setting the threshold for classifying results, HAS developers must consider the costs of false-positive and false-negative results. In short, the entire process of early detection, diagnosis, and treatment should be demonstrably more cost-effective than would be delaying treatment until the condition is symptomatic.

18.2 Information Systems to Support Health Assessment

An HAS requires an HAIS to collect, process, store, and retrieve patient information. In addition, the HAIS supports the operational tasks of the HAS, including tracking patients, scheduling appointments, and suggesting secondary tests and follow-up referrals.

The development of an HAIS is complicated by the varying objectives among different health-assessment programs, the lack of standardization of medical terms and procedures, and the ever changing state of medical knowledge and practice. Successful development of an HAIS requires the same considerations of system design, implementation, and evaluation that we discussed in Chapter 5. These considerations include choosing between vendor and inhouse development; defining functional and technical requirements and specifications; selecting competent personnel; obtaining funding; acquiring an appropriate hardware configuration; developing or acquiring necessary software; installing the system; orienting and training the users; and operating, evaluating, revising, and improving the system. Like any medical information system, an HAIS must be reliable, must have a mechanism for data recovery in the case of system failure, and must provide adequate security against unauthorized access to patient information. Furthermore, the system must be designed for ease of use. For example, the terminals must be conveniently located, the system must provide adequate response time, and the programs must be easy to learn and to operate.

18.2.1 Patient Registration and Identification

The HAIS must provide a means for identifying each patient at the time of registration, and for verifying the identification at subsequent stations. Positive identification requires agreement on four identifiers: a unique patient number, name, gender, and birthdate. Any identification procedure that uses less than all four of the identifiers will probably have a significant error rate in reporting tests for incorrectly identified patients. The patient number can be a sequential accession number, the patient's Social Security number, or some other unique medical-record number. Because this number serves as the basic linkage for all a patient's data, it should never be reassigned by the HAIS.

Patients' identifying data can be embossed or punched on paper, plastic, or metal cards, thus facilitating the identification process and reducing the chance of data-entry errors. Family members, however, may inadvertently exchange identification cards. Therefore, health-care staff at the registration station must verify that the card being used does in truth identify the person being tested. In facilities with online data acquisition and storage, patients can enter their identification numbers by inserting machine-readable cards in a card reader, or technicians can enter the numbers via terminals.

18.2.2 Operational Support

The appointment-scheduling component of an HAIS must identify unfilled appointment slots by criteria such as date, time of day, approximate waiting time, physician, and reason for the examination. It should post and cancel appointments, print appointment-verification notices to be sent to patients, and print personalized examination instructions. Based on scheduling information, the HAIS can generate daily working lists of patients, print specimen labels and patient-specific data-collection forms, and retrieve patients' computer-stored medical records for review prior to examinations.

An HAIS can help health-care personnel to monitor the quality of the HAS by performing data quality-control procedures, such as checking patient data for completeness, analyzing combinations of data for errors and inconsistencies, and notifying staff of erroneous and missing test results. The system should monitor the accuracy of automated testing devices by performing test quality-control procedures and tracking the results of analyses performed on standard samples; and it should signal needed equipment adjustment and maintenance. In addition, an HAIS should generate periodic reports of system utilization, costs, error rates, and other process measures of system performance.

18.2.3 Data Collection

During the health-assessment process, data are collected from a variety of sources: automated instruments, health-care providers, and patients. The HAIS can acquire many data directly through interfaces with automated testing equipment—for example, sphygmomanometers (which measure blood pressure), spirometers (which measure parameters related to pulmonary function), Coulter counters (which analyze blood samples), and automated chemical analyzers (which perform panels of clinical chemistry tests). Human intermediaries must manually enter via terminals the data gathered from standalone instruments.

Various health professionals participate in the health-assessment process—physicians, physicians' assistants, nurse practitioners, nurses, technicians, and counselors. All these health-care workers gather information that must be included in patients' medical records. For example, nurse practitioners must enter the results of physical examinations, and physicians must record their interpretations of X-ray films and ECG recordings. The vast majority of data collected during routine examinations are easily captured on coded encounter forms. All such data should be entered into the computer directly by the collector of the data, rather than by a data-entry intermediary. Real-time data entry allows the computer to analyze the information in the database while the patient is still present and to provide immediate feedback to health-care providers about unusual results, appropriate follow-up tests, and possible data-entry errors.

The capture of medical-history information is the most problematic component of the data-collection process in HASs. Physicians recognize the patient interview as an invaluable tool for diagnosis and as a crucial aspect of medical practice. Researchers studying the medical decision-making process generally agree that physicians apply an iterative approach to data collection and hypothesis refinement (see Chapter 2). Within this framework, however, individual practitioners tend to develop their own history-taking styles. Thus, standardization of the medical history poses a significant problem for AMHTs.

Physicians use a variety of techniques to save time in acquiring medical-history information. Many physicians use preprinted checklist forms or employ allied health personnel to gather routine background information, and thus to assume a portion of the data-collection burden. The use of self-administered questionnaires and automated history takers provides another solution to the problem. The lack of standardization of the patient's medical history, the difficulty of creating understandable and reliable sets of questions, and the challenge of designing acceptable human–machine interfaces complicate the task of collecting information automatically, directly from patients.

The medical history has two components (1) the *problem history,* and (2) the *database history,* or general review. The problem history contains information about current medical problems, symptoms, and complaints. The database history contains more general history information, including identification and demographic data; past history of patients' medical problems; background data on family, social, and occupational history; and the review of physiological systems (respiratory, gastrointestinal, reproductive, and so on).

It is unlikely that automated history takers will be able to replace physician interviews for gathering problem-specific data. The information contained in the problem history varies widely by individual patient. Furthermore, physicians acquire information about a patient's condition not only by listening to answers to direct questions, but also by observing the patient's appearance and interpreting subtle voice inflections and gestures. On the other hand, collection of the database history is amenable to automation and may be an effective method for saving physician time. These data are collected routinely for all patients. Because most patients in a health-assessment program are fairly healthy, they will answer "no" to the vast majority of questions posed in the general review.

There are two basic instruments for acquiring medical-history information directly from patients: batch-processed questionnaires and interactive history-taking programs. Approaches to the offline (batch) collection of data include completion of paper questionnaires or checklists and manual data entry by clerks; completion of machine-readable checklists that can be read by optical scanners or mark-sense readers; sorting of prepunched cards (patients respond to questions by sorting cards into either a "yes" or a "no" box) (Figure 18.4); and the use of programmed audio cassette tapes (patients respond to questions by pressing appropriate buttons on a keyboard). Offline collection of history data is economical. For some methods, patients can even complete the forms at home before a scheduled appointment. On the other hand, questionnaires are often long and tedious to complete. If they exceed about 200 questions or take longer than 30 minutes to complete, patients become tired and bored and the reliability of responses decreases. Furthermore, manual questionnaire forms do not readily permit branching questions, which could add detail and specificity.

Interactive history-taking programs can simulate the dialog between physician and patient more flexibly, and are less tedious than batch-processing methods of data collection. Typically, the computer displays questions on the screen of a video display terminal; patients respond by typing their answers using a keyboard, by pointing to answers on a touch-sensitive screen, or by selecting regions using a light pen or a mouse pointing device. Real-time interaction between user and computer makes it feasible to collect data using **branching questioning algorithms**—a patient's response to a question determines which question the system will ask next. Thus, the interaction is tailored to the individual patient. The program automatically omits irrelevant questions and gathers increasingly detailed information when patients give positive responses to more general questions.

Initially, the high computer-hardware and processing-time costs, large requirements for online data storage, poor system reliability, and slow response time inhibited the use of interactive history-taking programs. The development of powerful, reliable, and inexpensive microcomputers subsequently removed these barriers. Today, the largest problem to be solved is the development and validation of sophisticated branching programs that can collect information accurately and reliably.

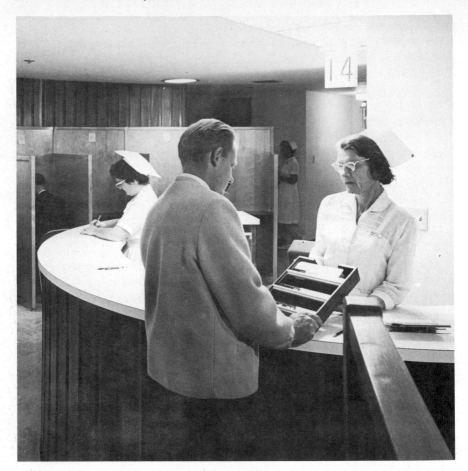

FIGURE 18.4 Multiphasic health-testing programs often automate the collection of general history information to save physician time. One early approach to completion of self-administered questionnaires was to have patients sort prepunched questionnaire cards into piles of "yes" and "no" box responses. (*Source:* Photograph courtesy of Kaiser-Permanente Hospitals.)

Each question must be unambiguous and easily understandable, so that patients can provide accurate and consistent answers. Ideally, patients should be able to respond to questions by indicating "yes" or "no," by choosing from a list of alternatives, or by entering a numeric response. If the program uses graphics to illustrate questions, patients should be able to point to locations on the display—for example, to indicate the location of pain in the body. The program should display a rephrasing of the question or provide a simple explanation if a patient responds to a question with "do not know," or "do not understand." In addition, the system might flag the responses to a question for later review by the health-care staff. Patients should be able to review previous responses and to revise answers—a subsequent question might, for example, stimulate the recall of information related to a previous question. In some institutions, foreign-language translations of the questionnaire should be available to meet the needs of patients who do not read English.

18.2.4 Report Generation and Data Retrieval

The summary report generated by the HAIS must be formatted to display important information clearly. It should present a list of the patient's current medical problems, and should provide detailed information about positive responses to medical-history questions (problems and symptoms) grouped by organ system; negative responses should be presented only briefly (Figure 18.5). In addition, the program should compare the patient's responses from the current and past examinations to identify new complaints and significant changes in the patient's health status. It should display laboratory-test results and measurements of physical parameters along with individualized (that is, by age and gender) normal values, highlight abnormal results, and present prior test results together with current results.

Many HASs now include a health-risk appraisal in their final reports. Clinical researchers have developed algorithms for estimating a patient's statistical probability of death within the next 10 years using mortality tables, such as those developed by the National Center for Health Statistics, and risk factors determined from clinical trials, such as the Framingham studies [Breslow, 1978; Goetz et al., 1980; Robbins and Hall, 1970]. The computer program calculates a patient-specific risk of death based on the data collected by the HAS—data on health habits and lifestyle, and the results of available tests. A typical printout for a health-risk appraisal lists the most common 10 to 15 causes of death within the patient's age and gender group, compares the patient's chances of dying from each cause to the average chances of dying for all patients in that age and gender group, and displays the achievable reduction in mortality risk if the patient changes eating habits, exercise patterns, or smoking behavior, according to a health-improvement program. This adjusted risk is often reported as the actuarial age that the patient can achieve by following the prescribed advice.

In addition to routine generation of summary reports, the HAIS should be able to support ad hoc requests for data and should generate special reports at the request of HAS administrators and other authorized users. Ideally, users should be able to retrieve any or all of a patient's medical data from the HAIS database, and to view those data in either a time-oriented or a problem-oriented format. HAS data also may be used to support clinical and epidemiologic research. Thus, an HAIS should be able to create machine-readable files containing selected subsets of patient data, and, ideally, to perform simple statistical calculations.

18.2.5 Data Processing Using Decision Rules

After the routine tests performed in an HAS have been completed, an onsite physician may review the final results of testing. If a patient's tests indicate an abnormality, a reviewer can arrange for additional testing to be performed *before* the patient

```
                    PERMANENTE MEDICAL GROUP - OAKLAND
        FINAL SUMMARY REPORT - MULTIPHASIC HEALTH CHECKUP - 2/24/65

    DOE, JANE                                    DR. SMITH J J
    M.R.NO. 9876543     BIRTHDATE 05-27  FEMALE  OAKL

       ANTHROPOMETRY: 127.5 LB.,  64.5 IN

    **ECG: LT.VENT.HYPERTROPHY
    **PHONOCARD: SYSTOLIC BASAL MURMUR
    **SUPINE BLOOD PRESSURE: 165/80        SUPINE BRACHIAL PULSE:  76.

       VITAL CAPACITY: 2.3 L 1 SEC              3.2 L TOTAL
    **CHEST XRAY: CARDIAC ENLARGEMENT HEART/CHEST RATIO =.52
       BREAST XRAY: NSA

       VISUAL ACUITY: R.E.20/40 OR BETTER    L.E.20/40 OR BETTER
       PUPILLARY ESCAPE: NO PUPILLARY ESCAPE
       OCULAR TENSION: R.E. NORMAL            L.E. NORMAL
    **RETINAL PHOTO: MINIMAL DIABETIC RETINOPATHY
       HEARING: NO CLINICALLY SIGNIF.HEARING DEFECT

    **URINE: PH 6    GLUCOSE MED.    PROTEIN 0    BLOOD 0      BACILLI NEG.
            CLINITEST 1+2+           ACETONE 0
       VDRL 0               BLOOD GROUP AB      LATEX AGGLUT. 0
       HEMOGLOBIN 12.3 GM (NORM.12.0-15.2)     WHITE COUNT  9,000

       SERUM:             (NORMAL)       SERUM:               (NORMAL)
    **GLUCOSE (1 HR.) 215  MG (UNDER 205)  CHOLESTEROL 195   MG (140-270)
    **GLUCOSE (2 HR.) 170  MG (UNDER 151)
       TOTAL PROT.     6.7 GM (5.8-7.8)    CALCIUM       9.5 MG (8.4-10.8)
       ALBUMIN         4.0 GM (3.4-5.0)    URIC ACID     3.9 MG (3.0-6.3)
       CREATININE      .90 MG (UNDER 1.3)  SGOT           21 U  (UNDER 50)
    * 2 HR.BLOOD DRAWN  10 MIN.LATE

    **PATIENT RECEIVED THE FOLLOWING (ADVICE RULE) DIRECTIONS:
       700-2 HR.BLOOD SUGAR              800-ROUTINE MEDICAL APPOINTMENT

    * CONSIDER REFER TO ASYMPT. DIABETES STUDY IF FOLLOW-UP CONFIRMS DIABETES.

    PATIENT ANSWERED YES TO THESE QUESTIONS ON 1964 FORM:
       249-HAD BAD REACTION OR SENSITIVITY TO PENICILLIN?
    IN THE PAST MONTH:
       434-THROAT BEEN SORE ALMOST EVERY DAY?
    IN THE PAST 6 MONTHS:
       450-SHORTNESS OF BREATH WITH USUAL WORK OR ACTIVITY?
    IN THE PAST YEAR:
       476-REPEAT PAIN,PRESSURE,TIGHT FEELING IN CHEST IN MIDDLE OF BREAST BONE?
       478-REPEAT PAIN,PRESSURE,TIGHT FEELING IN CHEST WHEN SITTING STILL?
       482-REPEATED PAIN OR PRESSURE, IN CHEST WHEN WALK FAST,LEFT ON REST?
       483-REPEATED PAIN,PRESSURE OR TIGHT FEELING IN CHEST FORCED STOP WALKING?
       484-REPEATED PAIN OR PRESSURE, IN CHEST LASTING MORE THAN 10 MINUTES?
       574-ALWAYS HAVE TO GET UP FROM SLEEP TO URINATE?




    ** CONSIDER ABNORMAL,OR POSSIBLE VARIATION FROM NORMAL
    NSA=NO SIGNIFICANT ABNORMALITY
    * NOTE
```

FIGURE 18.5 The summary report displays the results of multiphasic health testing, including laboratory-test results, measurements of physiological parameters, and positive answers to medical-history questions. Possible abnormalities are highlighted for review by the physician. (*Source:* Courtesy of Kaiser-Permanente Hospitals.)

is seen by a physician. As a result, the primary-care physician often can complete the health evaluation in a single office visit. Many of the decision rules that physicians apply manually can be programmed into a computer. Thus, sophisticated AMHTs assume some of the responsibilities of human reviewers by applying *advice rules* that analyze a patient's test results, and recommend additional diagnostic tests to order and refer patients for more extensive medical workups. For example, if the results of urinalysis show proteinuria, the computer can instruct the receptionist to ask the patient to return to the laboratory for retesting with a first-morning urine specimen. If the program detects a potentially urgent medical condition, it can advise the health-care staff to arrange for the patient to be seen immediately by a physician.

The benefits of computer-based review of HAS data using advice rules include

- Improved accuracy and decreased errors as a result of avoiding the tedium of routine manual review of summary reports
- Standardization of the ordering procedure for follow-up tests, and improved quality control, as a result of reviewing all cases using the same criteria
- Increased patient throughput, and more expedient treatment of patients with serious abnormalities, as a result of online processing

Researchers have demonstrated that computer-generated advice for follow-up testing can have a significant effect on the efficiency of the health assessment. One study compared the patterns of follow-up medical care for two groups of patients who were subjected to automated multiphasic health testing and who were found to have abnormal laboratory findings [Collen, 1975]. Both groups were eligible to receive computer-generated advice; however, the advice was given for one group, but not for the other (because of equipment failure or because the patient failed to wait). In the first group, 90 percent of all patients had their periodic health examinations completed in one physician office visit. In the other group, only 80 percent had just one visit; that is, approximately twice as many additional office visits occurred (20 percent versus 10 percent). The addition of online advice rules also decreased the number of patient-to-physician telephone calls and of physician-ordered laboratory tests that were relevant to the HAS checkup.

As the scope of testing in an HAS is broadened to include more tests, and more sensitive tests, it becomes possible for the computer to use information in the patient database not only to identify abnormal results, but also to suggest possible diagnoses. In essence, such diagnostic algorithms extend the concept of the advice rule. From a given set of signs, symptoms, and test results, the system may be able to suggest a preliminary diagnosis and to recommend additional tests that may help physicians to establish a firm diagnosis.

18.3 Historical Development of Health-Assessment Systems

The concept of health-assessment is not new. For decades, physicians have advocated periodic health examinations, such as the annual checkup. Over the past 45 years, the systematic, integrated, or multiphasic approach to health testing gradually evolved from individual screening programs.

Screening, as a public-health measure in the United States, began prior to 1900 with the screening of immigrants by the Marine Hospital Service to identify people with significant disease who might become a financial burden on the country. This activity was extended to the screening of communities for communicable diseases. Later, as serious communicable diseases gradually diminished in prevalence, the Public Health Service again expanded its attention to screening for chronic, noncommunicable diseases.

To decrease the costs of giving examinations to large numbers of people, researchers developed screening techniques that consisted of quick, simple tests that, with acceptable accuracy, identified persons likely to have the disease of interest. In 1948, multiphasic screening was introduced as an extension of the mass screening technique.

In 1951, the first multiphasic health-testing program within a comprehensive prepaid health plan was initiated in the Kaiser-Permanente Medical Care Program in its Oakland, California medical center. The advent of electronics and automation in medicine provided the opportunity to improve and augment screening techniques, so not only more tests, but also more accurate and quantitative measurements, could be used. In 1963, with the partial support of a grant from the Public Health Service, the multiphasic screening program already operational in the Kaiser-Permanente Oakland Medical Center was replaced by the first automated multiphasic health-testing program. In the first year, 35,000 patients received health-assessment examinations through the system. This program has operated continuously since that date and has provided more than 900,000 examinations.

Multiphasic testing programs proliferated throughout many of the developed countries of the world. In the early 1970s, there were about 300 programs in the United States [Schoen, 1973], 40 in Japan, 30 in Europe, and a few in Australia, Asia, Canada, and Latin America. Today, Japan and France continue to use automated multiphasic health testing to provide periodic health checkups. In Japan in 1980, there were more than 100 multiphasic testing centers [Yasaka et al., 1980]. The social-security system in France operates about 40 multiphasic testing programs; all French citizens are eligible for a free health checkup every 5 years. On the other hand, the number of multiphasic programs in the United States has been decreasing since the late 1970s. Most patients receive a panel of routine tests in conjunction with diagnostic workups when they visit physicians with specific medical complaints, a process called **case finding.** Currently, multiphasic testing is used primarily by HMOs that provide health checkups as a prepaid benefit of membership and by corporations that pay for employee checkups. In addition, some hospitals use multiphasic testing programs to perform preadmission workups and to categorize patients by diagnosis-related group (DRG).

The current public interest in personal health and self-care has stimulated public-health policy makers to reactivate voluntary mass testing programs; for example, "health fairs" sometimes are held at schools and shopping centers. These multiphasic testing programs focus on health-risk appraisal, health promotion, and patient education, rather than on early disease detection and subsequent medical treatment. This practice is supported by evidence that intervention to decrease bodily risk factors (for example, hypertension or high serum-cholesterol values) and behavioral risk factors (for example, cigarette smoking or insufficient exercise) can reduce mortality. Less than 15 causes of death constitute about two-thirds of a patient's total mortality risk, so health-risk appraisal programs estimate an individual's risk of dying from these common causes of death and recommend a health-improvement program to reduce these risks [Laszlo and Varga, 1981].

18.4   An Analysis of Health-Assessment Systems

Given the widespread acceptance of periodic health checkups, and the use of AMHTs in Japan and France, why are AMHTs not popular in the United States? Two factors contributed to the failure of multiphasic health-testing programs to achieve widespread acceptance in the United States. First, within the traditional health-care financing system, private fee-for-service physicians have little incentive to refer patients to multiphasic testing centers. Rather, they perform routine physical examinations or diagnostic workups for patients who present with specific medical complaints (and are paid for them by the patient or a third-party payer). Second, Medicare and indemnity insurance companies (such as Blue Cross and Blue Shield) do not reimburse patients for routine health testing, reasoning that the need for these services can be anticipated, and therefore are not insurable events.

Researchers have demonstrated that AMHTs are more economical than traditional methods for providing comprehensive screening examinations. For example, one study compared the costs of alternative modes of providing health examinations, including physician visits, laboratory tests, and X-ray examinations [Collen, 1984]. The study showed that, at Kaiser Hospitals in 1984, the average cost of a traditional physician examination with followup was $124. The average cost of multiphasic health testing followed by a brief physician examination was $89—a savings of 28 percent. Less clear was the benefit of early detection of disease in terms of mortality, morbidity, and total health-care costs. Critics of multiphasic testing programs argue that routine examinations of apparently healthy individuals represent an inefficient use of scarce health-care resources, because these programs are used for many people who do not currently require medical care.

The most well-known report of the effects of multiphasic health testing is based on a Kaiser-Permanente controlled trial that was initiated in 1964 [Friedman et al., 1986; Dales et al., 1979]. The study was designed to evaluate the effectiveness of annual multiphasic checkups in preventing or postponing morbidity, disability, and mortality. The study and control groups each were composed of about 5000 Kaiser members, aged 35 to 54 years at the initiation of the study. Researchers telephoned the members of the study group annually and urged them to schedule appointments for testing. The members of the control group were not urged to undergo multiphasic health testing, but could request an examination if they desired one.

After 11 years, the use of hospital and outpatient clinic services in the two groups was similar. Mortality from "potentially preventable" causes (in particular, death due to colorectal cancer and hypertensive cardiovascular disease) was significantly lower in the study group. There was, however, no difference in overall mortality rate (see Table 18.1), because both groups received the same overall care by primary physicians and because the potentially preventable conditions accounted for only 15 percent of all deaths. These conclusions were still valid 16 years into the study. Researchers also examined the economic effects of health-related events in a more limited analysis of men aged 45 to 54 years at the start of the study. The results of this analysis showed a significant savings due to the program—an estimated $2.6 million for the 1232 men in this age group, spread over the 11-year follow-up period. The primary monetary benefit of the program was increased earnings due to decreased disability. The medical costs were actually slightly higher in the study group (Table 18.2). Although the more detailed analysis was not performed for women or younger men, the health-outcome results indicate that there was no net savings associated with the multiphasic testing program for these subgroups.

This study suggests several important conclusions regarding multiphasic health testing. First, despite the objective to show that the early identification of physical abnormalities should lead to improvements in health, there were only a few conditions (hypertension and colorectal cancer) for which multiphasic testing had a demonstrable effect on health outcomes. In general practice, the failure to attain significant results may be due to the long chain of events that must take place between detection and cure; physicians must follow up on abnormal results and prescribe therapy, patients must comply with physicians' orders, and the therapy must be effective in treating the condition. Each of these links is imperfect; for example, physicians sometimes fail to follow up on abnormal results [Bates and Yellin, 1972]. Of course, as we discussed in Chapter 3, the failure to act on abnormal results may be a rational decision in many cases, because of the imperfect sensitivity of the tests and the low prior probability of disease in an asymptomatic population.

Second, the costs of health-care screening programs may exceed the benefits to institutions in terms of reduced medical costs. The results of the Kaiser study suggested that multiphasic health testing has significant benefits for middle-aged men in terms of increased lifetime earnings due to reduced disability and to lower mortality rate. These benefits can be captured by the health-care institutions that provide the care, to the extent that years of life saved generate dues payments by members of the health plans. Industrial corporations may benefit from the increased productivity of their workers and reduced expenditures for sick-leave pay, medical-care benefits, and training of new employees. Thus, it is understandable that company-sponsored multiphasic testing is one of the primary areas for application of this technology today.

Many people will continue to want some form of periodic health assessment. The current trend is to tailor the health-assessment process more specifically to the characteristics of individual patients, while still capturing many of the benefits of the automated health-testing process. As we have shown in this chapter, questions of cost-effectiveness, the structure of the health-care delivery system, and the nature of reimbursement for health services affected the availability of AMHTs in the United States. These same factors also influence the acceptance and diffusion of other health-care technologies. We shall provide a more general discussion of health-care financing in Chapter 19.

TABLE 18.1 Number of Deaths and Death Rates in Study- and Control-Group Subjects, 1965–1975

Cause of Death	No. of Deaths*		Death Rate* (per 1000 for the 11-year period)		Chi-Square Value†
	Study	Control	Study	Control	
Potentially Postponable Causes	44	73	8.6	13.2	5.25‡
Cancer of colon and rectum	5	18	1.0	3.3	6.43‡
Cancer of breast (women only)	14	14	5.0	4.8	0.01
Cancer of cervix and endometrium (women only)	1	4	0.4	1.4	1.68
Cancer of prostate (men only)	0	2	0.0	0.8	0.40
Cancer of kidney	1	0	0.2	0.0	0.00
Hypertension, hypertensive cardiovascular disease, and hemorrhagic cerebrovascular disease with hypertension	13	26	2.5	4.7	3.44
Hemorrhagic cerebrovascular disease without hypertension	10	9	2.0	1.6	0.15
Other Causes	309	320	60.1	57.8	0.26
Infectious and parasitic disease	5	2	1.0	0.4	1.52
Cancer of buccal cavity and pharynx	0	1	0.0	0.2	0.00
Cancer of esophagus	6	3	1.2	0.5	1.23
Cancer of stomach	5	6	1.0	1.1	0.03
Cancer of pancreas	8	10	1.6	1.8	0.09
Cancer of bronchus and lung	25	26	4.9	4.7	0.01
Cancer of ovary and tube (women only)	6	6	2.2	2.1	0.00
Cancer of brain	2	1	0.4	0.2	0.41
Metastatic cancer, primary site unknown	3	7	0.6	1.3	1.32
Lympho-hematopoietic cancer	15	5	2.9	0.9	5.79‡
Other cancer	7	5	1.4	0.9	0.50
Endocrine, nutritional and metabolic disease	5	5	1.0	0.9	0.01
Mental, nervous system, and sense organ disease	3	5	0.6	0.9	0.36
Ischemic heart disease	92	98	17.9	17.7	0.00
Non-hemorrhagic cerebrovascular disease	10	6	2.0	1.1	1.32
Other circulatory system disease	16	18	3.1	3.3	0.01
Respiratory system disease	10	18	2.0	3.3	1.73
Cirrhosis	26	36	5.1	6.5	0.96
Other gastrointestinal disease	6	9	1.2	1.6	0.40
Genitourinary system disease	8	8	1.6	1.5	0.02
Skin and subcutaneous tissue disease	0	1	0.0	0.2	0.00
Musculoskeletal system disease	4	3	0.8	0.5	0.22
Suicide	18	7	3.5	1.3	5.71‡
Other injuries and poisoning	29	34	5.6	6.1	0.11
All Causes	353	393	68.7	71.0	0.21

*Populations alive as of 1 January, 1965: Study—5138, Control—5536.
†Yates' continuity correction was applied when the expectation for the smallest cell was less than 1.0.
‡ $p < 0.05$.
Source: Reprinted with permission from Dales, L. G., Friedman, G. D., and Collen, M. F. Evaluating periodic multiphasic health checkups: A controlled trial. *Journal of Chronic Diseases*, 32:392, 1979.

TABLE 18.2 Economic Effects of Health-Related Events in Study- and Control-Group Men Ages 45 to 54 Years at Entry

Health Status and Costs for Control and Study Groups		1965	1966	1967	1968	1969	1970	1971	1972	1973	1974	1975	1965–1975 Total
A. Estimated proportions of initial populations with													
1. No disability	Control	0.87	0.84	0.81	0.79	0.76	0.73	0.70	0.68	0.65	0.64	0.63	
	Study	0.88	0.85	0.83	0.82	0.81	0.78	0.74	0.72	0.71	0.69	0.67	
2. Partial disability	Control	0.11	0.11	0.12	0.13	0.14	0.15	0.16	0.17	0.17	0.16	0.15	
	Study	0.10	0.11	0.12	0.11	0.11	0.11	0.12	0.13	0.13	0.13	0.13	
B. Economic equivalent proportions with no disability (A1 + 0.75 A2)	Control	0.95	0.93	0.90	0.89	0.87	0.84	0.82	0.80	0.77	0.76	0.74	
	Study	0.95	0.94	0.92	0.91	0.89	0.86	0.83	0.82	0.80	0.78	0.77	
C. Estimated average annual earnings per man, in dollars	Control and Study	7440	7710	8130	8870	9540	10270	11250	12210	13240	14370	15590	
D. Mean annual earnings per man, in dollars (B × C)	Control	7046	7132	7341	7859	8262	8668	9270	9756	10235	10878	11521	
	Study	7090	7224	7488	8045	8500	8863	9349	9976	10645	11266	11926	
E. Mean annual physician visit expense per man	Control	$29	$26	$26	$25	$27	$39	$35	$35	$33	$48	$41	
	Study	$25	$27	$26	$25	$29	$39	$41	$41	$34	$46	$43	
F. Mean annual laboratory expense per man	Control	$21	$18	$21	$21	$23	$36	$27	$30	$30	$40	$38	
	Study	$19	$24	$26	$21	$25	$38	$42	$38	$38	$44	$43	
G. Mean annual hospitalization expense per man	Control	$23	$24	$29	$46	$59	$79	$76	$104	$93	$94	$134	
	Study	$23	$21	$38	$31	$35	$69	$67	$77	$78	$108	$104	
H. Mean annual MHC expense per man	Control	$11	$11	$11	$11	$10	$10	$13	$10	$12	$13	$23	
	Study	$19	$32	$40	$45	$40	$41	$43	$41	$40	$32	$59	
I. Net difference in economic impact per man in initial population*	Study minus control	$42	$67	$104	$167	$228	$172	$37	$202	$388	$353	$392	$2152

*Study–control difference in earnings (Row D) minus net study–control difference in medical care expenses (Rows E through H).

[MHC = multiphasic health checkup.]

Source: Adapted with permission from Dales, L. G., Freidman, G. D., and Collen, M. F. Evaluating periodic multiphasic health checkups: A controlled trial. *Journal of Chronic Diseases*, 32:398, 1979.

Suggested Readings

Bates, B. and Yellin, J. A. The yield of multiphasic screening. *Journal of the American Medical Association,* 222:74, 1972.

> *This article reports the results of a study to evaluate physicians' responses to abnormal findings discovered through multiphasic screening. The authors conclude that the failure of physicians to follow up on abnormal results, the uncertain effects of therapy, and problems with patient compliance make it unlikely that studies of multiphasic screening will show demonstrable benefits in terms of reduced mortality and morbidity.*

Collen, M. F. (ed). *Multiphasic Health Testing Services.* New York: John Wiley & Sons, 1977.

> *This book provides a comprehensive review of Collen's 25 years of experience with multiphasic health testing.*

Dales, L. G., Friedman, G. D., and Collen, M. F. Evaluating periodic multiphasic health checkups: A controlled trial. *Journal of Chronic Diseases,* 32:385, 1979.

> *This article covers the 11-year follow-up results of a controlled study to measure the economic and health effects of multiphasic health testing at the Kaiser-Permanente Oakland Medical Center.*

DeFriese, G. H. (ed). A research agenda for personal health risk assessment methods in health hazard/health risk appraisal. *Health Services Research,* 22:442, 1987.

> *The articles in this special issue provide an excellent summary of health-risk appraisal.*

Friedman, G. D., Collen, M. F., and Fireman, B. H. Multiphasic health checkup evaluation: A 16-year follow-up. *Journal of Chronic Diseases,* 39:453, 1986.

> *This article presents results from a 16-year clinical trial to evaluate the effect of a multiphasic health-testing program on the mortality of a patient population at the Kaiser-Permanente Oakland Medical Center.*

Questions for Discussion

1. Develop a flowchart for an interactive, branching history taker designed to ask patients about the stress factors they face during a typical day.
2. Discuss three factors important in choosing which diagnostic tests to include in an HAS. What considerations are particularly relevant in deciding whether to include tests for high cholesterol level, hypertension, breast cancer, and presence of the AIDS antibody? For each condition, define the appropriate population for testing.
3. Despite the fact that AMHTs have been shown to be more economical than traditional methods for providing comprehensive screening examinations, AMHTs have not achieved widespread acceptance in the United States. Discuss the sociological and economic factors that have limited acceptance of these systems in this country.

III

Medical Informatics
in the Years Ahead

19

Health-Care Financing and Technology Assessment

Alain C. Enthoven and Nancy A. Wilson

After reading this chapter, you should know the answers to these questions:

- How has health-care insurance contributed to rapid growth in health-care spending during the 1970s and 1980s? How will insurance evolve in the decade ahead?
- What are health-maintenance organizations, prepaid group practices, and preferred-provider organizations? How do these groups provide incentives to reduce health-care costs?
- What are the goals and methods of cost–benefit analysis?
- What are the human-capital and willingness-to-pay approaches to valuation of human life?
- How may changes in fiscal constraints affect the development and adoption of medical-computing technology?
- How can medical-information systems help health-care institutions respond to the changing financial environment?

You may be wondering why a chapter on health-care financing and technology assessment is included in a book about computer applications in medicine. At first glance, this topic may seem to have little to do with medical computing. Yet many of the chapters in this book have mentioned fiscal issues that affect the development, implementation, and dissemination of new computing technologies for health-care applications. As we saw in Chapter 18, we clearly cannot study and understand new technologies independently of the economic realities that shape their design and influence the potential for their successful use in routine settings.

There are two reasons why you need to understand fiscal issues as they relate to medical informatics. First, it is important to know the ways in which funding from the public and private sectors leads to the development of new technologies. Many of the systems discussed in this book were originally conceived as research projects and were funded by government or private grants. The ultimate transition to routine function by some of these systems was not easy, and the determination of how the computers, staff, and servicing would be financed when the grants ran out often was a major issue in the technology-transfer process. The general argument has been that the costs of computer-based clinical services can be passed on to patients only to the extent that such services are shown to be cost-effective.

Many observers have suggested that it is the new technologies of medicine that account in large part for the increasing cost of health care. In light of the fiscal constraints under which hospitals, clinics, and physicians now operate, people are paying close attention to cost–benefit analysis for *all* new technologies, including computer-based information systems. Some information systems, such as automated billing systems, will be relatively unaffected because their costs are not tied directly to patient care and because they replace less efficient manual systems. The benefits of other systems, however, are not as easy to analyze. Patient-monitoring applications in the intensive-care unit (ICU), pharmacy systems that detect and alert staff to drug–drug interactions, clinical decision-support systems that give diagnostic and therapeutic advice—the cost-effectiveness of systems such as these will be subjected to close scrutiny in an attempt to curb the growth in health-care expenditures.

The second way in which fiscal issues are important to the study of medical informatics relates to the growing pressures on hospitals and other health-care providers to manage information more effectively, to collect cost-effectiveness data, to generate management reports, and to deal optimally with a complex array of reimbursement schemes. The computer has become an essential part of this monitoring and reporting function, and new integrated approaches to patient-data collection, diagnostic classification, cost allocation, and similar tasks will have a profound effect on the ability of the health-care community to respond to this increasingly challenging financial environment. On a more global level, modern health-care policy analysis would not be possible without computer systems that collect, store, and analyze enormous data sets.

In this chapter, we provide an overview of the U.S. health-care economy and describe how health-care institutions are reimbursed for the services they provide. The first part of the chapter provides a historical perspective and explains how the system has evolved to its current organization. The remainder of the chapter explores the issue of how managers of hospitals and other health-care institutions need to think about costs, technology assessment, and capital investments in the cost-contained health-care system. We provide a description of cost–benefit analysis, discuss cost concepts from the disciplines of accounting and microeconomics, and review methods for estimating costs. We close the chapter with a discussion of the implications of changes in health-care financing and, in particular, of how these changes may affect both the introduction of computer-based systems and the use of computers to assist with management functions.

19.1 The Era of Open-Ended Spending

The period from 1960 to 1980 can be characterized as the *open-ended era* in health-care financing. During these 2 decades, national health-care spending increased from about \$27 billion to nearly \$250 billion (Figure 19.1), from 5.3 percent of the gross national product (GNP) to 9.5 percent (Figure 19.2) [Gibson, 1984]. Public-sector spending on health care increased from \$6.6 billion to \$105.5 billion. Aggregate private health-care insurance premiums increased from \$5.8 billion, or 2.1 percent of wages and salaries, to \$63.6 billion, or 4.7 percent of wages and salaries. In this section, we consider the ways in which patients managed to pay for their care as costs soared dramatically during the 20-year period.

19.1.1 Private Health-Care Insurance

Although the antecedents to modern health insurance began in the nineteenth century, and several formative decisions were made in the 1930s, health insurance in the United States did not become a large-scale enterprise until World War II.

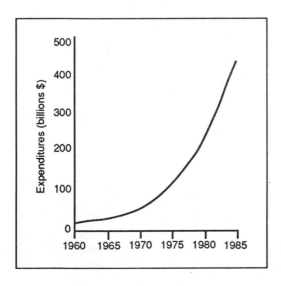

FIGURE 19.1 National health-care expenditures (in billions of dollars) grew at an increasing rate between 1960 and 1985. (*Source:* National Center for Health Statistics: *Health, United States, 1987.* DHHS Pub. No. (PHS) 88-1232. Public Health Service. Washington. U.S. Government Printing Office, March 1988. (Previous volumes in the series also used.))

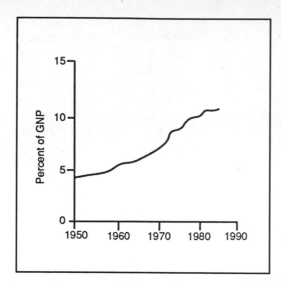

FIGURE 19.2 National health-care expenditures as a percent of gross national product (GNP) rose steadily during the period 1950 to 1985. (*Source:* National Center for Health Statistics: *Health, United States, 1987.* DHHS Pub. No. (PHS) 88-1232. Public Health Service. Washington. U.S. Government Printing Office, March 1988. (Previous volumes in the series also used.))

About 12 million people had insurance for hospital expenses in 1940; nearly 77 million had insurance by 1950 [Health Insurance Association of America (HIAA), 1983]. Several trends encouraged this development. Collective bargaining was an important factor, as union leaders considered employer-paid health insurance to be an attractive bargaining prize. Employers of nonunionized personnel also generally were willing to provide insurance, because they wished to avoid grievances that would encourage unionization. Perhaps the most influential factor was that employer-paid health insurance was excluded from the taxable incomes of employees; thus, health insurance was a form of tax-free compensation. Health insurance as a fringe benefit continued to grow rapidly in the 1950s. In 1959, legislation was enacted to cover all federal employees. By 1960, about 123 million people were covered, at least for hospital expenses.

During this period, health insurance generally was of two types. Commercial insurance companies offered *indemnity insurance,* modeled on casualty insurance. The typical form was payment of a specified amount for a hospital day, or for each of a list of surgical procedures. Commercial insurance companies had no contractual link to providers. Their role was to indemnify patients for medical expenses presumably beyond their control. Most of this insurance was sold to employers, usually as a part of a package that included group life and disability insurance. As time went by, the coverages became more comprehensive. Frequently, they were backed up by **major medical insurance** that paid 80 percent of all the patient's outlays after the patient had paid a specified amount.

The other major type of health insurance was called *service benefit,* offered by Blue Cross and Blue Shield. Blue Cross plans were offered by independent local nonprofit insurance companies sponsored by hospital associations. Blue Shield plans were sponsored by medical societies. These organizations were created to ensure that the providers would be paid in the manner most acceptable to those providers—that is, they could choose to be paid through cost reimbursement, or through payment of billed charges to hospitals and fee-for-service payment to physicians. Most hospitals and physicians participated in Blue Cross and Blue Shield (the "Blues"). In the former case, this usually meant hospitals would give Blue Cross a discount from the fees charged patients who were insured by other carriers. In the latter case, it usually meant agreement to accept Blue Shield fees as payment in full.

These insurance systems have certain features in common. First, they reimburse physicians for services based on **usual, customary, and reasonable** fees. They pay hospitals on the basis of billed charges or retrospective cost reimbursement. Thus, they assign providers no responsibility for the total cost of care. They do not create incentives to analyze or control costs. On the contrary, they pay providers more for doing more, whether or not more is necessary for or beneficial to the patient. If outlays exceed premium revenues, future premiums are raised to make up the difference.

Second, these insurance systems were based on the principle that at all times the patient must have free choice of provider. In many states, it was even against the law for the insurer to influence the patient's choice of provider. In such an arrangement, the insurer has no bargaining power with providers, and thus no way to control prices or costs.

Third, these financing systems generally covered entire employee groups. They were not conceived as competitors in situations in which individual employees would have a choice among health-care financing plans.

The most important exception to these systems of health-care finance was **prepaid group practice,** in which members paid a set annual fee in advance and received comprehensive health care during the year. In 1960, membership in prepaid group practice plans was very small (about 1 million nationwide). The plans' importance lay in the concepts on which they were based. Kaiser-Permanente, the largest and most successful of these organizations, adopted the following principles as its "genetic code" [Somers, 1971]:

- Multispecialty group practice
- Integrated inpatient and outpatient facilities
- Direct prepayment to the medical-care organization
- Reversal of economics: Providers are better off if the patients remain well or have their medical problems solved promptly
- Voluntary enrollment: Every enrollee should have a competing alternative
- Physician responsibility for quality and cost of care

The principle of voluntary enrollment was the beginning of the competition among health-care financing and delivery plans that became widespread by the mid-1980s. The principles of direct prepayment created a natural interest in evaluation of the costs versus the benefits of different uses of resources and patterns of care. This is important from the point of view of this chapter, because organizations of this type were the first to have a serious interest in cost–benefit analysis in medical care. In the future, the competition of such organizations is likely to increase that interest.

During the era of open-ended spending, the number of persons covered and the scope of private health-insurance coverage increased markedly. The number of people with private hospital-insurance protection increased from 123 million in 1960 to 189 million by 1980 [Health Insurance Association of America (HIAA), 1983]. This increase was encouraged by the tax laws. The inflation that started in the late 1960s and intensified in the 1970s pushed people into higher and higher income-tax brackets. As this shift occurred, it became increasingly advantageous for employer and employees to agree that the employer would pay for comprehensive health insurance with before-tax dollars, rather than paying the same amount in cash to employees and letting them pay for the insurance with net after-tax dollars. By 1980, the average federal taxpayer was in about the 40-percent marginal tax bracket, counting both income and payroll taxes. That is, of the last dollar earned by an average taxpayer, 40 percent went to income and payroll taxes. In 1981, this tax subsidy for health insurance (in which employers used nontaxed dollars to purchase insurance for employees) cost the federal government about $20 billion in foregone tax revenues [Ginsburg, 1982].

In the 1970s, high interest rates made employers more aware of the time value of money. Instead of paying a premium to an insurance company that would keep the money for perhaps 3 or 4 months before paying the bills, an increasing number of large employers decided to pay their employees' medical bills directly, to hire insurance companies to perform claims processing or **administrative services only (ASO)**, and perhaps to buy insurance for only truly catastrophic cases (minimum premium plan, or MPP). By 1981, about 31 million people were covered for hospital expense through ASO–MPP arrangements. In effect, this meant that many large employers took on the health-insurance function (and risk) directly.

19.1.2 Public Financing and Legislation

In 1965, Congress enacted the Medicare and Medicaid programs, Titles XVIII and XIX of the Social Security Act. Medicare is the federal program of hospital- and medical-insurance for Social Security retirees. In 1972, legislation added coverage for the long-term disabled and for patients suffering from chronic renal failure. By 1980, Medicare covered 25.5 million aged and 3 million disabled persons [Social Security Administration, 1983].

Medicare was based on the same principles of payment as were Blue Cross and Blue Shield (reimbursement of reasonable cost to hospitals and fees to physicians). Patients were given unlimited free choice of provider, so a Medicare beneficiary received no financial advantage from going to a less costly hospital. The Medicare law did provide for certain **deductibles** and **coinsurance** to be paid by the patient who was receiving services. For example, under today's Medicare system, the hospitalized patient is charged a deductible that approximates 1 day's cost at the average hospital's per diem rate. After an annual deductible, Medicare pays 80 percent of the doctor's usual and customary fee; the patient is responsible for the rest. The coinsurance, then, is the remaining 20 percent that the Medicare beneficiary is responsible for paying. However, any cost-consciousness that cost sharing might encourage is attenuated, because about 65 percent of Medicare beneficiaries purchase private supplemental insurance that helps to pay the coinsurance and deductibles. Another 11 percent have resources that place them below the federally defined poverty level, and thus are jointly covered by Medicaid, which has no coinsurance and deductibles [U.S. Department of Health and Human Services (DHHS), 1984].

Medicaid is a program of federal grants to help states pay for medical care of welfare recipients. Only about one-half of the low-income population is covered by Medicaid. For example, care for "medically indigent adults" has remained the responsibility of local, usually county governments. Under Medicaid, the federal government set elaborate standards that a state program must meet to be eligible for federal subsidies. The federal government paid a share of the cost (at least 50 percent, average 55 percent), depending on the state's per capita income. Like Medicare, Medicaid was based on the principles of fee-for-service, cost reimbursement, and free choice of provider. Many physicians, however, chose not to participate in Medicaid.

In an effort to slow the growth of federal and state health-care outlays, numerous regulatory restraints were tried during the 1970s, all with little success. Examples include institution of reimbursement limits on daily routine hospital care, creation of local nonprofit physicians' organizations called **Professional Standards Review Organizations (PSROs)** to review use of Medicare and Medicaid services and to deny payment for unnecessary services, and tying of growth in reimbursable physician fees to an index of wages. These restraints were ineffective; Medicare and Medicaid outlays grew by about 17 percent per year through the 1970s.

In 1973, Congress passed the Health Maintenance Organization (HMO) Act. The law defined two types of HMOs: group-practice models, based on prepaid group practices, and **independent-practice associations (IPAs).** In both kinds of organizations, the premiums or dues are paid directly to the provider organization in the form of a fixed periodic payment for comprehensive care, set in advance. (This reimbursement is sometimes called **per capita payment** or **capitation**). In the IPA model, physicians continue to practice on a fee-for-service basis in their own offices, but they agree to fee schedules, management controls, and risk-sharing arrangements to ensure that the care is delivered for the contractual amount.

The HMO Act provided grants and loans to help HMOs get started. It also mandated that employers of 25 or more employees, subject to the Fair Labor Standards Act, must offer a group practice and an individual practice HMO to their employees, if such organizations serve the areas where their employees live and if the HMO asks that its services be offered. These provisions helped to expand access to the HMO market, and thus the number of HMOs. From 1977 to 1983, HMO membership grew from 6.3 million to 12.4 million, an annual average growth rate of about 12 percent [InterStudy, 1985].

19.1.3 The Uninsured

Nonetheless, by the end of the 1970s, health insurance was far from universal. An analysis of 1977 data showed that about 8 percent of all Americans lacked either private health insurance or eligibility for public programs of health insurance [U.S. Department of Health and Human Services (DHHS), 1985]. These people were concentrated among the low-income, the young, and the unemployed populations. Concern over finding ways to continue coverage for people who had lost their jobs continued into the 1980s. In cases of serious illness, the uninsured have to pay for their own care until they have exhausted their assets. At that point, they may receive free care at community hospitals, or they can fall back on local government hospitals.

19.2 Health-Care Financing: The 1980s and Beyond

The early 1980s saw increasing strains on public finance. The taxpayer revolt, increases in spending for national defense, and interest on the national debt intensified the competition for public funds. Still, from 1980 to 1982, Medicare outlays grew from $36.8 billion to $52.2 billion, or 19 percent per year (Figure 19.3). Medicaid outlays grew from $26.8 billion to $34 billion, or 13 percent per year. Federal tax revenue losses from the favorable tax treatment of health insurance grew from about $17 billion to $23 billion, or about 16 percent per year. By comparison, the GNP grew about 8 percent per year. Pressures for change intensified accordingly.

19.2.1 1981 to 1983: The Turning Point in Public Finance

Fiscal pressures led to a great deal of legislative activity during 1981, 1982, and 1983, the general thrust of which was to change the government's commitment from open-ended cost-unconscious **retrospective payment** to limited, cost-conscious **prospective payment**. There was also a move from free choice of provider toward limited choice of provider, with limitations based on cost.

The Omnibus Budget Reconciliation Act of 1981 included many changes in Medicare and Medicaid. Two changes in Medicaid were particularly significant. First, the federal matching payments to each state were reduced. States could avoid a part of these

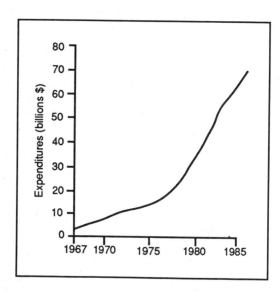

FIGURE 19.3 Increases in federal expenditures for Medicare (in billions of dollars) between 1967 and 1985 mirrored the growth in total national expenditures for health care during this period (Figures 19.1 and 19.2). (*Source:* National Center for Health Statistics: *Health, United States, 1987.* DHHS Pub. No. (PHS) 88-1232. Public Health Service. Washington. U.S. Government Printing Office, March 1988. (Previous volumes in the series also used.))

reductions if they took certain cost-control actions. Second, the Congress increased the flexibility of states to change their Medicaid programs to control costs. In particular, the law provided that the secretary of Health and Human Services (HHS) could waive the freedom of choice of provider provision in the Medicaid law and allow states to engage in selective provider contracting. This led some states, such as California, to enact legislation to require their Medicaid programs to contract selectively on the basis of price, and to seek competitive bids from hospitals.

The Tax Equity and Fiscal Responsibility Act of 1982 (TEFRA) put two new constraints on the all-inclusive cost per case for Medicare. First, it placed a limit on total inpatient operating costs, applied on a cost-per-case basis, adjusted for each hospital's severity of case mix. Second, it placed a new limit on each hospital's rate of increase in cost per case, based on an index of the wages and prices hospitals pay. The same law provided that Medicare could contract with HMOs or other "competitive medical plans" to care for Medicare beneficiaries. These plans are being paid by Medicare on the basis of a fixed prospective per capita payment equal to 95 percent of the adjusted average per capita cost to Medicare of similar patients who remain with fee-for-service providers.

In the Social Security Amendments of 1983, Congress enacted a new **prospective-payment system (PPS)** for Medicare inpatient cases. Hospitals are now being paid a uniform national fixed payment per case, based on about 468 **diagnosis-related groups (DRGs),** adjusted for area hospital wage levels. The DRG classification system was derived empirically; diagnoses were assigned to a group based on major diagnostic category, length of stay, secondary diagnosis, surgical procedure, age, and types of services required. Within each DRG, the average length of stay is expected to be similar. Figure 19.4 shows a subset of DRG categories. Initially, capital-related costs, direct medical-education costs, and outpatient services have been paid for on the basis of cost reimbursement, although Congress has directed the secretary of HHS to study and make recommendations on methods of including capital-related costs and inpatient physician services in the prospective payments.

19.2.2 Marketplace Changes

Parallel to these legislative changes, significant changes occurred in the marketplace. First, growth in HMO membership accelerated. By the end of 1987, there were 29.3 million HMO enrollees. Second, **preferred-provider organizations (PPOs)** formed at a rapid rate. Use of PPOs is a method of financing health care based on selective contracting in advance for the services of health-care providers. Because PPOs lack a specific legal definition, however, it is not possible to measure the number of people they insure with any precision. A PPO typically is composed of the following:
- A provider panel, presumably selected for cost-effectiveness
- A negotiated fee schedule that providers agree to accept as payment in full for their services
- Some form of utilization control
- Incentives for consumers to select providers from the panel, usually in the form of reduced coinsurance

MDC 04		Diseases & Disorders of the Respiratory System
075	P	Major Chest Procedures
076	P	O.R. Proc. on the Resp. System Except Major Chest with C.C.
077	P	O.R. Proc. on the Resp. System Except Major Chest w/o C.C.
078	M	Pulmonary Embolism
079	M	Respiratory Infections & Inflammations Age >= 70 and/or C.C.
080	M	Respiratory Infections & Inflammations Age 18–69 w/o C.C.
081	M	Respiratory Infections & Inflammations Age 0–17
082	M	Respiratory Neoplasms
083	M	Major Chest Trauma Age >= 70 and/or C.C.
084	M	Major Chest Trauma Age < 70 w/o C.C.
085	M	Pleural Effusion Age >= 70 and/or C.C.
086	M	Pleural Effusion Age < 70 w/o C.C.
087	M	Pulmonary Edema & Respiratory Failure
088	M	Chronic Obstructive Pulmonary Disease
089	M	Simple Pneumonia & Pleurisy Age >= 70 and/or C.C.
090	M	Simple Pneumonia & Pleurisy Age 18–69 w/o C.C.
091	M	Simple Pneumonia & Pleurisy Age 0–17
092	M	Interstitial Lung Disease Age >= 70 and/or C.C.
093	M	Interstitial Lung Disease Age < 70 w/o C.C.
094	M	Pneumothorax Age >= 70 and/or C.C.
095	M	Pneumothorax Age < 70 w/o C.C.
096	M	Bronchitis & Asthma Age >= 70 and/or C.C.
097	M	Bronchitis & Asthma Age 18–69 w/o C.C.
098	M	Bronchitis & Asthma Age 0–17
099	M	Respiratory Signs & Symptoms Age >= 70 and/or C.C.
100	M	Respiratory Signs & Symptoms Age < 70 w/o C.C.
101	M	Other Respiratory Diagnoses Age >= 70 and/or C.C.
102	M	Other Respiratory Diagnoses Age < 70

FIGURE 19.4 A sampling of the 468 diagnosis-related group (DRG) categories. DRGs form the basis for reimbursement of Medicare hospital cases under the Prospective Payment System enacted in 1983. [MDC = major diagnostic category, O.R. Proc. = operating-room procedure, C.C. = complication or comorbidity (significant secondary conditions that are likely to increase length of stay), P = surgical case, M = medical case.]

For example, a PPO might pay 80 percent of the negotiated fee if the patient goes to a contracting doctor, but only 64 percent of the negotiated fee (which is likely to be a lower percent of the actual fee) if the patient uses a noncontracting doctor.

HMO providers differ from PPO providers in that the former bear the financial risk associated with members' use of services, whereas the latter do not. The HMO agrees to provide all necessary services for a comprehensive per capita payment set in advance, independent of the number of services actually used. PPO providers do not suffer financially if the use of services increases, and they are not directly rewarded for reducing the use of services or for treating patients in less costly ways. The HMO member agrees, for 1 year at a time, to receive all covered services from participating providers. By contrast, PPO members can elect to receive services, with less favorable insurance coverage, from nonparticipating providers.

From the point of view of economy, the PPO offers several important advances over traditional insurance. First, it is an attempt to select cost-effective providers and to reward insured patients, who otherwise would not be cost-conscious, for going to these providers for care. Second, the PPO includes contracting in advance for prices by someone who has bargaining power, knowledge, time to shop, and an incentive to make economical arrangements. Third, the PPO has the potential for ensuring quality control. If providers are selected based on the quality of care they provide, and not just by the prices they charge, a PPO might direct patients away from physicians who provide poor-quality care.

Selective contracting on the basis of quality and cost-effectiveness is a timely response to employer demands for cost control. In the long run, however, PPOs are likely to prove less effective than are prepaid group practices, the dominant and most effective model of HMO. The PPO format does not reward providers for keeping patients out of the hospital, which is the single most important source of cost savings in health care. PPOs do not organize the health-care system for efficiency; they merely try to shop for price in an inefficient system. PPOs may serve as a transition step. In the short run, with doctors and hospitals in excess supply, they are likely to obtain substantial price reductions.

19.2.3 A Look to the Future

These developments of the early 1980s point to likely trends for the rest of the century. First, the rapid growth of HMOs and PPOs is likely to continue. In the past, some critics suggested that HMOs showed lower costs because they served healthier people. However, 1983 saw the publication of the results of a controlled experiment in which people were assigned at random to fee-for-service or to membership in Group Health Cooperative of Puget Sound, a large prepaid group practice. Both groups were followed for 5 years. Those assigned to Group Health Cooperative incurred 28 percent fewer expenses and experienced 40 percent fewer days hospitalized than did those assigned to (free) fee-for-service care [Manning et al., 1984]. This study supported the findings of numerous other nonrandomized comparisons. This margin of economic advantage seems likely to lead to continued success in an increasingly competitive marketplace.

One market segment in which this development is likely to be pronounced is Medicare. The HMO format offers retirees both decreases in and increased predictability of health-care costs. The provision of the 1982 TEFRA legislation enables Medicare beneficiaries to realize for themselves the savings associated with joining an efficient HMO.

Second, employers are finding ways to return some cost-consciousness and responsibility for cost to employees. For example, one study of 250 major employers found that, from 1979 to 1983, the percentage of insurance plans charging no deductible for hospital room and board fell from 85 percent to 66 percent. This is likely to promote further the trend to establish more HMOs and PPOs.

Third, as competition intensifies, fee-for-service providers will find it increasingly necessary to engage in PPO contracts to attract patients. PPOs will find that they are less effective than are HMOs at controlling cost, however, because the providers retain fee-for-service incentives and are not financially constrained by a per capita budget. As a consequence, employers and other payers in PPO arrangements will increasingly insist that providers share at least part of the risk for per capita costs. Thus, PPOs will come to resemble HMOs in their financial aspects.

Fourth, the Medicare PPS, based on an all-inclusive price per case, represents a profound change from cost reimbursement and a step in the direction of economic efficiency. It has encouraged hospitals and their health-care staffs to cooperate in controlling costs. It has encouraged greater effort to relate clinical and financial information, to evaluate cost–benefit tradeoffs, to develop standards of care, to examine patterns of care critically, and to improve quality control. It remains, however, basically a fee-for-service system. Its goal is to bring the growth in cost per case into line with growth in the wages and other costs hospitals pay. In pursuing this goal, it does create incentives for hospitals and their medical staffs to assume some economically less desirable behaviors: to increase admissions of people who are less sick; to "unbundle" services (for example, to perform services on an outpatient basis where possible); and to classify patients into higher-paid DRGs. Some observers believe that, because it creates these incentives, this PPS is likely to fail to bring the growth in Medicare outlays into line with growth in tax revenues [Enthoven and Noll, 1984].

In the long run, employers and government will bring the growth of their outlays for health care into line with the growth in their revenues. Gradually, per capita cost—adjusted for age, gender, and other factors correlated with medical need—will prove to be the most important indicator used in setting the price for medical care. Per capita payment gives providers an incentive to solve the patient's medical problem in the least costly way and to keep patients out of the hospital. As HMO membership expands, and PPOs and PPSs evolve in the direction of per capita payment, providers will become increasingly interested in cost–benefit analyses of alternative medical treatments. This trend will of course have a major effect on the demand for computer-based tools that can be shown to save money, either by encouraging efficient use of other technologies or by providing data that support cost–benefit analyses.

What are the implications of these trends in health-care financing on technology assessment? In the era of open-ended health-care financing, providers of care could pass costs through to payers; thus, they did not have to think carefully about benefits versus costs. In the prospective-payment era, however, they must make these analyses. Investment decisions will have to be based on much more careful consideration of benefits versus costs, and of the implications for operating costs and return on investment. Health-care managers will have to do *make* versus *buy* analyses to evaluate, for example, whether they can obtain a test at less cost by contracting with an outside laboratory, rather than by purchasing the testing equipment. There will be more sharing of expensive capital equipment among hospitals. Physicians will have to consider whether new equipment will help to reduce costs per case (for example, by shortening hospital stays), rather than merely letting them perform a more expensive procedure. Cost–benefit analysis will play an increasing role in medical investment decision making, as it already does in many other industries.

19.3 Cost–Benefit Analysis

At the most general level, cost–benefit analysis can be defined as a systematic attempt to evaluate and compare all the costs and benefits of alternative ways of using resources to achieve an objective. Terminology is not completely standard in this field. The term **cost–benefit analysis (CBA)** generally refers to methods used when it is possible to assign dollar values to all the benefits and costs associated with alternative courses of action. The objective is to identify the alternative that yields the maximum net benefit. The term **cost-effectiveness analysis (CEA)** generally refers to methods used when it is not possible to measure benefits in dollar units. For example, given a budget for an immunization program, say we wish to determine what approach will save the most lives and reduce disability the most. We may not agree on how to assign dollar values to lives saved, but at least we can rank different programs by their effectiveness in saving lives, and can compare the costs of these programs. The objective is to identify either the alternative that yields the maximum effectiveness achievable for a given amount of spending, or the alternative that minimizes the cost of achieving a stipulated level of effectiveness. In a CBA, the optimum scale of the program or activity is an "output" of the analysis. In a CEA, the scale of the program is an "input," a starting assumption. Both CBA and CEA originated in applied economic analysis. We shall use the term *CBA*, referring to the general idea of evaluation of costs, risks and benefits, in the remainder of this chapter.

The Congressional Office of Technology Assessment (OTA) has identified 10 general principles of CBA methodology [Office of Technology Assessment (OTA), 1980]:

1. Define the problem
2. State the objectives
3. Identify the alternatives
4. Identify and analyze the benefits
5. Identify and analyze the costs
6. Differentiate the perspective of the analysis
7. Perform discounting
8. Analyze the uncertainties
9. Address the ethical issues
10. Interpret the results

Our discussion shall follow their outline, with special attention to the hallmarks of a good analysis.

19.3.1 Define the Problem

Explicitness in problem definition and a reasoned consideration of alternative definitions may be the most important part of the analysis. Exactly what is the problem to be solved? For example, is it "What can be done to improve the health of a given population?" or "How can diagnostic capabilities be improved?" or "How can we increase our census?" Broad ultimate objectives such as "improve health" do not provide useful guides to making resource-allocation decisions. Large problems must be broken down into manageable subproblems for people to be able to work on them— but this subdivision must be done with care. The laboratory manager told to reduce her budget might cut costs in a way that delays the reporting of test results and generates even greater costs elsewhere by causing longer hospital stays. Trying to minimize the laboratory's costs without considering the effects elsewhere would produce the wrong decisions.

19.3.2 State Objectives

A CBA evaluates alternative technologies in terms of their abilities to contribute to specific objectives, such as "reduce cancer mortality by detecting cancer earlier." The choice of objectives, and the methods by which these objectives are defined and measured, are worth much careful thought. Criteria should not be chosen casually. A good analysis will test the implications of apparently similar criteria, and will avoid errors in choice of criteria. The following are examples of errors made in choosing criteria:

- *Using ratios that do not relate well to the broader objectives being sought.* The government tried to control expenditures by limiting hospital reimbursement per patient day, ignoring the effect on total outlays. A hospital can reduce its average cost per day by keeping patients longer, which in turn increases total cost and reimbursement. So the government is now trying to control hospital reimbursement per case through the PPS. Such controls, however, create incentives for the hospital to reduce its average cost per stay by admitting more low-cost cases that otherwise could be treated less expensively on an outpatient basis. In fact, prepaid group practices lower total cost per capita by reducing hospital admissions and lengths of stay, even though that may increase costs per day and costs per stay (because either their typical inpatient is sicker, or more resources are consumed on a per day basis in an effort to shorten the patient stay).

- *Ignoring spillovers or unintended side effects.* One study of screening for hypertension found that identifying people as hypertensive increased their absenteeism from work [Haynes et al., 1978]. Being identified as hypertensive may have reduced these people's sense of well-being and caused them to consider themselves to be sick, whereas previously they considered themselves to be well. A similar error is the priority approach: "Nothing else matters until we have achieved our top-priority objective." This is the sort of reasoning that would lead public officials to reallocate funds from sanitation and education services to pay Medicaid bills in the name of increasing public health.

- *Confusing inputs with outputs.* If all patients stayed in the hospital 1 extra day, the GNP would increase, but average health status probably would not improve, because after a certain point, a patient can recuperate as well at home as in a hospital. Even counterproductive health care adds to the GNP.

19.3.3 Identify Alternatives

A good analysis identifies and evaluates the real alternatives, not mere "straw men" set up to be knocked down. Interested parties sometimes attempt to manipulate analyses by restricting the alternatives to be considered. A study might ask, "How large should our hospital-expansion program be to accommodate the increased needs of the population?"—and ignore alternatives such as dropping some services that duplicate similar services at other hospitals. Or an analysis might address the issue of, "Should we purchase laboratory equipment X or Y?"—and fail to consider contracting for some tests with an outside laboratory.

Although the methodology of CBA focuses on comparison of alternatives that are generated outside the process of evaluation, the most important results of CBA may be to design new alternatives based on insights derived from the analysis.

19.3.4 Identify and Analyze Benefits

In analyzing the benefits (or potential benefits) of, for example, a new diagnostic technology, we must ask the obvious questions: What will be the effect of having this additional information? Will it result in an altered course of medical treatment? Will it result in a shortened length of hospital stay? The benefits of computer-based information or decision-support systems often appear obvious, yet they are difficult to measure. Improvements in productivity associated with hospital information systems (HISs), for example, cannot be attributed to computers alone—they may have been achieved through improvements in methods and procedures that were implemented concurrent with the computer system (see Chapter 7). Similarly, computer-based systems installed without the support of appropriate procedures may not achieve the anticipated benefits.

Another issue to consider in assigning benefits is at what point in the technology's development the purchase decision is made. Often, the system will be used more as it is refined further and as new applications are discovered. The demand for CT scanners was dramatically underestimated in the early stages of the scanners' development. For innovative technologies, it is extremely difficult to forecast usage or to appreciate fully the potential for applications.

Even for stable technologies, there is the possibility of achieving benefits that were not anticipated prior to installation. For example, when a new appointment-scheduling system for a multispecialty practice was installed, the result was not only the predicted benefit of improved efficiency, but also the unexpected benefit of gaining access to better data on physicians' practice patterns.

After you have identified all foreseeable benefits or effects of each alternative, you need to measure and assign dollar values to them. In the easiest cases, market values exist and accurately reflect the social values of the benefits. This will be the case if the market is competitive—if effective markets exist for the benefits in question. As we have described, however, our health-care system is notorious for failing to satisfy the conditions for a normal competitive market.

Measuring and assigning values to the benefits of alternative health-care programs is usually made difficult by the lack of data linking health treatments and procedures with changes in outcomes. Many of the few available data come from observational studies, which are not controlled with regard to stratification of patients, randomization, and formal measurement criteria. When you use such data, you should remember that differences in outcomes may have been produced by bias in patient selection, rather than by differences in treatment. Randomized controlled trials (RCTs), which avoid biases due to patient selection, are relatively few. Ethical considerations may make it difficult to conduct RCTs to develop data relating different levels of health benefit to different amounts of spending. In general, it is considered ethical to perform an RCT comparing two treatments only if there is genuine uncertainty regarding which treatment produces a better outcome. Human subjects committees, responsible for ensuring the safety of experimental subjects, would not approve an RCT in which one treatment was known to produce an inferior outcome, even though at a much lower cost. For example, it is difficult to measure directly the benefits of hospitalization in ICUs, because most people believe that ICU care is valuable for critically ill patients and are unwilling to withhold this level of care from a random subpopulation of such patients. Thus, it is difficult to obtain reliable data relating costs and outcomes. However, the development of cost-conscious prospective-payment systems will increase the demand for data on the health effects of all medical and surgical interventions. Even if data were available that linked benefits with treatment, how could a dollar value be assigned, for example, to a life saved? We shall discuss this complex issue in Section 19.4.1.

19.3.5 Analyze Costs

Generally speaking, hospitals do not have *cost-accounting systems* in the sense that the term is used in most industries. That is, they do not have data systems that allow them to assign costs accurately to particular tests, procedures, and other units of care. The advent of cost-conscious prospective payment created a greatly increased demand for cost estimates, for cost-accounting systems, and for associated software to produce estimates systematically and reliably. The integration of such capabilities into medical information systems is likely to become an important motivation for introducing new computing technologies into health-care settings.

The most appropriate concept of cost in these settings is **economic cost** or **opportunity cost**—the value of the alternatives foregone that might have been produced with those resources. Economic costs are not necessarily the same as either charges or accounting costs. Because of the nature of the reimbursement system, hospitals have manipulated figures for charges and accounting costs to maximize reimbursement from insurers. Demand has not been cost-conscious and markets have not been competitive. Thus, there has been no market force to make charges reflect actual costs.

Cost concepts and methods of cost estimation are addressed in Sections 19.4 and 19.5.

19.3.6 Differentiate Perspective of Analysis

Whose costs? Whose benefits? CBA originally was developed to evaluate public programs. From that perspective, total social costs and benefits were considered. However, this may not be the appropriate perspective for a particular study in health care. A physician treating a well-insured patient may judge that, from the point of view of the patient, resource costs are irrelevant. As financing systems change, however, this perspective must change. Under prospective payment, a hospital may seek to maximize the health benefits it can produce for its patients, subject to the financial limits created by prospective payment, but without consideration of the costs imposed on the rest of the health-care sector (for example, on outpatient care), or on the patient (for example, reduced quality of care). An HMO will properly consider the benefits and costs to its own members. A county hospital may wish to focus on health benefits to the medically indigent population of its county, but it may be forced to consider "spillover" costs and benefits of its programs: An improved health-care program might attract patients from other counties, or a restricted health-care program might impose costs on other hospitals in the county. A good analysis will be explicit about whose costs and benefits are considered relevant.

19.3.7 Perform Discounting

How can we add equipment and building costs in 1990 and personnel expenses in each year from 1990 through 1995? How can we compare these expenses to revenues received during the years 1990 through 1995? We create comparable revenue and expense streams by first discounting the cash flows to their **present value (PV),** then subtracting the PV of the costs from the PV of the benefits, giving the **net present value (NPV).**

The concept of present value generally reflects the fact that $1 received 1 year from now is not worth as much as $1 received today. If the interest rate is 10 percent, the promise of $1 to be collected 3 years from today is worth 1.10^{-3} or 75 cents. (This assumes people are free to borrow and lend at 10 percent, that the interest payments can be reinvested at 10 percent, and that there are no transaction costs.) Because 75 cents invested at 10 percent will be worth $1 at the end of 3 years, we say that the present value of $1 received 3 years from now is 75 cents.

Choosing the appropriate interest rate to discount the cash flows can be a complex matter. In the case of public-sector investments, the appropriate interest rate is the opportunity cost—the rate of return that the resources used would otherwise yield in the private sector. Because of the distorting effects of different tax rates in different sectors, this value can be difficult to estimate. In the case of a private nonprofit institution that is able to borrow, the extra interest costs associated with the extra debt that would be incurred to finance the project in question would be the appropriate discount rate.

19.3.8 Analyze Uncertainties

Most CBAs are done in the face of significant uncertainties. There are no analytical methods to transform uncertainties into certainties. A good analysis will try to treat uncertainties explicitly, helping the decision maker to understand on what assumptions they depend. There are several techniques to help accomplish this task. The first step is to put bounds on the uncertainties; for example, to develop optimistic and pessimistic estimates, as well as best estimates, of each parameter. At the same time, it is useful to envision scenarios of the future that are worth considering. What will be the effect of the availability of magnetic-resonance imaging (MRI) on the demand for CT? We do not know, but we can begin to formulate an estimate by considering a range of possibilities. The next step we perform is to do **sensitivity calculations.** Which parameters, scenarios, and uncertainties have a significant effect on the outcome, and which do not? It is helpful to highlight key sensitivities for the decision makers, indicating which factors merit special attention. Another useful step is to perform **break-even calculations:** We estimate at what value of parameter X alternative A leads to a better outcome than does alternative B.

Sensible patterns of behavior under uncertainty include buying time or information. It might be wise to rent time at an MRI facility for 1 or 2 years, rather than to purchase the equipment, while waiting for the technology to evolve and for the costs of purchase to come down. Designing new alternatives (such as equipment rental) that perform better under unfavorable conditions allows us, in effect, to buy insurance.

Using another strategy, we might try to make a case for alternative A while making all the assumptions about uncertain values in favor of alternative B. If A emerges as preferred even under these conditions, it would certainly be preferred under more favorable assumptions.

In general, a good analyst will not look for an optimum choice under only one set of assumed conditions. The conditions of the future are unknown; therefore, a good analyst will look for a solution that performs well over a broad range of conditions, and that permits flexibility to adapt to new information and changing conditions.

19.3.9 Address Ethical Issues

Decision-making about tradeoffs between health benefits and resource costs must take place in the context of ethical values, and analyses should reflect that necessity. There are many ethical dimensions in these choices. For example, does the analysis ensure equity in access to services? A policy that eliminated all health insurance would remove incentives for overspending, but would leave many people unable to purchase medical care. Or, how does profitability weigh against objectives such as saving lives? The autonomy and intrinsic worth of each patient should be assigned value in the analysis. The physician is primarily responsible for the welfare of her patient. CBA, however, usually concerns actions by an institution for the benefit of a population. Decision makers must consider, for example, whether costly services should continue to be provided to prolong the life of a terminally ill patient, when such provision is made at the expense of other services that would relieve suffering or would prolong the productive lives of other patients.

19.3.10 Interpret Results

In real situations, there is no single formula to cover all circumstances. There is no mathematical substitute for common sense. A good analyst figures out what the problem is and applies careful thought and judgment to the specific circumstance. He must look at the actual situation and think about implementation. What is happening elsewhere may influence his decision. For example, the cost of giving X-ray examinations to an extra 100 patients will depend in large measure on whether the existing X-ray capacity is fully used.

A successful analysis usually will produce a few key insights that can and should be communicated clearly to decision makers. Analysis accordingly should be seen as the servant of judgment, not as a substitute for judgment.

19.3.11 Present Results

Once the CBA is completed, there remains the issue of presenting the results to those people whose actions may depend on the presentation's persuasiveness. The following are guidelines for making successful presentations:

• *Keep it simple:* The results will not influence people who cannot understand them
• *Do not overemphasize the quantitative aspects:* Do not ignore nonquantifiable costs and benefits
• *Make it open and explicit:* Analysis is not a substitute for debate; rather, it should provide a framework for constructive debate

19.4 Concepts of Valuation

Measuring the costs and putting a value on the benefits of health-care services are not straightforward tasks. They draw from a variety of disciplines. In this section, we shall examine the tools for valuing life and limb, and shall discuss several useful cost concepts from microeconomics and accounting.

19.4.1 Valuation of Life and Limb

What is it worth to save a life, to prevent or cure an illness, or to relieve suffering? Many people have grappled with such issues without producing entirely satisfactory answers. People have an understandable resistance to the idea of putting a dollar value on human life or suffering. Yet people must make resource-allocation decisions. Society is not willing or able to spend unlimited amounts on health care or on occupational health and safety, highway safety, and the like. People do not put an infinite value on avoiding risks to their own lives.

In thinking about this problem, you must bear in mind the distinction between an **identified life** and a **statistical life.** People's response to a decision that saves or kills a named individual is very different from that to a decision that saves or kills an anonymous "one in a thousand." The president can appear on television and appeal for funds to pay for a liver transplant that may save the life of a little girl in Detroit while at the same time recommending to Congress that it cut back on Medicaid appropriations, without appearing to be inconsistent. Most program decisions by institutions are concerned with statistical lives.

Human-Capital Approach

In the **human-capital approach** to valuation of life, persons are viewed as productive assets [Cooper and Rice, 1976]. The economic cost of illness, or the economic value of prevention, is measured by the sum of direct outlays for diagnosis and treatment of illness, and loss in productivity because of illness or premature death. In a competitive economy, the value of a person's contribution to total output is measured by her wage. So the value of a life lost is measured by the PV of the person's stream of earnings over her lifetime if she had not died prematurely.

The human-capital approach has retained its popularity despite having been subjected to cogent criticisms, primarily because it lends itself to producing a reasonably accurate and reproducible calculation. One frequent objection is that it discriminates against women, minority-group members, and poor people: The values of saving their lives are calculated to be lower because they earn less. The most fundamental objection is that the method ignores the valuations people put on their own lives. A person or his family might quite reasonably value a life at more or less than the PV of that person's earnings. A healthy retired 65-year-old man might have no expected future earnings but might nonetheless place a substantial value on things that enhance his health and safety. There is something profoundly wrong with a concept that places zero value on saving his life.

Willingness to Pay

These objections to the human-capital approach have led economists to recommend that a reduction in the probability of a person's death should be valued by the person's **willingness to pay** for that reduction [Mishan, 1971; Schelling, 1968]. In other words, people should be allowed to place a value on their own lives. Economists note that people put values on changes in their probabilities of living or dying every day. They take more or less risky jobs. They travel in more or less risky ways. They may choose not to have a periodic health examination because they do not believe the benefits, in terms of increased longevity, are worth the time and cost. If people are willing to pay only so much to prolong their own lives, these economists argue, then society should not place a higher valuation on those lives.

The main shortcoming of this approach is that in practice it has proved to be exceedingly difficult to obtain stable, reproducible estimates of people's willingness to pay for reductions in the probability of their own death. Some researchers have conducted interview surveys and have obtained widely differing answers. One difficulty is *strategic behavior.* For example, people have been asked what having a mobile coronary-care unit in their town would be worth to them. People's responses to such a question if they think they will have to pay the amount they answer are different from their responses if they think they will not have to pay. Another problem is that people find it difficult to understand and to respond meaningfully to changes in probabilities of improbable events. Suppose you are told that your chances of being killed in a motor-vehicle accident this year are 0.0004, and then are asked what you would be willing to pay to reduce this probability to 0.0003. Would you have confidence in your answer? Some researchers have examined the wage premiums required to induce people to work in risky occupations; others have examined what people are willing to pay for smoke detectors, for seat belts, and for houses in less polluted areas. Again, the estimates obtained have varied widely because of numerous measurement problems.

Because of these difficulties, another study focused on attempts to link human capital and willingness to pay by asking what rational individuals should be willing to pay to avoid small risks to life [Landefeld and Seskin, 1982]. The conclusion the investigators reached was that, under certain reasonable conditions, a rational individual should be willing to purchase an increased probability of survival at a cost of at least the PV of his expected future net income (earned and unearned), multiplied by a factor representing his risk aversion, multiplied by the change in his survival probability.

Suppose the PV of your expected lifetime income is $1 million. Now suppose that a new risk emerges that increases your chances of death this year by 0.0001. In this new state, the PV of the expected lifetime income you will enjoy is reduced to $999,900, because there is an increased 0.0001 chance you will not be around to enjoy the $1 million. The argument is that you should be willing to pay at least $100 to avoid this new threat, because with the threat and your $100 both removed, the PV of your expected lifetime income remains $999,900. This approach may help to generate consensus on appropriate standards for investments in public safety. It remains to be seen whether it will find application in the evaluation of health-care programs.

Foregone Opportunities

Another approach that sometimes can be effective is to use opportunity costs, or foregone opportunities. For example, we might argue, "We should not pay for liver transplants at a cost of $500,000 per life saved if, at the same time, due to resource constraints, we are failing to avail ourselves of opportunities to save lives in other ways at a cost of $100,000 each."

Quality-Adjusted Life-Years

To do a CBA to determine whether the life-saving benefits of a program are worth that program's cost, we must find some way of putting a dollar value on the benefits. Because assigning this value is so difficult and controversial, some analysts have suggested a focus on CEA—how best to allocate a given budget for health services using quality-adjusted life-years (QALYs) [Zeckhauser and Shepard, 1976]. The idea begins with the sensible notion that "lives saved" is not an adequate criterion. Everyone will die eventually. So the product of health and safety programs is really *life-years* saved. The *quality* of the life-years saved needs to be considered as well. Prolonging the life of a comatose or gravely ill and suffering person for 1 year might seem to be a less worthy object of expenditure than is adding 1 year of healthy productive life to another person's lifespan.

A substantial problem with this approach is that it is difficult to determine the quality-adjustment weights. One approach taken has been to confront people with hypothetical gambles (in Chapter 3, we discussed this approach to utility assessment). A sample lottery in this case might assign to 1 full year of healthy life a weight of 1, and to 1 year without life a weight of 0. Suppose a person has a specific impairment that could be cured by surgery, but the surgery has an x percent chance of killing him. If x is 50 and the person is indifferent between having the operation and not having it, then we would infer that, on a scale of 0 to 1, the value he places on 1 year of life with that impairment is 50 percent of the value he places on 1 year of life without it.

Another approach has been to survey health professionals directly experienced in the care of patients with specific illnesses and disabilities, and to ask them what weights they would assign to 1 year of life under various conditions. This approach has produced some specific numerical estimates, but it has not escaped criticism. One objection is that this method assumes that the relative utility of two health states is the same for all people. Yet economists would argue that a "football knee" would have a different significance for a professional football player than it would for a corporate executive.

Summary of the Valuation Problem

Not one of these approaches is without shortcomings. Yet people must make allocation decisions, whether explicitly or implicitly. The disadvantages of the implicit approach include the inability of people to share the basis on which decisions are being made, which can result in serious misallocations. An open, explicit approach may expose painful choices, but it carries a better chance of avoiding bad decisions. People who must evaluate life-saving and health benefits should do so thoughtfully, paying great attention to the specific circumstances of application and maintaining sensitivity to ethical concerns.

19.4.2 Alternative Measures of Cost

In this section we shall examine various measures of cost. Definitions for different cost terms vary throughout the health-care industry (as well as in other industries); those we give here are simplified.

Variable, Fixed, Direct, and Indirect Costs

Costs that change with the volume of services produced during a given period are **variable costs.** They can be avoided if no services are produced. Thus, labor and supply costs are generally variable. A simple linear function for variable costs is shown in Figure 19.5. Variable-cost functions are not always linear; they may include steps (for example, labor costs may be added by 1 full-time equivalent (FTE), rather than by 0.1 or 0.5 FTE), or they may be semivariable (they may have both a fixed and a variable portion), as illustrated in Figure 19.6.

All costs that are not variable are fixed. **Fixed costs** do not vary with volume during a given period. Examples are plant and equipment and administrative salary expenses. A simple fixed-cost function is shown in Figure 19.7.

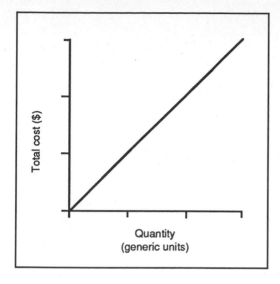

FIGURE 19.5 A simple linear-cost function. Each additional unit costs the same amount to produce as every other unit.

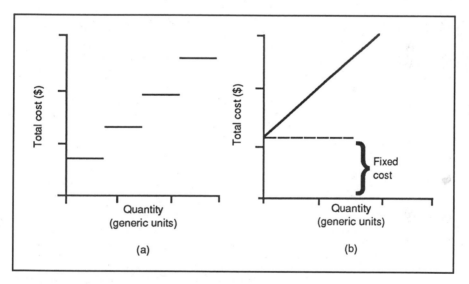

FIGURE 19.6 Variations on variable-cost functions: (a) step costs and (b) semivariable costs. The variable-cost function in (b) is linear starting at a basic fixed cost.

Direct costs are those costs that can be directly assigned to the production of services to patients. Direct costs in the laboratory would include the cost of the technician's salary, equipment, and supplies. Direct costs can be either variable or fixed. In the laboratory, equipment costs are likely to be fixed, whereas supply costs are likely to be variable.

All costs incurred in producing health services that are not direct costs are **indirect costs.** Indirect costs include those costs that cannot be attributed to a specific

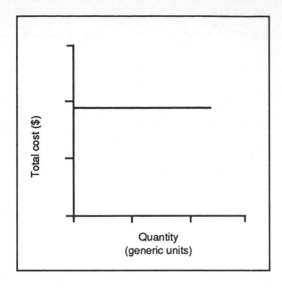

FIGURE 19.7 A fixed-cost function. The total cost does not
change, regardless of the quantity
of goods produced because the
cost of producing additional goods
is zero.

output. Examples in the laboratory include clerical supplies and the department manager's salary. Indirect costs may also be fixed or variable.

Traditionally, indirect costs included all costs incurred in those departments that did not produce services that could be billed to patients; such departments were called *cost centers* or *overhead departments*. Examples of overhead departments include data processing, administration, plant and maintenance, billing, admitting, and housekeeping. In this chapter, the terms **overhead** and *indirect costs* have been used interchangeably.

Marginal Costs

Marginal cost is defined as the increase in total cost associated with the production of one more unit per period of time. As you can see from the graph in Figure 19.7, the marginal cost of producing one more unit for a fixed-cost service is zero. That is, there is no increase in cost associated with one more unit of production. For the linear variable-cost function in Figure 19.5, the marginal cost of producing one more unit would be equal to the total cost incurred, divided by the quantity produced (the average unit cost), which is equal to the incremental cost. For the semivariable-cost function in Figure 19.6, the marginal cost is equal to the incremental (or variable) cost associated with producing one more unit, but is not equal to the average unit cost because that includes a fixed-cost component.

In the production of health services, many different margins can be imagined: one more case, one more day of patient stay, one more laboratory test or X-ray examination. Is the marginal cost of performing one more laboratory test equal to the incremental cost associated with the laboratory test reagents, or does it include specimen collection, transportation of the specimen to the laboratory, some portion of laboratory technician time, and all other resources used? If these are resources that would not be used if the test were not performed, then all aspects of the process must be considered.

Although marginal cost often is the relevant cost for decision making, measuring it in practice is difficult and requires substantial judgment. The problems are that there are so many different margins to measure, that data are not collected routinely to support this kind of analysis, and that the hospital environment is a moving target—it does not hold still so that all the margins can be measured simultaneously. In developing marginal-cost figures, it is essential to identify explicitly which margin is being discussed and at what volume.

Average Costs

Average cost is defined as the total cost of producing a service divided by the number of units of service produced per period of time. As with marginal cost, what is considered to constitute unit cost is not always clearly specified, and developing accurate estimates from existing data systems can be difficult. Hospitals have a high percentage of fixed costs; therefore, they generally experience declining average cost. That is, as volume increases, the fixed costs per patient are spread across more patients, thereby reducing the costs per patient. A decreasing average-cost function is depicted in Figure 19.8.

Although marginal costs usually are the most appropriate costs for making the purchase decision, it also is useful to know whether the project is profitable on an average-cost basis. After all, a hospital that does not cover its average costs cannot remain in business. For this reason, the hospital may require that a project cover its average costs in order to be approved. When you use average-cost figures, it is advisable to break out estimates into their indirect and direct, variable and fixed components. Because overhead costs can represent a large proportion of the average-cost figure, how overhead is assigned can greatly affect the NPV calculation for a project.

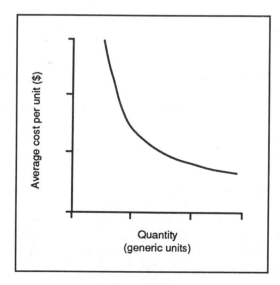

FIGURE 19.8 Decreasing average-cost function. (Note that the ordinate is average cost, not total cost, as in Figures 19.5 to 19.7.) As more goods are produced, the fixed costs of production are spread across more items, thereby reducing the average cost per unit produced.

Short- and Long-Run Costs

The concepts of **short-** and **long-run cost** need to be considered explicitly in CBA. In microeconomics, *short-run* and *long-run* do not refer to duration; the terms refer to the variability of certain factors of production. In the short-run, some factors of production are considered variable (for example, supplies, power, nursing hours), whereas others are considered fixed (plant and equipment). In reality, there are many "runs." In the short-run, we have a given amount of plant and equipment, and the decision we must make is at what level to operate it. Short-run variable costs do not include the costs associated with capital. In the long-run, the appropriate amount of plant and equipment is a variable to be decided. Which run makes sense within the context of a specific CBA should be discussed and established.

19.5 Guidelines for the Development of Estimates of Cost and Benefit

In this section, we discuss practical guidelines that you should keep in mind when you develop numerical estimates to assign to the costs and benefits identified in CBA.

19.5.1 Consistency with Definition of Hospital Product

It is important to ensure that an analysis of costs and benefits is consistent with the definition of hospital product. Under Medicare's PPS, hospitals are reimbursed by a set amount for each entire inpatient episode. This reimbursement has led to changes in the concepts of what it is that hospitals produce and in how costs are analyzed for CBA purposes.

Historically, administrators viewed hospitals as being in the business of producing services (for example, laboratory tests, X-ray examinations, nursing hours, hours of operating-room time), not cases. How these services related to one another and how they were further classified into *product groupings* varied throughout the industry. Generally, services were divided into revenue-center services and cost-center services. **Revenue centers** included departments that charged patients directly for the services provided (for example, X-ray examinations, laboratory tests, and physical therapy). **Cost centers** were those departments that did not have revenue associated with the services they provided (for example, administration, data processing, billing, and housekeeping). Cost-center services could be further refined on the basis of whether a direct patient service was provided. For example, direct-service cost centers included dietary and billing. Nondirect-service cost centers included plant and administration.

PPS has provided the hospital industry with uniform concepts and terminology to define what it is that hospitals produce for inpatients: The product is a patient episode, classified by DRG category. Under PPS, hospitals are paid for each Medicare inpatient case based on the DRG assigned to that patient. Each DRG is associated with an established price that represents Medicare's reimbursement for the total care of a patient. The amount paid does not vary with the length of stay or as a function of resources used.

What is the implication of this new product view for cost–benefit analysis and technology assessment? The answer depends on what, specifically, is being evaluated. Traditionally, the purchase of a piece of diagnostic equipment was evaluated on the basis of whether the revenue generated by the equipment would be sufficient to off-set the purchase and operating costs. Under prospective payment, it is the entire in-patient episode that is reimbursed—not particular services. Therefore, for Medicare inpatients, there will be no additional revenue received as a result of the purchase of the new equipment. If the hospital is considering buying a new piece of diagnostic equipment, it will want to assess how owning the equipment might affect the total amount of resources consumed for a patient stay. Will the equipment improve qual-ity of care? Will it decrease length of stay? Will it decrease total resources consumed? Will it decrease the total cost of care?

In contrast, consider the evaluation of capital equipment for an overhead depart-ment. Suppose a new computer system for financial accounting is being evaluated. This type of system neither has been associated with revenue, nor has been cost-justified based on use by a particular group of patients. It is not so important in this case to tie costs into the DRG product view, because we would not expect the system to affect the costs of one DRG more than it will those of another.

19.5.2 Models of Cost Flows

It also is important to track costs and benefits through models of expense flows within the hospital. For example, to develop accurate cost estimates of a particular DRG case, test, and so on, we need a model of the cost of the hospital's operation. This model should account for all costs and should allow them to be traced through the various services provided in a manner that reflects actual use of resources.

One way to model the flow of costs through the hospital is to consider DRG cases as final products. All direct services provided to patients are considered intermediate products, and all indirect services are considered overhead costs. (All department costs are considered either direct or indirect service costs.) This model of costs is illustrated in Figure 19.9.

19.5.3 The Role of Economic Costs in Performing CBAs

Accounting costs are measurements intended to answer questions such as, "Which of a hospital's revenues and expenditures are appropriately attributed to 1983?" "What share of a hospital's expenditures is attributable to Medicare patients?" Generally speaking, accounting costs contain many allocations that do not reflect actual resource use, but rather are calculated to maximize reimbursement from third-party payers. They also are aggregated, so the cost of a specific laboratory test or DRG case can-not be determined from accounting data alone. *Economic costs* are the value of the resources used in producing goods and services. In general, accounting costs are not a good proxy for economic costs.

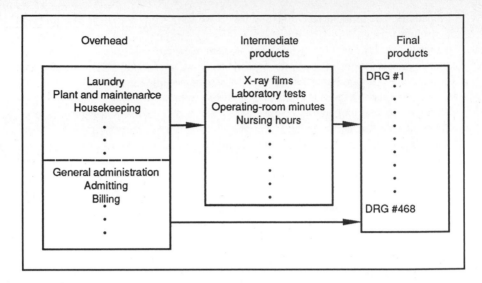

FIGURE 19.9 A product-cost model. To develop an accurate cost estimate for a DRG, we model the flow of expenses within the hospital by identifying the indirect services (overhead costs) and direct services (intermediate products) used in caring for a typical patient who is classified as being in the DRG.

Charges are the prices established for hospital services. It is not uncommon in health care to set prices without consideration for the cost of providing the service. The reimbursement and regulatory environments have contributed to this lack of cost-based pricing. As limits were imposed on reimbursement for routine care, hospitals found ways to allocate more overhead costs to the ancillary departments in order to maximize reimbursement. Private insurance also influenced pricing; demand has not been cost-conscious and markets have not been competitive. The hospitalized patient usually is not in the best position to question the need for tests or to inquire as to the appropriateness of the prices, and private insurance companies rarely questioned prices charged. So there has been no market force to ensure that charges approximate costs.

In estimating economic cost, you value all resources at their highest and best alternative use. For example, an MRI program uses floor space. The fact that the use of that floor space does not entail a current cash outflow does not mean that the space is free. If there is no alternative use for the floor space, then in the short-run this use is free. If there is an alternative use, then the space's value for that use is the economic cost of using the space for MRI.

19.5.4 Combinations of Techniques to Produce Estimates of Cost and Benefit

Because the health-care industry generally has not paid attention to costs and cost-accounting systems beyond what was required for reimbursement, the average cost and marginal cost of providing specific types of health-care services are rarely known. Therefore, deriving good estimates can be a time-consuming and costly task.

As a starting point, we recommend collecting whatever data are available. Such data might include hospital financial reports, department records and reports, industry reports, and vendor information. It is important to think carefully and critically about costs and about the cost data provided. Many of the data that are readily available are not usable for decision making. For example, the data may

- Be averaged, obscuring figures at a detailed level
- Contain arbitrary allocations
- Include charge as opposed to cost data
- Not be presented in a manner that is consistent with the current concept of what hospitals produce

As an alternative to using existing data, it may be possible to collect data. Conceptually, it is appealing to track all use of resources at a detailed, or microcosting, level. The variation in the distribution of nursing hours per patient day and the average length of stay are used to illustrate the value of microcosting for DRG 210 (fractured hip or femur), and DRG 122 (myocardial infarction) in Figure 19.10.

Administrators often view decreasing length of stay as a key method for reducing costs. In Figure 19.10, although the average hours of nursing care per patient day are not very different for the two DRGs, reductions in the length of stay for DRG 210 patients will result in significantly greater savings relative to reductions for DRG 122 patients. Administrators armed with these data would be in a better position to forecast potential savings through reductions in length of stay.

Although it is appealing to monitor all use of resources at a detailed level, the costs of doing this type of analysis, in comparison to the benefits, will make the exercise practical in only limited circumstances. The search for the average cost and marginal cost for a particular service or case in a hospital can prove to be extremely complex and expensive, depending on the level of accuracy desired. You must remember that cost estimates do not have to be perfect, and that the cost of gathering the data should not be greater than the benefits of having the information.

Because of the general dearth of good cost information, and the lack of (or inability to collect) data for new technologies, developing cost estimates often requires using a variety of methods that go beyond observation and use of historical cost and utilization figures. For example, you might seek the opinions of one or more experts, hire an outside consultant to evaluate the situation, consult professional standards, or perform statistical analyses.

19.5.5 Dealing with Nonquantifiable Benefits

Not all benefits and costs can be translated into numbers, yet it is essential that those that cannot be translated be explicitly considered and weighed in the analysis. One way of dealing with **nonquantifiable** or **intangible benefits** is at least to describe them explicitly so that decision makers can consider them. This approach makes the analysis and interpretation of results more difficult compared to a single NPV figure, but it encourages thoughtful consideration of significant factors.

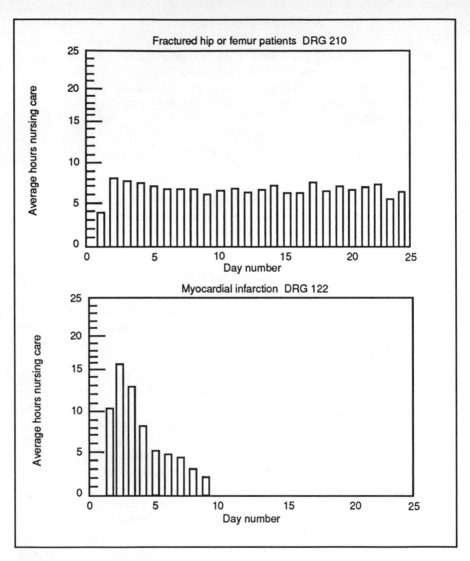

FIGURE 19.10 The distributions of nursing time per patient day for two DRGs. Analyzing the use of nursing resources at the microcosting level allows administrators to predict more accurately savings due to reductions in length of stay.

19.6 Medical Informatics and Health-Care Financing

As we indicated in the introduction to this chapter, the evolution of computer systems will be influenced increasingly by the relationship of those systems to issues in health-care financing. The links are largely inevitable and will take two forms: computer systems as *subjects* of CEA–CBA, and computer systems as *tools* for financial planning and decision making, and for health administration and management. No person involved in professional medical informatics, and no health-care provider or planner, will be able to ignore the key health-financing issues that will guide research and technology transfer for medical information systems, and that also will create a demand for new tools to assist with data collection and analysis.

19.6.1 Health-Care Financing and the Need for Computational Tools

The complex reporting and planning requirements outlined in this chapter cannot be met realistically without computational tools to assist with data collection, analysis, and report generation. Because of the rapid changes in health-care financing that occurred during the early 1980s, we now see the need for new systems in a number of areas:

- Under PPS, abstracted data from medical records are the basis for obtaining reimbursement. This arrangement creates a need to increase the timeliness and quality of these data. Systems have been developed that assist with coding while reducing coding errors, thereby facilitating maximum reimbursement under PPS.

- PPS for the first time links clinical and financial data through inpatient cases classified by DRG. The DRG system thus creates a need for health-care administrators and providers to study the relationship between resource use and outcomes, in order to examine and evaluate cost–benefit tradeoffs. It creates a need to develop product cost accounting by DRG, so that managers can tell whether the hospital is gaining or losing income on each DRG. This information helps decision makers to identify whether each service is being offered in an economically viable way. Computer-based systems are required to capture, link, store, and monitor this information.

- Information systems are being used to increase the productivity of high-cost professionals. A bedside charting system used by nursing staff would be an example of this type of system.

- Because hospitals must ensure cost recovery under prospective payment, and because in hospitals average costs generally decline, administrators have an incentive to increase occupancy. They may use information systems as strategic tools to attract a larger client base (by appealing to physicians, to patients, to third-party payers, and so on). For example, hospitals may attract local physicians by providing office terminals to assist with patient-care activities, so that these doctors can readily access current patient information and can order tests, medications, and procedures, or can arrange from their offices for the admission of a patient. Similarly, improved management of data for third-party payers can attract preferred-provider programs.

- Historically, capturing *lost charges* was a significant benefit of hospital financial systems, and was often used to justify the purchase of such systems. Under prospective payment, there is neither a charge-based nor a retrospective cost-based reimbursement system. This arrangement renders relatively unimportant the capability of systems to reduce the number of charges not captured. This decreased emphasis on the charge side is being replaced by the hospital administrator's need to understand costs and associated benefits, so that these people can make rational decisions on how best to use their limited resources.

19.6.2 The Increasing Use of Cost–Benefit Analysis

As we have described, recent trends indicate that payment from private insurance companies, as well as from the government, will be prospective and will cover global units of service such as hospital cases. Prospective-payment systems create economic incentives for hospitals to reduce their operating and capital expenditures. Thus, capital expenditures will be evaluated more stringently in the future.

Benefits of computer-based information systems will become even more difficult to quantify. For example, how can the strategic benefits of systems be quantified? How can dollars be attributed to technology that is implemented to attract physicians or third-party payers? Benefits such as this one are more difficult to quantify than is the benefit of a reduction in lost charges.

19.6.3 The Federal Government and Clinical Computing

Until recently, the role of the federal government in promoting research and development in clinical computing systems has been effected primarily through research grants (largely from the Division of Research Resources of the National Institutes of Health, the National Library of Medicine, and the National Center for Health Services Research and Technology Assessment). As medical information and decision-support systems mature and technology-transfer issues become of paramount importance, however, concerns about health-care financing will have an increasing influence on technology adoption. An unquantifiable claim of a beneficial effect on quality of care generally will not be persuasive to a hospital administrator who is facing tighter fiscal constraints and who accordingly requires that the cost-effectiveness of new technologies be demonstrated before she will make an investment. Similarly, office practitioners will be forced to consider cost–benefit tradeoffs, and will demand data on these issues, before investing in computing systems in an era with ceilings on reimbursement for the care they provide.

The federal government also may exert an important influence on the introduction and dissemination of computing technologies through the regulatory activities of the Food and Drug Administration (FDA). Thus far, the FDA has chosen to avoid involvement with validating or licensing new information-management or decision-support technologies, as long as the computer systems depend on the intervention of a competent health professional before the patient's management is affected [Young, 1987]. Rather than viewing such programs as medical devices subject to regulation (as is a monitoring instrument in an ICU), the FDA has ruled that computer systems are like textbooks and other information sources that have never been in the FDA's purview. If the FDA does regulate software, however, we still do not know whether it will assess whether a program is "safe and effective" (as it does, for example, in assessment of new drugs), or whether it will examine cost-effectiveness in its validation studies. What the appropriate mechanism is for validating and regulating medical software remains a highly controversial issue at present; that issue probably will be resolved over the next decade, as more medical information systems move from the research to the commercial world.

The role of medical computing applications in the future of medicine in the United States has been discussed extensively in the previous chapters. As we have noted, changes in the health-care economic environment have inevitably led to changes in system requirements. At this time, the information needs of hospitals are evolving and cannot be predicted with certainty. What *is* clear is that hospital decision makers need to understand how much provision of care costs, to establish standards and to improve controls over the cost and quality of care, and to learn how to collect and process efficiently the information they require. Computer systems will play a central role in this process. As information needs become more demanding and complex, computer systems will be implemented in a wide variety of health-care settings.

Suggested Readings

Enthoven, A. and Kronick, R. A consumer-choice health plan for the 1990s: Universal health insurance in a system designed to promote quality and economy. *New England Journal of Medicine,* 320:29–37, 94–101, 1989.

> *In this two-part article, the authors review the shortcomings of the current systems of health-care financing and propose a strategy for providing universal health insurance based on a system of managed competition. They describe the necessary characteristics of a plan that can gain broad acceptance, and discuss the potential effects of implementing the plan on medical practice, insurance coverage, employment, and wage rates.*

Fuchs, V. R. Paying the piper, calling the tune. In Fuchs, V. R. *The Health Economy.* Cambridge, MA: Harvard University Press, 1986.

> *This essay describes the pressures leading to changes in health-care financing in the 1980s. It considers the economic and ethical implications of these changes.*

Fuchs, V. R. *Who Shall Live?* New York: Basic Books, 1974, 1983.

> *The author presents an excellent introduction to the structure of the health-care delivery system. The roles of the main players and the relationship between medical care and health are discussed.*

Gilbert, J. P., Light, R. J., and Mosteller, F. Assessing social innovations: An empirical base for policy. In Zeckhauser, R., et al. (eds), *Benefit–Cost and Policy Analysis 1974.* Chicago: Aldine Publishing Co., 1975.

> *This article reviews the literature on evaluation of medical and social experiments. The authors find that many evaluations do not have randomized controls and are therefore subject to bias, or that the methods of randomization used are deficient. They explain the need for carefully designed randomized controls.*

Jencks, S. F. and Dobson, A. Refining case-mix adjustment: The research evidence. *New England Journal of Medicine,* 317:679, 1987.

> *This article summarizes research on case-mix adjustment—the process of adjusting for differences in patient cases to allow comparisons of costs and outcomes among cases and across hospitals. The authors examine the Medicare system of prospective payment, which*

relies on case-mix adjustment to determine payments. They also review current systems for categorizing cases by severity of illness.

Lipscom, J., Raskin, I. E., and Eichenholz, J. The use of marginal cost estimates in hospital cost-containment policy. In Zubkoff, M., Raskin, I. E., and Hanft, R. S. (eds), *Hospital Cost Containment*. New York: Prodist, 1978.

This paper surveys the literature on attempts to measure the marginal cost of a patient day or a patient stay. The authors show that investigators have derived widely varying estimates of the ratio of marginal cost to average cost of a patient stay.

Office of Technology Assessment (OTA). *The Impact of Randomized Clinical Trials on Health Policy and Medical Practice*. Washington, D.C.: Congress of the United States, U.S. Government Printing Office, August 1983.

This OTA report gives an overview of the status of systematic evaluation of medical practices.

Office of Technology Assessment (OTA). *The Implications of Cost-Effectiveness Analysis of Medical Technology,* Chapters 1–4. Washington, D.C.: Congress of the United States, U.S. Government Printing Office, August 1980.

This OTA report provides a good introductory overview of cost-effectiveness analysis applied to medical technology.

Schelling, T. C. The life you save may be your own. In Chase, Jr., S. B. (ed), *Problems in Public Expenditure Analysis*. Washington, D.C.: The Brookings Institution, 1968.

This article is a classic statement of the conceptual basis for valuing life and limb. Schelling argues that people put valuations on changes in the risks they face of death and illness, and that these valuations are not necessarily the same as changes in the expected value of their future earnings. He draws interesting distinctions, such as the difference between an identified life and a statistical life. The article is one of the basic statements of the economist's case for public policy valuing lives in the same way that people value their own lives.

Weinstein, M. C. and Stason, W. Foundations of cost-effectiveness analysis for health and medical practices. *New England Journal of Medicine,* 296:716, 1977.

The authors provide a concise overview of cost-effectiveness analysis of medical practices.

Zeckhauser, R. and Shephard, D. Where now for saving lives? *Law and Contemporary Problems* (Duke University School of Law), 40:5, 1976.

This article notes the serious conceptual and methodological difficulties associated with assigning a dollar value to changes in the probability of death or suffering. It offers an alternative measure for cost-effectiveness evaluation, which the authors call quality-adjusted life-years.

Questions for Discussion

1. Define the following terms, each of which is relevant to current health-care financing:
   a. Usual, customary, and reasonable (UCR) fees
   b. Professional standards review organization (PSRO)
   c. Health-maintenance organization (HMO)
   d. Diagnosis-related group (DRG)
   e. Preferred-provider organization (PPO)
   f. Quality-adjusted life-year (QALY)

2. Distinguish cost–benefit analysis (CBA) from cost-effectiveness analysis (CEA). For each method, describe a sample problem that you might solve by performing this type of analysis, drawing on your knowledge of medical-computing applications.

3. Distinguish hospital *cost centers* from *revenue centers*. Select three of the hospital-based medical-computing services discussed earlier in this book, and indicate in which kind of center they are likely to be classed.

4. Define the term *net present value*. Explain why it is important to perform discounting when evaluating a program for which costs are incurred in the present and benefits are realized in the future.

5. Distinguish between the *human-capital* and *willingness-to-pay* methods for placing a value on human life. Are these techniques more relevant for identified-life or for statistical-life problems? Which technique, if either, do you believe is more appropriate for assigning this valuation? Explain your answer. If you were asked to place a dollar value on a human life, how would you make the assignment?

6. Compare HMOs and PPOs. What are the strengths and potential limitations of each with respect to cost and quality of care?

7. How will the differences in incentives for providers under each of the following payment systems affect providers' assessments of new medical technologies, such as patient-monitoring systems?
   a. An HMO
   b. An individual physician participating in a PPO agreement
   c. A hospital with a large number of patients treated under Medicare's prospective-payment system
   d. A standard fee-for-service arrangement

8. You are the new administrator of the Health Care Financing Administration, the agency responsible for Medicare and for the federal component of Medicaid. You are about to authorize a new program for health-care financing for the elderly. The program is a capitated physician-payment system in which each Medicare enrollee chooses a primary-care physician who is paid a fixed annual fee by Medicare. The program will reimburse for the services of other physicians only if the primary-care physician authorizes those services. The primary-care physician must pay for all the services he provides to the patient from the revenues of the fixed annual fee.
   a. What data would you want to collect to evaluate the performance of this program?
   b. What mechanisms would you implement to collect these data?
   c. For how long would you have to collect the data to obtain meaningful information?

20

The Future of
Computer Applications
in Health Care

Lawrence M. Fagan and Leslie E. Perreault

In this book, we have summarized the current state of medical informatics in a variety of application areas, and have reflected on the development of the field during the past 30 years. To provide a background for our discussions, we opened the book with a glimpse into the future—a vision of medical practice when individual physicians routinely and conveniently use computers to help with information management, communication, and clinical decision making. In this chapter, we again look forward, this time concentrating on likely trends in medical applications of computers, on current avenues of research, and on the issues that will determine along which paths medical informatics will develop.

We begin by presenting two scenarios from the not-too-distant future—possible scenes that we can extrapolate from the current status of medical computing and that provide perspective on the ways that computers may someday pervade medical practice. A key aspect of these scenarios is the extent to which, unlike most specialized medical paraphernalia of today, medical-computing applications are integrated into routine medical practice, rather than used on an occasional basis. The realization of a highly integrated environment depends on the solution of technological challenges, such as integrating information from multiple data sources and making the integrated information accessible to health professionals when, and where, and in the form that it is needed. Integration of medical information also encompasses social issues, such as defining the appropriate role of computers in the workplace, resolving questions of legal liability and ethics related to medical computing, and assessing the effects of computer-based technology on health-care costs. The chance that our hypothetical scenarios will become reality thus depends on the resolution of a number of technological and social issues that will be debated during the coming years.

20.1 Two Scenarios from the Future

The following situations might well occur in the year 2010. In the first, we learn about a patient who undergoes heart surgery and recovers in an intensive-care unit (ICU). In the second, we follow a patient who has a chronic disease and receives intermittent care, provided primarily in an outpatient setting. For another view of what medical computing might be like in the future, you can consult the report of the National Library of Medicine's 1986 planning panel on medical informatics [National Library of Medicine, 1986b]. This report describes a hypothetical situation from the year 2006, in which victims of chemical exposure are transported to a hospital, evaluated, and treated.

20.1.1 Heart Surgery and Recovery

A 54-year-old man is admitted to the hospital for coronary-artery bypass graft (CABG) surgery. When he is brought into the operating room (OR), his bar-coded identification bracelet is passed under an optical scanner. Once this identifying information has been entered, the OR computer begins to retrieve, from various HIS computers on the network, the patient's medical record, including results of recent radiographic studies, physiological measurements, current problem list, current medications, and drug allergies. When the surgeon and anesthesiologist identify themselves to the system, the information in the records is configured in the various formats typically requested by each of them for this specific operation. The information is then displayed on wall monitors throughout the surgical suite, as well as on the anesthesiologist's console display.

The patient is connected to a variety of computer-based monitoring devices, which measure and record his blood pressure, respiratory rate, blood oxygen content, and other parameters of physiological status. The anesthesiologist has primary responsibility for tracking these variables during the procedure. She selects which of the many channels of measurements available from transducers are to be charted automatically on her flowsheet display, and the flowsheet is initialized with the static patient data. In addition to physiological measurements, therapeutic interventions also are recorded automatically. To simplify the recording of the treatments administered to the patient, the anesthesiologist connects a measuring device to each intravenous line as she sets it up; the fluid type and drip rates are transmitted over the OR medical bus and are recorded as elements of the flowsheet display. The types and doses of the nonintravenous drugs administered are recorded manually. Prior to administering each drug, the physician or nurse verifies its identity by scanning the drug's barcoded label.

During surgery, the anesthesiologist monitors the online data, comparing this patient's actual responses to an anesthesia plan that encodes the expected responses. The anesthesiologist entered the patient-specific plan (a tailored version of her prototypical plan) into the system via a voice interaction during the preoperative evaluation. At that time, the system critiqued the plan and presented pertinent elements of the patient's history to support that critique. Now, the software supporting the anesthesiologist's charting system tracks the anesthesia plan and uses it to anticipate possible side effects and to detect unexpected deviations. For example, the system contains knowledge about how long the anesthetic effect will last and how it will affect blood pressure over time.

As measurements are continuously recorded from the patient, the system compares the data to estimates of the patient's expected response at each phase of the operative procedure; the estimates are derived from mathematical models, and the parameters of these models slowly adapt to the patient-specific measurements. Rather than sounding alarms when values exceed preset thresholds, the monitoring devices generate alarms only when the measurements have moved beyond the acceptable range, as determined for this specific patient and in response to the current clinical context. The monitoring program highlights the set of measurements that is most important for assessing the problem, and generates probable explanations for the situation. As the anesthesiologist adjusts the settings of the machines controlling administration of drugs and oxygen, the system calculates the time when the alarm situation is expected to be resolved, then updates the mathematical model by observing the actual time of resolution. If the patient does not respond to therapy, then a list of the possible reasons is determined and displayed. The results of laboratory tests performed during surgery are also fed back electronically to the anesthesiologist's display and are integrated into the model of the current clinical situation.

The surgeon also has access to the anesthesiologist's display of measurement trends and to a high-level summary of the patient's status during surgery. He can retrieve radiological images and other important elements of the patient's records, such as the results of recent laboratory tests. In addition, he is automatically notified as new information, such as biopsy results or measures of hematological status, becomes available. To display this information, the surgeon uses structured speech commands, thereby maintaining sterility of his hands.

After surgery, the clinicians verbally present the case history of the patient to the ICU team. The programs that supported the anesthesiologist's display electronically transfer patient information to the ICU patient-monitoring programs. A list of the important events during the surgery is included in the transfer, as is a description of the patient-specific mathematical-model parameters that define how this patient differs from the typical cardiac-surgery patient. A textual report that summarizes physiological changes during surgery, particularly the patient's responses to various stresses (for example, change in blood pressure with blood loss), is created and is given to the anesthesiologist for review and correction. The surgeon dictates an operative report, which is automatically transcribed for his signature.

Meanwhile, the ICU monitoring program has adapted its range of expected values for each of the measurements that is monitored during the postoperative period, and has computed the time that it expects to elapse before the patient emerges from anesthesia. It provides suggestions for controlling the mechanical ventilator, taking into account the standard protocols for ventilator weaning and the patient's underlying problems—for example, his chronic lung disease as well as cardiac disease. As in the operating room, alarms sound when measurements exceed the ranges established for this particular patient. The patient-monitoring system is completely integrated with the ICU charting system and produces text summaries of patient status, both on demand and automatically at the beginning of each nursing shift.

When the patient's condition improves to the point that the patient can be transferred to a regular treatment unit, a therapy-planning program helps the ICU physicians to plan follow-up treatments and tests. After approval by the physician, the test requests are forwarded to the appropriate locations in the hospital, along with a brief summary of the patient's care to date. At the time of discharge, a summary of the patient's hospital stay, discharge medications, and updated problem list is automatically forwarded in both paper and electronic form to the office of the physician who will provide outpatient care.

20.1.2 Chronic Treatment for a Patient with Rheumatological Disease

The second scenario follows a patient through the diagnostic and therapeutic stages of a chronic medical condition. The case begins as a 34-year-old woman visits her family doctor, an internist, complaining of symptoms of a persistent facial rash, pain and swelling in her joints, weight loss, and fatigue. The physician interviews the patient to gather a history of the present illness, and performs a physical examination. As she conducts her history interview and examination, the physician forms a provisional diagnosis of systemic lupus erythematosus, an autoimmune disorder. To review this and other possible diagnoses, she consults a computer-based clinical decision-support system that covers the breadth of internal medicine and includes a program that specializes in rheumatological diseases. The programs evaluate the patient's online history information and the data collected during the current visit, generate a differential diagnosis, compare the differential to the physician's working diagnosis, and provide a critique for evaluation by the physician. They also recommend appropriate diagnostic tests and explain the implications of the results for alternative diagnoses.

The consultation programs and test results support the physician's diagnosis, so the physician refers the patient to a rheumatologist for treatment. She sends electronic mail to the specialist, describing the case and summarizing the patient's diagnostic workup. Additional information, including the patient's past medical history, current medications, and pertinent laboratory findings, is recorded on a medical information card that was created by a laser digital-encoding device. The patient carries the card with her to her appointment; thus, the specialist has immediate access to the patient's detailed medical record.

To verify the working diagnosis, the rheumatologist orders additional tests. The new laboratory findings and their interpretation are included in a computer-stored record that describes the specialist's overall assessment. This information is communicated back to the referring physician by electronic mail, and the medical information card is updated. The patient's record is then added to the national database of records of patients with rheumatological diseases. Most of the data needed to establish this record are selected automatically from the patient's workup to date, including the patient's demographic data, diagnosis, and key laboratory data.

The national database combines the records from many practitioners throughout the country, and provides a vehicle for the retrospective analysis of hypotheses about diagnostic and therapeutic decisions, along the lines of today's ARAMIS project (see Chapter 16). The database also acts as a clearinghouse for the enrollment of patients in research protocols. The system automatically searches all the current national research protocols for which this patient may be eligible, using the data that have been transferred to the national database. The list of applicable protocols is sent back to the rheumatologist to help him decide whether to enroll this patient in an experimental study.

In this case, the rheumatologist identifies an appropriate protocol for administration of medications, and the protocol guidelines are transferred from the central database to the physician's computer in two forms. A hypertext version of the protocol is available for browsing during treatment, and a decision-support system that encodes the protocol in logical statements is activated to provide advice for each patient visit. Had the physician chosen to treat the patient using a standard therapeutic regimen, he could have queried the database for a summary of the treatment history and course of disease for patients who have similar characteristics.

Two months after her enrollment in the experimental protocol, the patient develops a severe toxic reaction to her medications. She is rushed to a hospital emergency room (ER). When she arrives, the ER physicians display the information encoded on her medical information card to find clues about her condition. They review the most recently collected information, then examine the medical record by major problem area. The record also includes a list of current medications and dosages, and identifies the patient's physician, who is notified immediately. Once the patient's condition has been stabilized, the woman is admitted to the hospital.

Some patients may have an unusual form of a disease, or—like this woman—an unexpected response to treatment, such that neither clinical protocols nor standard regimens are completely satisfactory for determining the next therapeutic step. The rheumatologist performs a search of the medical literature to find the information he needs to evaluate her response to the medication. The computer program proposes a search strategy of the literature databases based on the typical searches undertaken by this physician in the past, and using disease descriptors gleaned from the patient's electronic medical record. Based on the information reported in recent studies, the rheumatologist chooses to take his patient off protocol and to modify her treatment. When the woman is discharged from the hospital, the ER and inpatient summary notes are encoded on the patient's medical information card.

During subsequent follow-up visits, the rheumatologist examines the patient, and—using a clipboard-sized computer display and stylized speech input—records relevant data. He is especially careful to enter the key signs and symptoms as defined by the national disease committee, which was formed to produce a standardized terminology to support rheumatological research. At the conclusion of each visit, the data are encoded onto the medical card; at night, the rheumatologist's computers forward the data collected from all the day's patients to the national database. As the patient's disease status changes over time, the computer system provides summary reports, and suggests when various measurements indicate a possible complication or exacerbation.

20.1.3 Assumptions Underlying the Scenarios

To help you evaluate these scenarios of the future, we must make explicit the assumptions on which these speculations are based. In particular, we assume that health-care workers will work increasingly with computers in their daily lives, and that improvements in computer technology will continue, independent of technological advances in medical science. Furthermore, we assume that concerns about health-care cost containment and the threat of malpractice litigation will not be resolved in the near term.

The technological development of medical computing depends in large part on advances in general computing capabilities. Except in the area of medical imaging, little computer technology is first developed for medical applications and then applied to the rest of industry. This is especially true now that a few general-purpose microprocessors have become standard for all personal computers. Specialized computer chips will continue to be created for computationally intensive medical applications, such as signal processing. In these image-processing applications, rotation, filtering, enhancement, and reconstruction algorithms must handle more data than can be processed with the standard microprocessors; thus, a market exists for specialized machines.

It is difficult to predict whether the development of new general-purpose computer products will continue to follow an evolutionary trend, or will undergo a *paradigm shift*—defined by Kuhn in his book on the nature of scientific discovery as a complete change in perspective, such as occurred with the revelation that the earth is not flat [Kuhn, 1962]. Computer processing has gone through some major shifts in direction over the last 30 years: from single-user batch processing, to time-sharing on a central resource, then back to single-user processing, this time on local machines with access to specialized machines through a network. The human–machine interaction style has changed dramatically, with graphical interfaces for novices replacing typing and command-line interfaces. There also has been a gradual change from electrical to optical methods of network transmission (fiberoptic cables) and storage (CD-ROM and writable laser discs), as well as a steady progression from analog to digital recording of information. The latter is best illustrated by the slow switch from film to digital images in radiology, and the digitization of measurements taken in ICUs so that numeric information can be provided to clinicians, as well as the analog waveforms. For the purposes of this chapter, we shall assume the continued progression of current trends, rather than a significant paradigm shift. An unanticipated discovery that is just around the corner could, of course, quickly invalidate the assumption.

Another subtle, but pervasive, assumption underlies this book, much of which has been written by researchers in medical informatics. We tend to believe that more technology, thoughtfully introduced, is usually better, and that computers can enhance almost any aspect of medical practice—especially information access and the diagnostic and therapeutic components of the decision-making process. For example, there exist record-keeping systems, such as the RMRS system described in Chapter 6, that currently function effectively using paper encounter forms that are generated by computer, filled out by hand, and later processed again by machine. Still, we strive to eliminate the paper-based step, and assume that a well-designed interface (for example, one that allows continuous-speech input) applied to a sufficiently fast computer can significantly improve the overall process. This assumption, however, has yet to be verified.

People frequently criticize medical professionals for being technocrats—for encouraging an increase in mechanization and electronic gadgetry that tends to alienate both workers and patients. Such increases fuel the concern that modern medicine is becoming increasingly impersonal and sterile. How do we meld the automated environments proposed in this chapter's introductory scenarios with our wistful memories of kindly family doctors making house calls and attending their patients' weddings, christenings, bar mitzvahs, and the like? The reality, of course, is that the trend away from such traditional images predated the introduction of computers in medicine and has resulted more from modern pressures on health-care financing and the need for subspecialization to deal with an increasingly complex subject area. The role for computers and other information technologies results as much from these pressures as it does from a blind faith that all technology is good, useful, and worth the associated costs.

Once medical-computing applications have been shown to be effective, the technologies will need to be evaluated carefully and consistently prior to their routine adoption. We need to know that the benefits exceed the costs, both financial and sociological. The debate about where and how computers should be used is even more complex in developing countries, where advanced technology might partially compensate for shortages in medical expertise, but where scarce health-care resources might be more effectively employed to provide sanitation, antibiotics, and basic medical supplies. Nonetheless, the scenarios were painted with the assumption that there will be an increased application of computers in all aspects of medicine, and that the key difference between the future and today will be that computers will become ubiquitous, and will be highly interconnected.

20.2 Integration of Computer-Based Technologies

Most of the individual capabilities described in the preceding scenarios exist today in prototype form. What does not exist is an environment that *integrates* a large variety of computer-based support tools. The removal of barriers to integration requires both technological advances, such as the development of common hardware-communication protocols, and a better understanding of sociological issues, such as when computer use may be inappropriate or how the need for coordinated planning can overcome logistical barriers to connecting heterogeneous resources in a seamless fashion. In this section, we shall address issues related to system integration, and shall describe current national programs to develop standards that will enhance our ability to introduce computers to medical practice. These proposed standards cover, for example, determining the way that data measured at the bedside will be sent along wires to data-management computers; creating a common terminology for all aspects of biomedicine; and integrating components of a medical center via electronic means.

We can begin to assess the degree of connectivity in a medical center by asking simple questions. Can the laboratory computer communicate results to the computer that provides decision support, without a person having to reenter the data? Do the programs that provide decision support use the same terms to describe symptoms as do those that professionals use to perform electronic searches of journals in the local medical library? Do physicians use computers to get information without thinking about the fact that they are using a computer system, just as they pick up a medical chart and use it without first thinking about the format of the paper documents?

Computer systems must be integrated into the medical setting in three ways. First, applications must fit the existing information flow in the settings where they are to be used. If the terminal sits in a corner of the clinic, out of the normal traffic flow, and if there is another way to accomplish the specific task, then the computer system is likely to be ignored. Likewise, programs that arbitrarily constrain physicians to unnatural procedures for entering and accessing information are less likely to be used. User interfaces should be flexible and intuitive; just as the fields of a paper medical form can be completed in an arbitrary order, data-entry programs should allow users to enter information in any order.

Second, computer systems should provide common access to all computer-based resources, so a user cannot tell where one program ends and another starts. In this book, we have described such diverse applications as CT scanning and bibliographic searching. Many of these systems have been developed independently, and most are completely incompatible. In the future, the radiologist's PACS workstation should deliver more than just images—for example, a radiologist may wish also to search easily for references on unusual presentations of a specific disease process and to include these references in a paper that he is composing with a text editor. Ideally, users should not have to switch between computers, to stop one program and to start another, or even to use different sets of commands to obtain all the information they need. That the desired information resources may exist on multiple machines in different parts of the medical center or the country should be invisible to the user.

Third, the user interface must be both consistent across applications and easy to use, which may require multiple interface modalities, such as pointing, flexible spoken natural-language interfaces, and text input. Both at the user interface and internally, programs should use a common terminology to refer to frequently used concepts, such as a diagnosis, a symptom, or a laboratory-test value. The development of standards is essential for integrating computer systems in medical settings.

20.2.1 System Integration and the Development of Standards

In some respects, our HISs have taken a step backward since the 1960s. In the systems designed before 1970, a single mainframe computer ran all the applications, and used display terminals that had only minimal computing power to deliver the information. In the few installed systems, everyone had the same equipment; because the programs were written by one group, information sharing was easy. In the late 1970s and 1980s, many individual systems were created in response to specialized needs— for example, the PACS system was designed to store and retrieve radiologic images, and the laboratory system was designed to improve efficiency and accuracy of specimen handling and data management in the clinical laboratory. These specialized systems were developed on a variety of computers and typically functioned independently of other systems. Some hospitals now have a bank of terminals at each medical station, one for each source of information—which is certainly not the best way to provide computer support!

Ideally, all applications should be accessible from a single workstation via a uniform interface. The task of integrating the large number of incompatible hardware and software systems, however, currently is a time-consuming and extraordinarily costly endeavor. It typically requires custom design of myriad connections and internal interfaces. If standards existed for physical hardware connections, data-transmission protocols, and data formats, and if developers conformed to such standards, the task of integration would be greatly simplified. Just as people can purchase household appliances without worrying about the power requirements or the shape of the electrical plugs, standards for computer systems make it easier for institutions to acquire and combine special-purpose programs to produce integrated information systems.

The usual approach to standardization is to impose national or international conventions based on the recommendations of a committee of interested parties. The standardization process can be highly political; companies that are already producing a particular type of product have large vested interests in encouraging the committees to set standards that match their existing products. Furthermore, the timing of standard setting is crucial. If a standard is created too early in the development of a technology, then artificial limitations may be cemented in place. Examples are the 640-kilobyte memory limitation in the IBM-compatible PC standard (a standard set by a manufacturer, rather than a standards committee) and the 78-rpm (revolutions per minute) phonograph record. On the other hand, if a standard is created too late, then incompatible formats may have become established; examples are the VHS and BETA (and now 8-millimeter) formats for videotape.

In medical computing, people are attempting to set standards at different levels of specificity. At the lowest level, researchers are working to develop a medical information bus (MIB), a project designed to standardize the hardware and software protocols used by medical instruments, such as the equipment used in the ICU (see also Chapter 12). At a higher level, investigators are developing a Unified Medical Language System (UMLS) that can provide a common terminology for medical records systems, diagnostic programs, and bibliographic retrieval systems. At the most general level, researchers are responding to a need for communication and common terminology among different components of the medical center, such as between the library's online catalog and the computers used on the wards for medical record keeping and decision support. This third level is being addressed by research programs aimed at creating integrated academic information-management systems (IAIMS).

20.2.2 MIB: Connecting the Instruments

As we discussed in Chapter 12, researchers currently are working to define standards for an MIB to facilitate data integration at the bedside [Hawley et al., 1988]. In ORs and ICUs, patients frequently are connected to multiple monitoring devices, ventilators, infusion pumps, and other medical devices. These machines are produced by independent manufacturers that used different standards for hardware interfaces and data representation. Typically, they run as standalone equipment, and health-care personnel must manually enter data into the paper-based or computer-based medical records. Automated acquisition of data from medical devices would improve the timeliness and accuracy of data capture, and would allow many more data to be captured. The data could be presented in a common format in a convenient location, and interpretation programs could access all the data, thus improving the possibility of sophisticated evaluation and computer-based decision support.

Currently, each new device must be wired into the data-collection system according to its own particular wiring pattern, and special programs must interpret and translate the data transmitted by the device. (Some of the early wiring conventions did not define the voltages on all the attached wires, making it possible to destroy equipment by connecting two devices wired according to the RS-232 standard.) Once the wiring conventions have been worked out, then specific protocols for data transmission must be specified. The next step is to decide on conventions for naming variables and representing data. If one device uses "HR" to specify heart rate and a second device uses "pulse rate" to identify the same measure, then information will be lost if there is no mapping mechanism to relate the two variables. Independent systems also must use the same standard units of measurement (for example, is weight recorded in pounds, ounces, kilograms, or grams?) and standards for representing date and time (for example, is the time recorded as 29MAR1990 4:00PM, 29MAR90 16:00, 0329901600, or in some other format?).

Prototype versions of the developing MIB define standards at each of three levels: physical connections, data-communication protocols, and medical terminology (Figure 20.1). Up to 255 devices can easily be attached to the MIB using a standard hardware interface. A master communication controller (MCC) processes and relays information between the MIB and a host computer. It checks continuously for connection and disconnection of instruments and polls each instrument several times per second, collecting and transferring pertinent data to the host. Device communication controllers (DCCs) provide interfaces between the MIB and medical instruments, converting instrument outputs into the MIB standard protocol, and converting MIB instructions into device-specific codes. An important function of a DCC is to filter instrument output, sending only pertinent clinical information, and thus avoiding the collection and storage of large numbers of meaningless data. For example, the DCC can be programmed to specify how often data are sent and what the magnitude of clinically

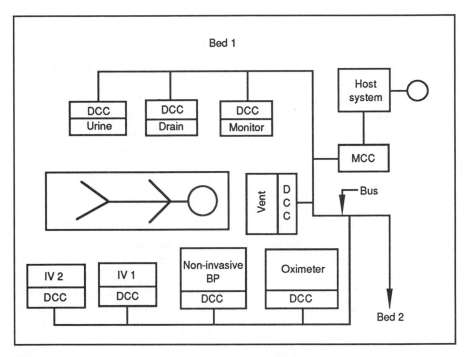

FIGURE 20.1 The medical information bus (MIB) facilitates automated collection and integration of data from independent bedside instruments by providing a standard hardware interface and data-communication protocol. Device communication controllers (DCCs) convert instrument outputs into the MIB protocol and MIB instructions into device-specific codes. A master communication controller (MCC) processes and relays information between the MIB and a host computer. Note that all the monitoring devices shown here are attached to a single patient. [IV = intravenous line, BP = blood pressure.] (*Source:* Reprinted with permission from Gardner, R. M. and Hawley, W. L. Standardizing communications and networks in the ICU. In *Patient Monitoring and Data Management.* Association for Advancement of Medical Instrumentation [AAMI], 1985.)

significant changes is. The DCC also contains memory and a power supply, so it can continue to store data for later transmission if the instrument is disconnected from the network. Once the MIB standard specifications are completed and accepted, manufacturers will be expected to conform to them when designing new systems.

Various groups are working on similar projects to define standards in other areas of medicine. For example, a committee of the American Society of Testing Materials (ASTM) has defined standards for the representation, storage, and transmission of clinical laboratory data [McDonald and Hammond, 1989], and work is underway to extend these standards to other types of clinical data. Health Level Seven (HL-7), a group of hospitals, consultants, and information-system vendors, has worked closely with ASTM to define standards for transmitting data for billing, updating the hospital census (ADT), order entry, and results reporting within hospital networks of many computers. Likewise, the American College of Radiology and the National Electronic Manufacturers' Association (ACR-NEMA) have developed a standard for storing digital radiographic images.

20.2.3 UMLS: Fusing the Terminology

In many respects, the UMLS starts where the MIB leaves off, at the level of defining common medical terminology. A variety of information sources currently is used by health-care personnel, including computer-based resources, such as clinical databases, bibliographic databases, and decision-support systems. Although use of electronic resources is growing (as evidenced by the increasing number of computer-assisted literature searches), a significant barrier to widespread acceptance is lack of integration among systems; a more fundamental problem is the lack of common terminology for accessing data and information.

Existing sources employ a variety of quasistandard and ad hoc schemes to identify concepts, such as diseases, diagnoses, symptoms, and findings. Common examples are MeSH, CPT, ICD, and SNOMED (see Chapter 2); DRGs (see Chapter 19); and special-purpose vocabularies, such as that created for Internist-1/QMR (see Chapter 15). As we discussed in Chapter 2, none of the existing coding systems is sufficiently general to support all applications. Users who consult systems with different underlying coding schemes will find that the systems often use different terminology to express the same concepts, or use the same words to express similar— but not identical—concepts. Some concepts may be entirely missing or may be expressed at the wrong level of detail.

To address the lack of a uniform medical terminology, the National Library of Medicine (NLM) is sponsoring research to build a Unified Medical Language System, or UMLS [Humphreys, 1989; McCray, 1989]. The researchers are not attempting to create a single standard vocabulary and to impose it on the medical community. Rather, the goal of the UMLS is to accommodate the diversity of existing systems. The UMLS will encompass an explicit machine-readable representation of the various biomedical coding schemes and their relationships to one another, to existing applications, and to the vocabularies used by health professionals and biomedical researchers. Thus, it will facilitate the retrieval and integration of information from diverse sources. For example, a common terminology would allow a patient-information system to communicate with a bibliographic-search system. A diagnostic program that produced a differential diagnosis that included a rare disease could use the UMLS structure to help formulate a MEDLINE search to determine whether the unusual patient presentation had been described previously in the literature.

In late 1988, following several years of background research and exploratory studies, researchers began to build and test prototypes of basic UMLS components (Figure 20.2). The UMLS, as currently envisioned, will comprise two classes of components: knowledge sources (Metathesaurus, semantic network, and information sources map) and functional features (such as query-interpreter and search-formulator programs). The *Metathesaurus* is the central vocabulary representation for each medical concept. Rather than attempting to build a definitive biomedical taxonomy from scratch, researchers plan to create the Metathesaurus using automated lexical-matching techniques combined with manual review and editing. Thus, the Metathesaurus will contain terms from existing vocabularies and will record the relationships among the various terms used to express the same concepts (Figure 20.3).

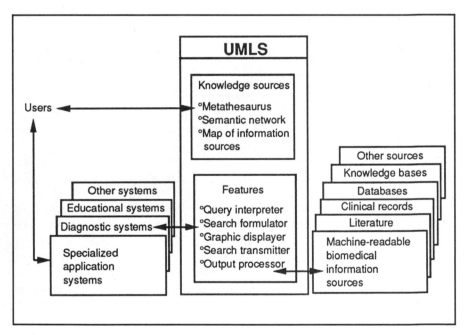

FIGURE 20.2 As currently envisioned, the Unified Medical Language System (UMLS) will comprise knowledge sources (Metathesaurus, semantic network, information sources map) and functional features (for example, the query-interpreter and search-formulator programs). Users will be able to access these components directly or via special-purpose application systems. (*Source*: Courtesy of Donald A. B. Lindberg, M.D. and Betsy L. Humphreys. Modification of Figure 3 in their article: Computer systems that understand medical meaning. In Scherrer, J. R., Côté, R. A., and Mandil, S. D. (eds), *Computerized Natural Medical Language Processing for Knowledge Representation*. Amsterdam: Elsevier Science Publishers, 1989, p. 9.)

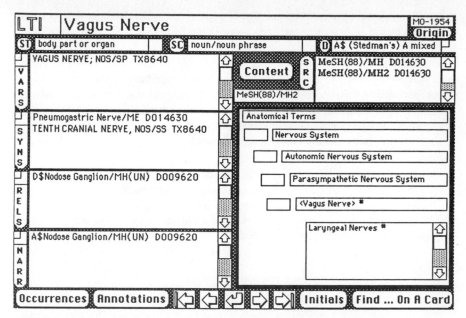

FIGURE 20.3 This screen from Meta-0, a 2000-entry prototype of the UMLS Metathesaurus, displays one possible view of the entry "vagus nerve." "Vagus nerve" has semantic type (ST) "body part or organ" and syntactic classification (SC) "noun/noun phrase." A text definition (D) of "vagus nerve" can be viewed on another screen. The left of the screen displays the term's lexical variants (VARS) and synonyms (SYNS), related terms (RELS), and narrower terms (NARR). The right side of the screen displays the MeSH hierarchy for the second of the two places where the term appears in the hierarchy. (*Source:* Courtesy of M. S. Tuttle and D. D. Sherertz, Lexical Technology, Inc. [supported by NLM Contract N1-LM-8-3512].)

Another knowledge structure, the *semantic-type network,* will represent the relationships among the basic concepts included in the Metathesaurus. For example, the semantic type "virus" has an *is-a* relationship to the semantic type "organism" and a *can-cause* relationship to the semantic type "disease." An *information sources map* will contain information about the scope, location, vocabulary, syntax rules, and access conditions of publically available information resources. The UMLS will also include functional features, such as a query interpreter to analyze users' input, an interactive search formulator to aid in refinement and translation of users' queries, and a presentation system to organize and display the information retrieved. Users will be able to access the UMLS directly or via special-purpose application systems.

20.2.4 IAIMS: Coalescing Information Flow in the Medical Center

We mentioned at the beginning of this chapter that much of the work in medical informatics has focused on the development of individual applications. Since the early 1980s, however, there has been increasing recognition that optimal use of resources in health institutions requires integration of computer applications, as well as information exchange among organizational units. In medical centers, integration of information is necessary to support patient care, education, research, and administration. There is also increasing recognition of the evolving role of academic libraries in dealing with new forms of information—for example, knowledge bases, bibliographic databases, and online references—and mechanisms for communication of information. Consequently, increasing attention has been devoted to the development of integrated academic information management systems (IAIMS). A primary concern in IAIMS research is the establishment of electronic networks to support such integration and communication of information (Figure 20.4).

As described in an NLM-sponsored symposium on IAIMS,

> The IAIMS concept is to use computer and communication technologies to bring together a health institution's various information resources into a unified, easily accessible system. The goal is to integrate library systems with the multitude of individual and institutional working information files, such as clinical, administrative, research and educational databases. [National Library of Medicine, 1986a, foreword]

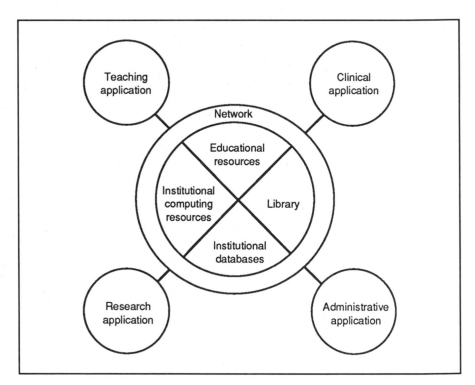

FIGURE 20.4 A schematic representation of the relationship between IAIMS infrastructure and applications. A primary goal of IAIMS research is to integrate teaching, clinical, research, and administrative applications by providing convenient access through an electronic network to a wide variety of information resources. (*Source:* Reprinted with permission from Hendrickson, G., et al. The role of IAIMS in stimulating educational change at the Columbia-Presbyterian Medical Center. *Proceedings of IAIMS and Health Sciences Education,* March 12, 1986.)

Clearly, if we are to integrate these diverse resources fully, we will have to address the same standardization issues faced in MIB and UMLS research. An equally difficult problem is the development of organizational and administrative infrastructures for creating and managing IAIMS. Administrative units must agree on common needs for information handling; on responsibility for purchasing, installing, and maintaining hardware and software; and on procedures for conversion from paper-based systems. In most academic medical centers, the number of academic and hospital functional units that must cooperate is large, and the units usually do not have the unified administrative structures or information policies required to achieve such coordination [Piemme and Ball, 1984].

In 1984, the NLM began to provide research support to foster the development of IAIMS. Funding was aimed at promoting the institutionwide use of communications and information-processing technologies and at preparing medical libraries to expand and develop services to support the new computer-based information technologies. A few medical centers that already had an HIS and an online library card catalog in place were given Phase I contracts to facilitate the administrative planning process and to develop a medical-information policy. In 1985, grants were awarded for Phase II, based on proposals for prototype projects of information integration in various parts of the medical center and the demonstration of significant internal support for the IAIMS concept from the medical-center administration. Often, Phase I and II grants were given to medical centers where local-area networks (LANs) were being installed to provide the backbone of the communication activities. Recently, Phase III awards were provided to stimulate full-scale development of IAIMS implementations. A variety of organizational and technical challenges is being addressed in these projects, including the development of information-management policies; user education and promotion of computer-based technologies; acquisition and development of electronic workstations for clinicians, researchers, and managers; and evaluation and selection of communication protocols to support diverse sets of existing hardware and software.

20.3 Computers in Health Care: Finding a Happy Medium

The opening scenarios in this chapter highlight the extent to which the computer will need to be integrated with medical practice. As we discussed in the previous section, fulfillment of the scenarios will require significant technological changes. Equally important are the organizational and attitudinal changes that will be necessary to implement the new technologies as they emerge. Health professionals, health institutions, medical-system developers, and society as a whole must carefully consider the appropriate role of computers in medicine and assess the potential benefits of computers in terms of improved access to information, enhanced communication, increased efficiency of health-care delivery, and higher quality of medical care.

Although the potential benefits of using computers are many, there are also potential costs, only some of which are monetary. For example, computer-based medical-record systems will never exactly replicate the flexibility of current paper-based systems.

This flexibility includes the ability to create progress notes about patients, using any words in any order and in any format, with or without diagrams, to record the information. Computer-based systems limit flexibility in return for increased legibility and access to the information and for the ability to use the information for other purposes, such as clinical research studies that use multiple patient databases. We see the same pattern in the use of automated bank-teller machines. There is only one way to complete a cash-withdrawal transaction through a sequence of button pushes, but there is a large number of ways in which we can make this request of a human teller. Automated tellers, however, are available at 3:00 in the morning; human tellers are not.

The notion that computer approaches would require the additional structuring of medical records was perceived by Lawrence Weed more than 20 years ago [Weed, 1969]. Weed noted that, for medical records to be useful, they had to be indexed such that important information could be extracted. In particular, he proposed that the medical record be organized according to the patient's current problems—the problem-oriented medical record (POMR). Variations on the POMR have become a standard feature of medical record keeping, regardless of whether computers are used. In PROMIS, a computer-based implementation of the POMR (see Chapter 7), such rigid and time-consuming indexing of patient problems was required that clinicians ultimately proved reluctant to use the system. Standardization provides benefits, but exacts costs in terms of decreased flexibility; it makes information more accessible, but restricts freedom to pursue alternate means to accomplish the same result. It is unlikely that new computer innovations will ever eliminate this tradeoff.

Similarly, the use of computers requires tradeoffs with respect to confidentiality of medical information. Legitimate users can more conveniently access computer-based records in well-designed systems. Without sufficient security measures, however, unauthorized users may threaten the confidentiality and integrity of databases. Fortunately, with adequate attention to security issues, modern methods can ensure that patient data are kept with greater confidentiality in computer systems than they are in paper charts on hospital wards.

Earlier fears that computers could replace physicians have not been borne out, and computers are likely to remain decision-support tools rather than substitute decision makers [Shortliffe, 1989]. It is more likely that computers will be used increasingly to monitor the quality of health care delivered and to help evaluate physician performance. Greater automation will therefore change the nature of medical practice in nontrivial ways. The challenge for system developers and users will be to identify the solution that provides the optimal balance between flexibility and standardization.

20.4 Forces Affecting the Future of Medical Computing

In this book, we have identified several important factors that affect the current and future roles of computers in medicine. These factors include advances in biotechnology and computer hardware and software, changes in the backgrounds of health professionals, changes in the medicolegal climate, and changing strategies for health-care reimbursement. The relative strengths of these forces will determine how likely it is that the scenarios we proposed will take place and how quickly we can expect such changes to occur.

20.4.1 Changes in Computers and Biomedical Technology

Modern computers are smaller, less expensive, and more powerful than were their predecessors. Although microchip designers are approaching the physical limits of how close together electronic elements can be placed, these trends will continue. By the time a new microprocessor chip or memory chip is adapted for use in new computer systems, manufacturers are creating samples of the next generation of chips. The most important ramification of current trends in microcomputer technology is that it is now possible to include a small microprocessor and memory in most sophisticated pieces of medical equipment. Thus, the many individual devices used in a setting such as an ICU could be connected to one another and to a central repository of clinical data, which the proposed MIB standard is designed to facilitate.

The ability to connect multiple devices over high-speed networks is foreshadowing a dramatic change in the way medical computer systems are designed. It is now practical to consider systems in which multiple data-storage devices may be accessed by complex computers that sort and abstract the numerous patient data that are generated. This design contrasts with the traditional approach in which health professionals would need to gather information from many different devices or locations in the medical center to obtain a complete picture of a patient's status. We have many more data to transmit over the network, such as those from digitized radiology images, online reports, and computer-based charting of the patient's condition. Faster networks, based on fiberoptics, and larger storage devices, based on writable optical discs, may be necessary to manage the overwhelming volume of data that will be created by all-digital medical data systems. Low-cost computer workstations allow information to be manipulated at each patient's bedside, as well as at central nursing stations.

The advent of high-speed telephone networks will allow physicians in private offices to connect to computers in the hospitals where these professionals admit patients or in the laboratories that process the patients' specimens. In situations where it is not practical to connect all the practitioners in a communication network, it may be possible to exploit medical data cards (as described in the second scenario) that can store a large amount of information via optical or magnetic memory, and that can be updated by an output device using a laser or a magnetic field.

20.4.2 Changes in the Background of Health Professionals

Computers will continue to be made faster and less expensive, and will have more features; however, sufficient computing power now exists for many applications. Thus, the limitations on the pervasiveness of computers in medicine do not hinge as crucially on the development of new hardware as they did in the past. The availability of relatively inexpensive and powerful computers is changing health-care workers' familiarity with machines by exposing these people to computers in all aspects of their daily lives. This increased familiarity in turn increases acceptance of computers in the workplace, another crucial determinant of how computers will fare in the next 20 years.

Since the early 1970s, people have increasingly interacted with computers in their daily lives to perform financial transactions, to make travel arrangements, and even to purchase groceries. In many situations, people do not use the computer themselves, but rather talk to an intermediary, such as an airline-reservation agent or bank clerk. Large computer systems are so deeply integrated into the many business practices that it is not uncommon to hear, "I can't help you—the computer is down." This switch to computer-based record keeping for most financial transactions is so pervasive that you would be surprised and concerned if you were to receive a monthly bank statement that was written out in longhand.

Within the last 10 years, many mediated computer-based transactions have slowly been replaced by direct contact between a consumer and a computer system. We can withdraw cash from automated bank tellers, request a trip routing from a computer at the rental-car stand, or obtain an account balance by touch-tone telephone. Thus, health-care professionals are certainly aware of the pervasiveness of computers outside of medical settings. Although this exposure guarantees that health-care professionals are familiar with computers, it does not mean that they want to use computers in medical practice. Physicians are particularly resistant to using computers for tasks that are far removed from the familiar numeric or financial applications.

The following quote, taken from a recent survey of the use of computers in medical care, is typical of this type of reaction:

> I would find a computer useful in pointing out potential pitfalls—drug interactions that I didn't remember, for example, or detailed contraindications to specific drugs (especially new ones). As far as pushing in numbers or buttons and [being told] you should do this or that, I think that takes a little too much of the feel away from the physician who is calling the shots. . . . I guess if it was a field I knew nothing about, then certainly an expert (even if he didn't agree with all the other experts) could help more than my own database, which might be close to zero. [Shortliffe, 1989, p. 2]

Furthermore, physicians are reluctant to invest time and money to adopt innovative (but unproven) technologies that significantly alter practice patterns.

> The paperless office is too radical a concept for us in practice today. And it's unnecessary and expensive. I don't really see an improvement. Can you imagine walking into a paperless office—no notes, everything that happens you type it in and it goes into memory . . . ! [Shortliffe, 1989, p. 2]

Young health-care workers today have been exposed to computers throughout their education. Some college courses assign projects that must be carried out using the computer. As in the everyday environment, the use of computers in schools is likely to increase. It is difficult to determine how the current hodgepodge of computers in the medical setting will bias its users. It may be that, when the integrated system becomes available, health-care professionals will not use the system fully because of previous negative experiences in less sophisticated environments. On the other hand, familiarity with computers and with their operation may prepare users to accept well-designed, easy-to-use systems.

20.4.3 Legal Considerations

The number of malpractice lawsuits and the size of the settlements have increased in recent years. Today, the specter of potential legal action hangs over every medical interaction. Computers can either exacerbate or alleviate this situation. The computer-based diagnostic system may provide a reminder of a rare but life-threatening disease that might have been overlooked in the differential diagnosis. On the other hand, decision-support systems might generate warnings that, if ignored by health-care workers, could be used as evidence against those workers in a court action.

In Chapters 5 and 15, we discussed legal issues that affect the design and regulation of computer systems designed to support information management and clinical decision making. Increasingly, complex software directly controls medical hardware, such as mechanical ventilators and radiation-therapy devices. The development and use of such systems raise additional questions: When is a product safe enough to place on the market? Who should be held responsible when system errors result in injuries? Instances of accidental death and injury resulting from errors in control software have probably played a role in the FDA's decision to regulate software in medical equipment. More stringent requirements in turn may slow the development of computer-based systems.

Safety measures on mechanical devices have often included checks to ensure that all actions are really intended—for instance, a plastic cover over a crucial switch will ensure that a person cannot trip the switch accidentally, but must lift the cover before consciously flipping the switch. Similar controls are necessary when mechanical methods for controlling medical devices are replaced by computer methods because operators rely on the computer to control hazardous machinery. This need was highlighted in a series of incidents in which software failure in the control system of a particular type of radiation-therapy machine resulted in many times the prescribed dose of radiation therapy being administered to patients [Jacky, 1989].

Computer-controlled radiation machines called *linear accelerators* can generate two types of radiation beams: electron beams and X-ray beams. Electron beams may be used to irradiate patients directly. X-ray beams are produced by aiming an electron beam at a metal target. As electrons are absorbed, X rays are produced. Because this process is inefficient, however, a much higher-intensity electron beam must be used. Irradiating the patient directly with the high-intensity beam can be fatal. In the faulty machine, both target position and beam intensity were controlled by a computer; when the operator selected a mode, the computer moved the target and set the beam intensity accordingly. In unusual circumstances when the operator selected the X-ray mode in error, then quickly switched to the other mode, the computer removed the metal target without reducing the intensity of the beam. This series of events happened several times, and the patients received severe radiation overdoses.

This situation represents a clear-cut software error. In addition, the problem was exacerbated by a poorly designed user interface, which encouraged operators to ignore potential safety hazards, rather than reporting the incidents for investigation. This particular machine indicated the malfunction by displaying a nonintuitive numeric code. It often displayed a similar code when the actual beam intensity did not exactly match the expected intensity, usually a relatively unimportant and benign situation.

In such cases, the operators simply overrode the computer alarm by typing "p" (for proceed). Because of the use of nonintuitive alarm codes, the ease with which the system was overridden, and the rarity of actual malfunctions, the overdose situations were not recognized immediately. These incidents led to lawsuits, and to discontinuation of this model of linear accelerator. The full effects on software design and regulation are not yet clear.

Just as manufacturers may be liable for the malfunction of a computer device, physicians may someday be liable if they fail to take advantage of computer aids. Physicians are expected to treat patients according to the *standard of care* in the community. For example, a CT scan has become a standard test for diagnosis of severe head injuries. Failure to obtain a CT scan when a scanner is available can be used as evidence of malpractice against a doctor who has failed to diagnose an internal head injury. Should computer-based diagnostic and therapeutic systems become popular, many physicians may be forced by the legal situation to use computer-based technology, even if they do not believe such procedures or devices are warranted. As will health-care financing (discussed in the next section), legal issues will dramatically influence the future role of medical informatics.

20.4.4 Health-Care Financing

Some people assume that the continuing evolution of computer hardware and software is the most important force influencing the development of medical computing. Social issues such as health-care financing and the legal aspects of medicine, however, probably outweigh the technological factors. Perhaps the strongest force at work today is the pressure to control health-care costs. Health-care financing influences all choices regarding the acquisition and maintenance of high-technology equipment.

As we saw in Chapter 19, health-care costs have grown rapidly in recent decades. Current schemes for health-care financing have been designed to slow the rate of growth of these costs. These policies translate into pressure to reduce costs in every aspect of medical diagnosis and treatment, such as to shorten hospital stays, to select less expensive surgical procedures, and to order fewer laboratory tests. As incentives for making optimal decisions in these areas increase, there is a greater need for computers that can collect, store, interpret, and present data during the decision-making process. A laboratory system might screen test orders against criteria for test ordering and question or cancel tests that do not meet the criteria. A more sophisticated application might serve as an adjunct to a laboratory-data system, assessing which tests are most appropriate to order for specific patients who require expensive workups (for example, custom-tailored evaluation of thyroid function). Such a program could specify the sequence of tests to be administered during the diagnostic phase and the optimal timing of tests in the monitoring phase of inpatient care. A pharmacy system might evaluate drug orders and suggest less expensive substitutes that are equally effective, could check for drug–drug interactions, and so on.

It is possible that hospital administrators will require clinicians to use computer programs if the clinicians are allowed access to hospital resources. It is even more probable that computers will be used by insurance companies to enforce a particular style of care through concurrent or post hoc review of the medical decision-making process, including decisions about length of stay and tests performed. Insurance companies are not currently using computers for decision support, but many of the impediments to hands-on use by health-care workers do not apply to employees of insurance companies who do not directly treat patients. Thus, one force promoting the use of computers by clinicians may be the knowledge that computers will be used by insurers to review these clinicians' decisions after the fact. The clinicians may prefer to know what the computer system will advise beforehand, so that they can be prepared to justify intentional deviations from the norm.

Although the use of computer technology can help health professionals to cope with the growing complexity of medical practice, it can also contribute to the increasing cost of health care, and demonstrating corresponding benefits is not always easy. It is difficult to show that use of computers can lead to a decrease in patient morbidity or mortality, especially in complex environments such as operating rooms or ICUs. Large numbers of devices are already being used in these settings, and patients are often treated for multiple concurrent problems. Even if patient-monitoring equipment could help health-care workers to recognize potentially dangerous situations earlier than they otherwise would, showing that the computer system affected the outcome would be difficult. At the other extreme are devices that can be shown to make a difference, but whose cost is very high, such as CT and MRI systems. Because they replace invasive techniques (which have a significant potential for causing harm) or provide information that is available from no other source, there has been little debate about the utility of these new modalities. Instead, the high cost of this equipment has focused attention on how best to distribute these new resources. No matter how computer systems are used in the future, we will need to evaluate the influence of the computer application on health-care financing, and to assess the new technology in light of alternative uses of resources.

20.5 Looking Back: What Have We Learned?

An introductory book can only scratch the surface of a field as varied and complex as medical informatics. In our discussions of each topic, we have examined technical questions about how a system works (or ought to work); we must also view each area in light of the health-care trends and the social and fiscal issues that shape the ways in which medical care is delivered now and in the future. In this chapter, we have emphasized the rich social and technological context in which medical informatics moves ahead, both as a scientific discipline and as a set of methodologies, devices, and complex systems that serve health-care workers and, through them, their patients. Glimpses of the future can be at once both exciting and frightening—exciting when we see how emerging technologies can address the frequently cited problems that confound current health-care practices, but frightening when we realize that methodologies must be applied wisely and with sensitivity if patients are to receive the humane and cost-sensitive health care that they have every right to expect. The question is not whether computer technologies will play a pervasive role in the health-care environment of the future, but rather how we can ensure that future systems are designed and implemented effectively to optimize technology's role as a stimulus and support for the health-care system and for individual practitioners. The outcomes of the process will depend as much on health-care planners, practitioners, and policy makers as they will on system developers and medical-informatics professionals.

Suggested Readings

Anderson, J. G. and Jay, S. J. (eds). *Use and Impact of Computers in Clinical Medicine.* New York: Springer-Verlag, 1987.

> *This collection of papers presents research on the factors that affect the adoption, diffusion, and utilization of clinical information systems in hospitals. It includes chapters on the attitudes of health professionals toward computers, the diffusion of medical computer applications, and the probable effects of computer systems on medical practice.*

Greenes, R. A. (ed). *Proceedings of the Twelfth Annual Symposium on Computer Applications in Medical Care.* New York: IEEE Press, 1988.

> *The Unified Medical Language System (UMLS) project is best described in terms of the individual research programs. A selection of papers is published in this volume, as well as in each subsequent year's conference proceedings. The article by Hawley and associates describes MIB research that has been conducted by investigators at the LDS Hospital since 1985. The experience of the researchers in developing and testing a prototype MIB has provided valuable insights to the Institute of Electrical and Electronic Engineers (IEEE) MIB standards committee.*

Miller, R. A., Schaffner, K. F., and Meisel, A. Ethical and legal issues related to the use of computer programs in clinical medicine. *Annals of Internal Medicine,* 102:529, 1985.

> *This paper describes the ethical and legal issues that underlie the development of computer-based decision-support tools. It discusses the proper balance between confidentiality of patient information and shared access to medical records by authorized health-care personnel. Also addressed is the question of how regulatory agencies, physicians, and patients can evaluate the safety of medical programs. Finally, the legal status of computer programs that provide medical advice is examined.*

National Library of Medicine. *IAIMS and Health Sciences Education.* Bethesda, MD: U.S. Department of Health and Human Services, Public Health Service, National Institutes of Health, March 1986.

> *This volume, the proceedings of the second NLM-sponsored IAIMS symposium, contains reports from institutions receiving NLM funding to support IAIMS planning, development, and testing.*

National Library of Medicine. *NLM Long Range Plan.* Bethesda, MD: U.S. Department of Health and Human Services, Public Health Service, National Institutes of Health, January 1987.

> *This volume of reports describes potential research directions for the NLM over the next 20 years. Volume 4, dealing with medical informatics research, includes a scenario that might take place in the year 2006.*

Schwartz, W. B. Medicine and the computer: The promise and problems of change. *New England Journal of Medicine,* 283(23):1257, 1970.

The author speculates about the effects on medical practice of advances in medical computing, and discusses potential psychological, organizational, legal, and economic costs of the increasing use of computers in health-care settings. Although the paper was written 20 years ago, many of the issues are still relevant.

Shortliffe, E. H. Testing reality: The introduction of decision-support technologies for physicians. *Methods of Information in Medicine,* 28:1, 1989.

This paper provides commentary by physicians on their views of the role of computers in decision support for medicine. It identifies and describes a number of problems and concerns about computer systems that are commonly voiced by physicians, including fear of loss of rapport with patients, fear of loss of control, and reluctance to embrace new technologies that could radically alter practice styles.

Questions for Discussion

1. Select an area of medicine with which you are familiar, but that is different from the intensive-care unit and chronic-care setting described at the beginning of this chapter. Based on what you have learned in this book, propose a scenario for that area that takes place 20 years in the future. Be sure to think about how issues of system integration and networking will affect the evolution of computers in the setting you describe.

2. Select a field of medicine with which you are familiar, and identify examples of terminology that illustrate redundancy (two or more terms that denote the same object) and ambiguity (one term that denotes more than one object). Many medical concepts can be organized hierarchically to indicate varying levels of abstraction. For example, a *poliovirus* is a type of *enterovirus,* which is a type of *virus,* which is a type of *organism.* Identify examples of concept hierarchies with at least three levels of nesting. Consider other medical fields that use the same terms. Do the terms you have chosen have precisely the same meanings and implications in all the areas? How might you deal with the problem of standardizing the terminology, given the strong pressures to use existing terms?

3. Consider an academic health-science center that wishes to tie together its hospital information system, medical-library computer system, clinical-research databases, financial-management systems, and applications running on the computer at the associated medical school. Describe the logistical and political problems that you envision a person would face were she to attempt coordinating these diverse systems. How would you deal with the problems? In medical centers with which you are familiar, are there individuals who have both the expertise and the authority to design and implement such coordinated systems?

4. Imagine that you are a patient visiting a health-care facility at which the physicians have made a major commitment to computer-based tools. How would you react to the following situations?
   a. Before you are ushered into the examining room, the nurse takes your blood pressure and pulse in a work area. He then enters the information into a computer terminal located in the nursing station adjacent to the waiting room.

b. While the physician interviews you, she occasionally types information into a computer terminal that is facing her; you cannot see the screen.

c. While the physician interviews you, she occasionally uses a mouse pointing device to enter information into a computer terminal that is facing her; you cannot see the screen.

d. While the physician interviews you, she occasionally uses a mouse pointing device to enter information into a computer terminal that you both can see. As she does so, she explains the data she is reviewing and entering.

e. While the physician interviews you, she enters information into a clipboard-sized computer terminal that responds to finger touch and requires no keyboard typing.

f. While the physician interviews you, she occasionally stops to dictate a phrase. A speech-understanding interface processes what she says and stores the information in a medical-record system.

g. There is no computer in the examining room, but you notice that between visits, the physician uses a terminal in her office to review and enter patient data.

What do your answers to these questions tell you about the potential effect of the use of computers on patient–physician rapport? What insight have you gained regarding how interactive technologies could affect the patient–physician encounter? Did you have different reactions to the scenarios in parts (c) and (d)? Do you believe that most people would respond to these two situations as you did?

Glossary

(The bracketed number(s) following each definition indicate the chapter(s) where the key term is referenced.)

Accounting costs: In health-care institutions, the recorded costs of providing health-care services, as defined by the laws of taxation, the rules of corporate accounting, and the reimbursement guidelines of third-party payers. [19]

Active storage: In a hierarchical data-storage scheme, the devices used to store data that have long-term validity and that must be accessed rapidly. [4]

Address: In a computer system, a number or symbol that identifies a particular cell of memory. [4]

Administrative services only (ASO): The practice by employers of paying their employees' medical bills directly (self-insurance), and hiring insurance companies only to process claims. [19]

Admission-discharge-transfer (ADT): The core component of a hospital information system that maintains and updates the hospital census. [7]

Algorithm: A well-defined procedure or sequence of steps that solves a problem and terminates given any set of inputs. [1]

Ambulatory medical record: A paper-based or computer-stored document in which are recorded the data gathered during a patient's encounters with the health-care system, other than records created during hospital admissions. [6]

American Standard Code for Information Interchange (ASCII): A 7-bit code for representing alphanumeric characters and other symbols. [4]

Analog signal: A signal that takes on a continuous range of values. [4]

Analog-to-digital conversion: Conversion of sampled values from a continuous-valued signal to a discrete-valued digital representation. [4]

Anchoring and adjustment: A heuristic used when estimating probability, in which a person first makes a rough approximation (the anchor), then adjusts this estimate to account for additional information. [3]

Angiography: A technique used to increase the contrast resolution of X-ray images of the blood vessels by injection of radiopaque contrast material into the vessels. [11]

Application program: A computer program designed to accomplish a user-level task. [4]

Applications research: Systematic investigation or experimentation with the goal of applying knowledge to achieve practical ends. [1]

Archival storage: In a hierarchical data-storage scheme, the devices used to store data for backup, documentary, or legal purposes. [4]

Artificial intelligence (AI): The branch of computer science concerned with endowing computers with the ability to simulate intelligent human behavior. [1,15]

Assembler: A computer program that translates assembly-language programs into machine-language instructions. [4]

Assembly language: A low-level language for writing computer programs using symbolic names for operations and addresses. [4]

Authoring system: In computer-aided instruction, a specialized, high-level language used by educators to create computer-based teaching programs. [17]

Automated multiphasic health-testing services (AMHTS): An expanded automated multiphasic health-testing program that provides adjunctive services, including patient triaging, health counseling, and patient education. (See multiphasic health-testing program.) [18]

Automated multiphasic health-testing system (AMHT): A multiphasic health-testing program that uses automated instruments to analyze laboratory specimens collected at individual testing stations, and that uses a computer-based information system to maintain medical records, to assist in data interpretation, to provide decision support using advice rules, to generate summary reports, and to facilitate operational tasks, such as appointment scheduling, patient recall, and patient registration. (See multiphasic health-testing program.) [18]

Auxiliary memory: The devices for storing data and programs that are not currently being used in main memory. [4]

Availability: A heuristic method by which a person estimates the probability of an event based on the ease with which he can recall similar events. [3]

Average cost: The total cost of producing a good or service divided by the number of units of goods or service produced. [19]

Averaging out at chance nodes: The process by which each chance node of a decision tree is replaced in the tree by the expected value of the event that it represents. [3]

Back-projection: A method for reconstructing images, in which the measured attenuation along a path is distributed uniformly across all pixels along the path. [11]

Bandwidth: The capacity for information transmission; the number of bits that can be transmitted per unit of time. [4]

Baseband transmission: A data transmission technique in which bits are sent without modulation. (See modem.) [4]

Baseline, population: The prevalence of the condition under consideration in the population from which the subject was selected; **individual:** The frequency, rate, or degree of a condition before an intervention or other perturbation. [2]

Basic research: Systematic investigation or experimentation with the goal of discovering new knowledge. [1]

Basic science: The enterprise of performing basic research. [1]

Batch mode: A noninteractive mode of using a computer, in which users submit jobs for processing and receive results on completion. (See time-sharing mode.) [4]

Baud rate: The rate of information transfer; in practice, baud rate is equal to the number of bits per second being sent. [4]

Bayes' theorem: An algebraic expression for calculating posttest probability of a condition (a disease, for example) if the pretest probability (prevalence) of the condition, as well as the sensitivity and specificity of the test, are known (also called *Bayes' rule*). [3]

Bayesian diagnosis program: A computer-based system that uses Bayes' theorem to assist a physician in developing and refining a differential diagnosis. [15]

Bibliographic database: A file composed of a set of records, each of which characterizes a document in terms of author, title, publication source, and subject matter. [14]

Biomedical computing: The use of computers in biology or medicine. [1]

Biomedical engineering: An area of engineering concerned primarily with the research and development of medical instrumentation and medical devices. [1]

Bit: A digit that can assume the values of either 0 or 1. [4]

Bit-map: A digital representation of an image in memory, in which there is a one-to-one correspondence between bits and pixels of a displayed image. [4]

Bit-mapped display: A display screen that is divided into a grid of tiny areas (pixels), each associated with a bit that indicates whether the area is on (black) or off (white). [4]

Blinding: A technique to hide membership in a study group from the subject or from the observers to avoid biasing treatment response or evaluation of results. [16]

Bootstrap: A small set of initial instructions that is stored in read-only memory and executed each time the computer is turned on. Execution of the bootstrap is called *booting* the computer. By analogy, the process of starting larger computer systems. [4]

Branching questioning algorithm: A procedure for asking questions and collecting information, in which a person's response to a question determines which question the system will ask next; for example, allows an educational system to tailor its teaching to a student's level of knowledge. [17]

Branching questionnaire: A procedure for asking questions and collecting information, in which a person's response to a question determines which question the system will ask next. [18]

Break-even calculation: A calculation performed to determine at what value of parameter x alternative A does better than alternative B. [19]

Broadband transmission: A data-transmission technique in which multiple signals may be transmitted simultaneously, each modulated within an assigned frequency range. [4]

Byte: A sequence of 8 bits, often used to store an ASCII character. [4]

Capitation: In health-care financing, the payment of premiums or dues directly to the provider organization in the form of a fixed periodic payment for comprehensive care, set in advance (also called *per capita payment*). [19]

Case finding: The traditional method for health examination, in which a patient receives a panel of routine tests in conjunction with a diagnostic workup when she visits her physician with a specific medical complaint. [18]

Cathode-ray tube (CRT): A data-output device that displays information by projecting streams of electrons onto a fluorescent screen to create programmed patterns of light and dark, or color. [4]

Central computer system: A single system that handles all computer applications in an institution using a common set of databases and interfaces. [7]

Central processing unit (CPU): The "brain" of the computer. The CPU executes a program stored in main memory by fetching and executing instructions in the program. [4]

Chance node: A symbol that represents a chance event. By convention, a chance node is indicated in a decision tree by a circle. [3]

Charges: In a health-care institution, the established prices for services. Often, charges do not reflect the cost of providing the service. [19]

Clinical decision-support system: A computer-based system that assists physicians in making decisions about patient care. [15]

Clinical prediction rule: A rule, derived from statistical analysis of clinical observations, that is used to assign a patient to a clinical subgroup with a known probability of disease. [3]

Clinical research: The collection and analysis of medical data collected during patient care to improve medical science and the knowledge physicians use in caring for patients. [16]

Clinical subgroup: A subset of a population in which the members have similar characteristics and symptoms, and therefore similar likelihood of disease. [3]

Clinically relevant population: The population of patients that is seen in actual practice. In the context of estimating the sensitivity and specificity of a diagnostic test, that group of patients in which the test actually will be used. [3]

Closed-loop control device: A computer-based device that regulates a physiological variable, such as blood pressure, by monitoring the value of the variable and altering therapy without human intervention. (See open-loop control system.) [12]

Closest-match search: A statistical approach to information retrieval in which documents containing all or some of user-defined search terms are displayed in order of likelihood of relevance. [14]

Coding scheme: A system for classifying objects and entities (such as diseases, procedures, or symptoms) using a finite set of numeric or alphanumeric identifiers. [2]

Cognitive science: Area of research concerned with studying the processes by which people think and behave. [1]

Coinsurance: The percentage of charges that are paid by the insuree rather than by the insurance company once the deductible has been satisfied. [19]

Compact-disc read-only memory (CD-ROM): An optical-disc technology for storing and retrieving large numbers of prerecorded data. Data are permanently encoded through the use of a laser that marks the surface of the disc, then can be read an unlimited number of times using a finely focused semiconductor laser that detects reflections from the disc. [4]

Compiler: A program that translates a program written in a high-level programming language to a machine-language program, which can then be executed. [4]

Computed tomography (CT): An imaging modality in which X rays are projected through the body from multiple angles and the resultant absorption values are analyzed by a computer to produce cross-sectional slices. [11]

Computer-aided instruction (CAI): The application of computer technology to education. [17]

Computer architecture: The basic structure of a computer, including memory organization, a scheme for encoding data and instructions, and control mechanisms for performing computing operations. [4]

Computer-based bibliographic-retrieval system: A system composed of indexed online databases of bibliographic information and programs to search these databases to retrieve relevant information. [14]

Computer-based patient monitor: A patient-monitoring device that also supports other data functions, such as database maintenance, report generation, and decision making. [12]

Computer program: A set of instructions that tells a computer which mathematical and logical operations to perform. [4]

Computer system: An integrated arrangement of computer hardware and software, operated by users to perform prescribed tasks. [5]

Conditional independence: Two events, *A* and *B*, are conditionally independent if the occurrence of one does not influence the probability of the occurrence of the other, when both events are conditioned on a third event *C*. Thus, $p[A|B,C] = p[A|C]$ and $p[B|A,C] = p[B|C]$. The conditional probability of two conditionally independent events both occurring is the product of the individual conditional probabilities: $p[A,B|C] = p[A|C] \times p[B|C]$. For example, two tests for a disease are conditionally independentwhen the probability of the result of the second test does not depend on the result of the first test, given the disease state. For the case in which disease is present, p[second test positive | first test positive and disease present] $= p$[second test positive | first test negative and disease present] $= p$[second test positive | disease present]. More succinctly, the tests are conditionally independent if the sensitivity and specificity of one test do not depend on the result of the other test. (See independence.) [3]

Conditional probability: The probability of an event, contingent on the occurrence of another event. [3]

Consulting system: A computer-based system that develops and suggests problem-specific recommendations based on user input. (See critiquing system.) [15]

Contingency table: A 2 × 2 table that shows the relative frequencies of true-positive, true-negative, false-positive, and false-negative results. [3]

Continuity of care: The coordination of care received by a patient over time and across multiple health-care providers. [2,6]

Contrast radiography: A technique used to increase the contrast resolution of X-ray images by injection of radiopaque contrast material into a body cavity or blood vessels. [11]

Contrast resolution: A measure of the ability to distinguish among different levels of intensity (indicated in a digital image by the number of bits per pixel). [4,11]

Convolution: In image processing, a mathematical edge-enhancement technique used to sharpen blurred computed-tomographic images. [11]

Cooperative clinical trials: Research studies conducted by multiple institutions. Larger and broader patient populations can be studied in this way. [16]

Core memory: Random-access memory that can be accessed directly by the central processing unit. [4]

Cost–benefit analysis (CBA): An analysis of the costs and benefits associated with alternative courses of action that is designed to identify the alternative that yields the maximum net benefit. CBA is generally used when it is possible to assign dollar values to all relevant costs and benefits. [19]

Cost center: A department that does not have revenue associated with the services it provides (for example, administration, data processing, billing, and housekeeping). [19]

Cost-effectiveness analysis (CEA): An analysis of alternative courses of action, the objective of which is to identify either the alternative that yields the maximum effectiveness achievable for a given amount of spending, or the alternative that minimizes the cost of achieving a stipulated level of effectiveness. CEA is generally used when it is not possible to measure benefits in dollar units. [19]

Critiquing system: A computer-based system that evaluates and suggests modifications for plans or data analyses already formed by a user. (See consulting system.)[15]

Cross-validation: Verification of the accuracy of data by comparison of two sets of data collected by alternative means. [12]

Cursor: A blinking region of a display monitor, or a symbol such as an arrow, that indicates the currently active position on the screen. [4]

Custom-designed system: A computer system designed and developed within an institution to meet the special needs of that institution. [5]

Data bus: An electronic pathway for transferring data—for instance, between a CPU and memory. [4]

Data capture: The acquisition or recording of information. [6]

Data compression: A mathematical technique for reducing the number of bits needed to store data, with or without loss of information. [11]

Data independence: The insulation of applications programs from changes in data-storage structures and data-access strategies. [4]

Data overload: The inability to access crucial information due to the overwhelming number of irrelevant data, or due to the poor organization of data. [12]

Data transcription: The transfer of information from one data-recording system to another. Typically, the entry into a computer by clerical personnel of the handwritten or dictated notes or datasheets created by a health professional. [6]

Database: A collection of stored data—typically organized into fields, records, and files—and an associated description (schema). [2,4]

Database-management system (DBMS): An integrated set of programs that manages access to databases. [4]

Datum: Any single observation or fact. A medical datum generally can be regarded as the value of a specific parameter (for example, red-blood-cell count) for a particular object (for example, a patient) at a specific time. [2]

Debugger: A system program that provides traces, memory dumps, and other tools to assist programmers in locating and eliminating errors in their programs. [4]

Decision analysis: A methodology for making decisions by identifying alternatives and assessing them with regard to both the likelihood of possible outcomes and the costs and benefits of the outcomes. [15]

Decision node: A symbol that represents a choice among actions. By convention, a decision node is represented in a decision tree by a square. [3]

Decision tree: A diagrammatic representation of the outcomes associated with chance events and voluntary actions. [3]

Deductible: A set dollar amount of covered charges that must be paid by the insuree before the insurance company begins to reimburse for outlays. [19]

Degrees of freedom: The number of the independent variables that determine an observed, dependent value. [16]

Dependent variable: In a statistical analysis, the variable that measures experimental outcome. Its value is assumed to be a function of the experimental conditions (independent variables). [16]

Derived parameter: A parameter that is calculated indirectly from multiple parameters that are measured directly. [12]

Diagnosis-related group (DRG): One of 468 categories based on major diagnosis, length of stay, secondary diagnosis, surgical procedure, age, and types of services required. Used to determine the fixed payment per case that the Health Care Financing Administration will reimburse hospitals for providing care to Medicare patients. [19]

Differential diagnosis: The set of active hypotheses (possible diagnoses) that a physician develops when determining the source of a patient's problem. [2]

Digital image: An image that is stored as a grid of numbers, where each picture element (pixel) in the grid represents the intensity of a small area. [11]

Digital radiography: The process of producing X-ray images that are stored in digital form in computer memory, rather than on film. [11]

Digital radiology: The use of digital radiographic methods for medical imaging. [11]

Digital signal: A signal that takes on discrete values from a specified set of values. [4]

Digital subtraction angiography (DSA): A radiologic technique for imaging blood vessels in which a digital image acquired before injection of contrast material is subtracted pixel by pixel from an image acquired after injection. The resulting image shows only the differences in the two images, highlighting those areas where the contrast material has accumulated. [11]

Direct cost: A cost that can be directly assigned to the production of goods or services. For example, direct costs in the laboratory include the cost of the technician's salary, equipment, and supplies. [19]

Direct data entry: The entry of data into a computer system by the individual who personally made the observations or electronically from automated instruments. [6]

Display monitor: A device for presenting output to users through use of a screen. (See cathode-ray tube.)[4]

Distributed computer system: A collection of independent computers that share data, programs, and other resources. [7]

Drill and practice: An approach to teaching in which students are presented with a small amount of information, then are asked questions about the material, and thus receive immediate feedback to support the learning process. [17]

Drug formulary: An institution-specific or program-specific document that specifies which drugs are to be kept in the pharmacy's inventory and describes any restrictions on the use of these drugs. [10]

Drug-use control: The drug-related knowledge, ethical constraints, and procedures that guide health professionals in providing drug therapies safely and effectively. [10]

Economic cost: See opportunity cost. [19]

End-user searcher: In the context of bibliographic searching, a person who formulates his own search request and performs his own search of the literature, rather than using a search intermediary. [14]

Encounter form: See structured encounter form. [13]

Epidemiology: The study of the incidence, distribution, and causes of disease in a population. [1]

Expected value: The value that is expected on average for a specified chance event or decision. [3]

Expected-value decision making: A method for decision making in which the decision maker selects the option that will produce the best result on average (that is, the option that has the highest expected value). [3]

Experimental bias: A systematic difference in outcome between groups that is caused by a factor other than the intervention under study. [16]

Experimental science: Systematic study characterized by posing hypotheses, designing experiments, performing analyses, and interpreting results to validate or disprove hypotheses and to suggest new hypotheses for study. [1]

Expert system: A program that symbolically encodes concepts derived from experts in a field and uses that knowledge to provide the kind of problem analysis and advice that the expert might provide. [15]

Extended Binary Coded Decimal Interchange Code (EBCDIC): An 8-bit code for representing alphanumeric characters and other symbols. [4]

Extralaboratory cycle: The portion of the specimen-testing process that takes place outside the laboratory. Steps in this cycle include ordering of tests, collection and identification of specimens, and communication of test results to the ordering physicians. [9]

False-negative rate (FNR): The probability of a negative result, given that the condition under consideration is true—for example, the probability of a negative test result in a patient who has the disease under consideration. [3]

False-negative result (FN): A negative result when the condition under consideration is true—for example, a negative test result in a patient who has the disease under consideration. [3]

False-positive rate (FPR): The probability of a positive result, given that the condition under consideration is false—for example, the probability of a positive test result in a patient who does not have the disease under consideration. [3]

False-positive result (FP): A positive result when the condition under consideration is false—for example, a positive test result in a patient who does not have the disease under consideration. [3]

Feature classification: The categorization of segmented regions of an image based on the values of measured parameters, such as area and intensity. [11]

Feature detection: In image processing, determination of parameters, such as volume or length, from segmented regions of an image. In signal processing, identification of specific waveforms or other patterns of interest in a signal. [11,12]

Field: The smallest named unit of data in a database. Fields are grouped together to form records. [4]

File: In a database, a collection of similar records. [4]

File server: A computer that is dedicated to storing shared or private data files. [4]

Fixed cost: A cost that does not vary with the volume of production during a given period. Examples are expenses for plant, equipment, and administrative salaries. [19]

Flowsheet: A tabular summary of information that is arranged to display the values of variables as they change over time. [6]

Follow up: Long-term data collection to determine the long-term effects of the variables under study. [16]

Free text: Unstructured, uncoded representation of information in text format; for example, sentences describing the results of a patient's physical examination. [6]

Full-text database: A bibliographic database that contains the entire text of journal articles, books, and other literature, rather than only citations. [14]

Functional image: An image, such as a computed-tomographic image or a digital subtraction angiogram image, which is computed from derived quantities, rather than measured directly. [11]

Gatekeeper: A person who keeps abreast of current information in an area of expertise and who keeps colleagues informed of new developments. [14]

Gateway: A computer that resides on multiple networks and that can forward and translate message packets sent between nodes in networks running different protocols. [4]

Global image processing: Any image-enhancement technique in which the same computation is applied to every pixel in an image. [11]

Gold-standard test: The test or procedure whose result is used to determine the true state of the subject—for example, a pathology test used to determine a patient's true disease state. [3]

Gray scale: A scheme for representing intensity in a black-and-white image. Multiple bits per pixel are used to represent intermediate levels of gray. [4]

Hardware: The physical equipment of a computer system, including the central processing unit, data-storage devices, terminals, and printers. [4]

Health assessment: A survey examination of a presumably well person to evaluate health status, to identify health risks, and to detect abnormalities that may indicate undiagnosed disease. [19]

Health-assessment information system (HAIS): A computer system that supports the operation of a multiphasic health-testing program by maintaining computer-based medical records and facilitating operational tasks, such as appointment scheduling, patient recall, and patient registration. [18]

Health-assessment system (HAS): A systematic approach to providing health assessments to a patient population. [18]

Health Insurance Claim Form (HICF): A standard billing form accepted by many third-party payment programs. [13]

Health-maintenance organization (HMO): A group practice or affiliation of independent practitioners that contracts with patients to provide comprehensive health care for a fixed periodic payment specified in advance. [19]

Heuristic: A rule of thumb; a cognitive process used in learning or problem solving. [2,3,15]

High-level process: A complex process comprising multiple lower-level processes. [1]

Host system: In bibliographic-retrieval systems, the system on which the databases and search programs reside. [14]

Human-capital approach: An approach to valuing life or illness in which people are viewed as productive assets. The value of a life lost is measured by the present value of the person's remaining lifetime earnings, had he not died prematurely. The economic cost of illness, or the economic value of prevention, is measured by the sum of direct outlays for diagnosis and treatment of illness, and loss in productivity because of illness or premature death. [19]

Hypothetico-deductive approach: In clinical medicine, an iterative approach to diagnosis in which physicians perform sequential, staged data collection, data interpretation, and hypothesis generation to determine and refine a differential diagnosis. [2]

Icon: In a graphical interface, a pictorial representation of an object or function. [4]

Identified life: A named individual who is affected by the outcome of a policy or other decision. (See statistical life.)[19]

Imaging modality: A method for producing images. Examples of medical applications are X-ray imaging, computed tomography, echosonography, and magnetic resonance imaging. [11]

Indemnity insurance: A type of insurance modeled on casualty insurance. Typically, an insuree is reimbursed a specified amount for a hospital day, or for each of a list of surgical procedures. [19]

Independence: Two events, A and B, are considered independent if the occurrence of one does not influence the probability of the occurrence of the other. Thus, $p[A|B] = p[A]$. The probability of two independent events A and B both occurring is given by the product of the individual probabilities: $p[A,B] = p[A] \times p[B]$. (See conditional independence.) [3]

Independent-practice association (IPA): A type of health-maintenance organization in which physicians continue to practice on a fee-for-service basis in their own offices. Patient members pay premiums or dues directly to the provider organization in the form of a fixed periodic payment, set in advance, for comprehensive care. Physician members agree to fee schedules, management controls, and risk-sharing arrangements. [19]

Independent variable: A variable believed to affect the outcome (dependent variable) of an experiment. [16]

Index test: The diagnostic test whose performance is being measured. [3]

Indexing: In bibliographic retrieval, the assignment to each document of specific terms that indicate the subject matter of the document and that are used in searching. [14]

Indirect cost: A cost incurred in producing goods or services that cannot be attributed to a specific output. Examples in the laboratory include clerical supplies and the department manager's salary (also called *overhead*). [19]

Information: Organized data or knowledge that provide a basis for decision making. [2]

Information science: The field of study concerned with issues related to the management of both paper-based and electronically stored information. [1]

Information-synthesis database: An information base containing indexed summaries of current literature on particular topics that have been created by experts—essentially, an online review article. [14]

Information theory: The theory and mathematics underlying the processes of communication. [1]

Input: The data that represent state information, to be stored and processed to produce results (output). [5]

Intangible benefits and costs: Benefits and costs that cannot be translated into numbers, yet must be explicitly considered and weighed in an analysis. [19]

Intelligent terminal: A terminal that can perform limited processing to arrange and display data for input and output. [4]

Intensive-care unit (ICU): A hospital unit in which critically ill patients are monitored closely. [12]

Intermittent monitoring: The periodic measurement of a physiological parameter. [12]

Interpreter: A program that converts each statement in a high-level program to a machine-language representation, then executes the binary instruction(s). [4]

Interventional radiology: The use of needles, catheters, biopsy instruments, or other invasive methodologies with the aim of producing a diagnostic or therapeutic, or possibly palliative, effect. Examples are balloon angioplasty for coronary stenosis and cyst aspiration and drainage. [11]

Intralaboratory cycle: The portion of the specimen-testing process that takes place within the laboratory. Steps in this cycle include assignment of unique accessioning number to specimens, performance of tests, and preparation of reports of test results. [9]

Invasive monitoring: A method for measuring a physiological parameter that requires breaking the skin or otherwise entering the body. [12]

Ionizing radiation: X rays and other forms of radiation that penetrate cells, and, when sufficiently intense, inhibit cell division, thereby causing cell death. [11]

Joystick: A leverlike device (like the steering stick of an airplane) that a user moves to control the position of a cursor on a screen. [4]

Kardex: A patient-care control document; for example, a nurse's Kardex contains physicians' orders and nursing care plans for each client. [8]

Keyboard: A data-input device used to enter alphanumeric characters through typing. [4]

Key field: A field in the record of a file that uniquely identifies the record within the file. [4]

Knowledge: Relationships, facts, assumptions, heuristics, and models derived through the formal or informal analysis (or interpretation) of data. [2]

Knowledge base: A collection of stored facts, heuristics, and models that can be used for problem solving. [2]

Laboratory information system (LIS): A computer-based information system that supports laboratory functions for collecting, verifying, and reporting test results. [9]

Light pen: A penlike photosensitive device with which a user can select and enter data by pointing at the screen of a video display terminal. [4]

Likelihood ratio (LR): A measure of the discriminatory power of a test. The LR is the ratio of the probability of a result when the condition under consideration is true to the probability of a result when the condition under consideration is false (for example, the probability of a result in a diseased patient to the probability of a result in a nondiseased patient). The LR for a positive test is the ratio of true-positive rate (TPR) to false-positive rate (FPR). [3]

Local-area network (LAN): A network for data communication that connects multiple nodes—all typically owned by a single institution and located within a small geographic area. [4]

Long-run cost: The cost of producing a good or service once the producer has employed the most economical mix and proportion of input resources (plant, equipment, labor, supplies, and so on). (See short-run cost.)[19]

Low-level process: An elementary process that has its basis in the physical world of chemistry or physics. [1]

Lump-sum bill: A single, unitemized bill; for example, a bill for all drugs received by a patient during a hospital admission. [6]

Machine language: The set of primitive computer instructions represented in binary code. [4]

Magnetic disk: A round, flat plate of material that can accept and store magnetic charge. Data are encoded on magnetic disk as sequences of charges on concentric tracks. [4]

Magnetic resonance imaging (MRI): A modality that produces images by evaluating the differential response of atomic nuclei in the body when the patient is placed in an intense magnetic field. [11]

Magnetic tape: A long ribbon of material that can accept and store magnetic charge. Data are encoded on magnetic tape as sequences of charges along longitudinal tracks. [4]

Mainframe computer: A large, multiuser computer, typically operated and maintained by professional computing personnel. [4]

Major medical insurance: Comprehensive insurance for medical expenses. Typically, the insurer pays a certain percentage of covered charges once the insuree has satisfied the deductible. [19]

Marginal cost: The increase in total cost associated with the production of one more unit of a good or service. [19]

Medical computer science: The subdivision of computer science that applies the methods of computing to medical topics. [1]

Medical-history form: A paper form used to record information about a patient's family history, social history, and past medical events. [13]

Medical image generation: The production of images of the body's structure and functions. [11]

Medical informatics: A field of study concerned with the broad range of issues in the management and use of biomedical information, including medical computing and the study of the nature of medical information itself. [1]

Medical information bus (MIB): A data-communication system that supports data acquisition from a variety of independent devices. [12]

Medical information science: The field of study concerned with issues related to the management and use of biomedical information. (See medical informatics.) [1]

Medical subject heading (MeSH): One of some 15,000 medical terms used to identify the subject content of the medical literature. The National Library of Medicine's MeSH vocabulary has emerged as the de facto standard for biomedical indexing. [14]

Medication profile: A record of a patient's past and current drug orders, including type of drug, dose amount, dosing frequency, and route of administration. [10]

Memory: Areas that are used to store programs and data. The computer's working memory comprises read-only memory (ROM) and random-access memory (RAM). [4]

Menu: In a user interface, a displayed list of valid commands or options from which a user may choose. [4]

Microcomputer: A small, single-user computer. [4]

Minicomputer: A multiuser computer of moderate size. [4]

Mixed-initiative system: An educational program in which user and program share control of the interaction. Usually, the program guides the interaction, but the student can assume control, and can digress when new questions arise during a study session. [17]

Modem: A device used to modulate and demodulate digital signals for transmission to a remote computer over telephone lines; a modem converts digital data to audible analog signals, and analog signals to digital data. [4]

Modular computer system: A system composed of separate units, each of which performs a specific set of functions. [7]

Mouse (input device): A small boxlike device that is moved on a flat surface to position a cursor on the screen of a display monitor. A user can select and mark data for entry by depressing buttons on the mouse. [4]

Multiphasic health-testing program: A system for providing health assessments to a patient population. Patients visit a series of stations, each of which is set up to collect medical-history information, to perform selected tests and procedures, or to conduct physical examinations. [18]

Multiprocessing: The use of multiple processors in a single computer system to increase the power of the system. (See parallel processing.) [4]

Multiprogramming: A scheme by which multiple programs simultaneously reside in the main memory of a single central processing unit. [4]

Mutually exclusive: A state in which one, and only one, of the possible conditions is true; for example, either A or not A is true, and one of the statements is false. When using Bayes' theorem to perform medical diagnosis, we generally assume that diseases are mutually exclusive, meaning that the patient has exactly one of the diseases under consideration. [3]

Negative predictive value (PV−): The probability that the condition of interest is false if the result is negative—for example, the probability that the disease is absent given a negative test result. [3]

Net present value (NPV): The difference between the present value of benefits and the present value of costs. (See present value.) [19]

Network node: One of the interconnected computers or devices linked in a communications network. [4]

Network protocol: The set of rules or conventions that specifies how data are prepared and transmitted and that governs data communication among the nodes of a network. [4]

Network topology: The configuration of the physical connections among the nodes of a computer communication network. [4]

Ninth International Classification of Diseases–Clinical Modification (ICD-9-CM): A coding system for medical diagnoses, symptoms, and nonspecific complaints. It is frequently used on insurance claim forms to identify the reasons for providing medical services. [13]

Noise: The component of acquired data that is attributable to factors other than the underlying phenomenon being measured (for example, electromagnetic interference, inaccuracy in sensors, or poor contact between sensor and source). [4]

Nomenclature: A system of terms used in a scientific discipline to denote classifications and relationships among objects and processes. [2]

Noninvasive monitoring: A method for measuring a physiological parameter that does not require breaking the skin or otherwise entering the body. [12]

Nonionizing radiation: Radiation that does not cause damage to cells; for example, the sound waves used in echosonography. (See ionizing radiation.) [11]

Nonquantifiable benefits and costs: See intangible benefits and costs. [19]

Nonquantifiable benefits and costs: See intangible benefits and costs. [19]

Nuclear-medicine imaging: A modality for producing images by measuring the radiation emitted by a radioactive isotope that has been attached to a biologically active compound and injected into the body. [11]

Nursing care plan: A proposed series of nursing interventions based on nursing assessments and nursing diagnoses. It identifies nursing care problems, states specific actions to address the problems, specifies the actions taken, and includes an evaluation of a client's response to care. [8]

Nursing information system (NIS): A computer-based information system that supports nurses' professional duties in clinical practice, nursing administration, nursing research, and education. [8]

Nursing intervention: Any of a variety of interactions between nurse and client, including physical care, emotional support, and client education. [8]

Nyquist frequency: The minimum sampling rate necessary to achieve reasonable signal quality. In general, it is twice the frequency of the highest-frequency component of interest in a signal. [4]

Odds: An expression of the probability of the occurrence of an event relative to the probability that it will not occur [3]:

$$\text{Odds} = \frac{p[\text{event}]}{1 - p[\text{event}]}$$

Odds-likelihood form: See odds-ratio form. [3]

Odds-ratio form: An algebraic expression for calculating posttest odds of a disease or other condition of interest if the pretest odds and likelihood ratio are known (an alternative formulation of Bayes' theorem, also called the *odds-likelihood form*). [3]

Offline device: A device that operates independently of the processor—for example, a card-to-tape converter. [4]

Online bibliographic searching: The use of computers to search electronically stored databases of indexed literature references. [14]

Online device: A device that is under the direct control of the processor; for example, a magnetic-disk drive. [4]

Open-loop control: A computer system that assists in regulation of a physiological variable, such as blood pressure, by monitoring the value of the variable and reporting measured values or therapy recommendations. Health-care personnel retain responsibility for therapeutic interventions. (See closed-loop control device.) [12]

Operating system: A program that allocates computer hardware resources to user programs and that supervises and controls the execution of all other programs. [4]

Opportunity cost: When resources are utilized, the value of the alternatives foregone that might have been produced with those resources (also called the *economic cost*). [19]

Optical disc: A round, flat plate of plastic or metal that is used to store information. Data are encoded through the use of a laser that marks the surface of the disc. [4]

Order entry: In a hospital information system, online entry of orders for drugs, laboratory tests, and procedures, usually performed by nurses or physicians. [7]

Outcome measure: A parameter for evaluating the success of a system; the parameter reflects the top-level goals of the system. [5]

Output: The results produced when a process is applied to input. Some forms of output are hardcopy documents, images displayed on video display terminals, and calculated values of variables. [4,5]

Overhead: See indirect cost. [19]

Parallel processing: The use of multiple processing units running in parallel to solve a single problem. (See multiprocessing.)[4]

Pathognomonic: Distinctively characteristic, and thus uniquely identifying, of a condition or object (100-percent specific). [2]

Patient monitor: An instrument that collects and displays physiological data, often for the purpose of watching for and warning against life-threatening changes in physiological state. [12]

Patient monitoring: Repeated or continuous measurement of physiological parameters for the purpose of guiding therapeutic management. [12]

Pattern recognition: The process of organizing visual, auditory, or other data and identifying meaningful motifs. [11,12]

Per capita payment: See capitation. [19]

Personal computer (PC): A small, relatively inexpensive, single-user computer. [4]

Phantom: In image processing, an object of known shape, used to calibrate imaging machines. The reconstructed image is compared to the object's known shape. [11]

Pharmacokinetic parameters: The drug-specific and patient-specific parameters that determine the mathematical models used to forecast drug concentrations as a function of drug regimen. [10]

Pharmacokinetics: The study of the routes and mechanisms of drug disposition over time, from initial introduction into the body, through distribution in body tissues, biotransformation, and ultimate elimination. [1,10]

Pharmacology: The study of the properties, uses, and actions of drugs. [10]

Pharmacy information system: A computer-based information system that supports pharmacy personnel. [10]

Phased installation: The incremental introduction of a system into an institution. [5]

Picture-archiving and communication system (PACS): An integrated computer system that acquires, stores, retrieves, and displays digital images. [11]

Pixel: One of the small picture elements that makes up a digital image. The number of pixels per square inch determines the spatial resolution. Pixels can be associated with a single bit to indicate black and white or with multiple bits to indicate color or gray scale. [4,11]

Point-of-care system: A hospital information system that includes bedside terminals or other devices for capturing and entering data at the locations where patients receive care. [7]

Positive predictive value (PV+): The probability that the condition of interest is true if the result is positive—for example, the probability that the disease is present given a positive test result. [3]

Posterior probability: The updated probability that the condition of interest is present after additional information has been acquired. [3]

Posttest probability: The updated probability that the disease or other condition under consideration is present after the test result is known (more generally, the *posterior probability*). [3]

Precision: The degree of accuracy with which the value of a sampled observation matches the value of the underlying condition, or the exactness with which an operation is performed. In bibliographic searching, a measure of a system's performance in retrieving relevant information (expressed as the ratio of relevant records to irrelevant records retrieved in a search). [4,14]

Predictive value: The posttest probability that a condition is present based on the results of a test. (See positive predictive value and negative predictive value.) [2]

Preferred-provider organization (PPO): A method of health-care financing based on selective contracting in advance for the services of health-care providers. A PPO typically is composed of a panel of providers, a negotiated fee schedule that providers agree to accept as payment in full for their services, a mechanism for utilization control, and incentives for consumers to select providers from the panel, usually in the form of reduced coinsurance. [19]

Prepaid group practice: An affiliation of health-care providers that agrees to provide comprehensive health care to members for a fixed annual fee set in advance. [19]

Present value (PV): The current value of a payment or stream of payments to be received in the future. The concept of present value generally reflects the fact that $1 received 1 year from now is not worth as much as $1 received today, because the money is not available to earn interest over the course of 1 year. [19]

Pressure transducer: A device that produces electrical signals proportional in magnitude to the level of a pressure reading. [12]

Pretest probability: The probability that the disease or other condition under consideration is present before the test result is known (more generally, the *prior probability*). [3]

Prevalence: The frequency of the condition under consideration in the population. For example, we calculate the prevalence of disease by dividing the number of diseased individuals by the number of individuals in the population. Prevalence is the prior probability of a specific condition (or diagnosis), before any other information is available. [2,3]

Primary care: The level of care normally provided by a personal physician or walk-in clinic. [7]

Prior probability: The probability that the condition of interest is present before additional information has been acquired. In a population, the prior probability also is called *prevalence.* [3]

Private branch exchange (PBX): A telephone switching center. PBXs can be extended to provide a local-area network in which digital data are converted to analog signals and are transmitted over an existing telephone system. [4]

Probability: Informally, a means of expressing belief in the likelihood of an event. Probability is more precisely defined mathematically in terms of its essential properties. See any introductory statistics textbook for details. [3]

Problem-oriented medical record: A clinical record in which the data collected, the physician's assessment, and the proposed therapeutic plans are grouped by association with the patient's specific medical problems. [6]

Process measure: A parameter for evaluating the success of a system; the parameter measures a byproduct of the system's function. [5]

Production rule: A conditional statement that relates premise conditions to associated actions or inferences. [15]

Professional Standards Review Organization (PSRO): A physicians' organization created to review use of Medicare and Medicaid services and to deny payment for unnecessary services. [19]

Prospective payment: A method of health-care reimbursement in which providers receive a set payment specified in advance for providing a global unit of care, such as a hospitalization for a specified illness or a hospital day. [19]

Prospective-payment system (PPS): A scheme for health-care financing enacted by Congress in 1983, in which hospitals receive from Medicare a fixed payment per hospital admission, adjusted for diagnosis-related group. [19]

Prospective study: An experiment in which researchers, before collecting data for analysis, define study questions and hypotheses, the study population, and data to be collected. [2,16]

Prosthesis: A device that replaces a body part—for example, an artificial hip or heart. [1]

Prototype system: A working model of a planned system that demonstrates essential features of the operation and interface. [5]

Proximity searching: A technique used with full-text databases that retrieves documents containing the specified words when they are adjacent in the text, or when they occur within a certain number of words of each other. [14]

Quality-adjusted life-year (QALY): A measure of the value of a health outcome that reflects both longevity and morbidity; it is the expected length of life in years, adjusted to account for diminished quality of life due to physical or mental disability, to pain, and so on. [3]

Quality assurance (QA): A means for monitoring and maintaining the goodness of a service, product, or process. [7]

Quality control (QC): See quality assurance. [9]

Query: In a database system, a request for specific information that is stored in the computer. [6]

Queue: In a computer system, an ordered set of jobs waiting to be executed. [4]

Radiography: The process of making images by projecting X rays through the patient onto X-ray–sensitive film. [11]

Radiology information system (RIS): A computer-based information system that supports radiology department operations; includes management of the film library, scheduling of patient examinations, reporting of results, and billing. [11]

Random-access memory (RAM): The portion of a computer's working memory that can be both read and written into. It is used to store the results of intermediate computation, and the programs and data that are currently in use (also called *variable memory* or *core memory*). [4]

Randomization: A research technique for assigning subjects to study groups without a specific pattern. The approach is designed to minimize experimental bias. [16]

Randomized clinical trial (RCT): A prospective experiment in which subjects are randomly assigned to study subgroups to compare the effects of alternate treatments. [2,16]

Raster-scan display: A pattern of closely spaced rows of dots that forms an image on the cathode-ray tube of a video display monitor. [4]

Read-only memory (ROM): The portion of a computer's working memory that can be read, but cannot be written into. [4]

Real-time data acquisition: The continuous measurement and recording of electronic signals through a direct connection with the signal source. [4]

Recall: In information retrieval, the ability of a system to retrieve relevant information (expressed as the ratio of relevant records retrieved to all relevant records in the database). [14]

Receiver operating characteristic (ROC) curve: A curve that depicts the tradeoff between the sensitivity and specificity of a test. [3]

Record: In a data file, a group of data fields that collectively represent information about a single entity. [4]

Register: In a computer, a group of electronic switches used to store and manipulate data. [4]

Remote access: Access to a system or to information therein, typically by telephone or communications network, by a user who is physically removed from the system. [6]

Representativeness: A heuristic by which a person judges the probability that a condition is true based on the degree of similarity between the current situation and the stereotypical situation in which the condition is true. For example, a physician might estimate the probability that a patient has a particular disease based on the degree to which the patient's symptoms match the classic disease profile. [3]

Requirements analysis: An initial analysis performed to define a problem clearly and to specify the nature of the proposed solution (for example, the functions of a proposed system). [5]

Research protocol: In clinical research, a prescribed plan for managing subjects that describes what actions to take under specific conditions. [2]

Results reporting: In a hospital information system, online access to the results of laboratory tests and other procedures. [7]

Retrospective chart review: Extraction and analysis of data from medical records to investigate a question that was not a subject of study at the time the data were collected. [2,16]

Retrospective payment: A method of health-care financing in which providers are reimbursed based on charges for the services delivered. [19]

Retrospective study: An analysis of existing sets of data to answer experimental questions. [16]

Revenue center: In a health-care institution, a department that charges patients directly for the services provided. (See cost center.) [19]

Review of systems: The component of a typical history and physical examination in which the physician asks general questions about each of the body's major organ systems to discover problems. [2]

RS-232-C: A commonly used standard for serial data communication that defines the number and type of the wire connections, the voltage, and the characteristics of the signal, and thus allows data communication among electronic devices produced by different manufacturers. [4]

Sample attrition rate: The proportion of the sample population that drops out before the study is complete. [16]

Sampling rate: The rate at which the continuously varying values of an analog signal are measured and recorded. [4]

Schema: In a database-management system, a machine-readable definition of the contents and organization of a database. [4]

Search intermediary: In bibliographic searching, a specially trained information specialist who interprets users' requests for information, formulates search requests in terms of the commands and vocabulary of the search systems, and carries out the search. [14]

Secondary care: The level of care normally provided by a hospital. [7]

Segmentation: In image processing, the extraction of selected regions of interest from an image using automated or manual techniques. [11]

Selection bias: An error in the estimates of disease prevalence and other population parameters that results when the criteria for admission to a study produces systematic differences between the study population and the clinically relevant population. [3,16]

Semantics: The meanings assigned to symbols and sets of symbols in a language. [4]

Sensitivity (of a test): The probability of a positive result, given that the condition under consideration is true—for example, the probability of a positive test result in a person who has the disease under consideration (also called the *true-positive rate*). [2,3]

Sensitivity analysis: A technique for testing the robustness of a decision analysis by repeating the analysis with a range of probability and utility estimates. [3]

Sensitivity calculation: An analysis to determine which parameters, scenarios, and uncertainties affect a decision, and what the degree of that effect is. [19]

Service bureau: A data-processing business that produces bills, third-party invoices, and financial reports for medical practices from information recorded on encounter forms. [13]

Short-run cost: The cost of producing a good or service when the levels of some inputs (for example, plant and equipment) remain fixed. (See long-run cost.)[19]

Signal artifact: A false feature of the measured signal caused by noise or other interference. [12]

Simulation: A system that behaves according to a model of a process or another system; for example, simulation of a patient's response to therapeutic interventions allows a student to learn which techniques are effective without risking human life. [17]

Simultaneous access: Access to shared computer-stored information by multiple concurrent users. [6]

Software engineering: The discipline concerned with organizing and managing the software-development process (the process of creating computer programs and documentation) to facilitate production of high-quality systems in a timely and cost-effective manner. [5]

Spatial resolution: A measure of the ability to distinguish among points that are close to each other (indicated in a digital image by the number of pixels per square inch). [4,11]

Specificity (of a test): The probability of a negative result, given that the condition under consideration is false—for example, the probability of a negative test result in a person who does not have the disease under consideration (also called the *true-negative rate*). [2,3]

Spectrum bias: Systematic error in the estimate of a study parameter that results when the study population includes only selected subgroups of the clinically relevant population—for example, the systematic error in the estimates of sensitivity and specificity that results when test performance is measured in a study population consisting of only healthy volunteers and patients with advanced disease. [3]

Spirometry: Evaluation of the air capacity and physiologic function of the lungs. [6]

Staged evaluation: Incremental evaluation of a system, in which different criteria for success are applied at successive stages of development. [5]

Statistical error: In a model relating x to y, the portion of the variance in the dependent variable that cannot be explained by variance in the independent variables. [16]

Statistical life: An anonymous individual, such as a person affected by a policy that saves "one life in a thousand." (See identified life.) [19]

Statistical package: A collection of programs that implement statistical procedures. It is used to analyze data and report results. [16]

Structured encounter form: A form for collecting and recording specific information during a patient visit. [6,13]

Structured programming: The composition of computer programs using only sequences of statements and formal constructs for iteration (*do while*) and selection (*if . . . then . . . else*); implies modularity, absence of *go to* statements, and the use of stylistic conventions, such as indentation and the use of meaningful variable and subroutine names. [5]

Study population: The population of subjects—usually a subset of the clinically relevant population—in whom experimental outcomes (for example, the performance of a diagnostic test) are measured. [3]

Study protocol: A prescribed plan for managing experimental subjects that describes what actions to take under what conditions. [16]

Superbill: An itemized bill that summarizes the financial transactions occurring during a patient–physician encounter, including specification of the type of visit and a listing of the procedures performed and drugs administered; also, a checklist form for generating such a bill. [6,13]

Surveillance: In a computer-based medical-record system, systematic review of patients' clinical data to detect and flag conditions that merit attention. [6]

Syntax: The rules that specify the legal symbols and constructs of a language. [4]

System: A set of integrated entities that operates as a whole to accomplish a prescribed task. [5]

System programs: The operating system, compilers, and other software that are included with a computer system and that allow users to operate the hardware. [4]

System-review form: A paper form used during a physical examination to record findings related to each of the body's major systems. [13]

Temporal resolution: The time between acquisition of each of a series of images. Limited by the time needed to produce each image. [11]

Terminal interface processor (TIP): A utility communications computer that is used to attach video display terminals and other communications devices to a local-area network. [7]

Tertiary care: The level of care normally provided by a specialized medical center. [7]

Test-interpretation bias: Systematic error in the estimates of sensitivity and specificity that results when the index and gold-standard test are not interpreted independently. [3]

Test-referral bias: Systematic error in the estimates of sensitivity and specificity that results when subjects with a positive index test are more likely to receive the gold-standard test. [3]

Text editor: A program used to create files of character strings, such as other computer programs and documents. [4]

Text-word searching: In a bibliographic database, retrieval of relevant articles based on the words that appear in titles and abstracts, rather than the index terms that have been assigned to each entry. [14]

Time-sharing mode: An interactive mode for communicating with a computer in which the operating system switches rapidly among all the jobs that require CPU services. (See batch mode.) [4]

Touch screen: A display screen that allows users to select items by touching the corresponding areas on the screen. [4]

Transducer: A device that produces electrical signals proportional in magnitude to the level of a measured parameter, such as blood pressure. [1,12]

Treatment-threshold probability: The probability of disease at which the expected values of withholding or giving treatment are equal. Above the threshold, treatment is recommended; below the threshold, treatment is not recommended, and further testing may be warranted. [3]

True-negative rate (TNR): The probability of a negative result, given that the condition under consideration is false—for example, the probability of a negative test result in a patient who does not have the disease under consideration (also called *specificity*). [3]

True-negative result (TN): A negative result when the condition under consideration is false—for example, a negative test result in a patient who does not have the disease under consideration. [3]

True-positive rate (TPR): The probability of a positive result, given that the condition under consideration is true—for example, the probability of a positive test result in a patient who has the disease under consideration (also called *sensitivity*). [3]

True-positive result (TP): A positive result when the condition under consideration is true—for example, a positive test result in a patient who has the disease under consideration. [3]

Turnaround document: A form that serves first as a summary form for presenting results and, subsequently, as a data-collection form. [6]

Turnkey system: A computer system that is purchased from a vendor and that can be installed and operated with minimal modification. [5]

Ultrasound imaging: The production of images by transmission of sound waves through the body and analysis of the returning echos. [11]

Unit-dose dispensing: An approach to the distribution of drugs, whereby patients' drugs are packaged on a unit-of-dose basis to reduce wastage and to control drug use. [10]

Usual, customary, and reasonable fee: The typical fee used as the basis for billed charges and retrospective cost reimbursement. [19]

Utility: A number that represents the value of a specific outcome to a decision maker. (See, for example, quality-adjusted life-year.) [3]

Utilization review: In a hospital, inspection of patients' medical records to identify cases of inappropriate care, including excessive or insufficient use of resources. [7]

Validation: Verification of correctness. [6]

Validity check: In a database system or computer-based medical-record system, a test (such as a range check or a pattern check) that is used to detect invalid data values. [6]

Variable cost: A cost that changes with the volume of goods or services produced during a given period. [19]

Variable memory: See random-access memory. [4]

Vendor system: A host computer owned by a third party that provides users with access to multiple databases or other services. [14]

Video display terminal (VDT): An input–output device that is used for communication with a remote computer and that has a cathode-ray–tube display for viewing output and a keyboard for entering data. [4]

View: In a database-management system, a logical submodel of the contents and structure of a database used to support one or a subset of applications. [4]

Virtual memory: A scheme by which users can access information stored in auxiliary memory as though that information were in main memory. Virtual-memory addresses are translated into actual addresses automatically by the hardware. [4]

Vital signs: A person's core temperature, pulse rate, respiratory rate, and arterial blood pressure. [12]

von Neumann machine: A computer architecture that comprises a single processing unit, computer memory, and a memory bus. [4]

Voxel: A volume element, or small cubic area of a three-dimensional digital image. (See pixel.) [11]

Waveform template: A wave pattern that is stored in a computer and compared to collected waveforms, such as those acquired from patients. It is used to identify and classify abnormal wave patterns. [12]

Weak model: A model of relation in which the independent variables are insufficient to predict the outcome (dependent variable). [16]

Wide-area network: A network that connects computers owned by independent institutions and distributed over long distances. [4]

Willingness to pay: An approach to valuing human life based on the values implied by the choices people make every day to change their probabilities of living or dying. For example, a person's implicit valuation of life could be calculated based on how much she is willing to pay for a car airbag that will reduce her chance of death by a specified incremental amount. [19]

Word: In computer memory, a sequence of bits that can be accessed as a unit. [4]

Workstation: A powerful desktop computer system designed to support a single user. Workstations provide specialized hardware and software to facilitate the problem-solving and information-processing tasks of professionals in the latters' domains of expertise. [4]

Write-it-once system: A type of paper-based billing system that uses carbon paper or photocopying to generate bills from patient-encounter information that has been transcribed onto ledger cards. [13]

References

Abdulla, A., Watkins, L., and Henke, J. (1984). The use of natural language entry and laser videodisk technology in CAI. *Journal of Medical Education*, 59:739.

Abraham, I. (1986). Diagnostic discrepancy and clinical inference: A social-cognitive analysis. *Genetic, Social, and General Psychology Monographs*, 112:43–102.

Abraham, I., et al. (1984a). A multivariate mathematical algorithm for diagnostic information systems: I. Data-acquisition and storage procedures. In *Proceedings of the European Federation for Medical Informatics*, Berlin. Springer.

Abraham, I., et al. (1984b). A multivariate mathematical algorithm for diagnostic information systems: II. Procedures for clinical inference. In Cohen, G. (ed), *Proceedings of the Eighth Annual Symposium for Computer Applications in Medical Care*, Silver Spring, MD. IEEE.

Adams, I., Chan, M., Clifford, P., et al. (1986). Computer-aided diagnosis of acute abdominal pain: A multicentre study. *British Medical Journal*, 293:800–804.

Aikins, J., Kunz, J., Shortliffe, E., et al. (1983). PUFF: An expert system for interpretation of pulmonary function data. *Computers and Biomedical Research*, 16:199–208.

American College of Pathologists (1982). *SNOMED*. Skokie, IL: College of American Pathology.

American Nurses' Association (1980). *Nursing: A Social Policy Statement*. Kansas City, MO: American Nurses' Association.

American Society for Testing and Materials (1988). *ASTM E 1238-88, Standard Specification for Transferring Clinical Laboratory Data Messages Between Independent Computer Systems.* Philadelphia, PA: ASTM.

Anbar, M. (ed) (1987). *Computers in Medicine.* Rockville, MD: Computer Science Press.

Anderson, J. and Jay, S. (1983). Utilization of computers in clinical practice—the role of physician networks: Preliminary communication. *Journal of the Royal Society of Medicine,* 76:45–52.

Andrews, R., et al. (1985). Computer charting: An evaluation of a respiratory care computer system. *Respiratory Care,* 30:695.

Arenson, R. (1984). Automation of the radiology management function. *Radiology,* 153:65.

Arenson, R., et al. (1982). The formation of a radiology computer consortium. In Bauman, R. (ed), *Proceedings of the 7th Conference on Computer Applications in Radiology,* Boston. American College of Radiology.

Arenson, R., et al. (1988). Clinical evaluation of a medical image management system for chest images. *American Journal of Roentgenology,* 150:55.

Association of American Medical Colleges (1984). Physicians for the twenty-first century (Report of the Project Panel on the General Professional Education of the Physician and College Preparation for Medicine). *Journal of Medical Education,* 59(11):(Part 2)1–208.

Association of American Medical Colleges (1986). *Medical Education in the Information Age* (Proceedings of a symposium on medical informatics). Washington, D.C.: AAMC.

Ayers, S., et al. (1983). NIH consensus conference: Critical care medicine. *Journal of the American Medical Association,* 250:798.

Bailey, J., McDonald, F., and Claus, K. (1972). *An Experiment in Nursing Curriculum at a University.* Belmont, CA: Wadsworth.

Banaham, B. (1987). Computer use by Mississippi pharmacies. *Bulletin of the Bureau of Pharmaceutical Services,* 23:6.

Barnes, D. (1986). Promising results halt trial of anti-AIDS drug. *Science,* 234:15.

Barnett, G. (1984). The application of computer-based medical-record systems in ambulatory practice. *New England Journal of Medicine,* 310:1643.

Barnett, G., Cimino, J., Hupp, J., et al. (1987). DXplain: An experimental diagnostic decision-support system. *Journal of the American Medical Association,* 257:67.

Barnett, G., et al. (1979). COSTAR—A computer-based medical information system for ambulatory care. *Proceedings of the IEEE,* 67:1226.

Barrett, J., Hersch, P., and Caswell, R. (1979). *Evaluation of the Impact of the Implementation of the Technicon Medical Information System at El Camino Hospital, Part II: Economic Trend Analysis.* Columbus, OH: Battelle Columbus Laboratories. NTIS report number PB 300 869.

Bates, B. and Yellin, J. (1972). The yield of multiphasic screening. *Journal of the American Medical Association,* 222:74.

Bauman, R., Arenson, R., and Barnett, G. (1975a). Computer-based master folder tracking and automated file room operations. In *Proceedings of the Fourth Conference on Computer Applications in Radiology,* Las Vegas, NV. American College of Radiology.

Bauman, R., Arenson, R., and Barnett, G. (1975b). Fully automated scheduling of radiology appointments. In *Proceedings of the Fourth Conference on Computer Applications in Radiology,* Las Vegas, NV. American College of Radiology.

Bauman, R., et al. (1972). Further development of an on-line computer system for radiology reporting. In Lodwick, G. (ed), *Proceedings of the Conference on Computer Applications in Radiology,* Washington, D.C. U.S. Government Printing Office. DHEW publication number (FDA) 73-8018.

Benson, D., et al. (1986). Developing tools for online medical reference works. In Salamon, R., Blum, B., and Jørgensen, M. (eds), *MEDINFO 86.* Amsterdam: Elsevier North-Holland.

Berenson, R. (1984). *Health Technology Case Study 28: Intensive Care Units (ICUs)—Clinical Outcomes, Costs and Decisionmaking.* Washington, D.C.: Office of Technology Assessment.

Bergeron, B. and Greenes, R. (1989). Clinical skill-building simulations in cardiology: HeartLab and EKGLab. In Kingsland III, L. (ed), *Computer Methods and Programs in Biomedicine,* Special Issue SCAMC Student Paper Competition 1987-1988, 30:111.

Bernstein, L., Siegel, E., and Goldstein, C. (1980). The Hepatitis Knowledge Base: A prototype information transfer system. *Annals of Internal Medicine,* 93:169.

Bernstein, L. and Williamson, R. (1984). Testing of a natural language retrieval system for a full text knowledge base. *Journal of the American Society for Information Science,* 35:235.

Bitzer, M. and Boudreaux, M. (1969). Using a computer to teach nursing. *Nursing Forum,* 8:234.

Blaine, G., et al. (1983). PACS workbench at Mallinckrodt Institute of Radiology (MIR). In Dwyer, S. (ed), *Proceedings of SPIE Vol. 418 (PACS II),* Kansas City, MO. IEEE Computer Society.

Bleich, H. (1972). Computer-based consultation: Electrolyte and acid–base disorders. *American Journal of Medicine,* 53:285-291.

Bleich, H., et al. (1985). Clinical computing in a teaching hospital. *New England Journal of Medicine,* 312:756.

Blois, M. (1984). *Information and Medicine: The Nature of Medical Descriptions.* Berkeley and Los Angeles: University of California Press.

Blois, M., Tuttle, M., and Sherertz, D. (1981). RECONSIDER: A program for generating differential diagnoses. In *Proceedings of the Fifth Annual Symposium on Computer Applications in Medical Care,* Washington, D.C. IEEE Computer Society Press.

Blum, B. (1986a). *Clinical Information Systems.* New York: Springer-Verlag.

Blum, B. (1986b). Clinical information systems: A review. *Western Journal of Medicine,* 145:791.

Bradshaw, K., et al. (1984). Physician decision-making: Evaluation of data used in a computerized ICU. *International Journal of Clinical Monitoring and Computing,* 1:81.

Bradshaw, K., et al. (1988). Improving efficiency and quality in a computerized ICU. In Greenes, R. (ed), *Proceedings of the Twelfth Annual Symposium on Computer Applications in Medical Care,* Washington, D.C. IEEE.

Braunwald, E., et al. (eds) (1987). *Harrison's Principles of Internal Medicine.* 11th ed. New York: McGraw-Hill.

Breslow, L. (1978). Prospects for improving health through reducing risk factors. *Preventive Medicine,* 7:449.

Brimm, J. (1987). Computers in critical care. *Critical Care Nursing Quarterly,* 9(4):53.

Brinkley, J. (1985). Knowledge-driven ultrasonic three-dimensional organ modelling. *IEEE Transactions on Pattern Analysis and Machine Intelligence,* PAMI-7(4):431.

Brinkley, J., et al. (1982). Fetal weight estimation from ultrasonic three-dimensional head and trunk reconstructions: Evaluation in vitro. *American Journal of Obstetrics and Gynecology,* 144:715.

Brodie, D. (1966). *The Challenge to Pharmacy in Times of Change.* Washington, D.C.: American Society of Hospital Pharmacists.

Bronzino, J. (1982). *Computer Applications for Patient Care.* Menlo Park, CA: Addison-Wesley.

Brown, T. and Smith, M. (1986). *Handbook of Institutional Pharmacy Practice.* 2nd ed. Baltimore, MD: Williams & Wilkins.

Brown, V., Mason, W., and Kalzmarski, M. (1971). A computerized health information service. *Nursing Outlook,* 19:158.

Burke, D., Brundage, J., Redfield, R., et al. (1988). Measurement of the false positive rate in a screening program for human immunodeficiency virus infections. *New England Journal of Medicine,* 319:961–964.

Burton, M., Cobb, R., and Fink, J. (1986). Use of computers in community pharmacies in Kentucky. University of Kentucky School of Pharmacy. Unpublished manuscript.

California Medical Association (CMA) (1969). *1969 California Relative Value Studies.* 5th ed. San Francisco, CA: CMA.

Campbell, J. (1986). An ambulatory information system serving the needs of clinical practice: COSTAR V. In Orthner, H. (ed), *Proceedings of the Tenth Annual Symposium on Computer Applications in Medical Care,* Washington, D.C. IEEE.

Carl, F., English, W., and Burr, B. (1978). Evaluation of mouse, rate-controlled, isometric joystick, step-keys and text keys for text insertions on a CRT. *Ergonomics,* 21:601.

Chard, T. (1988). *Computing for Clinicians*. London: Elmore-Chard.

Clancey, W. (1984). Use of MYCIN's rules for tutoring. In Buchanan, B. and Shortliffe, E. (eds), *Rule-Based Expert Systems*. Reading, MA: Addison-Wesley.

Clancey, W. (1986). From GUIDON to NEOMYCIN and HERACLES in twenty short lessons: ORN final report 1979–1985. *AI Magazine,* 7(3):40.

Clancey, W. and Shortliffe, E. (eds) (1984). *Readings in Medical Artificial Intelligence: The First Decade*. Reading, MA: Addison-Wesley.

Clyman, S. and Melnick, D. (1987). The computer-based examination (CBX)—A clinical simulation by the National Board of Medical Examiners. In *Demonstration Digest of the Eleventh Annual Symposium on Computer Applications in Medical Care (SCAMC)*, Washington, D.C. SCAMC.

Coffman, G., et al. (1987). A subject tracking system for a randomized trial. In Stead, W. (ed), *Proceedings of the Eleventh Annual Symposium on Computer Applications in Medical Care,* Los Angeles. IEEE Computer Society Press.

Collen, M. (1975). Computer algorithms for clinical data collection. In Kallstrom, M. and Yarnall, S. (eds), *Design and Use of Protocols*. Seattle, WA: Medical Computer Services Association.

Collen, M. (1984). The cost-effectiveness of health checkups—an illustrative study. *Western Journal of Medicine,* 141:786.

Collen, M. (1986). Origins of medical informatics. *Western Journal of Medicine,* 145:778.

Connor, R. (1960). *A Hospital Inpatient Classification System*. Ph.D. thesis, Johns Hopkins University. University Microfilms (No. 60-3319). Ann Arbor, MI.

Cook, M. and Mayers, M. (1981). Computer-assisted data base for nursing research. In Werley, H. and Grier, M. (eds), *Nursing Information Systems*. New York: Springer.

Cooper, B. and Rice, D. (1976). The economic cost of illness revisited. *Social Security Bulletin,* 39(2):21.

Côté, R. and Robboy, S. (1980). Progress in medical information management: Systematized nomenclature of medicine (SNOMED). *Journal of the American Medical Association,* 243:756.

Covell, D., Uman, G., and Manning, P. (1985). Information needs in office practice: Are they being met? *Annals of Internal Medicine,* 103:596.

Cox, Jr., J., Nolle, F., and Arthur, R. (1972). Digital analysis of the electroencephalogram, the blood pressure wave, and the electrocardiogram. *Proceedings of the IEEE,* 60:1137.

Crouse, L. and Wiederhold, G. (1969). An advanced computer system for real-time medical applications. *Computers and Biomedical Research,* 2:582–598.

Cuadra/Elsevier (1988). *Directory of Online Databases*. New York: Cuadra/Elsevier.

Cuddigan, J., et al. (1987). Validating the knowledge in a computer-based consultant for nursing care. In Stead, W. (ed), *Proceedings of the Eleventh Annual Symposium for Computer Applications in Medical Care,* Washington, D.C. IEEE.

Cushing, H. (1903). On routine determination of arterial tension in operating room and clinic. *Boston Medical Surgical Journal,* 148:250.

Dales, L., Friedman, G., and Collen, M. (1979). Evaluating periodic multiphasic health checkups: A controlled trial. *Journal of Chronic Diseases,* 32:385.

Day, H. (1963). An intensive coronary care area. *Diseases of the Chest,* 44:423.

de Dombal, F., Leaper, D., Staniland, J., et al. (1972). Computer-aided diagnosis of acute abdominal pain. *British Medical Journal,* 1:376–380.

DeJong, G. (1983). Artificial intelligence implications for information retrieval. *Proceedings of the Sixth Annual International ACM SIGIR Conference on Research and Development in Information Retrieval,* 17(4):10.

De Solla Price, D. (1981). The development and structure of the biomedical literature. In Warren, K. (ed), *Coping with the Biomedical Literature.* New York: Praeger Publishers.

de Zegher-Geets, I., et al. (1988). Summarization and display of on-line medical records. *M.D. Computing,* 5(3):38.

Dewing, S. (1962). *Modern Radiology in Historical Perspective.* Springfield, IL: Charles C. Thomas.

Donabedian, A. (1966). Evaluating the quality of medical care. *Milbank Memorial Fund Quarterly,* 44:166.

Donabedian, D. (1976). Computer-taught epidemiology. *Nursing Outlook,* 24:749.

Doszkocs, T. (1983). Natural-language searching in an online catalog. *Information Technology and Libraries,* 2:364.

Downs, S., Walker, M., and Blum, R. (1986). Automated summarization of on-line medical records. In Salamon, R., Blum, B., and Jørgensen, M. (eds), *MEDINFO 86.* Amsterdam: Elsevier North-Holland.

Drazen, E. (1980). Methods for evaluating costs of automated hospital information systems. In O'Neill, J. (ed), *Proceedings of the Fourth Annual Symposium on Computer Applications in Medical Care,* Washington, D.C. IEEE.

Duda, R. and Shortliffe, E. (1983). Expert systems research. *Science,* 220:261–268.

Dwyer, S., et al. (1982). The cost of managing digital diagnostic images. *Radiology,* 144:313.

Edwards, W. (1968). Conservatism in human information processing. In Kleinmutz, B. (ed), *Formal Presentation of Human Judgment.* New York: Wiley.

Elstein, A., Shulman, L., and Sprafka, S. (1978). *Medical Problem Solving: An Analysis of Clinical Reasoning.* Cambridge, MA: Harvard University Press.

Enthoven, A. and Noll, R. (1984). Prospective payment: Will it solve Medicare's financial problem? *Issues in Science and Technology,* 1(1):101.

Erickson, B. and Robb, R. (1987). A desktop computer based workstation for display and analysis of 3-D and 4-D biomedical images. In Stead, W. (ed), *Proceedings of the Eleventh Annual Symposium on Computer Applications in Medical Care,* Los Angeles. IEEE.

Evans, R. (1987). A computerized approach to monitor prophylactic antibiotics. In Stead, W. (ed), *Proceedings of the Eleventh Annual Symposium on Computer Applications in Medical Care,* Los Angeles. Computer Society of the IEEE.

Evans, R., Larsen, R., Burke, J., et al. (1986). Computer surveillance of hospital-acquired infections and antibiotic use. *Journal of the American Medical Association,* 256:1007–1011.

Fagan, L. (1985). Extensions to the rule-based formalism for a monitoring task. In Buchanan, B. and Shortliffe, E. (eds), *Rule-Based Expert Systems.* Reading, MA: Addison-Wesley.

Finkel, A. (ed) (1977). *CPT4—Physician's Current Procedural Terminology.* 4th ed. Chicago: American Medical Association.

Finlayson, H. (1976). Numbers approach to nursing management. *Dimensions in Health Service,* 53(5):39.

Fischer, P., et al. (1980). User reaction to PROMIS: Issues related to acceptability of medical innovations. In O'Neill, J. (ed), *Proceedings of the Fourth Annual Symposium on Computer Applications in Medical Care,* Washington, D.C. IEEE.

Flexner, A. (1910). *Medical Education in the United States and Canada: A Report to the Carnegie Foundation for the Advancement of Teaching.* Boston, MA: Merrymount Press.

Flynn, F., et al. (1968). Data processing in clinical pathology. *Journal of Clinical Pathology,* 21:231.

Franklin, D. (1988). Secretary of IEEE P1073 Medical Information Bus (MIB) committee. Address: Southern Technical Institute, 112 Clay Street, Marietta, GA 30060.

Freedman, S. (1989). Personal communication. Advanced Media Research Group, Division of Human Anatomy, Stanford University School of Medicine, Stanford, CA.

Freund, L. and Mauksch, I. (1975). *Optimal Nursing Assignments Based on Difficulties.* Springfield, VA: U.S. Department of Commerce.

Friedman, B. and Dieterle, M. (1987). The impact of the installation of a local area network on physicians and the laboratory information system in a large teaching hospital. In Stead, W. (ed), *Proceedings of the Eleventh Annual Symposium on Computer Applications in Medical Care,* Washington, D.C. IEEE Computer Society Press.

Friedman, B. and Martin, J. (1987). Hospital information systems: The physician's role. *Journal of the American Medical Association,* 257:1792.

Friedman, G., Collen, M., and Fireman, B. (1986). Multiphasic health checkup evaluation: A 16 year follow-up. *Journal of Chronic Diseases,* 39:453.

Friedman, R. (1973). A computer program for simulating the patient–physician encounter. *Journal of Medical Education,* 48:92.

Friedman, R. and Gustafson, D. (1977). Computers in clinical medicine: A critical review. *Computers and Biomedical Research,* 8:199.

Friedman, R., et al. (1978). Experience with the simulated patient–physician encounter. *Journal of Medical Education,* 53:825.

Fries, J. (1974). Alternatives in medical record formats. *Medical Care,* 12:871.

Fries, J. and McShane, D. (1986). ARAMIS (The American Rheumatism Association Medical Information System)—A prototypical national chronic-disease data bank. *Western Journal of Medicine,* 145:798.

Gabbert, C., et al. (1975). *Nursing Utilization Management Information System.* Ann Arbor, MI: CSF.

Gall, Jr., J. (1976). Computerized hospital information systems cost effectiveness: A case study. In van Egmond, J., deVries Robbe, P., and Levy, A. (eds), *Information Systems for Patient Care: Review, Analysis, and Evaluation.* Amsterdam: North-Holland.

Gardner, R. (1989). Personal communication. LDS Hospital, Salt Lake City, UT.

Gardner, R. and Hawley, W. (1984). Standardizing communications and networks in the ICU. In *Patient Monitoring and Data Management.* AAMI (Association for Advancement of Medical Instrumentation) Technology Analysis and Review. TAR No. 11-85. Alexandria, VA: AAMI.

Gardner, R., Monis, S., and Oehler, P. (1986). Monitoring direct blood pressure: Algorithm enhancements. *IEEE Computers in Cardiology,* 13:607.

Gibson, R. (1984). National health expenditures, 1983. *Health Care Financing Review,* 6:1.

Ginsburg, P. (May 1982). *Containing Medical Care Costs Through Market Forces.* Washington, D.C.: Congressional Budget Office.

Goetz, A., Duff, J., and Bernstein, J. (1980). Health risk appraisal: The estimation of risk. *Public Health Reports,* 2(95):119.

Goldman, L., et al. (1977). Multifactorial index of cardiac risk in noncardiac surgical procedures. *New England Journal of Medicine,* 297:845.

Goodwin, J. and Edwards, B. (1975). Developing a computer program to assist the nursing process: Phase I—From systems analysis to an expandable program. *Nursing Research,* 24:299.

Gorry, G. (1973). Computer-assisted clinical decision making. *Methods of Information in Medicine,* 12:45–51.

Gorry, G., Kassirer, J., Essig, A., et al. (1973). Decision analysis as the basis for computer-aided management of acute renal failure. *American Journal of Medicine,* 55:473–484.

Gould, J., et al. (1986). Why is reading slower from CRT displays than from paper? In *Proceedings of Human Factors Society Thirtieth Annual Meeting,* Dayton, OH. Human Factors Society.

Gould, J. and Grischkowsky, N. (1984). Doing the same work with hardcopy and with cathode ray tube (CRT) computer terminals. *Human Factors,* 26:323–338.

Gouveia, W., Neal, T., and Nold, E. (1986). *1986 Report: Hospital Pharmacy Computer Systems.* Bethesda, MD: American Society of Hospital Pharmacists.

Grams, R. and Peck, G. (1986). National survey of hospital data processing—1985. *Journal of Medical Systems,* 10:423.

Greenes, R. (1982). OBUS: A microcomputer system for measurement, calculation, reporting, and retrieval of obstetrical ultrasound examinations. *Radiology,* 144:879.

Greenes, R. (1986). Knowledge management as an aid to medical decision making and education: The EXPLORER-1 system. In Salamon, R., Blum, B., and Jørgensen, M. (eds), *MEDINFO 86.* Amsterdam: Elsevier North-Holland.

Greenes, R., et al. (1970). Recording, retrieval, and review of medical data by physician-computer interaction. *New England Journal of Medicine,* 282:307.

Greenes, R., et al. (1978). Immediate pathologic confirmation of radiologic interpretation by computer feedback. *Radiology,* 127:381.

Grimm, R., Shimoni, K., Harlan, W., et al. (1975). Evaluation of patient-care protocol use by various providers. *New England Journal of Medicine,* 292:507–511.

Grobe, S. (1983). Nursing process algorithm used for a nursing CAI authoring system. In van Bemmel, J., Ball, M., and Wigertz, O. (eds), *MEDINFO 83.* Amsterdam: Elsevier North-Holland.

Harless, W., et al. (1971). CASE: A computer-aided simulation of the clinical encounter. *Journal of Medical Education,* 46:443.

Harless, W., Zier, M., and Duncan, R. (1986). Interactive videodisc case studies for medical education. In Orthner, H. (ed), *Proceedings of the Tenth Annual Symposium on Computer Applications in Medical Care,* Washington, D.C. IEEE.

Hatchell, J. and Winsten, D. (1987). Laboratory system review. *Healthcare Computing and Communications,* 4(3):26.

Hawley, W., Tariq, H., and Gardner, R. (1988). Clinical implementation of an automated medical information bus in an intensive care unit. In Greenes, R. (ed), *Proceedings of the Twelfth Annual Symposium on Computer Applications in Medical Care,* Washington, D.C. IEEE Computer Society Press.

Hayes-Roth, F., Waterman, D., and Lenat, D. (eds) (1983). *Building Expert Systems.* Reading, MA: Addison-Wesley.

Haynes, R., et al. (1978). Increased absenteeism from work after detection and labelling of hypertensive patients. *New England Journal of Medicine,* 299:741.

Health Care Financing Administration (1980). *The International Classification of Diseases, 9th Revision, Clinical Modification, ICD-9-CM.* Washington, D.C.: U.S. Department of Health and Human Services. DHHS publication number (PHS) 80-1260.

Health Insurance Association of America (HIAA) (1983). *Source Book of Health Insurance Data 1982–1983.* Washington, D.C.: HIAA.

Heckerman, D., Horvitz, E., and Nathwani, B. (1989). Update on the Pathfinder project. In Kingsland III, L. C. (ed), *Proceedings of the Thirteenth Annual Symposium on Computer Applications in Medical Care,* Washington, D.C. IEEE Computer Society Press.

Henderson, V. (1960). *ICN Basic Principles of Nursing Care.* London: International Council of Nurses (ICN) House.

Henley, R., Wiederhold, G., et al. (1975). *An Analysis of Automated Ambulatory Medical Record Systems.* University of California San Francisco Medical Center. Technical Report 13, vols 1 and 2.

Hickam, D., Shortliffe, E., Bischoff, M., et al. (1985a). The treatment advice of a computer-based cancer chemotherapy protocol advisor. *Annals of Internal Medicine,* 103:928–936.

Hickam, D., Sox, H., and Sox, C. (1985b). Systematic bias in recording the history in patients with chest pain. *Journal of Chronic Diseases,* 38:91.

Higgins, M. (1976). An application of computer technology to rural health care delivery. In *Proceedings of the Twenty-Ninth Annual Conference on Engineering in Medicine and Biology,* Boston. IEEE Press.

Hoffer, E. (1975). Computer-aided instruction in community hospital emergency departments: A pilot project. *Journal of Medical Education,* 50:84.

Hoffer, E., et al. (1975). Use of computer-aided instruction in graduate nursing education: A controlled trial. *Journal of Emergency Nursing,* 1:27.

Hoffer, E., et al. (1986). Computer-aided instruction in medicine: 16 years of MGH experience. In Salamon, R., Blum, B., and Jørgensen, M. (eds), *MEDINFO 86.* Amsterdam: Elsevier North-Holland.

Horn, B. and Swain, M. (1978). *Criterion Measures of Nursing Care Quality: A Health Status Instrument.* Bethesda, MD: National Center for Health Services Research.

Hudson, L. (1985). Monitoring of critically ill patients: Conference summary. *Respiratory Care,* 30:628.

Humphreys, B. and Lindberg, D. (1989). Building the Unified Medical Language System. In Kingsland III, L. (ed), *Proceedings of the Thirteenth Annual Symposium on Computer Applications in Medical Care,* Washington, D.C. IEEE Computer Society Press.

InterStudy (1985). *National HMO Census, 1984.* Excelsior, MN: InterStudy.

Jacky, J. (1989). Programmed for disaster. *The Sciences,* 29(5):22–27.

James, B., et al. (1986). PSM: A system for protocol selection and eligibility verification in clinical trials. In Salamon, R., Blum, B., and Jørgensen, M. (eds), *MEDINFO 86.* Amsterdam: Elsevier North-Holland.

Javitt, J. (1986). *Computers in Medicine: Applications and Possibilities.* Philadelphia, PA: W. B. Saunders.

Jelinek, R., Zinn, T., and Brya, J. (1973). Tell the computer how sick the patients are and it will tell you how many nurses they need. *Modern Hospital,* 121(December):81.

Jelliffe, R., Buell, J., and Kalaba, R. (1972). Reductions of digitalis toxicity by computer-assisted glycoside dosage regimens. *Annals of Internal Medicine,* 77:891.

Johnson, D. and Razenberger, J. (1981). A computer-based system for hospital-wide patient monitoring. In Werley, H. and Grier, M. (eds), *Nursing Information Systems.* New York: Springer.

Jost, R. (1986). Radiology reporting. *The Radiology Clinics of North America,* 24(1):19.

Jost, R., et al. (1982). A computer system to monitor radiology department activity: A management tool to improve patient care. *Radiology,* 145:347.

Jydstrup, R. and Gross, M. (1966). Cost of information handling in hospitals. *Health Services Research,* 1:235.

Kassirer, J. and Gorry, G. (1978). Clinical problem solving: A behavioral analysis. *Annals of Internal Medicine,* 89:245.

Kennedy, G., et al. (1987). Computers and software: Special report. *Hospitals,* 61(August 5).

King, C. (1986). Data management systems in clinical research. In Javitt, J. (ed), *Computers in Medicine: Applications and Possibilities.* Philadelphia: W. B. Saunders.

Knaus, W., et al. (1986). An evaluation of outcome from intensive care in major medical centers. *Annals of Internal Medicine,* 104:410.

Komaroff, A. (1979). The variability and inaccuracy of medical data. *Proceedings of the IEEE,* 67:1196.

Komaroff, A., Black, W., and Flatley, M. (1974). Protocols for physician assistants: Management of diabetes and hypertension. *New England Journal of Medicine,* 290:307–312.

Kritek, P. (1984a). Report of the group work on taxonomies. In Kim, M., McFarland, G., and McLane, A. (eds), *Classification of Nursing Diagnoses: Proceedings of the Fifth National Conference,* St. Louis, MO. Mosby.

Kritek, P. (1984b). Personal communication. Center for Nursing Research and Evaluation, University of Wisconsin–Milwaukee, Milwaukee, WI.

Kuhn, I., et al. (1982). *Automated Ambulatory Medical Record Systems in the U.S.* Department of Computer Science. Stanford University, Stanford, CA. Technical Report STAN-CS-82-928.

Kuhn, T. (1962). *The Structure of Scientific Revolutions.* Chicago: University of Chicago Press.

Kuipers, B. and Kassirer, J. (1984). Causal reasoning in medicine: Analysis of a protocol. *Cognitive Science,* 8:363–385.

Kuperman, G. and Gardner, R. (1988). *The HELP System: A Snapshot in Time.* Salt Lake City, UT: Department of Biophysics, LDS Hospital.

Lagina, S. (1971). A computer program to diagnose anxiety levels. *Nursing Research,* 20:484.

Landefeld, J. and Seskin, E. (1982). The economic value of life: Linking theory to practice. *American Journal of Public Health,* 72:555.

Langlotz, C. and Shortliffe, E. (1983). Adapting a consultation system to critique user plans. *International Journal of Man–Machine Studies,* 19:479–496.

Larsen, J. and Jenkins, J. (1987). Computerized arrhythmia monitoring. *Journal of Cardiovascular Nursing,* 2:58.

Laszlo, C. and Varga, L. (1981). A computerized health hazard appraisal system (CHAMP). *Methods of Information in Medicine,* 20:147.

Ledley, R. (1965). *Use of Computers in Biology and Medicine.* New York: McGraw-Hill.

Ledley, R. and Lusted, L. (1959). Reasoning foundations of medical diagnosis. *Science,* 130:9–21.

Leeming, B. and Simon, M. (1982). CLIP: A 1982 update. In Bauman, R. (ed), *Proceedings of the Seventh Conference on Computer Applications in Radiology,* Boston. American College of Radiology.

Leeming, B., et al. (1981). Computerized radiologic reporting with voice data-entry. *Radiology,* 585:138.

Lehr, J., et al. (1973). Experience with MARS (Missouri Automated Radiology System). *Radiology,* 106:289.

Lenert, L., Sheiner, L., and Blaschke, T. (1988). Improving drug dosing in hospitalized patients: Automated modeling of pharmacokinetics for individualization of drug dosage regimens. In Greenes, R. (ed), *Proceedings of the Twelfth Annual Symposium on Computer Applications in Medical Care,* Washington, D.C. IEEE.

Light, N. (1983). Computers in nursing practice: On-line nursing care plans. *Computers in Nursing,* 1(3):4.

Lincoln, M., Turner, C., Hesse, B., and Miller, R. (1988). A comparison of clustered knowledge structures in Iliad and in Quick Medical Reference. In Greenes, R. (ed), *Proceedings of the Twelfth Annual Symposium on Computer Applications in Medical Care,* Washington, D.C. IEEE Computer Society Press.

Lindberg, D. and Humphreys, B. (1989). Computer systems that understand medical meaning. In Scherrer, J., Côté, R., and Mandil, F. (eds), *Computerized Natural Medical Language Processing for Knowledge Representation.* Amsterdam: North-Holland.

Lodwick, G. (1984). The ACR-NEMA standardization effort. In Jost, R. (ed), *Proceedings of the Eighth Conference on Computer Applications in Radiology,* St. Louis, MO. American College of Radiology.

Loop, J., et al. (1988). Evaluation of a digital imaging network: A multidisciplinary approach. In Chiesa, A., Gasparotti, R., and Marololi, R. (eds), *Proceedings of the Fifth International Symposium on the Planning of Radiological Departments,* Florence, Italy.

Lundsgaarde, H., Fisher, P., and Steele, D. (1981). *Human Problems in Computerized Medicine.* University of Kansas, Kansas City, MO. Technical Report Publications in Anthropology No. 13.

Maloney, Jr., J. (1968). The trouble with patient monitoring. *Annals of Surgery,* 168:605.

Manning, W., et al. (1984). A controlled trial of the effect of a prepaid group practice on use of services. *New England Journal of Medicine,* 310:1501.

Margulies, S. and Wheeler, P. (1972). Development of an automated reporting system. In Lodwick, G. (ed), *Proceedings of the Conference on Computer Applications in Radiology,* Washington, D.C. U.S. Government Printing Office. DHEW Pub No. (FDA) 73-8018.

McCain, R. (1965). Nursing by assessment—not intuition. *American Journal of Nursing,* 65(4):82.

McCray, A. (1989). The UMLS semantic network. In Kingsland III, L. (ed), *Proceedings of the Thirteenth Annual Symposium on Computer Applications in Medical Care,* Washington, D.C. IEEE Computer Society Press.

McDonald, C. and Hammond, W. (1989). Standard formats for electronic transfer of clinical data. *Annals of Internal Medicine,* 110:333–335.

McDonald, C. and Tierney, W. (1986a). The medical gopher—A microcomputer system to help find, organize and decide about patient data. *Western Journal of Medicine,* 145:823.

McDonald, C. and Tierney, W. (1986b). Research uses of computer-stored practice records in general medicine. *Journal of General Internal Medicine,* 1(supplement):S19.

McDonald, C., et al. (1983). Data base management, feedback control, and the Regenstrief medical record. *Journal of Medical Systems,* 7:111.

McDonald, C., et al. (1984). Reminders to physicians from an introspective medical record: A two year randomized trial. *Annals of Internal Medicine,* 199:130.

McDonald, C., et al. (1988). The Regenstrief medical records. *M.D. Computing,* 5(5):34.

McFadden, E. (1988). Personal communication. Dana Farber Cancer Institute, Harvard School of Public Health, Cambridge, MA.

McShane, D. and Fries, J. (1988). The chronic disease data bank: The ARAMIS experience. *Proceedings of the IEEE,* 76:672.

Medical Economics Company (1988). *Physician's Desk Reference.* 42nd ed. Oradell, NJ: Medical Economics Company.

Miller, P. (1986). *Expert Critiquing Systems: Practice-Based Medical Consultation by Computer.* New York: Springer-Verlag.

Miller, P. (1988). *Selected Topics in Medical Artificial Intelligence.* New York: Springer-Verlag.

Miller, R., McNeil, M., Challinor, S., et al. (1986). The INTERNIST-1/Quick Medical Reference project: Status report. *Western Journal of Medicine,* 145:816–822.

Miller, R., Pople, Jr., H., and Myers, J. (1982). INTERNIST-1: An experimental computer-based diagnostic consultant for general internal medicine. *New England Journal of Medicine,* 307:468–476.

Miller, R., Schaffner, K., and Meisel, A. (1985). Ethical and legal issues related to the use of computer programs in clinical medicine. *Annals of Internal Medicine,* 102:529.

Miller, R., Steinback, G., and Dayhoff, R. (1980). A hierarchical computer network: An alternative approach to clinical laboratory computerization in a large hospital. In O'Neill, J. (ed), *Proceedings of the Fourth Annual Symposium on Computer Applications in Medical Care,* New York. IEEE Computer Society.

Mishan, E. (1971). Evaluation of life and limb: A theoretical approach. *Journal of Political Economy,* 9(4):687.

Mohr, D., et al. (1986) Asymptomatic microhematuria and urologic disease. *Journal of the American Medical Association,* 256:224.

Moliver, N. and Coates, A. (1987). Decision support for medical treatment: A TPN prescription system on a central hospital computer. In Stead, W. (ed), *Proceedings of the Eleventh Annual Symposium on Computer Applications in Medical Care,* Los Angeles. IEEE.

Munnecke, T. and Kuhn, I. (1989). Large-scale portability of hospital information system software within the Veterans Administration. In Orthner, H. and Blum, B. (eds), *Implementing Health Care Information Systems.* New York: Springer-Verlag.

Musen, M., Fagan, L., Combs, D., et al. (1987). Use of a domain model to drive an interactive knowledge-editing tool. *International Journal of Man–Machine Studies,* 26:105–121.

National Center for Health Statistics (1978). *The International Classification of Diseases, 9th Revision, Clinical Modification.* Ann Arbor, MI: Commission on Professional and Hospital Activities.

National Center for Health Statistics (1988). The National Ambulatory Medical Care Survey, United States, 1975–1981 and 1985 trends. In *Vital and Health Statistics,* Series 13, Number 93. Washington, D.C.: U.S. Government Printing Office, Public Health Service. DHHS Publication number (PHS) 88-1754.

National Library of Medicine (1986a). *IAIMS and Health Sciences Education.* Bethesda, MD: U.S. Department of Health and Human Services, Public Health Service, National Institutes of Health. Proceedings of a symposium sponsored by the National Library of Medicine.

National Library of Medicine (1986b). *Long Range Plan: Medical Informatics (Report of Panel 4).* Bethesda, MD: U.S. Department of Health and Human Services, Public Health Service, National Institutes of Health.

National Library of Medicine (1987). *NLM Long Range Plan.* Bethesda, MD: U.S. Department of Health and Human Services, Public Health Service, National Institutes of Health.

Nightingale, F. (1860). *Notes on Nursing: What It Is and What It Is Not.* New York: Appleton. Republished in 1969, New York: Dover.

Office of Technology Assessment (OTA) (1980). *The Implications of Cost-Effectiveness Analysis of Medical Technology.* Washington, D.C.: Congress of the United States, U.S. Government Printing Office.

Orem, D. (1980). *Nursing: Concepts of Practice.* 2nd ed. New York: McGraw-Hill.

Ozbolt, J. (1982). A prototype information system to aid nursing decisions. In Blum, B. (ed), *Proceedings of the Sixth Annual Symposium on Computer Applications in Medical Care,* Washington, D.C. IEEE Computer Society.

Ozbolt, J., et al. (1984). Developing an expert system for nursing practice. In Cohen, G. (ed), *Proceedings of the Eighth Annual Symposium on Computer Applications in Medical Care,* Silver Spring, MD. IEEE.

Packer, C. (1986). Hospital pharmacy automation skyrockets 21 percent. *Hospitals,* 60(August 20):90.

Packer, C. (1987a). Data processing budgets jump during 1987. *Hospitals*, 61(December 20):60.

Packer, C. (1987b). Lab software vendors expand market share. *Hospitals*, 61(April 20):126.

Packer, C. (1987c). Local area networks increase 500 percent in 1986. *Hospitals*, 61(January 20):110.

Packer, C. (1988). Software, staff dominate '88 hospital budgets. *Hospitals*, 62(January 20):70.

Park, B. (1982). Computerized medical records in private practice. In Blum, B. (ed), *Proceedings of the Sixth Annual Symposium on Computer Applications in Medical Care*, Washington, D.C. IEEE.

Pauker, S. and Kassirer, J. (1981). Clinical decision analysis by computer. *Archives of Internal Medicine*, 141:1831–1837.

Pauker, S., et al. (1976). Towards the simulation of clinical cognition: Taking a present illness by computer. *American Journal of Medicine*, 60:981.

Peabody, G. (1922). The physician and the laboratory. *Boston Medical Surgery Journal*, 187:324.

Peacock, A., et al. (1965). Data processing in clinical chemistry. *Clinical Chemistry*, 11:595.

Peck, C. (1989). *Bedside Clinical Pharmacokinetics*, Revised Edition. Vancouver, WA: Applied Therapeutics, Inc.

Peterson, W. and Birdsall, T. (1953). *The Theory of Signal Detectability.* Electronic Defense Group, University of Michigan, Ann Arbor. Technical Report No. 13.

Piemme, T. and Ball, M. (1984). *Executive Management of Computer Resources in the Academic Health Centers: A Staff Report.* Washington, D.C.: Association of Academic Health Centers.

Pople, H. (1982). Heuristic methods for imposing structure on ill-structured problems: The structuring of medical diagnosis. In Szolovits, P. (ed), *Artificial Intelligence in Medicine.* Boulder, CO: Westview Press.

President's Science Advisory Committee (1963). *Science, Government, and Information: The Responsibilities of the Technical Community and the Government in the Transfer of Information.* Washington, D.C.: U.S. Government Printing Office.

Pryor, D., et al. (1983a). Estimating the likelihood of significant coronary artery disease. *American Journal of Medicine*, 75:771.

Pryor, D., et al. (1987). The changing survival benefits of coronary revascularization over time. *Circulation*, 76(supplement V):V–13.

Pryor, T., et al. (1983b). The HELP system. *Journal of Medical Systems*, 7:87.

Quigley, E. (1984). Writing practice systems without programming. *M.D. Computing*, 1:18.

Ransahoff, D. and Feinstein, A. (1978). Problems of spectrum and bias in evaluating the efficacy of diagnostic tests. *New England Journal of Medicine*, 299:926.

Rapp, B., et al. (1989). MEDLINE on CD-ROM: Summary report of a nationwide evaluation. In Woodsmall, R., Lyon-Hartmann, B., and Siegel, E. (eds), *MEDLINE on CD-ROM: National Library of Medicine Evaluation Forum.* Medford, NJ: Learned Information.

Raub, W. (1984). Uses of the PROPHET system to model the kinetics of biologically active substances. In Nicolini, C. (ed), *Modeling and Analysis in Biomedicine.* Singapore: World Scientific.

Reggia, J., Tabb, O., Price, T., et al. (1984). Computer-aided assessment of transient ischemic attacks. *Archives of Neurology,* 41:1248–1254.

Reggia, J. and Tuhrim, S. (eds) (1985). *Computer-Assisted Medical Decision Making* (2 vols). New York: Springer-Verlag.

Rennels, G. (1987). *A Computational Model of Reasoning from the Clinical Literature.* New York: Springer-Verlag.

Richart, R. (1976). Evaluations of a medical data system. *Computers and Biomedical Research,* 3:417.

Robb, R. (1982). The dynamic spatial reconstructor: An X-ray video fluoroscopic CT scanner for dynamic volume imaging of moving organs. *IEEE Transactions in Medical Imaging,* MI-1(1):22.

Robbins, A., et al. (1987). Speech-controlled generation of radiology reports. *Radiology,* 164:569.

Robbins, L. and Hall, J. (1970). *How to Practice Prospective Medicine.* Methodist Hospital of Indiana, Indianapolis.

Rodolitz, N. and Clancey, W. (1989). GUIDON-MANAGE: Teaching the process of medical diagnosis. In Evans, D. and Patel, V. (eds), *Cognitive Science in Medicine: Biomedical Modeling,* Chapter 8. Cambridge, MA: MIT Press.

Rogers, M. (1970). *An Introduction to the Theoretical Basis of Nursing.* Philadelphia: Davis.

Rosati, R., et al. (1975). A new information system for medical practice. *Archives of Internal Medicine,* 135:1017.

Roy, Sr., C. (1982). Theoretical framework for classification of nursing diagnoses. In Kim, M. and Moritz, D. (eds), *Classification of Nursing Diagnoses: Proceedings of the Third and Fourth Conferences,* New York. McGraw-Hill.

Rubenstein, E. and Federman, D. (eds) (1988). *Scientific American Medicine.* New York: Scientific American.

Ryan, S. (1985). An expert system for nursing practice. *Journal of Medical Systems,* 9:29.

Saba, V. (1982). Computers in public health: Today and tomorrow. *Nursing Outlook,* 9:510–511.

Saba, V. (1983). How computers influence nursing activities in community health. *First National Conference on Computer Technology in Nursing.* USPIHS Pub. No. 83-2142. Bethesda, MD: National Institutes of Health.

Safran, C., Porter, D., Lightfoot, J., et al. (1989). ClinQuery: A system for on-line searching of data in a teaching hospital. *Annals of Internal Medicine,* 111:751–756.

Salton, G. (1971). *The SMART Retrieval System.* Englewood Cliffs, NJ: Prentice-Hall.

Sartorius, N. (1976). I. Methodological problems of common terminology, measurement, and classification. II. Modifications and new approaches to taxonomy in long-term care: Advantages and limitations of the ICD. *Medical Care,* 14:109.

Schelling, T. (1968). The life you save may be your own. In Chase, Jr., S. (ed), *Problems in Public Expenditure Analysis.* Washington, D.C.: Brookings Institution.

Schneider, R. and Dwyer, S. (eds) (1988). *Medical Imaging II: Image Data Management and Display.* Proceedings of the Society of Photo-Optical Instrumentation Engineers (SPIE), Vol. 914 (Part B). Newport Beach, CA: IEEE.

Schoen, A. (1973). *AMHT Program Directory, International 1972–73,* 3rd ed. Burbank, CA: Bioscience Publications.

Schoolman, H. (1982). Information transfer: Past, present and future. *Mobius,* 2:38.

Schultz II, S. (1978). A critical analysis of methodology for monitoring quality of nursing care (HEW, Rush-Medicus). Paper presented at the First Annual Symposium on the Appraisal of Quality of Nursing Care Measures, Buffalo, NY.

Schwartz, R., Weiss, M., and Buchanan, A. (1985). Error control in medical data. *M.D. Computing,* 2:19.

Schwartz, W. (1970). Medicine and the computer: The promise and problems of change. *New England Journal of Medicine,* 283(23):1257.

Schwartz, W., Patil, R., and Szolovits, P. (1987). Artificial intelligence in medicine: Where do we stand? *New England Journal of Medicine,* 316:685–688.

Senior Medical Review (1987). Urinary tract infection. *Senior Medical Review.*

Severinghaus, J. and Astrup, P. (1986). History of blood gas analysis. VI. Oximetry. *Journal of Clinical Monitoring,* 2:270.

Shabot, M. (1989). Standardized acquisition of bedside data: The IEEE P1073 medical information bus. *International Journal of Clinical Monitoring and Computing* (in press).

Shabot, M., Leyerle, B., and LoBue, M. (1987). Automatic extraction of intensity-intervention scores from a computerized surgical intensive care unit flowsheet. *American Journal of Surgery,* 154:72.

Shani, U. (1981). *Understanding Three-Dimensional Images: The Recognition of Abdominal Anatomy from Computed Axial Tomograms (CAT).* Ph.D. thesis, Department of Computer Science, University of Rochester, Rochester, NY.

Sheiner, L. (1975). Improved computer-assisted digoxin therapy: A method using feedback of measured serum digoxin concentrations. *Annals of Internal Medicine,* 82:619.

Sheppard, L. (1980). Computer control of infusion of vasoactive drugs. *Annals of Biomedical Engineering,* 8:431.

Sheppard, L. and Sayers, B. (1977). Dynamic analysis of blood pressure response to hypotensive agents, studied in post-operative cardiac surgery patients. *Computers and Biomedical Research,* 10:237.

Shneiderman, B. (1986). *Designing the User Interface: Strategies for Effective Human–Computer Interaction.* Reading, MA: Addison-Wesley.

Shortliffe, E. (1976). *Computer-Based Medical Consultations: MYCIN.* New York: Elsevier/North Holland.

Shortliffe, E. (1982). The computer and clinical decision making: Good advice is not enough. *IEEE Engineering in Medicine and Biology Magazine,* 1:16–18.

Shortliffe, E. (1984a). Coming to terms with the computer. In Reiser, S. and Anbar, M. (eds), *The Machine at the Bedside: Strategies for Using Technology in Patient Care.* Cambridge, MA: Cambridge University Press.

Shortliffe, E. (1984b). The science of biomedical computing. *Medical Informatics,* 9:185.

Shortliffe, E. (1986). Medical expert systems: Knowledge tools for physicians. *The Western Journal of Medicine,* 145:830–839.

Shortliffe, E. (1989). Testing reality: The introduction of decision-support technologies for physicians. *Methods of Information in Medicine,* 28:1.

Shortliffe, E. and Buchanan, B. (1984). The problem of evaluation. In Buchanan, B. and Shortliffe, E. (eds), *Rule-Based Expert Systems.* Reading, MA: Addison-Wesley.

Shortliffe, E., Buchanan, B., and Feigenbaum, E. (1979). Knowledge engineering for medical decision making: A review of computer-based clinical decision aids. *Proceedings of the IEEE,* 67:1207–1224.

Shortliffe, E. and Fagan, L. (1989). Research training in medical informatics: The Stanford experience. In Salamon, R., Protti, D., and Moehr, J. (eds), *Proceedings of the 1989 International Symposium on Medical Informatics and Education,* Victoria, B.C., Canada. School of Health Information Science, University of Victoria. Republished in *Academic Medicine,* 64(10):575–578.

Shubin, H. and Weil, M. (1966). Efficient monitoring with a digital computer of cardiovascular function in seriously ill patients. *Annals of Internal Medicine,* 65:453.

Simborg, D. (1984). Networking and medical information systems. *Journal of Medical Systems,* 8:43.

Simborg, D., et al. (1983). Local area networks and the hospital. *Computers and Biomedical Research,* 16:247.

Sittig, D. (1987). Computerized management of patient care in a complex, controlled clinical trial in the intensive care unit. In Stead, W. (ed), *Proceedings of the Eleventh Annual Symposium on Computer Applications in Medical Care,* Washington, D.C. IEEE.

Slack, W. (1984). A history of computerized medical interviews. *M.D. Computing,* 5:52.

Smith, Jr., J. (1984). Using expert systems for interpretive reporting. *Journal of Medical Technology,* 1(5):366.

Smith, Jr., J., et al. (1985). RED: A red-cell antibody identification expert module. *Journal of Medical Systems,* 9:121.

Smith, L. (1985). Medicine as an art. In Wyngaarden, J. and Smith, L. (eds), *Cecil Textbook of Medicine.* Philadelphia: W. B. Saunders.

Social Security Administration (1983). *Social Security Bulletin.* Annual Statistical Supplement. Washington, D.C.: U.S. Department of Health and Human Services.

Somers, A. (1971). *The Kaiser Permanente Medical Care Program: A Symposium.* New York: The Commonwealth Fund.

Sox, Jr., H., et al. (1988). *Medical Decision Making.* Boston: Butterworths.

Speedie, S., et al. (1988). MENTOR: Integration of an expert system with a hospital information system. In Stead, W. (ed), *Proceedings of the Eleventh Annual Symposium on Computer Applications in Medical Care,* Washington, D.C. IEEE.

Stead, W., Garrett, L., and Hammond, W. (1983). Practicing nephrology with a computerized medical record. *Kidney International,* 24:446.

Stead, W. and Hammond, W. (1988). Computer-based medical records: The centerpiece of TMR. *M.D. Computing,* 5(5):48.

Stolar, M. (1988). ASHP National Survey of Hospital Pharmaceutical Services—1987. *American Journal of Hospital Pharmacy,* 45:801.

Swets, J. (1973). The relative operating characteristic in psychology. *Science,* 182: 990.

Szolovits, P. (ed) (1982). *Artificial Intelligence in Medicine.* Boulder, CO: Westview Press (AAAS Symposium Series).

Tatro, D., et al. (1975). Online drug interaction surveillance. *American Journal of Hospital Pharmacy,* 32:417.

Teach, R. and Shortliffe, E. (1981). An analysis of physician attitudes regarding computer-based clinical consultation systems. *Computers and Biomedical Research,* 14:542.

Templeton, A., Cox, G., and Dwyer, S. (1988). Digital image management networks: Current status. *Radiology,* 169:193.

Tolbert, S. and Pertuz, A. (1977). Study shows how computerization affects nursing activities in ICU. *Hospitals,* 51(17):79.

Tversky, A. and Kahneman, D. (1974). Judgment under uncertainty: Heuristics and biases. *Science,* 185:1124.

Tymchyshyn, P. (1982). An evaluation of the adaptation of CAI in a nursing program. In Blum, B. (ed), *Proceedings of the Sixth Annual Symposium on Computer Applications in Medical Care,* Los Angeles: IEEE.

U.S. Bureau of the Census (1987). *Statistical Abstract of the United States: 1988,* 108th edition. Washington, D.C.: U.S. Government Printing Office.

U.S. Department of Health and Human Services (DHHS) (1984). *Private Health Insurance Coverage of the Medicare Population.* Data Preview 18, NCHSR National Health Care Expenditures Study, Publication No. (PHS) 84-3362. Washington, D.C.: DHHS.

U.S. Department of Health and Human Services (DHHS) (1985). *Private Insurance and Public Programs: Coverage of Health Services.* Data Preview 20, NCHSR National Health Care Expenditures Study, Publication No. (PHS) 85-337. Washington, D.C.: DHHS.

Walker, D. (1982). The cost of nursing care in hospitals. In Aiken, L. (ed), *Nursing in the 1980's: Crisis, Opportunities, Challenges.* Philadelphia: Lippincott.

Walker, M. and Blum, R. (1986). Toward automated discovery from clinical databases: The RADIX project. In Salamon, R., Blum, B., and Jørgensen, M. (eds), *MEDINFO 86.* Amsterdam: Elsevier North-Holland.

Wallingford, K., et al. (1989). *Survey of Individual Users of MEDLINE on the NLM System.* NTIS Technical Report No. PB89-133722/GBB. Bethesda, MD: National Library of Medicine.

Walton, J., Musen, M., Combs, D., et al. (1987). Graphical access to medical expert systems: III. Design of a knowledge acquisition environment. *Methods of Information in Medicine,* 26:78–88.

Warner, H. (1979). *Computer-Assisted Medical Decision-Making.* New York: Academic Press.

Warner, H., Gardner, R., and Toronto, A. (1968). Computer-based monitoring of cardiovascular functions in postoperative patients. *Circulation,* 37 & 38(Supplement II):II–68.

Warner, H., Haug, B., Bouhaddou, O., et al. (1988). ILIAD as an expert consultant to teach differential diagnosis. In Greenes, R. (ed), *Proceedings of the Twelfth Annual Symposium on Computer Applications in Medical Care,* Washington, D.C. IEEE.

Warner, H., Toronto, A., and Veasy, L. (1964). Experience with Bayes' theorem for computer diagnosis of congenital heart disease. *Annals of the New York Academy of Science,* 115:2–16.

Weed, L. (1969). *Medical Records, Medical Education and Patient Care: The Problem-Oriented Record as a Basic Tool.* Chicago: Year Book Medical Publishers.

Weinberg, A. (1973). CAI at the Ohio State University College of Medicine (1973). *Computers in Biology and Medicine,* 3:299.

Weinstein, M. and Fineberg, H. (1980). *Clinical Decision Analysis.* Philadelphia: W. B. Saunders.

Weiss, S., Kulikowski, C., and Galen, R. (1981). Developing microprocessor-based expert models for instrument interpretation. In *Proceedings of the Seventh International Joint Conference on Artificial Intelligence,* Los Altos, CA. Morgan-Kaufman.

Weiss, S., et al. (1985). Screening test for HTLV-III (AIDS agent) antibodies. *Journal of the American Medical Association,* 253:221.

Weyl, S., Fries, J., Wiederhold, G., et al. (1975). A modular self-describing clinical database system. *Computers and Biomedical Research,* 8(3):279–293.

Whiting-O'Keefe, Q., et al. (1985). A computerized summary medical record system can provide more information than the standard medical record. *Journal of the American Medical Association,* 254:1185.

Whiting-O'Keefe, Q., Whiting, A., and Henke, J. (1988). The STOR clinical information system. *M.D. Computing,* 5(5):8.

Wirtschafter, D., Carpenter, J., and Mesel, E. (1985). A consultant-extender system for breast cancer adjuvant chemotherapy. In Reggia, J. and Tuhrim, S. (eds), *Computer-Assisted Medical Decision Making,* Vol. 1, New York: Springer-Verlag.

Wyngaarden, J. and Smith, L. (1988). *Cecil Textbook of Medicine,* 18th edition. Philadelphia, PA: W. B. Saunders.

Yachida, M., Ikeda, M., and Tsuji, S. (1980). A plan-guided analysis of cineangiograms for measurement of dynamic behavior of heart wall. *IEEE Transactions on Pattern Analysis and Machine Intelligence,* PAMI-2(6):537.

Yasaka, T., et al. (1980). Distribution types: Population and intra- and inter-individual distributions. In Lindberg, D. and Kaihara, S. (eds), *MEDINFO 80.* Amsterdam: Elsevier North-Holland.

Young, F. (1987). Validation of medical software: Present policy of the Food and Drug Administration. *Annals of Internal Medicine,* 106:628.

Yu, V., Buchanan, B., Shortliffe, E., et al. (1979a). Evaluating the performance of a computer-based consultant. *Computer Programs in Biomedicine,* 9:95–102.

Yu, V., Fagan, L., Wraith, S., et al. (1979b). Antimicrobial selection by a computer: A blinded evaluation by infectious disease experts. *Journal of the American Medical Association,* 242:1279–1282.

Zeckhauser, R. and Shepard, D. (1976). Where now for saving lives? *Law and Contemporary Problems* (Duke University School of Law), 40(4):5.

Zeichick, A. (1988). An apple a day. *CD-ROM Review,* 3:42.

Zucconi, G. (1986). An introduction to PILOT. *M.D. Computing,* 3(3):31.

Name Index

Subject Index